Books are to be returned on or before
the last date below.

T
D

LIBREX-

Textbook of Drug Design and Discovery

Third edition

Povl Krogsgaard-Larsen,
Tommy Liljefors and
Ulf Madsen

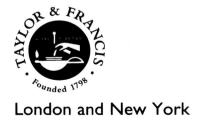

London and New York

First published 2002
by Taylor & Francis
11 New Fetter Lane, London EC4P 4EE

Simultaneously published in the USA and Canada
by Taylor & Francis Inc,
29 West 35th Street, New York, NY 10001

Taylor & Francis is an imprint of the Taylor & Francis Group

© 2002 Povl Krogsgaard-Larsen

Typeset in Baskerville by
Integra Software Services Pvt. Ltd, Pondicherry, India
Printed and bound in Malta by
Gutenberg Press Ltd.

British Library Cataloguing in Publication Data
A catalogue record for this book is available from the British Library

Library of Congress Cataloging in Publication Data
A catalog record for this book has been requested

ISBN 0–415–28287–X HB
ISBN 0–415–28288–8 PB

Contents

14 Design and application of prodrugs

CLAUS S. LARSEN AND JESPER ØSTERGAARD

15 Peptides and peptidomimetics

KRISTINA LUTHMAN AND ULI HACKSELL

Contributors

Anderson, Paul S.
Chemical and Physical
  Sciences R&D
Bristol-Myers Squibb Company
P.O. Box 80500
Wilmington
DE 19880-0500
USA

Andrews, Peter
Centre for Drug Design and
  Development
The University of Queensland
Brisbane
Queensland 4072
Australia

Bang-Andersen, Benny
H. Lundbeck A/S,
Department of Medicinal
  Chemistry
9, Ottiliavej
DK-2500 Valby
Denmark

Bräuner-Osborne, Hans
Royal Danish School of Pharmacy,
Department of Medicinal
  Chemistry
2, Universitetsparken,
DK-2100 Copenhagen Ø
Denmark

Bøgesø, Klaus P.
H. Lundbeck A/S
9, Ottiliavej
DK-2500 Valby
Denmark

Copeland, Robert A.
Chemical Enzymology
Bristol-Myers Squibb Company
P.O. Box 80400
Wilmington
DE 19880-0400, USA

De Clercq, Erik
Rega Institute
Katholieke Universiteit Leuven
10, Minderbroedersstraat
B-3000 Leuven, Belgium

Dooley, Michael
Centre for Drug Design
  and Development
The University of Queensland
Brisbane
Queensland 4072
Australia

Farver, Ole
Royal Danish School of Pharmacy
Department of Analytical and
  Pharmaceutical Chemistry
2, Universitetsparken
DK-2100 Copenhagen Ø
Denmark

Frydenvang, Karla
Royal Danish School of Pharmacy
Department of Medicinal Chemistry
2, Universitetsparken
DK-2100 Copenhagen Ø
Denmark

Frølund, Bente
Royal Danish School of Pharmacy
Department of Medicinal Chemistry
2, Universitetsparken
DK-2100 Copenhagen Ø
Denmark

Hacksell, Uli
Acadia Pharmaceuticals Inc.
3911 Sorrento Valley Blvd.
San Diego
CA 92121-1402
USA

Halldin, Christer
Department of Clinical NeuroScience
Psychiatry Section
Karolinska Hospital
S-17176 Stockholm
Sweden

Herdewijn, Piet
Rega Institute
Katholieke Universiteit Leuven
10, Minderbroedersstraat
B-3000 Leuven
Belgium

Högberg, Thomas
7TM Pharma A/S
2, Rønnegade
DK-2100 Copenhagen
Denmark

Jane, David E.
Department of Pharmacology
School of Medical Sciences
University of Bristol
University Walk
Bristol BS8 1TD
UK

Kastrup, Jette Sandholm
Royal Danish School of Pharmacy
Department of Medicinal Chemistry
2, Universitetsparken
DK-2100 Copenhagen Ø
Denmark

Kennedy, Ian J.
Department of Pharmacology
School of Medical Sciences
University of Bristol
University Walk
Bristol BS8 1TD
UK

Krogsgaard-Larsen, Povl
Royal Danish School of Pharmacy
Department of Medicinal Chemistry
2, Universitetsparken
DK-2100 Copenhagen Ø
Denmark

Larsen, Claus S.
Royal Danish School of Pharmacy
Department of Analytical and
   Pharmaceutical Chemistry
2, Universitetsparken
DK-2100 Copenhagen Ø
Denmark

Larsen, Ingrid Kjøller
Royal Danish School of Pharmacy
Department of Medicinal Chemistry
2, Universitetsparken
DK-2100 Copenhagen Ø
Denmark

Liljefors, Tommy
Royal Danish School of Pharmacy
Department of Medicinal Chemistry
2, Universitetsparken
DK-2100 Copenhagen Ø
Denmark

Luthman, Kristina
Göteborg University
Department of Chemistry
Medicinal Chemistry
S-412 96 Göteborg
Sweden

Madsen, Ulf
Royal Danish School of Pharmacy
Department of Medicinal Chemistry
2, Universitetsparken
DK-2100 Copenhagen Ø
Denmark

Mitscher, Lester A.
University of Kansas
School of Pharmacy
Department of Medicinal Chemistry
Lawrence, Kansas 66047-2101
USA

Norinder, Ulf
AstraZeneca R&D
Discovery
Medicinal Chemistry
S-15185 Södertälje
Sweden

Pettersson, Ingrid
Novo Nordisk A/S
Novo Nordisk Park G8
DK-2760 Måløv
Denmark

Triggle, David J.
University at Buffalo
State University of New York
415 Capen Hall
Buffalo
NY 14260-1608
USA

Østergaard, Jesper
Royal Danish School of Pharmacy
Department of Analytical and
 Pharmaceutical Chemistry
2, Universitetsparken
DK-2100 Copenhagen Ø
Denmark

Preface

The field of medicinal chemistry and drug design is in a state of swift development and is at present undergoing major restructuring. The molecular biological revolution and the progressing mapping of the human genome have created a new biochemical and biostructural 'world order'. These developments have provided new challenges and opportunities for drug research in general and for drug design in particular. The major objectives of the medicinal chemists are transformation of pathobiochemical and – physiological data into a 'chemical language' with the aim of designing molecules interacting specifically with the derailed or degenerating processes in the diseased organism.

Potential therapeutic targets are being disclosed with increasing frequency, and this exponential growth will continue during the next decades. In this situation, there is a need for rapid and effective target validation and for accelerated lead discovery procedures. Consequently, most industrial medicinal chemistry laboratories have built up new technologies in order to meet these demands. Key words in this regard are construction of compound libraries, high or ultrahigh throughput screening, accelerated ADME and toxicity tests, and automatized cellular assay systems.

In parallel with this development, biostructure-based drug design and intelligent molecular mimicry or bioisosterism are areas of growing importance in the medicinal chemistry 'playing field'. Structural biology is becoming an increasingly important part of molecular biology and biochemistry, and, furthermore, organic chemists are increasingly directing their attention towards synthetic aspects of biomolecules and biologically active compounds biosynthesized by plants and animals. Thus the borderland between biology, biochemistry, and chemistry is rapidly broadening and is becoming the most fruitful working field for innovative and intuitive drug design scientists.

Where are the academic medicinal chemistry and drug design departments in this area of drug research, which is moving towards an increasing degree of integration of scientific disciplines? Furthermore, how should medicinal chemistry teaching programmes be organized and taught in this highly dynamic research area? These burning questions need to be effectively addressed. In order to attract the attention of intelligent students, the creative and fascinating nature of drug design must be the underlying theme of basic and advanced student courses in medicinal chemistry. In relation to industrial screening programmes and 'hit-finding' procedures, students should be taught that the conversions of 'hits' into lead structures and further into drug candidates require advanced synthetic chemistry supported by computational chemistry. Furthermore, these medicinal chemistry approaches should be integrated with molecular pharmacology studies using cloned target receptors, ion channels, or enzymes, expressed in appropriate model systems.

It is beyond doubt that a steadily increasing number of biomolecules will be subjected to X-ray crystallographic structural analysis. The number of enzymes with established three-dimensional structure is now increasing exponentially, and this growth will continue during the next decades. Even oligomeric membrane-bound receptors can now be crystallized and subjected to X-ray crystallographic analysis, but such analyses of mono- or oligomeric receptors are still hampered by major experimental difficulties. In recent years, however, biostructural scientists have succeeded in crystallizing recombinant versions of the binding domains of a G protein-coupled receptor as well as a ligand-gated ion channel. Structural analyses of these binding domains co-crystallized with agonist and antagonist ligands have already provided insight into the structural basis of receptor–ligand interactions and of receptor activation and blockade.

These breakthroughs in biostructural chemistry have opened up new avenues in drug design. Structural information derived from X-ray analyses of enzyme-inhibitor conglomerates has been and continues to be very valuable for the design of new types of inhibitors. Similar pieces of information derived from studies of receptor binding domains co-crystallized with different types of competitive or noncompetitive ligands undoubtedly will be of key importance in receptor ligand design projects. These approaches which are in the nature of drug design on a rational basis will become important parts of student teaching programmes in medicinal chemistry.

In academic research and teaching, biologically active natural products probably will play a progressively important role as lead structures. Not only do such compounds often possess novel structural characteristics, but they also frequently exhibit unique biological mechanisms of action, although naturally occurring 'toxins' typically show nonselective pharmacological effects. By systematic structural modification, including molecular mimicry approaches, it has been possible to 'tame' such 'toxins' and convert them into leads with specific actions on biofunctions of key importance in diseases. Biologically active natural products undoubtedly will continue to be important starting points for academic drug design projects, and such approaches will continue to be exciting case stories in student medicinal chemistry courses.

In this third edition of the textbook, all of these aspects of academic and industrial medicinal chemistry and drug design are dealt with in an educational context.

Povl Krogsgaard-Larsen
Tommy Liljefors
Ulf Madsen

Chapter 1

Drug design and discovery: an overview

Lester A. Mitscher

1.1 INTRODUCTION

Drugs are chemicals that prevent disease or assist in restoring health to diseased individuals. As such they play an indispensable role in modern medicine.

Medicinal chemistry is that branch of science that provides these drugs either through discovery or through design. The classical drugs of antiquity were primarily discovered by empirical observation using substances occurring naturally in the environment. In the last two centuries, drugs increasingly were also prepared by chemical alteration of natural substances. In the century just past many novel drugs were discovered entirely by chemical synthesis. An ever increasing understanding of the nature of disease, how cells work, and how drugs influence these processes has in the last two decades led increasingly to the deliberate design, synthesis and evaluation of candidate drug molecules. In the third millennium, all of these techniques are in use still and the student of drug design and development must appreciate their relative value. Added to this picture are novel opportunities made possible by deeper understanding of cell biology and genetics.

Contemporary medicinal chemistry draws upon many disciplines so that its students and practitioners must have a broad working knowledge above all of organic chemistry but in addition, the student must be comfortable with significant elements of biochemistry, molecular biology, pharmacology, neurobiology, toxicology, genetics, cell biology, biophysics, quantum mechanics, anatomy, physiology, pathology, clinical medicine, computer technology, and the like. This is a tall but manageable order.

The central objective of each branch of chemistry is to possess such an understanding of the relationship between chemical structure and molecular properties that given a set of desired characteristics, a molecule can be proposed and prepared that should come close to possessing them. Next should follow, without undue experimentation, a testing and molecular refining cycle until a satisfactory molecular solution to the problem is at hand. A mature chemical science is efficient in achieving these characteristics. The reader will readily appreciate the complexity of the task in the case of medicinal chemistry and that the subject is still adolescent. A daunting feature is the number of properties that a candidate substance must possess in order to function therapeutically in the human body and so to become a drug. We also have much to learn about pathophysiology. Despite all this, a remarkable range of pharmaceuticals has been developed successfully and the pace of new entity introduction is gratifyingly rapid.

This textbook describes the manner in which medicinal chemists utilize the various fields upon which they draw and the specific stratagems that they employ to advance promising molecules into clinical use for the alleviation of disease and the betterment of mankind. This chapter is intended to introduce briefly some important topics not covered significantly elsewhere in this book and to provide a contextual framework especially for those comparatively new to the study of drug seeking.

1.2 HISTORICAL PERSPECTIVE

From prehistoric times until well into the twentieth century the vast majority of organic drugs originated from natural materials, often in crude mixtures. In early times, there was no possibility of understanding the nature of disease. Rather discoveries were made and preserved based upon observations of natural phenomena and the consequences of consumption of materials that alleviated distress. Of necessity, progress was disjointed and empirical. The use of opium, licorice, ephedra, marijuana, camellia, alcohol, digitalis, coca, quinine and a host of others still in use long predates the rise of modern medicine. It is interesting to note that the uses of these materials often are for diseases that are chronic and prevalent and are based upon responses that are observable in healthy individuals. These natural products are surely not elaborated by plants for our therapeutic convenience. We believe that they have survival value for the plants in dealing with their own ecological challenges and that only a small subset are found to have activity that can be co-opted for human or animal chemotherapy.

About 100 years ago, the mystery of why only certain molecules produced a specific therapeutic response was satisfactorily rationalized by the idea of Langley and Ehrlich that only certain cells contained receptor molecules that served as hosts for the drugs. The resulting combination created a new super molecule that had characteristically new properties producing a response of therapeutic value. One extension of this view was that the drug was a key that fit the target specifically and productively like a corresponding lock. When the fit was appropriate, a positive (agonist) pharmacological action followed analogous to opening a door. In other cases, a different kind of fit blocked the key so that the naturally intended key could not be inserted and antagonist action resulted so that the figurative door could not be opened. Thus, if one had found adventitiously a ligand for a receptor, one could refine its fit by opportunistic and systematic modification of the drug's chemical structure until it functioned very well. This productive idea hardly changed for the next half century and assisted in the preparation of many useful drugs. A less fortunate corollary of this useful picture is that it led to some restriction of imagination in drug design. The drug and its receptor (whose molecular nature was unknown when the theory was promulgated) were each believed to be rigid molecules precrafted to fit one another precisely. Most commonly, receptors are transmembranal glycoproteins accessible from the cell surface whose drug compatible region contains certain specific amino acids arranged in 3D-space.

Since the receptor surface is chiral, it is not surprising that chirality in the drug structure often plays an important role in cellular responses. This important topic is the subject of Chapter 3. Predicting an optimal ligand fit from structure–activity data through mathematical analytical methods is the subject of Chapter 5. These receptor surfaces are often present in molecular clefts such that they create a special local environment that is somewhat protected from the bulk solvent but accessible to substances present in it. The intricacies of interactions in this special environment is treated in Chapter 2. The active site is assembled from non-adjacent amino acid residues as a consequence of the 3D folding of the protein. Non-covalent bonds are formed with the appropriate ligand that indeed produce a temporary new macromolecule that usually signals other macromolecules deeper in the cell that satisfactory occupancy has taken place and the cell responds to this signal by taking the appropriate action.

Further complexities are uncovered continually. For example, a number of receptors are now known that consist of clusters of proteins either preassembled or assembled as a consequence of ligand binding. The component macromolecules can either be homo- or heterocomplexes. The complexity of finding specific ligands for systems of this complexity readily can be imagined (Milligan and Rees 2000).

The main modern difference from the classical picture, other than identifying specifically the chemical nature of the receptor and how it interacts with its ligand, is the realization that neither drug nor receptor need to be rigid. The opposite extreme to lock and key is the zipper model. In this view, a docking interaction takes place (much as the end of a zipper joins the talon piece) and, if satisfactory complementarity is present, the two molecules progressively wrap around each other and accommodate to each others steric needs. The reader will appreciate that all possible intermediate cases (rigid drug/flexible receptor; flexible drug/rigid receptor, etc.) are now known. A consequence of this mutual accommodation is that knowledge of the ground state of a receptor may not be particularly helpful when it adjusts its conformation to ligand binding. Thus, in many cases one now tries to determine the 3D aspects of the receptor–ligand complex. In those cases where X-ray analysis remains elusive, modeling the interactions involved is appropriate. This is the subject of Chapter 4. Further details of this marvelously complex system are presented in Chapter 6.

Earlier it was also noted that enzymes could be modulated for pharmacological benefit. Enzymes share many characteristics with glycoprotein receptors except that they assist in the performance of chemical reactions on their substrates so that the interaction is intrinsically more information rich than is the receptor–ligand interaction (which leaves the ligand unchanged). Until very recently, it was usually only possible to inhibit enzyme action rather than to promote it. Disease frequently results from excessive enzymatic action so selective inhibition of these enzymes is therapeutically useful. These interactions are covered in Chapter 12.

Much later it was discovered that other classes of receptors existed. For example, the highly lipophilic steroid hormones are able to cross the cell membrane and find their receptors in the cytoplasm. Receptor occupation is followed by migration of the new complex into the nucleus followed by selective gene activation. A third class of receptors consists of clusters of proteins assembled such as to create a specific transmembranal central pore. This channel permits the selective directional passage of specific ions in or out of the cell. These ion channels can be ion ligated or current sensitive. The ion flux creates a current that signals for the performance of specific work by the cell. New information involving this complex communication system appears almost daily. Chapter 7 discusses this field.

Over time, it became apparent that DNA and RNA also can be receptors and that the technology needed in order to design ligands for these macromolecules differs in detail from that needed to design ligands for receptors. The earliest applications of DNA liganding lie in inhibiting its formation and function so that cell death was the expected result. Since rapid uncontrolled cell growth is characteristic of cancer, this sort of methodology, starting in about 1940, led to the first successful chemical treatments of this dreaded disease. Revolutionary treatments for cancer are within our grasp based upon novel discoveries in cell biology and genomics. This will be presented in detail in Chapter 17.

Much greater therapeutic safety attends inhibition of the enzymes that are involved in DNA synthesis and its processing. This has led to recent remarkable advances in the chemotherapy of viral diseases. Until quite recent times, viral diseases were extremely difficult to treat but this picture has now changed remarkably as will be described in Chapter 16.

RNA is responsible for the biosynthesis of proteins and use of species specific inhibitory ligands for it results in cell death or stasis. This phenomenon is responsible for the therapeutically useful selective toxicity of many antibiotics.

Interestingly, until the mid 1970s known drug targets were primarily neuro-transmitter receptors on cell surfaces. Since that time, a wealth of information has been uncovered and many other choices are now available. In this context, it is interesting therefore to consider the molecular targets for which drugs are contemporarily crafted even though this is shifting rapidly (Drews 2000):

1	Cellular receptors	45%
2	Enzymes	28%
3	Hormones and factors	11%
4	Ion channels	5%
5	DNA	2%
6	Nuclear receptors	2%
7	Unknown	7%

Clearly, cellular receptors and enzymes make up the bulk of the targets favored at this time.

That it took so long to work out the details that we presently understand about drug action is not surprising. When the receptor theory was first advanced, no protein structure would be known for at least 50 years on. Furthermore, in contrast to enzymes, the receptor binds the ligand with temporary non-covalent bonds and does not process its ligand. Thus, one could only infer what intermolecular forces were operating and what could be the molecular and biological consequences of the interaction. Striking advances in molecular spectroscopy have led to the identification of the 3D-structure of many enzymes and their substrates and inhibitors and, indeed, for a few receptors and their ligands. Increasingly nuclear magnetic resonance methods are also producing detailed structural information. The use of computer graphic techniques allows for virtual screening of candidates for synthesis. By this, a given ligand can be subtracted from a 3D-picture of a drug ligand interaction and a new ligand can be fitted in instead. If suggestive, the new ligand can be synthesized and tested. It is also possible to screen actually or virtually through a collection of available molecules to find substances that will fit into the active site in place of a known ligand and then to test it for efficacy. The methodology is still empirical but the time investment is machine time rather than synthesis time so, aside from the cost of the machinery and the development of the sophisticated software, time is saved.

Even this complex picture is greatly simplified. It is now well recognized that most receptors exist as families of subreceptors and that further specificity of action results from ligands that occupy only a specific one of the subreceptors and not the others. Doing this effectively became widely practiced from about 1965. A well-known example of this that illustrates the concept is that norepinephrine exerts a variety of effects in the body by virtue of its occupying all three of the families of adrenergic sub receptors (Figure 1.1). Further complexities arise from there being many subclasses of receptors within each family. Each of these has its own

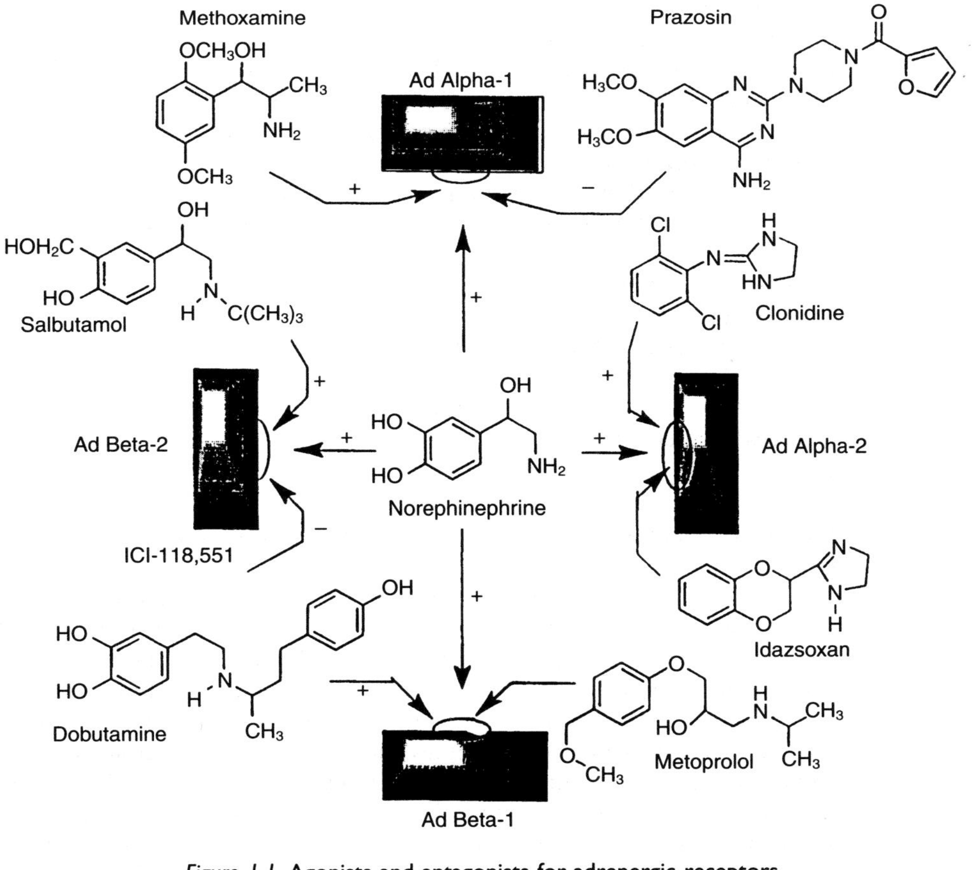

Figure 1.1 Agonists and antagonists for adrenergic receptors.

structural requirements. The body deals with this problem by secreting this neurotransmitter near a specific type of receptor so as to get a specifically desired response and then either destroying the transmitter promptly or reabsorbing it and putting it back into storage for future use once the stimulus that led to neurotransmitter release is over. An added virtue of this means of action is that the action of the drug is temporary so that it has a start point and a stop point of satisfactory length and that it does not migrate far away to occupy unintended receptors and so produce side actions. Through molecular manipulation, specific agonists and antagonists have been prepared for all of these adrenergic subreceptors (Figure 1.1). Thus, through creative analoging fine control of the specific pharmacological response can be obtained.

The devilish complexity of the process of drug design and development will be readily appreciated by considering also that the processes just described deal only with potency and selectivity. Suitable toxicological, pharmacokinetic, pharmacodynamic, pharmaceutical and commercial factors must also be built into the substance before marketing can take place.

Even with the advantage of all this accumulated knowledge it is certain that a great many molecules must be investigated before a marketable version can be found. It is estimated that in 1997 about US$6 billion were spent worldwide on screening technologies and about 100 000 compounds are screened per day. The numbers are truly daunting. Several million compounds must be screened in order to find a thousand or so that have approximately correct characteristics and only a few of these successfully advance through analoging and biotesting to produce a dozen agents suitable for clinical study. Only six of these on average progress into clinical trials and just one reaches the market. Those new to the field may be surprised to learn that terms implying deliberately rational drug design came into general acceptance only in the last 20 years! In this context, the view advanced at that time that X-ray and computer techniques would allow one to prepare only a few dozen substances before finding a marketable substance now appear incredibly naive. It is clear in retrospect that the barriers represented by pharmacokinetic problems had been very significantly underestimated. The appeal of rational drug design is obvious in that it promises to reduce the empiricism of drug seeking enhancing the satisfaction of the practitioners and promising rapid economic returns to their sponsors. Fortunately, the field moves ever closer to the realization of this dream.

The pace of screening has accelerated dramatically in recent years. The application of high throughput screening methods has required rapid synthesis of large arrays of compounds suitable for screening. This in turn has led to the introduction and wide spread acceptance of combinatorial chemical methods.

The remainder of this chapter and, indeed, the book will assume that the reader is familiar with modern synthesis and will therefore address the questions of design and optimization. What molecules should be made, how should they be evaluated, and how should they be advanced to clinical use is our topic. It is important at this stage also to emphasize that priority of discovery is essential not only for very valid commercial reasons but also because drugs relieve suffering and delay is undesirable for humanitarian reasons. Thus, we rarely are able to pursue perfection. We only find it in the dictionary anyhow. The medicinal chemists motto is, instead, 'good enough – soon enough'.

1.3 WHAT KINDS OF COMPOUNDS BECOME DRUGS?

In order to be successful, one should know what gold looks like before panning. Drug seeking is analogous – it is essential to have a good idea of what kind of molecules are likely to become successful drugs before beginning. The normally preferred means of administration of medicaments is oral. Whereas there are no guarantees and many exceptions, the majority of effective oral drugs obey the Lipinski rule of fives. The data upon which this rule rests is drawn from 2500 entries extracted from the US Adopted Names, the World Drug lists, and the internal Pfizer compound collections. There are four criteria:

1   The substance should have a molecular weight of 500 or less.
2   It should have fewer than five hydrogen-bond donating functions.
3   It should have fewer than ten hydrogen-bond accepting functions.
4   The substance should have a calculated $\log P$ ($c \log P$) between approximately -1 to $+5$.

In short, the compound should have a comparatively low molecular weight, be relatively non-polar and partition between an aqueous and a particular lipid phase in favor of the lipid phase but, at the same time, possess perceptible water solubility. There are many biologically active compounds that satisfy these criteria that fail to become drugs but there are comparatively few successful orally active drugs that fail to fit (Lipinski *et al.* 2001). Thus, this is a helpful guide but not a law of nature.

These criteria put in semi-quantitative terms a great deal of accumulated observations and rationalizations. For absorption and tissue distribution, a drug must be absorbed through a succession of lipid bilayers before reaching its target. Drugs must be able to pass through these barriers rapidly enough to allow therapeutic concentrations to build up. As diffusion is a logarithmic function of size and shape, comparatively compact molecules of modest molecular weight are most suitable. There must, in addition, be sufficient water solubility for dissolution and transport to take place. This correlates reasonably well with the capacity to donate and to accept a moderate number of hydrogen bonds. There must also be sufficient lipid solubility to allow the drug to enter and pass out of a lipid environment. The semi-quantitative aspects of the Lipinski rules address the question of how much is enough. In this sense, the rules embody useful aspects of the Hansch quantitative structure–activity equations that will be covered extensively in Chapter 5. It is also apparent that the pK_a of the molecule in question is also critical because it reflects the polarity of a substance as a function of the pH of its environment. Acids, bases and amphoteric molecules have strong polarities, hence partitioning behavior, that are strongly influenced by this. The more salt-like they become the poorer is their ability to be absorbed through lipid bilayers. Likewise, if they are too non-polar they will dissolve in the lipid bilayers and remain there.

Some of these considerations can be made clearer by the use of a simple cartoon (Figure 1.2). (1) Some small and rather water soluble substances pass in and out of cells through water lined transmembrane pores. Many salts fit into this category. (2) Other agents that are significantly polar are conducted into

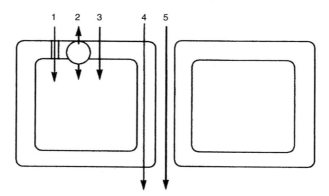

Figure 1.2 Means of cellular uptake and passage by drugs: (1) Passage through porins; (2) active uptake/ejection; (3) passive diffusion into cytoplasm; (4) passive diffusion through the cell; and (5) pericellular passage.

or out of cells by membrane associated and energy consuming proteins. Polar nutrients that the cell requires, such as glucose and many amino acids fit into this category. More recently drug resistance by cells has been shown to be mediated in many cases by analogous protein importers and exporters. (3) Those molecules that are partially water soluble and partially lipid soluble can pass through cell membranes by passive diffusion and are driven in the direction of the lowest concentration. (4) In cells lining the intestinal tract, it is possible for such molecules to pass into the body through the cell membrane alone. (5) Finally, it is also possible for molecules with suitable water solubility, small size and compact shape to pass into the body between cells. This last route is generally not available for passage into the central nervous system (CNS) because the cells are pressed closely together closing off these junctions. This tight capillary junction in aggregate is known as the blood–brain barrier. (6) If all else fails, hypodermic injection is the answer.

For drugs to become successful parenteral agents administered by hypodermic needle, satisfactory water solubility is an overridingly important criterion and a low to moderate molecular weight is much less important. Insulin and some glycopeptide antibiotics such as vancomycin exemplify these substances.

Other routes of administration (transdermal, sublingual, pulmonary, vaginal, rectal, e.g.) are much less frequently used. Each has special features requiring adjustment of molecular properties for optimization. Unfortunately, this fascinating topic would require too much space to explore here.

1.4 PREPARATION AND ORGANIZATION FOR DRUG SEEKING

Flowchart 1.1 synopsizes the stages through which the work passes from inception to marketing and beyond in drug seeking. From this the complexity of the task of finding new medications is readily apparent.

COMMON STAGES IN THE DRUG SEEKING CAMPAIGN

Year 0–1	Identify a suitable disease; Assemble a multi-disciplinary team; Select a promising approach; Obtain a satisfactory budget
	Start the chemistry (collect natural product sources; synthesize or purchase chemicals)
	Start the pharmacology (devise and perfect a suitable screen; select 'hits')
Year 1–2	Confirm potential utility of 'hits' in animals (potency; selectivity; acceptable toxicity)
Year 3–5	Analog around the most promising 'hits'; Ascertain freedom to operate (examine patents/literature); Detailed pharmacology (potency; mode of action; acute and chronic toxicity; reproductive toxicity; genotoxicity); Adjust absorption, distribution, metabolism and excretion characteristics; Devise large scale synthesis; Formulation studies; Stability studies; Apply for patent protection
Year 4–9	Phase I clinical studies (Safety; Dosage; Blood Levels)
	Phase II clinical studies (Effectiveness; Side Effects)
	Phase III clinical studies (Range of effectiveness; Long-term and rare side effects)
Year 8–11	Regulatory review
Year 10–15	Marketing and Phase IV clinical studies (Monitor safety; Very large scale chemistry; Distribution; Advertising; Education)
Year 17–20	Patent protection expires; Generic competition

Flowchart 1.1 The time course and the various stages through which a drug seeking campaign usually passes.

Once organizational and fiscal considerations have been accomplished the project can begin. These decisions are non-trivial and are usually made by committee. They require a great deal of judgement because there are rarely enough resources and talent to do all of the things one would like to do. Whereas the rewards for success are great, the consequences of failure are often devastating. This is a heavy responsibility.

Contemporarily important disease targets are typically CNS derangements, cancer, infectious diseases, degenerative diseases and cardiovascular problems. The pharmaceutical industry is still in the process of centripetal separation into fewer but much larger firms on the one hand and a number of much smaller specialized firms on the other. The large firms carry on drug discovery and development the whole way from inception to marketing. They become increasingly risk averse as a consequence and only drugs promising to earn major sales can be justified to the share holders. One consequence is that the category of orphan diseases, that is diseases with too fewer affluent sufferers to warrant attention, is expanding rapidly and increasingly includes diseases present in the developed countries where big pharma lies. The smaller firms lack the resources to accomplish this by themselves so specialize in serving the process through specialization in a narrower range of higher risk research. Development of novel screens, production of compound collections for screening, exploration of unusual means of administration, and the like, characterize their activity. They must of necessity pursue niche markets unattractive to big pharma, identify partners with deeper pockets, or be absorbed by them in order to survive.

The project team must examine the theories of disease causation and pick a likely approach that has not been thoroughly examined already, for which suitable therapy is not already available, and which one believes one has the resources to address. As an increasingly common alternative, a novel gene or gene product is selected that appears to be involved in the pathology of a disease. Successful knock-out mouse studies often enhance confidence that a novel cause-and-effect relationship exists involving the selected target and that the patient could tolerate the treatment.

With this in hand, it is possible to assemble a team of scientists with all of the necessary skills needed to address the problem. The team will then select an interesting molecule from which to proceed or will devise a suitable high through-put molecular screen to detect molecules with the needed characteristics and collect molecules to screen from which these can reasonably be expected to emerge. From the compounds found to be active in the screen, suitable molecules will be selected to advance. These 'hits' may be substances that are in the literature, a collection of compounds in one's retained sample collection, a collection of molecules available for purchase (often a diverse combinatorial library), a collection of extracts of natural origin, or a series of molecules speculatively synthesized on the belief that one or more might be active, and the like. This selection is often a very challenging part of the whole process.

Proof of concept is obtained from animal studies when the hit substance is shown to be active in whole cell or organ systems in model diseases. Next the initial lead molecules are modified synthetically to identify the pharmacophore and to enhance potency and selectivity. Then, other imperfections in the lead are solved by synthetic modification to elevate the lead into candidate drug status. The many problems beyond potency, selectivity and safety that must be overcome are listed in Section 1.6 of this chapter. Next, detailed pharmacological study in more than one species identify the likely utility and safety of the candidate drug in model diseases. Suitable back-up substances are prepared and brought forward as insurance against unexpected failure of the candidate to survive the development sequence. This happens all too often and then an alternative candidate must be brought forward. It is prudent to have more than one such back-up substance available and it is wise if their chemical structures differ significantly from the structure of the primary candidate. Suitable formulations and an economically attractive chemical synthesis is developed. Finally, clinical trials are undertaken.

This listing implies that these stages are completed in sequence. Unfortunately, however, it is often the case that difficulties in a later stage require the group to retreat to an earlier stage and bring alternative molecules forward again. As much of the early work as possible is carried out in parallel. This back and forth work is frustrating and consumes considerable time. Overall completion of the process normally consumes 8–12 years and costs between 0.3–0.5 billion dollars. At an estimated average profit return, firms often expect approximately 5 years of sales before the first profit is returned. With this extraordinary level of investment and commitment it is not surprising that drug houses merge with regularity and that they are intensely interested in methods promising to reduce the risks involved and in shortening the time between conception and marketing. Commercial viability contemporarily requires the introduction of 1–3 such substances each year and stock valuation is significantly affected by guesstimates of the quality and quantity of a firm's pipeline of promising molecules.

1.5   SOURCES OF HITS, LEADS AND CANDIDATE DRUGS

Once suitable biological screens have been set up, collections of promising molecules are passed through them. The initial screens often have high throughput but limited information content. Molecules which attach themselves significantly to selected enzymes or receptor preparations are called 'hits'. A necessary gating level of affinity is usually settled upon. This is often 50 micromolar or stronger. From the list of hits, drug-like molecules are selected that appear free from potentially toxic moieties, untoward reactivity or other undesirable features. The survivors of this screen are then tested in ever more elaborate biological assays, usually involving whole cell systems, to verify that affinity reflects potentially useful activity. Those surviving molecules that warrant the time, costs and effort of analog preparation to further enhance their desirable properties are called 'leads'. One generally tries to reach single digit micromolar potency or stronger with such compounds. When the leads have been refined further so that satisfactory potency, selectivity, freedom from toxicity, chemical novelty, suitable pharmacokinetic and pharmacodynamic properties, etc. are present in animal models of disease, the survivors are elevated to the status of 'candidate drugs' suitable for extensive biological evaluation up to and including clinical trials in humans. Single digit nanomolar potency is usually sought for these compounds. It will be seen that the biological tests become ever more content rich, challenging, and time consuming. The costs escalate dramatically as the experimentation proceeds. It is also clear that the number of substances that satisfy these ever more stringent requirements falls off dramatically with time. It is often estimated that for each 7000 substances that start, only one comes through to the end and that up to a dozen years often elapses from start to finish. The statistics are even more discouraging in the age of combinatorial chemistry where the numbers of compounds screened for each success is even larger.

Knowing what kinds of molecules make useful drugs, one needs to know where to find them. The possibilities are in theory infinite. In practice, however, suitable sources are well recognized.

1.5.1   Natural products

1.5.1.1   Higher plant and animal products

As described in Section 1.2, prehistoric drug discovery started with higher plant and animal substances and this continues to this day to be a fruitful source of biologically active molecules belonging to unanticipated structural types. Adding to the long list of classical plant products that have survived into modern medicine, one can list many substances of more recent origin including the antibiotics (penicillins, cephalosporins, tetracyclines, aminoglycosides, glycopeptides, etc.), anticancer agents (taxol, camptothecin, vinca alkaloids, doxorubicin, bleomycin, etc.), the immunosuppressant drugs cyclosporin and tacrolimus, and a variety of other pharmacological agents such as compactin, asperlicin, etc. In addition, natural products have provided the structural pattern that has led to the synthesis of valuable medications (snake venom peptides that led to orally active angiotensin converting enzyme inhibitors, cocaine which led to local anesthetics, willow bark glycosides led to aspirin and then to the COX-II inhibitors, and so on). The continuing encroachment of human habitation raises legitimate fears of extinction of important potential sources of drugs that are yet to be discovered in tropical regions. In many cases, as in traditional Chinese medicine and Ayurveda, a great deal of ethnobotanical medicine also exists to be mined. There is reason for haste in bioprospecting. These materials have the potential advantage of having had informal clinical trials before analoging begins. This lessens the chance that a nasty toxicological surprise awaits, as too often it does, at the end of long and expensive evaluation of a synthetic substance. The current commerce in herbal medicines in Europe and the United States of America is very substantial. Some of these herbals will in time be the source of new medications, some will remain in use in their present form and some will fade away as a consequence of scientific scrutiny. It is most likely that the successful materials will be suitable for chronic or preventative medicine rather than for rapid cure of florid conditions.

Animal products have also led to important medications. Porcine insulin, for example, is only one of a variety of hormones used in replacement therapy or, in modified form, for other therapeutic purposes. Genetic engineering techniques have had a significant impact here. Human insulin is now readily available from fermentation sources following transfection of the genes needed for its production and development of techniques for expression, excretion and isolation. Likewise available is human growth hormone. This list will expand dramatically in the years just ahead. A somewhat analogous promising developing technology is the production of genetically modified crops as a source of pharmaceuticals. This promises to be an economic resource at least partially divorced from national boundaries (Gruber and Theisen 2000).

One can also cite the anti-inflammatory uses of analogs of cortical hormones when given in suprahormonal doses made possible as a consequence of partial synthesis. The antifertility and anticancer properties of sex hormone analogs, and the like, have also benefitted from this work.

One of the primary values of natural products in drug seeking is the impressive molecular complexity and novelty that they possess. Very few chemists are imaginative enough to compete successfully with the structural diversity found in nature. Indeed, few synthesis chemists would be bold enough to make them if nature had not provided the pattern first. This process of drug discovery is useful but slow. It can, however, stimulate an enormous additional effort when a useful new structural type is identified. Large scale directed industrial screening of natural products from fermentations and the deliberate search for anticancer chemotherapy under the sponsorship of federal agencies represent modern variants of this ancient process.

A promising future avenue for drug discovery using natural products lies in the new field of combinatorial biosynthesis. Here manipulation of the genes involved in biosynthetic pathways are assembled in novel combinations leading to forced evolution and the artificial generation of novel structures that have yet to be found in nature.

Whereas the use of animal products in medicine is easy to rationalize, the reader may wonder how it is that higher plant products have useful pharmacological properties. In those comparatively few cases where we have convincing evidence, it appears that plant products occasionally have sufficient topographic similarity to indigenous mammalian chemicals that they can substitute topologically for them at their receptors. One cites ephedrine and epinephrine, morphine and enkephalins, and tetrahydrocannabinol and anandamide as pairs that illustrate this point. Thus, we believe that plants make these compounds for their own purposes but their biological activity is sufficiently broad that they can be co-opted for human medicinal chemical purposes also. As far as is known, the human receptors have no obvious counterpart in plants so the mutual fit is fortuitous.

1.5.1.2 Arthropod and insect products

Arthropod and insect products have yet to produce many significant medicinal agents but they show significant promise. The alkaloids in the skin of certain colorful tropical tree frogs show profound biological activity (rationalizing their ethnic use as arrow and dart poisons) and batracotoxin, for example, is under serious study for its cardiovascular properties. Intensive study has shown that these compounds are not produced directly by the frogs but rather are accumulated from digestion of arthropods that make up much of their diet. The florid appearance of the frogs seems to be an advertisement. Rather than seeking concealment they are clearly visible so that potential predators are warned not to eat them by mistake.

1.5.1.3 Fermentation products

Soil micro-organisms produce a wide variety of compounds when grown on complex media. This takes advantage of their versatile natural role in converting dead plants and animals into compost and their ability to exist on soil detritus as a consequence of their amazing intrinsic biosynthetic versatility. The first medicinal products from soil streptomycetes, bacteria and fungi, aside from alcohol, were powerful antibiotics that provided them with safety in their natural habitat but could also be used to combat human infections. Some of the more cytotoxic agents found are used in treatment of tumors. More recently, they have proven a valuable source of a wide variety of structures with general physiological activity that does not depend upon killing cells for their action. The use of fermentation products related to mevalonin and compactin, for example, to inhibit 3-hydroxy-3-methyl-glutaryl coenzyme A reductase and so reduce plasma cholesterol levels is a striking example. These and related agents have generated billions of dollars in revenue to their discoverer's firms.

1.5.1.4   Marine products

The Seven Seas were among the last regions of the earth to see extensive natural product exploration and have proven to be a rich source of unusual chemical structures. Most have proven to be too toxic or too narrow in spectrum to find use in human medicine but some, such as briostatin and dolestatin, have astonishing potency as cytotoxic agents and are under intensive clinical examination as potential antitumor agents. More recent compounds of this type showing anti-cancer promise include eleutherobin (a microtubule stabilizing compound from a soft coral), discodermolide and the sponge product mycalamide B. Marine gorgonians have proven to be comparatively rich sources of prostaglandins although other sources have proven to be more convenient in practice. The search goes on and practical results seem probable.

1.5.1.5   Pre-existing substances

Hundreds of thousands of organic chemicals have been synthesized for non-drug purposes. A number of these, when examined in appropriate test systems turn out to have useful pharmacological properties. For example, p-aminobenzenesulfonamide, found to be an antimicrobial agent of sufficient value to earn a Nobel prize in the 1930s had actually been synthesized in 1908 by Gelmo in Vienna but was not known at the time to be a biologically active substance. It is probably not useful to speculate about the toxicity and morbidity that could have been avoided during the First World War years if only it had been suitably tested in a timely manner! A more recent example involves the non-neutrative sweetner aspartame. The great economic utility of this compound as a sucrose substitute was discovered serendipitously when it was found to be exceptionally sweet tasting in the course of being weighed as a chemical intermediate in a synthetic project having a very different objective.

1.5.1.6   Compounds prepared by speculative syntheses

Once a popular avenue towards drug discovery, many compounds of unusual but suggestive structure have been synthesized so that they could be evaluated as potential drugs. Historically these were provided to pharmacologists in the hope that a useful biological property would be found during the course of general biological evaluation. The benzodiazepines were made in this mode and were found to be of outstanding medicinal value in the treatment of psychoses. This was not suspected in advance of their preparation and evaluation. An instructive and entertaining account of the work that led to this wonderful discovery is available (Sternbach 1979). This mode of drug discovery fell very much out of favor during the computer assisted drug design decades but is making a strong come back in the days of combinatorial chemistry.

1.5.1.7   Compound collections

Most firms archive samples of unsuccessful substances prepared in various drug-seeking campaigns. These are then subjected to each new screen that is developed and it is remarkable how often this turns up unsuspected activities that ultimately lead to useful new agents following further structural manipulation.

1.5.1.8 Combinatorial libraries

Because this methodology has become so prominent in such a short time, it deserves more extensive treatment than the other topics in this section can receive. Classically, chemists have prepared substances one at a time and took pride in using novel reactions and reactants to obtain the highest possible yield in the greatest possible purity. No matter how satisfying this is to its practitioners it is time consuming and expensive. As long as the rate of construction of new substances was faster than the time required for biological evaluation, there was no motivation for change. The development of many new tests and of high throughput screening methods in the 1980s, however, created a demand for more compounds to test. Chemists responded to this need by developing methods for multiple parallel synthesis and combinatorial chemistry. Now it is possible in favorable cases to prepare hundreds to thousands of compounds in very short time and synthesis and testing are back in phase with each other.

Combinatorial chemistry has consequently become a method of choice for the rapid construction of large arrays of drug-like molecules. It had its beginnings with the Merrifield resin-based peptide syntheses which were so useful that they were rewarded with a Nobel prize. The iterative nature of protein synthesis and the ready availability of the component parts made this methodology particularly apt and the explosion of information in cell biology made it particularly timely. Given that there are approximately the same number of amino acids commonly found in proteins as there are letters in the Latin alphabet and how many languages have been constructed from this alphabet, one readily appreciates the astronomical numbers of peptides that could in principle be prepared in a combinatorial mode by assembling all conceivable combinations of amino acids into peptides. To be sensible, smaller combinatorial arrays are made. By single compound synthesis, just making all of the possible tripeptides alone would be a life-time labor. Use of combinatorial methodology to be explicated below makes this a reasonably trivial undertaking.

Biochemists rapidly embraced this resin-based chemistry as did firms developing bioassays that did not have chemical libraries on hand or synthetic chemists to prepare them. Peptides are the normal means with which cells conduct their inter- and intracellular business. They are often biosynthesized near the site of their action so specificity of action is managable. The situation is different when they must be administered to patients for they must survive digestive processes and have a long way to travel and many cell membranes to cross before they reach their site of action. They often make satisfactory drugs if one is prepared to inject, but their polarity and digestibility make them poor drugs for oral therapeutic purposes. An enormous effort has been expended to overcome these natural drawbacks but the results have not yet been impressive. Still, they make convenient hits and methods for converting peptides into more drug-like molecules (peptidomimetics) are gradually being developed. This topic is treated extensively in Chapter 15.

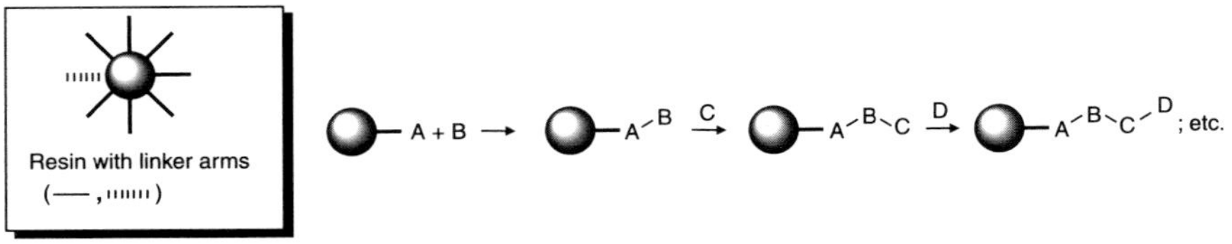

Figure 1.3 Single resin/single peptide (Merrifeld style) methodology.

Generally speaking only microgram to milligram quantities of peptides are prepared for biological evaluation using resin methods because of the limited loading capacity of the resins. These are often tested in mixtures that must be deconvoluted later to identify the active components. Many ingenious methods have been developed to tag these resin bound peptides so that their chemical history (and putative structures) can be determined without needing to separate them from the resin and determine their chemical structure by laborious micro methods.

Some of the methodologies used for the construction of very large arrays (libraries) of compounds preparable by iterative chemistry can be illustrated by the following examples.

1.5.1.8.1   Single resin/single peptide (Merrifeld style)

In this case (Figure 1.3), an insoluble resin (**r**) contains a number of linker arms (—), functionalized at the end so that an amino acid, represented by a capital letter (A, B, C, etc.) can be attached to each one and then reacted sequentially with additional amino acids to form peptide bonds. A different linker arm (----) can be present to which a signal sequence can be attached. The chemical nature of the two different types of linker arms differs so that they can be individually reacted and their contents detached independently from each other. At the end of the reaction sequence, the linker arm in most cases is selectively severed to release the peptide for analysis and testing and the resin and its arm can be recycled.

1.5.1.8.2   Combinatorial mode: mix and split style

In this case (Figure 1.4), an amino acid is linked to arms on a reaction inert resin and then split into two equal portions. One of these is reacted with amino acid A and the other with B to produce resins with two different dipeptides attached.

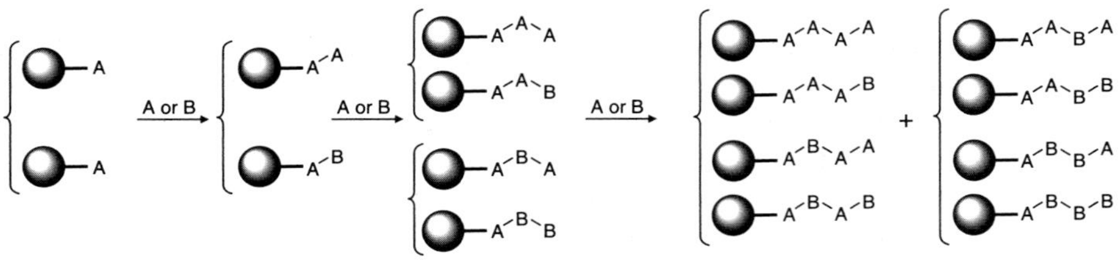

Figure 1.4 Combinatorial synthesis. Mix and split style.

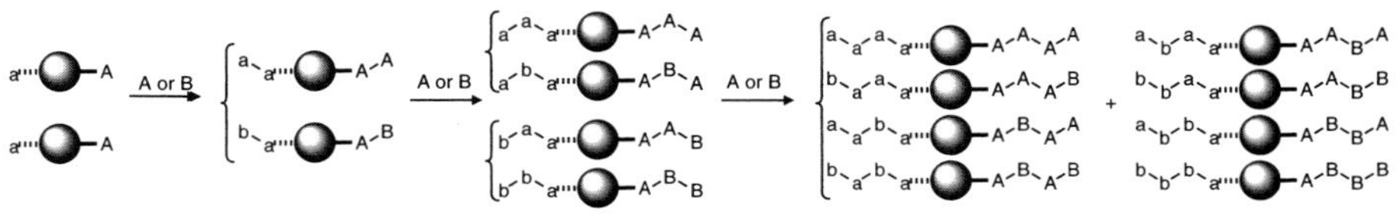

Figure 1.5 Combinatorial synthesis. Label, mix, and split style.

These are mixed and split again into two equal piles. Amino acid A is added to the first pile and B to the second. This produces two mixtures each containing two different tripeptides. Repetition produces two different resin mixtures each containing four different tetrapeptides. This process can be repeated indefinitely.

1.5.1.8.3   Combinatorial mode: label, mix and split style

In this example (Figure 1.5), the capital letters stand for one of two different amino acids while the small letters stand for one of two different but corresponding nucleotide or some other type of monomer. Each time amino acid A is added, code nucleotide a is also added. Likewise with B and b. The two kinds of linker arms are chemically distinct so that the code sequence and the peptide sequence can be removed independently for analysis. In this way, the history of the bead can be ascertained. Knowing this one knows what peptide should be on the bead.

1.5.1.8.4   Radiofrequency detection

It is possible to place a tunable radio signal-generator in the resin. In this way, the active compound on a resin can be determined by identifying the signal that it generates.

1.5.1.8.5   Deconvolution

The chemical labor of adding a signal sequence, detaching it and analyzing it can be avoided by use of biological deconvolution methods.

1.5.1.8.6   Iterative deconvolution

In this process, one does not mix the resins after the last reaction but keeps the resins terminating in A separate from those terminating in B and then mixes these into groups (Figure 1.6a). Each of these is tested separately and let us say that the mixture of tetrapeptides terminating in A is active (boxed in the figure). Next one synthesizes two mixed resins in which the penultimate amino acid is A in one and B in the other (Figure 1.6b). These are tested separately and, say, the group with amino acid B in the third position is active (boxed in the figure). Another iteration in which **r**-A-A-B-A and **r**-A-B-B-A are individually prepared and tested reveals that the active component responsible for activity in this whole series was **r**-A-B-B-A. This process is dependent on biological rather than chemical analysis for success. The more complex the library of compounds is, the more useful this process is.

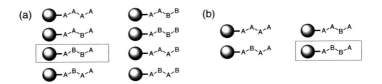

Figure 1.6 Iterative convolution: first (a) and second phase (b).

1.5.1.8.7   Positional deconvolution

In this process (Figure 1.7a), a series of sublibraries are prepared whose composition is systematically varied. In this manner, all C-terminal amino acids are the same whereas the remaining positions can have any of the possible compositions. If tripeptides consisting of all possible combinations of three amino acids are involved, 27 different peptides will be produced. In the example given (Figure 1.7a), the first amino acid is A, B, or C. One presumes that activity is found for this library. In this case, a second library (Figure 1.7b) is produced which contains A, B, or C as the first amino acid but always contains A as the last amino acid. Next (Figure 1.7c), a third library is produced which contains only A as the second amino acid. The fourth library (Figure 1.7d) has all the cases in which only A is the first amino acid. The fifth library (Figure 1.7e) has all the cases in which the third amino acid is B. The sixth library (Figure 1.7f) has all the cases in which the second amino acid is B. The seventh library (Figure 1.7g) has all the cases in which the first amino acid is B. The eighth library (Figure 1.7h) has all the cases in which the third amino acid is C. The ninth library (Figure 1.7i) has all the cases in which the second amino acid is C. The tenth and last library (Figure 1.7j) has all the cases in which the first amino acid is C.

Each of these libraries is tested. In this example libraries one, three, seven and eight are active. The only way in which this result could be obtained is if the sequence of the one active constituent is B-A-C. This example looks more laborious than it actually is although complex libraries with many components require the preparation and testing of a large number of sublibraries.

1.5.1.8.8   Omission and tester libraries

Another deconvolution method is to make a set of sublibraries where no component contains amino acid A, another without B and another without C. These omission libraries are tested. A tester library contains all of the peptides missing from the tester libraries. One of these has A peptides added, another B added and a third has C added. Testing of these libraries reveals the active sequence.

1.5.1.8.9   The Pasteur-like method

In a limited number of cases where the peptide still bound to the resin is biologically active in this form and the result of the activity is generation of a color or a zone of inhibition, it is possible to distribute the individual resin particles on a seeded solid surface such as an agar plate. After the test is complete the active

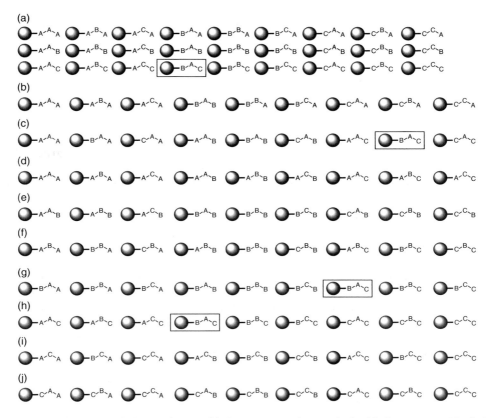

Figure 1.7 (a) Positional deconvolution; (b) Sequences ending with A; (c) Sequences with A in the middle; (d) Sequences starting with A; (e) Sequences ending with B; (f) Sequences with B in the middle; (g) Sequences starting with B; (h) Sequences ending with C; (i) Sequences with C in the middle; and (j) Sequences beginning with C.

resins are visible on inspection of the plate and can be picked off of the agar surface using tweezers and analyzed. Alternatively, the active beads may become colored in solution as a consequence of their activity and can be picked out on this basis. Another method involves the presence of a code residue that is colored. When tested in collections of beads in wells, the ones that are active are associated with a particular color. The components of that well can be tested individually in a separate series and the one that produces that color is the active one. This provides a confirmatory test and reveals the identity of the active product.

1.5.1.8.10   Spatially addressed libraries

PHOTOLITHOGRAPHIC METHOD

In this method (Figure 1.8), the resin is affixed to a solid support so as to form a coated layer, analogous to the surface of a credit card or a thin layer plate. The amino

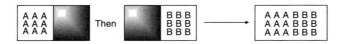

Figure 1.8 Photolithographic synthesis of peptide arrays. In this illustration, one field is covered while the other is reacted with A. Next, the mask is shifted and the uncovered field is reacted with B. Many different patterns can be used so that at the end of an iterative process each location has a different peptide. Thousands of different peptides can be generated in an amazingly small area.

acids to be affixed are derivatized with a photolabile protecting group. The surface of the resin bed is partially protected by a series of opaque filters. Irradiation with light deprotects the amino acid in question which is then bound to the surface of the resin bed. A second amino acid can be bound to a different region by use of another opaque filter protecting another region. A second amino acid can be joined to each of these first amino acids to form a group of dipeptides and this process can be repeated many times. The nature of the peptides found depends upon the number and the pattern of the successive filters. The result is that each address on the resin bed surface can be occupied by a different peptide whose identity is revealed by its X/Y co-ordinates. Testing consists of washing the surface with the test solution and observing a visible response.

PIN METHOD

In this experiment, a different peptide is generated on the end of each of a rank of pins affixed to a block. The peptide-containing pins can then be inserted in a 96 well plate (or larger) such that a single or a collection of different peptides is present in each well. Testing ensues and the identity of the actives comes from the identity of the peptide generated on the tip of the corresponding pin.

TEA BAG METHOD

In this method, a collection of resins is placed in each of a collection of porous plastic bags whose holes are sufficiently small to retain the resins but large enough to allow access to solutions into which the bags can be dipped. In this way, each bag can be made to contain an individual peptide or a collection of peptides whose identity is ascertained from the label on the bag.

The previous examples are but a selection of the many ingenious methods that have been developed for solid phase organic synthesis (SPOS) in a combinatorial or multiple parallel synthesis mode. For simplicity, the reactions have been illustrated using amino acid conversions to peptides. Oligonucleotides, oligosaccharides and many other kinds of organic molecules can be made in a similar manner. The power of the methodology is clear.

The reactions are generally driven to completion by use of excess reagents and long reaction times so that deletion errors are minimized. The excess reactants are removed by filtration and washing away the unwanted materials. Several components can be attached to each resin so as to saturate all of the available attachment

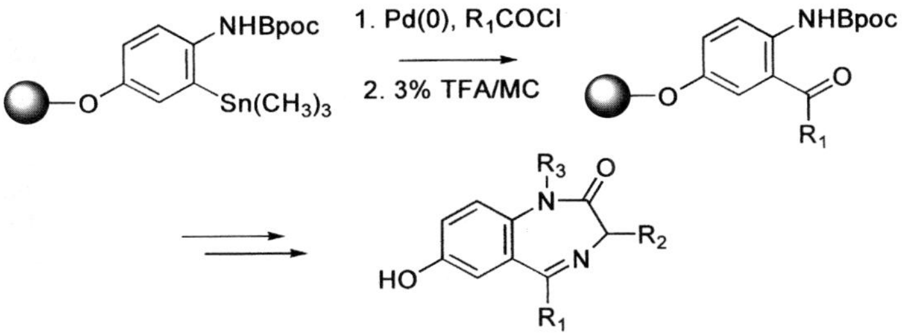

Figure 1.9 Combinatorial mode synthesis of hydroxylated benzodiazepines.

arms. This loading, however, is limited by the need to avoid interference with the chemistry by adjacent molecules. In principle, porous beads can be more heavily loaded than solid beads. In some instances, the compounds can be evaluated while still attached to the beads but in many cases, the compounds must be detached for analysis/identification and for pharmacological testing. For this to work, obviously the chemistry involved in linking the first component to the resin must differ from that involved in linking subsequent molecules to the first component. This kind of chemistry is termed 'orthogonal'.

Before long combinatorial libraries of DNA and RNA molecules were also prepared by iterative methods. Carbohydrate libraries have been the slowest of the informational macromolecules to be synthesized successfully by combinatorial methods. A principal barrier to be solved here is the necessity of controlling the stereochemistry of the anomeric center and its comparative chemical fragility.

The first drug-like heterocycles to be made in a combinatorial resin-based mode were the benzodiazepines (Figure 1.9). In this work, three different small organic molecules were combined using resin technology to produce a modest library of benzodiazepines which were screened for biological activity. The initial benzodiazepine libraries suffered from the defect that the attachment point to the resin arm required that the final products have a polar phenolic hydroxyl group following removal from the resin. The polarity of this functional group would inhibit penetration into the CNS (Bunin and Ellman 1992). Subsequent modifications led to the development of traceless linkers wherein the attachment point to the resin was lost upon cleavage from the resin without leaving behind a function in the products (Figure 1.10). The final benzodiazepines were therefore identical with those prepared previously one at a time in solution. Indeed, this chemistry could have been performed in solution if preferred. Gratifyingly, biotesting revealed that classic medicinal chemistry had identified the most active compounds already, albeit more slowly. This and related works opened a flood gate and within 5 years examples of most common drug-like molecules were synthesized and the methodology became increasingly divorced from resin methods and solution based methods, often termed multiple parallel synthesis (MPS), became increasingly popular. It was somewhat slow to take hold in drug preparation because the chemistry involved in the construction of small non-peptides is often much more idiosyncratic than peptide chemistry. By the year 2001, an average of three papers a day devoted to combinatorial and multiple parallel synthesis methods appeared in the chemical

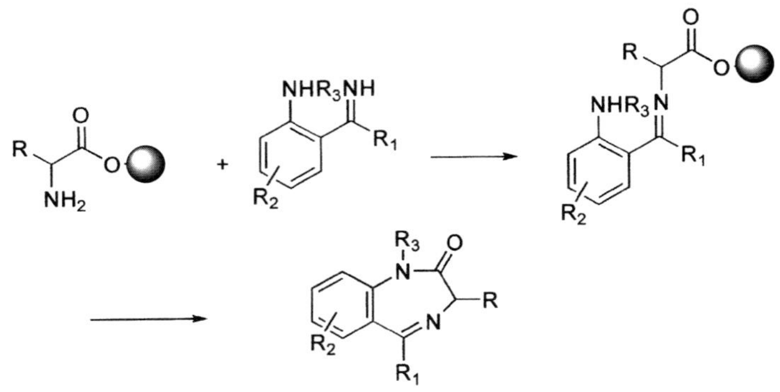

Figure 1.10 Combinatorial mode of traceless linker synthesis of benzodiazepines.

literature (not all of it devoted to drug seeking) and hundreds of different chemical libraries have been reported (Bunin, Dener and Livingston, 1999).

The combinatorial nature of this chemistry can be seen in that four variable positions are involved. Considering that the position of aromatic substitution involving R_2 is also variable, the reader can appreciate that thousands of analogs can be prepared quickly by simple variants of this process. Additional features of interest highlight the particular aptness of this example and illustrate important considerations in doing analogous work. The basic nucleus/core/centroid, where $R=R_1=R_2=R_3=H$, has a molecular weight of 160. This leaves 340 a.m.u. (500 − 160) to distribute amongst the four variable parts or an average of 85 a.m.u. that can be attached to each without getting the molecular weight too high. This would allow six methylenes or a benzene ring, etc. at each place. The projections from the centroids cover roughly the four cardinal points of the compass allowing significant exploration of space. The functional groups to which the R groups are attached are rather different from one another allowing flexibility and orthagonality in construction chemistry. The final products can readily be prepared so that they satisfy all of the Lipinski-rule characteristics and they are accordingly drug-like. The centroid has an amide and an imine function that can contribute to pharmacokinetic properties and even contribute to receptor binding so the centroid does not represent dead weight.

The speed with which a great number of analogs can be constructed can be illustrated by considering the result of starting with just 10 different variations of the R_2 in the aromatic ring. Ten different acyl side chains raises the number of analogs to 100 (10×10) and ten different groups attached to the anilino nitrogen leads to 1000 ($10 \times 10 \times 10$) variants. Use of 10 different amino acids in the condensation step produces 10 000 members in this small library alone. If each analog is chosen with some care using medicinal chemical logic, an enormous amount of useful knowledge emerges from testing such a library. Of course, if one does dumb things, then a large number of useless molecules emerge! Doing the work in successive pulses – that is, making smaller probing libraries, testing and using the results to define what should be in the next small library – is safer and more efficient than making all the possible analogs at once. Many hundreds of additional examples could be presented, including many in which the chemistry is performed in solution in individual reactors but there is not space enough for this.

The term combinatorial implies all conceivable arrangements of the available units. Since this would be very inefficient, but take nothing for granted, it is the antithesis of structure-based drug design where one presumes to understand the task sufficiently that only one or at most a few analogs need to be made in order to be successful. Neither extreme turns out to be realistic at this time. In fact, current trends show that the partisans for these extremes are coming ever closer in their views. Focused libraries, that is, smaller collections of promising molecules are now increasingly the objective of work in this field and it is becoming ever more intellectually satisfying to pursue.

In terms of speed, one can ask what one is talking about. The traditional mode of drug preparation is one at a time (usual speed analoging = usa) and the compound is not tested until available in significant quantity and demonstrable purity. A skilled medicinal chemist in a forgiving series can generally prepare between 50 and 100 compounds yearly. When drug evaluation was comparatively slow, this was sufficient to keep one's pharmacological colleagues quite busy. In the days of high throughput screening, this disincentive to preparing more compounds in unit time has been swept away. A combinatorial or multiple parallel synthesis chemist can now prepare this many analogs in a matter of a few days. Having made this analysis, however, one must point out that this is true but somewhat misleading. What is not stated is the time required to develop and rehearse the chemistry to be employed. This can take a matter of a few days to a year or more depending upon the state of the literature and the complexity of the targets. Nonetheless, the point is clear. Employment of combinatorial chemistry is essential for success in a competitive world.

Another factor which is not much discussed in the literature is the comparative costs of making combinatorial libraries. The purchase or synthesis of the component parts is often rather steep if very large libraries consisting of palpable quantities of each product are required. In industry, this is often less than the labor costs so may actually not be a major factor. The cost of automated equipment and the housing of complex synthesizers with large 'footprints' is itself not trivial. In talking with various firms, the number of about US$20 per analog seems not unreasonable. Thus making quite large libraries is expensive. The effective cost is reduced somewhat by archiving the materials and testing them in subsequent drug seeking campaigns when novel tests become available. The relative price of time and the value of the products appears to be the key consideration in judging the comparative value of this methodology.

Another important question is the level of purity one should aim for. In earlier times, this factor was all too often neglected and many examples have been discussed informally where worthless biological results were obtained from grossly impure products. Sometimes, in fact, the activity came from the impurity, or even that the substance in the vial was not the one on the label. Much greater care is now expended on quality assurance and commonly one expects at least 80–90% purity for each library component.

The question often arises as to how many compounds should be in a drug-seeking library. The ideal answer would be one. This is almost always impossible to realize. On the other hand, a skillful medicinal chemist who must make a hundred thousand compounds in order to get a candidate drug should be shot for incompetence. The usual answer is that somewhere between a hundred and a thousand substances will generally suffice. This is particularly true when uses the technique of pulsed libraries. Here one makes a limited number of structurally diverse molecules whose properties give them a chance of having useful pharmacokinetic and pharmacodynamic properties. The testing results suggest the next group to be prepared and evaluated. Each pulse then leads to a progressively more suitable collection of molecules from which the winners emerge expeditiously.

The question of whether to perform combinatorial or MPS chemistry on resins or in solution is partly a question of taste. Resin chemistry is not as familiar to the average chemist and requires attachment–detachment sequences analogous to protection–deprotection sequences resulting in unavoidable lengthening of the construction chemistry. The chemistry of the various attachments also must be compatable with the various linkers and the detachments must take place in the appropriate sequence. The resins must also be stable to the reagents and the reaction conditions and should not leave traces in the final products. Precedent chemistry is usually optimized in solution and so the reactions have to be adapted to the solid phase environment's needs. These disadvantages are balanced in part by the ease of purification of the products. Resin methodology is particularly useful for long sequences (more than five steps) and for very large libraries of comparatively small quantities (mgs at most) prepared by iterative processes. Solution methods are less limited in quantities to be prepared and conditions to be employed. They are also more familiar to the average chemist and many choices of reaction chambers are now available from which to choose.

Special applications of resins in solution phase organic synthesis (SnPOS) have also proven popular. For example, reagents can be present on resins. Following reaction, the excess or exhausted reagents can be removed by filtration and washing thereby simplifying workup. The synthesis of the adrenergic β-blocker propranolol serves as an example (Figure 1.11). Here, a six-step sequence was employed in which three of the steps utilized resin supported reagents. To start an amberlyst supported carbonate ion and iodine reacted with isopropylvinylamine salt and the resulting halide was transformed to the corresponding acetate ester with amberlyst supported acetate salt resin. Hydrolysis with potassium carbonate and ether formation with mesyl chloride was followed by a nucleophilic displacement with amberlyst-1-naphthoate resin and the carbonate protecting group was removed by KOH hydrolysis to produce propranolol. Obvious variants could be used to produce a library of analogs. Many other reactions have been performed with solid supported reagents (SSR) and this area has been nicely reviewed.

Resins can also be used to capture reaction by-products (e.g. basic resins to absorb acidic products) which can be separated by simple filtrations. These reactions can be worked up and the product isolated in pure form often by simple filtration and evaporation of solvents. Because the isolation of a large number of products resulting from combinatorial chemistry or multiple parallel synthesis can be exceedingly laborious and time consuming if performed in the traditional way, the convenience and time saving by using resin capture technology can be very

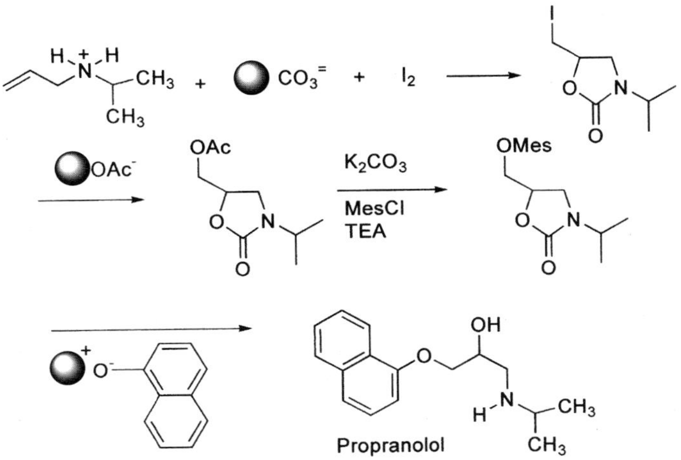

Figure 1.11 Solid phase organic synthesis of propranolol.

impressive. One certainly does not want to give back the time saved in construction by employing tedious separation operations! As an example of the utility of resin capture, a large collection of ureas was made by reacting an amine in solution with an excess of a substituted isocyanate to force the reaction to completion (Figure 1.12). The excess of isocyanate was captured by addition of a resin-immobilized amine to form an insoluble urea. The insoluble urea was removed by filtration and the desired urea in solution was obtained in pure form in high yield by filtration and washing.

In order for the combinatorial methods on resins to be useful, it is essential that suitable assays be developed and appropriate data handling methods be applied. In some cases, affinity chromatography using immobilized receptors/enzymes serves to separate beads containing active ligands. In others, soluble receptor/enzyme preparations bind to the tethered ligands on beads. Finally, one uses traditional solution methods in which soluble compounds are assayed alone or in

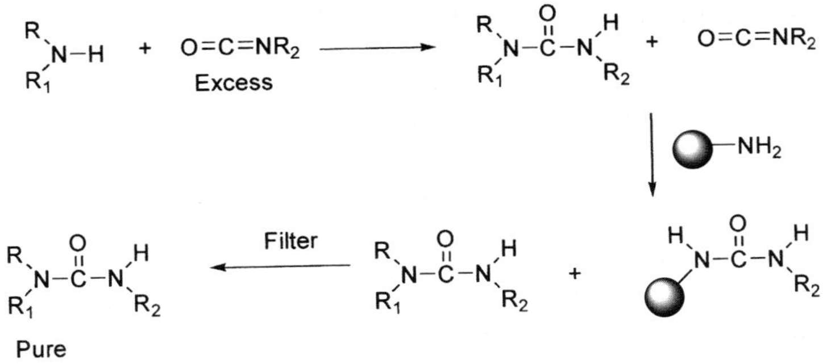

Figure 1.12 Resin capture methodology in the combinatorial synthesis of urea arrays.

combination with established ligands. Each of these devices possesses different requirements for success and must discriminate between specific and non-specific binding. Following up combinatorial hits in this way and progressing to candidate drugs is a form of chemical evolution and requires a combination of opportunism and the skillful application of drug design elements!

1.6 LEAD OPTIMIZATION

If potency, efficacy and selectivity were the only needed characteristics of a drug, the work of the medicinal chemist would be dramatically simplified. However, these characteristics are just the opening chapters in a long and complex saga. Many other factors must be built in before the job is done. The most important of these are summarized in the useful acronym ADME-To (absorption, distribution, metabolism and excretion as well as toxicity). Clearly, the drug must reach the site of action in a timely manner and in sufficient concentration to produce the desired effect.

The most common means of administration is oral and in this drug taking mimics eating. A degree of water solubility is required as only dissolved drug has a chance of being absorbed. Only highly lipophilic substances such as nitrogly-cerine and cocaine are significantly absorbed during the comparatively short time that substances are present in the mouth. The drug must next survive the acidic environment of the stomach and pass into the small intestine where the bulk of absorption takes place. Here the pH is neutral to slightly acidic. Although the upper part of the small intestine is fairly short, it is highly convoluted and highly vascularized. These factors promote absorption. Metabolism can take place here as a consequence of digestive enzymes (which create a particular problem for polypeptides) and because the gut wall is fairly rich in oxidative enzymes. As time for absorption is fairly short as the gut contents pass downstream, lipophilic small molecules are better absorbed than large molecules reflecting their comparative ease of diffusion. The pH of the small intestine is nearly neutral and the cells lining it are surrounded by the lipid bilayer of the cell surface. Thus, unless the drug benefits from active energy-requiring uptake mechanisms that primarily facilitate uptake of amino acids and glucose, the drug must be significantly unionized to penetrate into the body. Neutral substances and tertiary amines benefit from this. The Lipinski rule of fives puts this requirement into semi-quantitative terms.

Following absorption, the blood rapidly presents the drug to the liver. The liver is like a grease trap in the sense that it retards passage of lipophilic molecules and is rich in metabolizing enzymes that enhance the polarity of many foreign bodies. This causes their release as metabolically transformed molecules into the general circulation and facilitates their subsequent excretion in the urine. Oxidation, hydrolysis, reduction, etc. are Class I metabolic transformations introducing polar functions into many lipid molecules. When this is still insufficiently polarizing, Phase II metabolic transformations take place in which glucuronidation, sulfation and the like take place rendering the molecule still more polar. In some cases, the drug or its metabolite(s) are excreted in the bile back into the small intestine.

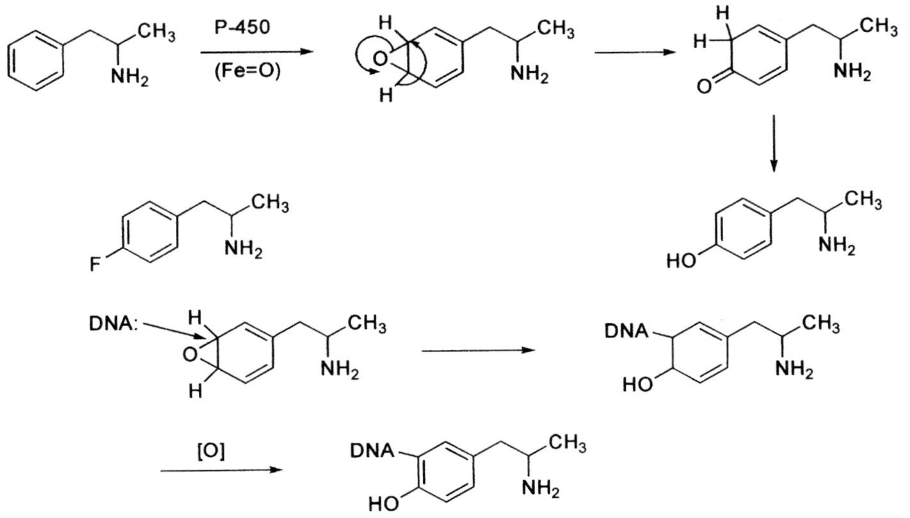

Figure 1.13 Oxidative metabolism of tyrosine.

In many cases, the drug then is excreted in the feces. In some cases, however, it undergoes further intestinal metabolism or in its own right is reabsorbed and presented again to the liver. This process is not common but is known as entero-hepatic cycling. An illustrative example of the process of polarizing metabolism is provided by amphetamine (Figure 1.13). This substance is hydroxylated to a more polar phenol by action of a heme containing P-450 enzyme. The intermediate is an arene oxide which undergoes rearrangement to the isolated product. This process can be blocked by installation of a *p*-fluoro substituent that deadens the aromatic ring to electrophilic substitution.

Occasionally, this well meant physiological process results in toxicity instead. Arene oxides are reactive species that can if long-lived, alkylate DNA, for example. If such adducts are not repaired in a timely manner, mutations can occur. Reactions of this type rationalize how apparently inert molecules such as certain polycyclic aromatic hydrocarbons (Figure 1.14) present in incompletely combusted materials present in chimney condensates, tobacco smoke, automobile exhausts, etc. can be carcinogenic. Epoxide hydrolase is but one of the mechanisms cells employ to intercept and detoxify such reactive molecules. Glutathione is yet another.

After release from the liver into the general circulation, the drug may or may not be bound to serum proteins. Molecules that undergo this binding are often acidic and lipophilic and in this are similar in properties to fatty acids. This is a normal means of transporting fatty acids without their salts (soaps) causing hemolysis of the fragile red-blood corpuscles. Drugs bound to serum proteins are often inhibited thereby from reaching their receptors in a timely manner although they are in equilibrium with them. They also remain longer in the body than otherwise as the

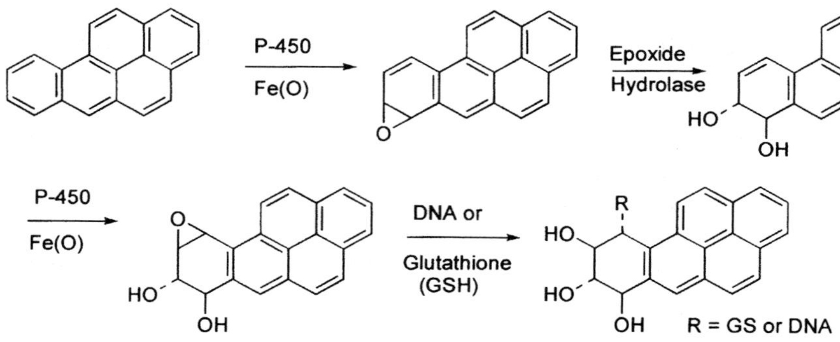

Figure 1.14 Oxidative metabolism of a polycyclic aromatic hydrocarbon (PAH).

urine is a protein-free filtrate. Most drugs, however, are not seriously protein bound so readily reach their receptors and interact with them. Organs are not uniformly supplied with blood but all organs and tissues are accessible, so most drugs can reach the site of action. The brain is unusual in that whereas it is richly supplied with blood, it is protected from the general circulation by the blood–brain barrier. In contrast to other organs where cells do not press closely together and therefore some passage of drugs can take place between cells, the cells lining the capillaries of the brain are tightly pressed together. The practical consequence of this is that drugs targeted to the brain are generally required to be more lipophilic than drugs targeted to other organs.

The kidneys serve to filter the blood and to retain essential molecules (certain salts and especially water) and to excrete waste materials. Thus, it is a selective clearing organ. This is the principal route of excretion of drugs and their metabolites. The product of the rate of absorption of drugs, their degree of metabolic transformation, their distribution in the body, and their rate of excretion is called pharmacokinetics. This is in effect the influence of the body on a drug as a function of time. The interaction of the drug with its receptors and the consequences of this as a function of time are pharmacodynamics. Both of these characteristics are strongly influenced by chemical structure and the skillful medicinal chemist must be able to optimize them through analoging. It is important to note in this respect that in doing this the parts of the drug molecule that are in direct contact with the receptor/enzyme may not be altered covalently without dramatically altering the potency of the molecule. This part of the molecule is defined as the pharmacophore. The rest of the molecule is molecular scaffolding and its structure is much less specifically demanding. It is in this part of the molecule that adjustments in ADME-To properties are more likely to be successful.

In favorable cases, it is possible to adjust molecular properties in a temporary manner by covering a misbehaving functional group by a moiety that is removed enzymically in the body once the problem area is bypassed. For example, a polar carboxylic acid moiety can be converted to an ester so that the resulting product undergoes enzymic hydrolysis in the liver or blood following efficient absorption. The product is the active drug which then proceeds to the receptor or target enzyme and functions as intended. This methodology is known as prodruging and is the topic of Chapter 14.

The medicinal chemist is expected to remedy any shortcomings by molecular manipulation. Bitter experience has shown that it is often easier to achieve potency, efficacy and selectivity in a molecule than it is to satisfy the ADME-To characteristics. Thus, it is usual to start with molecules that appear to be drug-like at the outset rather than to make a hit drug-like later. In addition to ADME-To, a number of other characteristics must also be satisfactory. These are listed below:

- Freedom from mutagenicity (in most cases mutagenicity is a show stopper if it is series general rather than molecule specific)
- Freedom from teratogenicity
- Chemical stability
- Synthetic or biological accessibility
- Acceptable cost
- Ability to patent
- Clinical efficacy
- Solubility
- Satisfactory taste
- Ability to formulate satisfactorily for administration
- Freedom from an idiosyncratic problem.

Toxicity is often difficult to control other than by the avoidance of the presence of functional groups that are known to be bad actors. Thioureas, aromatic nitro groups, furan rings, and electrophilic functions are well known to be problematic. This is not to say that there are no successful drugs with these functions present, but they always raise a red flag and require close examination in the testing phases because there are many precedent cases that engender concern. Functional groups that alter DNA are special problems. Flat three-ring containing aromatic molecules intercalate into DNA and are troublesome as they often cause frame shift mutations that, if not repaired, are self perpetuating when the DNA molecules are replicated. The resulting cells are transformed and will usually function poorly if not die or be cancerous.

Since the thalidomide disaster, drugs are closely monitored for safety in pregnant animals. This is particularly important for drugs that are likely to be administered chronically.

Failure to pass any of these challenges can be a show stopper. Getting a drug through to the market is equivalent to winning a lottery. All of the numbers must be correct and in the right sequence or one comes away only with a piece of non-negotiable paper.

Some insight into the popularity of particular drug design methods can be gained by considering just what chemists do when faced with the need to solve these problems. The following table results from an analysis of the frequency of particular drug design methods importantly utilized in the articles published in *The Journal of Medicinal Chemistry* during 1999 (Volume 21).

Technique	Number of articles wherein used
Bioisosteres	56
Natural product leads	49
Structure-based drug design	41
Prodrugs	32
Metabolism	31
Molecular rigidification	31
Peptidomimetics	27
Absolute configuration	26
Screening	21
Combinatorial libraries	19
DNA as a target	18
COMFA	15
Computer assisted drug design	12
Conformation	12

Some of these methods are under represented because of the existence of specialized journals dealing with particular methodologies (for example, several journals deal with combinatorial methods alone although these do not always focus specifically on drug discovery). The members of the list and the rank ordering varies from year to year but the practicing medicinal chemist must know when these methods are appropriate and when they are not and how to employ and to evaluate them.

Interestingly, the classical method of bioisosterism (or molecular mimicry) has led the list for nearly two decades so is worth singling out briefly. Bioisosteric atoms and groupings are those that have approximately the same size or molecular volumes so their interchange results in similarity in chemical, physical and notably biological properties of the resulting analogs. Classical isosteres include interchange of atoms in the same row of the periodic chart such as $-CH_2-$, $-NH-$, $-O-$ and $-F$. Note that hydrogen atoms are added to compensate for valence differences. This is known as the Grimm hydride displacement rule. Over time the definition of isosterism has broadened to include some isoelectronic interchanges as well. Examples of this phenomenon include $-S-$ and $-O-$ as well as $-F$, $-Cl$ and $-Br$. Bioisosteres include the classical isosteres, but bioisosteric atoms or groups of atoms do not nescessarily overlap. However, bioisosteres show sufficient steric, electronic or other properties to ensure biological activity similar to the parent. This widely employed drug design technique is covered in extenso in Chapters 9 and 10 to which the interested reader is directed.

Important additional insight can be gained from compilations of the reasons drugs fail in the clinic. Although there has not been a recent survey, experience indicates that the information that is available is not very different today. The data described in the following table comes from England and covers the years 1964–1985 (Prentis *et al.* 1988).

Problem	Instance	Percentage
Pharmacokinetic problems	78	39
Efficacy not proven	58	29
Toxicity	22	11
Adverse effects	20	10
Limited commercial interest	10	5
Replaced by improved candidate	4	2
Budget exhausted	2	1
Chemical problem	1	0.5
Unknown reason	3	1.5
Sum	198	100

Prudence requires that due attention be paid prospectively to avoiding structures likely to fall into one of these categories. One notes in particular the primacy of pharmacokinetic and toxicity problems.

1.7   CELL BIOLOGY AND GENOMICS AS A SOURCE OF DRUG TARGETS

The classical means of drug discovery involved finding a chemical that had a favorable influence on disease and, using this as a tool, eventually sorting out what its cellular target was and then figuring out how this could produce the observed effect. This has the character of a very involved detective story associated with few useful clues. Gradually this changed, as the result of increasing knowledge of cellular physiology, to understanding how a cell or organ system actually functioned and then finding a defective bit of cellular physiology associated with the cause of disease and then to searching for molecules that might rectify the situation. Clearly, this was a more gratifying and focused intellectual exercise but was by no means much simpler. In more recent years, increasing knowledge of cell biology converted an alphabet soup of vaguely characterized cellular factors into palpable molecules identified with particular signaling pathways involved in cellular responses to various external or internal stimuli. This led to the crafting of agents that could increase or decrease these signals in a therapeutically useful way.

New possibilities of increasing complexity continually open up as our knowledge of cell function and pathology becomes ever sophisticated. At the moment of this writing, the complete genome of *Homo sapiens* has just been published in two versions (The human genome, *Science* (2001) **291**; *Nature* (2001) **409**). We now know the 30 000 or so genes that lead to all of the proteins of which we are composed. Even with the added complication of post-translation modifications this is an unexpectedly finite number of informational macro-molecules with which to deal. Hurtful to our pride is the knowledge that genetically we are not much more complicated than a nematode! Many of the gene products made using these genes are receptors and enzymes of whose function we are presently unaware. This powerful new knowledge promises to define many new molecular targets for chemotherapy and gives us powerful tools for advancements in medicine undreamed of until very recent times. Indeed, this reverses the classical mode of drug seeking. Instead of proceeding from agent to target to knowledge of cellular physiology at the molecular level, we now are prepared to begin with knowledge of cellular factors, to trace their function, to determine what role, if any, they play in particular disease states, to devise molecular cures and then to search for molecules that will have these properties.

The days when a medicinal chemist need only have a knowledge of synthesis are rapidly passing away and contemporary drug seeking requires a knowledge of at least the application of high level chemistry to very sophisticated biological phenomena. The future involves mastery of important aspects of very new sciences.

Genomics is the comprehensive study of the interrelationships among families of genes. We already have at our disposal gene chips containing the mRNA produced by very large numbers of different DNA molecules in response to various cellular treatments. When quantitated as a function of time, this gives us powerful insights into how cells respond to particular stimuli and how they differ from diseased cells. Tracing back to the DNA involved and forward to the gene products increases our repertoire of targets for chemotherapy.

Functional genomics is the study of genomes to determine the biological function of all the genes and their products.

Proteomics is the study of the full set of proteins encoded by a genome.

Informatics is the study of the information storage and retrieval of information gathered from genomic and proteomic studies.

1.8   FUTURE DEVELOPMENTS

It is always perilous to predict the future in turbulent times. The unprecedented capabilities made possible by decoding of the genome not only for humans but for other life forms as well will surely transform the face of modern biology. Whereas for the majority of the century just past by and large chemistry put the ball in play in drug seeking, clearly the current century will be dominated as far as can be seen at this moment by biology. Medicinal chemistry lies at the interface between these two and cannot fail to be transformed as well. The art and science of medicine in the last century has been strongly influenced by the properties of small molecules. The years ahead will see a strong overlay associated with large molecules. In order to be functional, chemical education for those to practice medicinal chemistry must retain its traditional ability to predict the properties of molecules and to construct them efficiently but be expanded at the same time to include much more serious treatment of biological topics as well. The strain on the traditional curriculum will be substantial. Medicinal chemistry departments have made a strong start in this direction. Chemistry departments will need to join.

During the last century, every advance in organic chemistry has rapidly been incorporated into medicinal chemistry. One can cite advances in the understanding of reaction mechanisms, conformational analysis, host–guest interactions, quantum mechanics, spectroscopy, and so on. This is unlikely to change.

It is safe to predict that a more profound understanding of the factors involved in ADME-To lies just ahead. Understanding more perfectly the relationship between chemical structure and these factors will greatly facilitate drug design and discovery. Increasing use of structure-based drug design techniques will doubtless also take place enhancing our ability to craft more potent and more specific agents. These prospects are exhilarating.

The unraveling of the genome leads us to the identification of targets for chemotherapy not previously suspected and even allows us to dream of the possibility of correcting genetic defects, enhancing our prospects for a longer and more healthy life, and for devising drugs for specific individuals! Explanations for the perplexing phenomena of significantly varying responses of different individuals to the same treatment are likely to come from a better understanding of differing gene patterns in patients. Presuming that individual variations in response may often have a genetic basis, dividing populations into subgroups with similar genetic characteristics could allow us to prescribe drugs and even dosages within these groups so that a larger percentage would respond favorably. This form of individual gene typing is possible even now but would be very expensive. The costs could become manageable with time and effort. It is doubtful, however, if this could in the foreseeable future be brought within the reach of the very poor. The moral implications of this must be anticipated and settled. It is also likely that perplexing species differences in response to chemotherapy that complicate drug development may also be understood when the genomes of more species become available. Means of dealing with multidrug resistance will also depend upon this knowledge. Determination of the genome of pathogens, such as *Mycobacterium tuberculosis*, leads to the identification of novel targets for chemotherapy with the possibility of reducing resistance development and also to gene products that are associated with infection and pathogenicity.

The new biological capabilities raise many new prospects and problems for society. These not only open great scientific possibilities but also raise perplexing moral issues for which we are not yet prepared. Scientific knowledge by itself is morally neutral. What is done with it is not. It is imperative that we chose wisely and are reasonably tolerant when we occasionally put our feet wrong.

It is probably true that the majority of medicinal chemists who have ever lived are active when these lines are being written and it is certainly true that there has never been a more exciting time to take up the study of medicinal chemistry. In 1900, even far seeing geniuses such as Ehrlich could hardly imagine a small percentage of the wonders that are common place in 2000. It is very likely that wonders unimaginable today will be recounted in 2100. The techniques recounted in the remainder of this book represent the cutting edge of modern technology and represent the launching pad from which the wonders that lie ahead will be reached.

FURTHER READING

Annual Reports in Medicinal Chemistry. A yearly compilation of reviews on medicinal chemical topics organized by the Medicinal Division and published by The American Chemical Society. The current volume is no. 35.

Baichwal, V.R. and Baeuerle, P.A. (1998) Kinases in pro-inflammatory signal transduction pathways: new opportunities for drug discovery. *Annu. Repts. Med. Chem.*, **33**, 233.

Bailey, D.S. (1999) Pharmacogenomics and its impact on drug design and optimization. *Annu. Repts. Med. Chem.*, **34**, 339.

Black, J.W. (1989) Drugs from emasculated hormones: the principle of syntopic antagonism. *Science*, **245**, 486.

Brown, F.K. (1998) Chemoinformatics: what is it and how does it impact drug discovery. *Annu. Repts. Med. Chem.*, **33**, 375.

Flam, F. (1994) Chemical prospectors scour the seas for promising drugs. *Science*, **266**, 1324.

Gallop, M. *et al.* (1994) Applications of combinatorial technologies. I. Background and peptide combinatorial libraries. *J. Med. Chem.*, **37**, 1233.

Gordon, E. *et al.* (1994) Applications of combinatorial technologies. II. Combinatorial organic synthesis, library screening strategies and future directions. *J. Med. Chem.*, **37**, 1385.

Greer, J. *et al.* (1994) Application of the three-dimensional structures of protein target molecules in structure-based drug design. *J. Med. Chem.*, **37**, 1035.

Lau, K.F. and Sakul, H. (2000) Pharmacogenomics. *Annu. Repts. Med. Chem.*, **35**, 261.

Murcko, M.A., Caron, P.R.l. and Charifson, P.S. (1999) Structure-based drug design. *Annu. Repts. Med. Chem.*, **34**, 297.

Oldenberg, K.R. (1998) Current and future trends in high throughput screening for drug discovery. *Annu. Repts. Med. Chem.*, **33**, 301.

Stewart, B.H., Wang, Y. and Surendran, N. (2000) *Ex vivo* approaches to predicting oral pharmacokinetics in humans. *Annu. Repts. Med. Chem.*, **35**, 299.

Sweetnam, P.M. *et al.* (1993) The role of receptor binding in drug discovery. *J. Natural Products*, **56**, 441.

Trainor, G.L. (2000) Privileged structures – an update. *Annu. Repts. Med. Chem.*, **35**, 289.

Trivedi, B.K., Low, J.E., Carson, K. and LaRosa, G.J. (2000) Chemokines: targets for novel therapeutics. *Annu. Repts. Med. Chem.*, **35**, 191.

Weisbach, J. and Moos, W.H. (1995) Diagnosing the decline in major pharmaceutical research laboratories: a prescription for drug companies. *Drug Dev. Research*, **34**, 243.

REFERENCES

Bunin, B.A. and Ellman, J.A. (1992) A general and expedient method for the solid-phase synthesis of 1,4-benzodiazepine derivatives. *J. Am. Chem. Soc.*, **114**, 10997.

Drews, J. (2000) *Science*, **287**, 1962.

Gelmo, P. (1908) Über Sulfonamide der p-Amidobenzolsulfonsäure. *J. Pr. Chem.*, **N.S. 77**, 369–382.

Gruber, V. and Theisen, M. (2000) Genetically modified crops as a source for pharmaceuticals. *Annu. Repts. Med. Chem.*, **35**, 357.

Lipinski, C.A., Lombardo, F., Dominy, B.W. and Feeney, P.J. (2001) Experimental and computational approaches to estimate solubility and permeability in drug discovery and development settings. *Adv. Drug Deliv. Rev.*, **46**, 3.

Milligan, G. and Rees, S. (2000) Oligomerisation of G protein coupled receptors. *Annu. Repts. Med. Chem.*, **35**, 271.

Prentis, R.A., Lis, Y. and Walker, S.R. (1988) Pharmaceutical innovation by the seven UK-owned pharmaceutical companies. *British J. Clin. Pharmacol.*, **25**, 387.

Sternbach, L. (1979) The benzodiazepine story. *J. Med. Chem.*, **22**, 1.

Chapter 2

Role of molecular recognition in drug design

Peter Andrews and Michael Dooley

2.1 INTRODUCTION

Molecular recognition underpins every aspect of life, from the replication of the genome through genetic transcription and protein translation to the assembly and integrity of complex multicellular organisms such as humans. Drugs, which may modify any of these processes, also derive their actions by the absolute control of molecular recognition. Understanding the underlying physical basis for an association between drugs and their receptors is paramount to the ultimate task of drug design, that of *predicting* affinities of new drugs. This is a formidable challenge requiring a detailed knowledge of the physical forces that comprise drug–receptor interactions, and an understanding of the thermodynamic backdrop of the association, to ultimately determine the strength of drug–receptor interactions.

This chapter gives a basic understanding of the various types of non-bonded drug–receptor interactions and associated entropy terms, including a discussion of the various levels of approximation commonly used to calculate the overall strengths of the resulting intermolecular interactions from these components. It details some of the successes and pitfalls that go along with the use of various approximations in the prediction of drug affinity. It should leave the reader with no doubt that while the principles of molecular recognition are reasonably well understood, the business of predicting binding affinities between drugs and receptors is still far from an exact science.

2.2 THERMODYNAMIC CONSIDERATIONS OF DRUG BINDING

The interaction of a drug with its receptor may be written in the form of equation (2.1)

$$L:S_l + R:S_r + S_{bulk} \rightleftharpoons L^*:R^*:S_{lr} + S^*_{bulk} \tag{2.1}$$

where $L:S_l$ is the free ligand in solution surrounded by a perturbed solvation shell, $R:S_r$ is the free receptor together with a perturbed solvation shell and S_{bulk} is the bulk solvent. On the right hand side of the equilibrium, $L^*:R^*:S_{lr}$ represents the complex of ligand and receptor and a perturbed solvation shell and S^*_{bulk}

represents the bulk solvent. The ligand and receptor states and the solvation structure are all modified therefore nothing on the left hand and right hand sides can be considered equivalent (designated by *). The position of the equilibrium and therefore the affinity of the ligand are determined by the free energy difference (ΔG) between the two sides and this can be formally expressed in terms of equation (2.2). Here R is the gas constant, T is the temperature in Kelvin and K_d is the dissociation constant for the ligand. Optimally, in the context of drug design, there is a large negative free energy change in the right-hand direction of equation (2.1).

$$\Delta G = RT \ln K_d \qquad (2.2)$$

The great challenge for drug design is to determine the free energy change by computational means and therefore *predict* the binding affinity of a new drug. Calculation of the free energy change resulting from a ligand–receptor interaction can be used to predict the K_d of the ligand by equation (2.2). However, there is a very narrow margin for error since small variations in ΔG lead to large errors in K_d. Therefore, accurate predictions of affinity will require very accurate calculation of ΔG.

Free energy perturbation techniques are used to determine relative binding energies of ligands, however this method suffers from computational expense and the limitation that only very closely related ligands can be studied. Since the free energy change can also be related to the enthalpy (ΔH) and entropy changes (ΔS) for the equilibrium by equation (2.3), methods which approximate the free energy change by summing the component parts of molecular interactions have become popular.

$$\Delta G = \Delta H - T\Delta S \qquad (2.3)$$

The components of molecular interactions have typically been divided into entropic and enthalpic terms. The entropic contributions include the cost of reducing the rotational and translational entropy of the ligand, restricting rotation of internal rotors of the ligand and the receptor and the entropic cost or benefit of solvent reorganization. The enthalpic terms include the contributions of favorable and unfavorable non-bonded interactions and penalties for binding high-energy conformers. Several studies have used equations of a form similar to equation (2.4) to estimate ΔG

$$\Delta G = \Delta G_{t+r} + \Delta G_r + \Delta G_x + \Delta G_{conf} \qquad (2.4)$$

where ΔG_{t+r} is the cost of binding the ligand into the receptor, ΔG_r is the cost of restricting internal rotations, ΔG_x is the sum of the contributions of individual functional groups X, including weak intermolecular bonds such as hydrogen bonds and the free energy change associated with solvent reorganization (the hydrophobic effect), and ΔG_{conf} is the energy penalty for binding a high energy conformer.

2.3   THE PHYSICAL BASIS OF INTERMOLECULAR INTERACTIONS

2.3.1   Enthalpic contributions

2.3.1.1   *Electrostatic interactions*

Electrostatic interactions are the net result of the attractive forces between the positively charged nuclei and the negatively charged electrons of the two molecules. The attractive force between these opposite charges leads to three main bond types: charge–charge, charge–dipole and dipole–dipole interactions. The reader is directed to useful reviews on this topic by Bongrand (1999) and Glusker (1998).

2.3.1.1.1   *Ionic bonds*

The strength of any electrostatic (coulombic) interaction can be calculated from equation (2.5), where q_i and q_j are two charges separated by a distance r_{ij} in a medium of dielectric constant ε. This equation applies equally to ionic interactions, where the charges q_i and q_j are integer values, or to polar interactions, in which the total energy is summed over the contributions calculated from the partial charges on all the individual atoms.

$$E = \frac{q_i q_j}{\varepsilon r_{ij}} \tag{2.5}$$

It follows from equation (2.5) that the strength of an ionic interaction is inversely proportional to the distance separating the two charges and to the dielectric constant ε of the surrounding medium. The strength of an ionic interaction is thus dependent on its environment. In hydrophobic environments, like the interior of a protein molecule, the dielectric constant may be as low as 4, whereas in bulk phase water the corresponding value is 80. In other environments, intermediate values are appropriate e.g. for interactions occurring near the surface of a protein, an ε value of 28 is commonly used. Since the strength of coulombic interactions decays proportionally to the distance between the charges whereas other electrostatic interactions are even more sensitive to distance (decaying with the square, cube or sixth power of distance), they frequently dominate the initial long-range interactions between ligands and receptors. However, association does not require the ligand and receptor to have opposite net charges. For example, dihydrofolate reductase from *Escherichia coli* and superoxide dismutase from various species and their respective ligands each carry net negative charges.

2.3.1.1.2   *Charge–dipole and dipole–dipole interactions*

Although charge–dipole and dipole–dipole interactions are weaker than ionic bonds, they are nevertheless key contributors to the overall strengths of ligand–receptor interactions, since they occur in any molecule in which electronegativity differences between atoms result in significant bond, group or molecular dipole moments.

The key differences between ionic and dipolar interactions relate to their dependence on distance and orientation. For charge–dipole interactions, the strength of the interaction depends inversely on the square of the distance, while for dipole–dipole interactions, it reduces with the cube of the distance separating the dipoles. These interactions are also inversely proportional to the dielectric constant ε and they are therefore environmentally dependent.

Dipolar interactions may be either attractive or repulsive, depending on the relative orientation of the dipole moments. That is, there is a geometric dependence to the interaction.

2.3.1.1.3   Higher order multipole interactions

Ion–quadrupole and dipole–quadrupole interactions are known to be quite strong in the gas-phase and ion–quadrupole interactions in solution can be as strong as ion–dipole interactions (Dougherty 1996). As an example, interactions between aromatic rings and amine groups are observed in several crystal structures from the protein databank e.g. a thrombin complex (1uma), Lao-binding protein complexed with ornithine (1lah) and oligopeptide binding protein (2olb). Favorable interactions also arise from quadrupole–quadrupole interactions between aromatic rings. It has been shown that there is a statistical preference for particular contact geometries between aromatic rings that maximize this interaction (Hunter 1994).

2.3.1.1.4   Inductive interactions

The formation of a ligand–receptor complex is often accompanied by intramolecular and/or intermolecular redistributions of charge. In the intramolecular case, this redistribution is referred to as an induced polarization, whereas a redistribution of charge between two molecules is described as a charge transfer interaction. In either case, the resulting interactions are always attractive and strongly dependent on the distance separating the two molecules.

2.3.1.1.5   Dispersion forces

Dispersion or London forces are the universal forces responsible for attractive interactions between non-polar molecules. Their occurrence is due to the fact that any atom will, at any given instant, be likely to possess a finite dipole moment as a result of the movement of electrons around the nuclei. Such fluctuating dipoles tend to induce opposite dipoles in adjacent molecules, thus resulting in a net attractive force. Although the individual interactions between pairs of atoms is relatively weak and is inversely proportional to the sixth power of the distance between the atoms, the total contribution to binding from dispersion forces can be very significant if there is a close fit between ligand and receptor. The quality of the steric match is thus the dominant factor in non-polar interactions.

2.3.1.1.6 Hydrogen bonds

Hydrogen bonds are a complicated mix of electrostatic (coulombic) character, which makes them important in long range interactions, and dipolar character, which play an important role in aligning molecular components of biological systems. They are responsible for maintaining the tertiary structure of proteins and nucleic acids, as well as the binding of many ligands. The strongest hydrogen bonds are formed between groups with the greatest electrostatic character. Thus carboxylates are better acceptors than amides, ketones or unionized carboxyls, whilst substituted ammonium ions are better donors than unsubstituted ammonium ions or trigonal donors.

There is considerable evidence that burying unsatisfied hydrogen bond partners can be unfavorable. For example, McDonald and Thornton (1994) have performed a statistical analysis of high-resolution protein structures, which indicates that only 1.3% of amide NH groups and 1.8% of amide carbonyl groups are buried without forming hydrogen bonds. In the context of ligand–receptor interactions, Fersht *et al.* (1985) have shown that burying an unsatisfied donor or acceptor results in a $16 \, kJ \, mol^{-1}$ destabilization of the complex for a charged group and $4 \, kJ \, mol^{-1}$ for a neutral group.

N-methylacetamide has been used for some time as a prototypic model of protein backbone for the calorimetric and theoretical study of hydrogen bond formation during protein folding. The results of these studies may also be applicable where hydrogen bonds are formed between protein and ligand. Theoretical and experimental (Ben-Tal *et al.* 1997) studies both indicate that hydrogen bond formation between peptide bonds where the partners move from a solvated environment to a desolvated environment (either the interior of a protein or the interface between a ligand and the active-site) is energetically *unfavorable* (ΔG_8, Figure 2.1). The energetics of the system are best viewed as a thermodynamic cycle, as illustrated in Figure 2.1. A hydrogen bond is marginally stable in an aqueous environment (ΔG_4), but considerably more stable in a non-polar environment (ΔG_7). The result is that whilst burying a hydrogen bond might be energetically unfavorable, the burial of an unpaired hydrogen bond partner is around $5.7 \, kJ \, mol^{-1}$ *more unfavorable* (ΔG_5^*, ΔG_7^*, ΔG_8^*) than burying the hydrogen bond. If these results are generally applicable to various types of neutral hydrogen bond partners, then the implications for drug design are that while desolvating and burying a neutral hydrogen bond may be energetically *unfavorable*, failure to pair a hydrogen bond partner on the protein with one on the ligand, i.e. burying an unpaired hydrogen bond partner, may be even more energetically unfavorable. This is clearly an issue of ongoing debate in the field.

2.3.1.2 Steric interactions

2.3.1.2.1 Short-range repulsive forces

The short-range repulsive forces resulting from the overlap of the electron clouds of any two molecules increase exponentially with decreasing internuclear

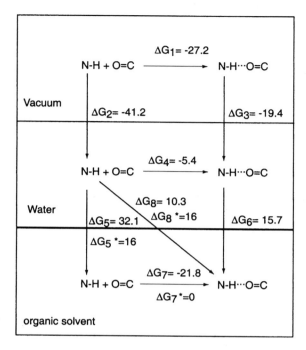

Figure 2.1 Thermodynamic cycle of hydrogen bond formation between N–H and C=O groups in different phases.

separation. The balance between these repulsive interactions and the dispersion forces thus determines both the minimum and the most favorable non-bonded separation between any pair of atoms. The equilibrium distance can be determined from crystal data, and is equivalent to the sum of the van der Waals radii of the two interacting atoms.

For non-polar molecules this balance between the attractive dispersion forces and the short range repulsive forces is generally defined in terms of the Buckingham (6-exp) potential given in equation (2.6) or the alternative Lennard-Jones 6–12 potential, given in equation (2.7). The extreme repulsive forces that develop as atoms approach closer than the sum of their van der Waals radii are perhaps the single most decisive influence on whether a molecule will bind to a receptor since very small steric clashes between molecules will abolish affinity.

$$E = \frac{Ae^{-Br}}{r^d} - \frac{C}{r^6} \tag{2.6}$$

$$E = \frac{A}{r^{12}} - \frac{C}{r^6} \tag{2.7}$$

2.3.2 Entropic contributions

2.3.2.1 Translational and rotational entropy

The formation of any ligand–receptor complex is accompanied by the replacement of the three rotational and three translational degrees of freedom of the ligand by six vibrational degrees of freedom in the complex ('residual motion'). The extent of this change is primarily dependent on the relative 'tightness' of the resulting complex. For a typical ligand–protein complex, the estimated change in free energy resulting from the loss of entropy on binding (at 310 K) ranges from $9 \, kJ \, mol^{-1}$ for a loose interaction to $45 \, kJ \, mol^{-1}$ for a tightly bound complex (Searle and Williams 1992).

In addition to this loss of rotational and translational freedom, there is a further entropy loss due to the conformational restriction that accompanies binding of flexible ligands. Based on the observed entropy changes accompanying cyclization reactions, the extent of this entropy loss is estimated at $5–6 \, kJ \, mol^{-1}$ per internal rotation, although the actual figure again depends on how tight a complex is formed between the ligand and the receptor. For bimolecular interactions that do not involve covalent bonds, a range of $1.6–3.4 \, kJ \, mol^{-1}$ per internal rotor has been proposed (Searle and Williams 1992). In the case of rigid analogs, for which there is no loss of conformational entropy on binding, this factor provides a free energy advantage relative to more flexible ligands and this is the basis of one of the central tenets of medicinal chemistry, that of conformational restriction.

In some cases, the bound conformation of a flexible molecule may also be its lowest energy conformation, in which the penalty for the resulting conformational constraint will be restricted to the loss of internal rotational entropy described above. In other cases, however, the optimal interaction between ligand and receptor will require a higher energy conformation, and this energy penalty will further reduce the net binding energy observed (for further discussions of conformational energy penalties see Chapter 4).

2.3.2.2 Hydrophobic effect

When a non-polar molecule is placed in water, stronger water–water interactions are formed around the solute molecule to compensate for the weaker interactions between solute and water. This results in an increasingly ordered arrangement of water molecules around the solute and thus a negative entropy of dissolution. The decrease in entropy is roughly proportional to the non-polar surface area of the molecule. The association of two such non-polar molecules in water reduces the total non-polar surface area exposed to the solvent, thus reducing the amount of structured water, and therefore providing a favorable entropy of association.

Although it can be determined theoretically from statistical mechanics calculations or free energy simulations, the hydrophobic effect is commonly estimated empirically. One of the methods used is measurement of the solubility of simple hydrocarbons in water (solvent transfer method). Estimates of the free energy required to transfer hydrocarbons from water into a hydrophobic environment range from 0.1 to $0.14 \, kJ \, mol^{-1}$ for every square angstrom of solvent-accessible hydrocarbon surface removed from exposure to water by the binding process (Williams and Bardsley 1999).

2.3.2.3 Solvent reorganization

In principle, the entropic component of the hydrophobic effect described in the previous section might be applied to a broad range of hydropathic types, not just non-polar molecules and surfaces. Thus, Klotz (1997) has made a theoretical derivation that electrostatic interactions (not only ionic) in water would have a large favorable entropic component. Intuitively this may be rationalized as similar to the entropic component of the hydrophobic effect. The solvation shell of the polar groups would be more ordered than the bulk solvent, and an interaction between two such polar groups would eliminate some of that water back to the bulk solvent with a favorable entropy gain. Klotz used the dissociation of acetic acid in water (ΔG 6.5 kcal mol^{-1} at 300 K, $\Delta H \sim 0$, $\Delta S - 22$ cal mol^{-1} K^{-1}) as an example. Negative entropies of transfer of ions and molecules from the gas phase to water also support this.

2.4   THE TOTAL ENERGY OF INTERMOLECULAR INTERACTION

2.4.1   Free energy perturbation

Free energy perturbation techniques are used to determine the difference in the free energy of binding between two ligands and a common receptor, or between the same ligands and solvent, by utilizing the concept of a thermodynamic cycle. This method has proved astoundingly accurate in predicting relative binding energies of ligand series, but still suffers from problems of computational expense. Its use is also limited to narrow structural changes between the two ligands. It does not require any partitioning of individual energetic components of the free energy change (Kollman 1993; Pang and Kollman 1995).

2.4.2   Partitioning methods

As noted earlier, the total free energy change ΔG resulting from a ligand–receptor interaction is the sum of the free energy changes associated with all of the electrostatic, inductive, non-polar and hydrophobic interactions listed in the previous sections, less any conformational energy and rotational, translational or conformational entropy costs associated with the interaction. Some of these terms can be calculated relatively simply using the equations given in the preceding pages. Others, such as the entropy terms, are much more complex, and are frequently handled empirically. It is important to avoid double counting these terms. The total free energy change can be calculated in a variety of ways, and the reader is directed to the review by Ajay and Murcko (1995), which gives a detailed account of the various methods.

Ultimately, a complete theoretical description of all of the energy contributions described above would require quantum mechanical treatment of the entire system, including solving the time-dependent Schrödinger equation for ligand, receptor, surrounding solvent and any other relevant solutes. The resulting free energy of interaction would be directly comparable, and hopefully in close agreement, with the observed dissociation constant for the ligand–receptor interaction. It is doubtful, however, if there is real benefit for the 3D QSAR or drug design practitioner in pursuing the calculation of intermolecular interactions to this level of complexity. The real question for us is not 'What is the total electrostatic or van der Waals, enthalpic or entropic, H-bond or hydrophobic, contribution to the intermolecular interaction?'. Rather, we want to know the answers to questions like 'What increase in binding could I expect if I add this functional group to my ligand?'.

2.5   ESTIMATING INDIVIDUAL GROUP COMPONENTS IN LIGAND–RECEPTOR INTERACTIONS AND CO-OPERATIVITY

The total free energy of interaction between a ligand and its receptor provides a measure of the strength of the association between the two molecules, but tells us little or nothing about the overall quality of their match. Does the observed binding reflect a composite of interactions between every part of the ligand and its receptor, or is it a case of one or two strong interactions contributing sufficient energy to disguise an otherwise mediocre fit? Is the observed increase in interaction energy resulting from the addition of a new functional group consistent with what might have been anticipated? To answer these questions we need some means of estimating the intrinsic binding strengths of individual functional groups, i.e. the free energy changes resulting (after allowance for any loss in translational or rotational entropy) when the specified functional groups are aligned optimally and without strain with corresponding functional groups in the receptor (Jencks 1981).

2.5.1   Intrinsic binding energies

Recall that the free energy of binding, ΔG, can be defined in terms of the binding energies for the individual functional groups which make up the ligand according to equation (2.4). The fourth term in equation (2.4) is the sum of the binding energies ΔG_x associated with each functional group X. In the ideal case, when the specified functional group is aligned optimally and without strain with the corresponding functional group in the receptor, ΔG_x is referred to as the intrinsic binding energy (Jencks 1981). In other cases, the term apparent binding energy is used. Page (1977) referred to this as the 'anchor principle', on the premise that the difference in binding of a ligand with or without the particular functional group incorporates only the factors associated with that group, i.e. the intrinsic binding energy ΔG_x of that group.

It should be noted that each binding energy ΔG_x incorporates a number of terms in addition to the obvious enthalpy of interaction between the functional group and its corresponding binding site on the receptor. These include the enthalpy changes associated with the removal of water of hydration from the functional group and its target site and the subsequent formation of bonds between the displaced water molecules, and the corresponding entropy terms associated with the displacement and subsequent bonding of water molecules.

The anchor principle assumes that intrinsic binding energies are properties of the functional group and are independent of the groups to which the particular functional group is attached. Such intrinsic binding potentials might thus reasonably be used in an additive manner to provide an overall estimate of the ligand–receptor interaction. The original application of the anchor principle described by Page (1977) related to data on the selectivity of amino acid-tRNA synthetases, from which he estimated intrinsic binding energies for the methylene group in the range $12–14\,kJ\,mol^{-1}$, and for carboxyl and amino groups of 18 and $>28\,kJ\,mol^{-1}$ respectively.

Intrinsic binding energies are not rigorously accurate, they are only useful approximations. If a molecule containing a particular functional group binds with a higher affinity than the corresponding molecule lacking that functional group, by definition there is a higher entropy cost to be paid by the higher affinity molecule. This is paid off against the intrinsic binding energy of the functional group resulting in an underestimation of the intrinsic binding. Conversely, the additional binding energy of the functional group may increase the enthalpy of neighboring interactions. This is paid into the intrinsic binding energy, leading to an overestimation. Other factors such as solvent effects and the conformational effect (Wiley and Rich 1993; Epps *et al.* 1990) of the functional group on the ligand are also buried in the intrinsic binding energy value and may not be easily predicted. Thus Williams and Bardsley (1999) showed that the enthalpy of interaction of a functional group is strengthened by an adjacent functional group in a manner that is separate from the well known entropically driven chelate effect. They suggest that this precludes the derivation of free energies of binding characteristic of common functional groups since these values must always be context dependent i.e. dependent on the molecular architecture of the ligand and probably the receptor.

The Williams and Bardsley (1999) study involved a series of ligands for the vancomycin antibiotics, which differ only by the presence or absence of a methyl group. The binding of *N*-acetyl-D-ala-D-ala, (**2.1**) (the truncated natural ligand for the vancomycin antibiotics from bacterial cell walls) was compared with ligands lacking methyl groups, i.e. glycine–alanine replacements of either or both positions (**2.2**, **2.3** and **2.4**). To a first approximation, the differences in binding affinities were attributed to the difference in hydrophobic surface area between the ligands: other factors such as conformational states were considered to be equivalent. The contribution of the hydrophobic effect was calculated to be $0.18–0.24\,kJ\,mol^{-1}\,\mathring{A}^{-2}$, which is larger than the values determined by solvent transfer. This inconsistency was traced to enthalpy–entropy compensation, which can negate prediction of binding affinities using partitioning of enthalpic and entropic components of the free energy change. At the molecular level, the motional restriction imposed by the favorable burial of the hydrophobic methyl group was transferred to a neighboring carboxylate, which strengthened the hydrogen bond this group made to the antibiotic. For systems that are networks of weak co-operative interactions (like ligand–protein interactions), any strengthening of one interaction necessarily strengthens linked interactions and essentially renders meaningless attempts to rigorously partition free energy. The same effect was noted for another series of vancomycin ligands (**2.5**, **2.6**, **2.1**) where the strength of the hydrogen bond

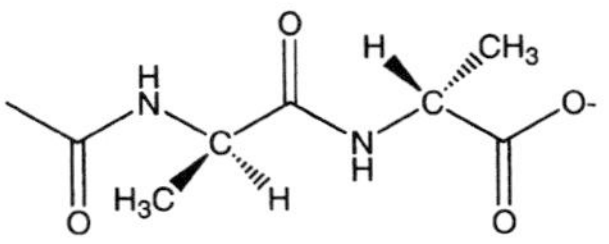

(2.1)

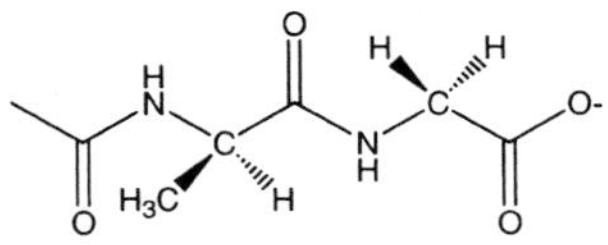

(2.2)

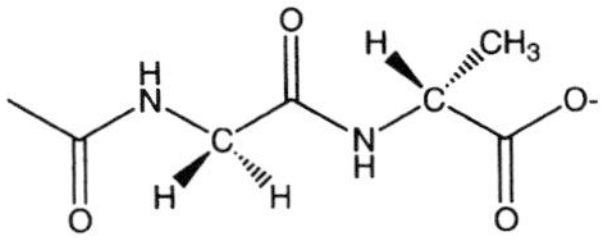

(2.3)

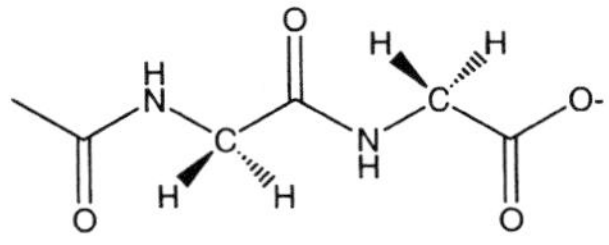

(2.4)

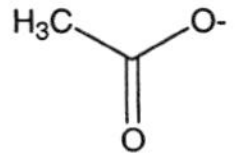

(2.5)

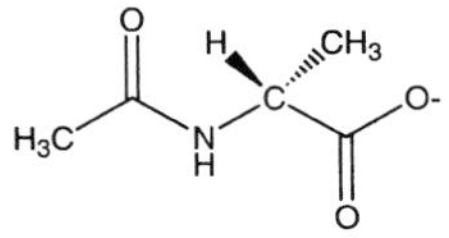

(2.6)

between the carboxylate of the ligand and vancomycin was found to increase through the series as adjacent co-operative networks of interactions increased.

Solvent effects may complicate derivation of intrinsic binding energies using the anchor principle. This is best illustrated by example. Morgan *et al.* (1991) has reported a series of thermolysin inhibitors in which a substrate peptide linkage is replaced by a phosphinate linkage $(-PO_2-CH_2-)$ and phosphonamide (PO_2-NH-) linkages. The crystal structures of the complexes between thermolysin and these two inhibitors show that they are essentially identical except for the presence of a single hydrogen bond from the phosphonamidate NH to the carbonyl oxygen of Ala 113. The methylene group of the phosphinate is unable to make this hydrogen bond. Surprisingly, the binding affinity of these two series is identical, resulting in a calculated intrinsic binding energy of $0\,kJ\,mol^{-1}$ for a neutral hydrogen bonding pair. In this case, it appears that any beneficial enthalpic component of the hydrogen bond is completely offset by other costs. It is likely that a major cost is desolvation energy that the phosphonamide must pay, but that the phosphinate does not (see Chapter 4). Recall from the discussion on hydrogen bond contributions above, that the phosphinate should be more unstable than the phosphonate since it buries the unpaired carbonyl oxygen of Ala 113. This example clearly illustrates that even if you can 'see' at atomic level the interface between ligand and receptor, indeed between a ligand series and a receptor, it is still very difficult to infer the important contributions to the ligand's affinity or predict the consequences of structural change on binding affinity.

Notwithstanding the above evidence that the anchor principle gives functional group contributions that are a complicated mix of enthalpic and entropic contributions that are context dependent, they are still useful in drug design. For example, the limiting contribution for a methyl group in many different systems appears to be a maximum of around $12–14\,kJ\,mol^{-1}$ which can be used to assess the effectiveness of the introduction of a methyl group into a drug.

2.5.2   Active site mutagenesis

Another measure of intrinsic binding energy based on the anchor principle is the impact of a single amino acid substitution in the active site of an enzyme on transition state stabilization, as determined by the change in either catalytic efficiency or inhibitor binding. As before, comparison of reaction rates or inhibitor dissociation constants with and without a single functional group in the active site will tend to overestimate the intrinsic binding energy (defined as including desolvation energies of the functional group and its partner in the transition state or an analogous inhibitor), but may nevertheless provide a useful measure of the increase in binding that might be targeted by the drug designer.

2.5.3   'Average' functional group contributions

An alternative to the anchor principle approach was developed by Andrews *et al.* (1984), who sought to average the contributions of individual functional groups to the observed binding energies of 200 ligand–protein interactions in aqueous solution. In effect, this approach combined the ideas of Page and Jencks (1971) with those of Beddell *et al.* (1979), who had earlier used a simple regression analysis to estimate the strengths of covalent (Schiff base) and ionic interactions between hemoglobin effector molecules and a variety of hemoglobin mutants lacking the corresponding binding groups.

Although the fit obtained by Beddell *et al.* (1979) was remarkably good, the calculated energies were much lower than those estimated using the anchor principle, primarily because no account was taken of the entropic costs of the interaction. In the subsequent work by Andrews *et al.*, this factor was taken into account, with the average loss of overall rotational and translational entropy accompanying ligand–receptor binding, ΔG_{t+r}, being estimated at $58.5\,kJ\,mol^{-1}$ ($14\,kcal\,mol^{-1}$) at $310\,K$. Regression analysis led to the 'average' values of the binding energies associated with each functional group in the 200 ligands, as follows: $C(sp^2$ or $sp^3)$, $3\,kJ\,mol^{-1}$; O, S, N, or halogen, $5\,kJ\,mol^{-1}$; OH and C=O, 10 and $14\,kJ\,mol^{-1}$, respectively; and CO_2^-, OPO_3^{2-}, and N^+, 34, 42 and $48\,kJ\,mol^{-1}$, respectively.

It should be stressed that these values are not intrinsic binding energies in the sense defined above: this would be the case only if each functional group in each ligand in the series was optimally aligned with a corresponding functional group in the receptor. In fact, since every functional group of every ligand was included in the analysis, the calculated values are averages of apparent binding energies, including those for some groups which may not interact with the receptor. This may apply particularly to the sp^2 or sp^3 carbons, many of which provide the structural framework for the ligands but are shielded from interaction with receptor groups by intervening functional groups of the ligand. The calculated averages might thus be expected to be smaller than the corresponding intrinsic binding energies, although the assumption of a constant rotational and translational entropy loss appropriate to a tightly bound complex will tend to operate in the other direction. In general, the magnitudes of the values for particular functional groups are in accord with the ranges derived from application of the anchor principle for different bond types (see below).

A further outcome of the preceding analysis was the finding of a negative coefficient for n_r, the number of degrees of internal rotational freedom. The loss of each internal rotation on receptor binding results in an entropy loss that reduces the free energy of binding by an average of $3 \, kJ \, mol^{-1}$, which may be compared to the estimated value for the total loss of conformational freedom around a single bond of $5–6 \, kJ \, mol^{-1}$ (Page and Jencks 1971). The smaller number obtained empirically implies that conformational freedom is not fully lost for all the bonds in an average ligand–receptor interaction, and is consistent with experimental estimates of $1.6–3.6 \, kJ \, mol^{-1}$ for the entropic cost of restricting rotations in hydrocarbon chains (Searle and Williams 1992).

These values have been used by Andrews (1986) and others to determine the quality of fit of a ligand to its receptor. This is done by comparing the observed binding constant to the average binding energy calculated from equation (2.4) by summing the binding energies of the component groups and then subtracting the two entropy related terms. Ligands that match their receptors exceptionally well have a measured binding energy that substantially exceeds this calculated average value. Conversely, if the observed binding energy is very much less than the calculated average value, then the ligand either matches its receptor less well than average, or binds to the receptor in a comparatively high energy conformation.

Although clearly useful guides, the application of these numbers in drug design is restricted by the fact that they are averages of apparent binding energies, rather than true measures of intrinsic binding activity. There are also concerns as to the statistical validity of the use of multiple regression to extract average values from the raw data, particularly with respect to the inclusion of the constant rotational and translational entropy term rather than an adjustable parameter.

In view of these problems, it would obviously be more useful if the true intrinsic binding energies of specified binding groups could be calculated directly from observations on well-defined interactions, including proper allowance for the rotational, translational and other entropy losses associated with the interaction.

2.5.4   The role of ΔG_{t+r}

The theoretical limit for the complete loss of rotational and translational entropy on the formation of a bimolecular complex in solution at a standard state of $1 \, mol^{-1}$ and 298 K has been calculated by several authors (Page 1977; Finkelstein and Janin 1989; Williams *et al.* 1991). For a ligand of average molecular weight (say 200 dalton) this figure is approximately $60 \, kJ \, mol^{-1}$. The question is, how much of this rotational and translational entropy is really lost on binding?

Calculations and experimental data cited by Page (1977) suggest that the net loss of rotational and translational entropy on formation of a 'tight' bimolecular complex, including allowance for residual motion, would be on the order of

45 kJ mol^{-1} at 310 K, compared to 12 kJ mol^{-1} for a very 'loose' complex. It follows that the net loss of rotational and translational entropy (including residual motion) on bimolecular complex formation cannot be regarded as a constant for any but the tightest ligand–receptor interactions, and even then the actual entropy loss is significantly less than the corresponding entropy of the free ligand. Much of the rotational and translational entopy is converted to vibrational entropy in the bound ligand. Based on the data of Williams and others, a reasonable estimate of ΔG_{t+r} for 'tight' complexes would appear to be about 75% of the entropy of the unbound ligand, in agreement with the original figure proposed by Page (1977) of 45 kJ mol^{-1} for an average-sized ligand. Williams argues that the overall loss of entropy of a bimolecular interaction is related to the enthalpy of interaction by a curve of the general form of Figure 2.2. Whatever the exact form of this curve, it clearly shows that ΔG_{t+r} should be a variable value that increases up to a limiting value of 45–50 kJ/mol at 298 K as the enthalpy of interaction increases. A sliding value for ΔG_{t+r} rather than the fixed value used in most approximation methods may be more useful and strictly more accurate.

The use of a constant figure of 58.5 kJ mol^{-1} (14 kcal mol^{-1}) rather than 45 kJ mol^{-1} for the average functional group binding energies calculated by Andrews *et al.* means these values are likely to be overestimated. Furthermore, the use of a constant rotational and translational entropy term to calculate average molecular binding energies from equation (2.4) will lead to a systematic error that underestimates weak interactions (for which a smaller value of ΔG_{t+r} should be used) and may overestimate stronger ones (for which a larger ΔG_{t+r} value may

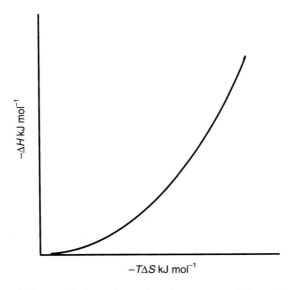

Figure 2.2 The general form of the relationship between enthalpy of association and the entropic cost of the interaction at room temperature. There is a limiting entropic cost that may be approached even when intermolecular associations are mediated by non-bonded interactions (Williams and Westwell 1998). The curve suggests that a sliding scale for ΔG_{t+r} (−TS) would be more appropriate than a constant value.

Table 2.1 Functional group contributions to ligand–receptor interactions (kJ mol^{-1})

Group type	Technique employed to determine contribution			
	Anchor principle	Site-directed mutagenesis	Average energy	Partition energy
Nonpolar (per CH$_2$)	12–14	1–3	3–6	
H-bond (uncharged)	16	2–6	5–14	1–12
H-bond (charge assisted)	20–42	15–19		
Ionic bond	18–28+	12–25	34–48	
ΔG_{t+r} (translation/rotation)	12–45		58.5*	
ΔG_r (internal rotation)	5–6		3	2–4

Note
* Assumed value.

be appropriate). Nevertheless, the numbers do provide the basis for some simple 'rules-of-thumb' that may be used by drug designers to answer practical design questions.

2.6   SOME RULES OF THUMB

The apparent contributions of different functional groups and/or bond types to overall binding energies derived from the various studies reviewed above are summarized in Table 2.1. Also included are corresponding values used or suggested for the overall loss of rotational and translational entropy, ΔG_{t+r}, and the loss of conformational entropy resulting from restriction of free rotation, ΔG_t.

Which of these numbers can most appropriately be used to explain the observed affinities of known ligands, or to *predict* the affinities of new ligands? The answer really depends on the question being asked.

2.6.1   What should this functional group do for my ligand?

If we wish to know what incremental binding contribution we might expect upon the addition of a functional group which is optimally aligned with a corresponding group in the receptor, then the numbers based on the anchor principle are probably the best bet, though co-operativity has to be born in mind. In particular, Wolfenden and Kati's (1991) observations in adenosine deaminase inhibitors of incremental binding energies of up to 42 kJ mol^{-1} (7 orders of magnitude increase in binding affinity) must be near the limit for charge-assisted hydrogen bonding by a hydroxyl group. As noted above, this and most other figures based on the anchor principle are not true intrinsic binding energies but a complicated mix of additional enthalpic and entropic terms. This is observed in the case of the adenosine deaminase study, where the hydroxyl not only forms a charge assisted hydrogen bond to a carboxylate, but also forms an additional charge interaction with a zinc atom and displaces a tightly bound water molecule already engaged in similar interactions with the enzyme. As an indication of potential incremental binding, however, these apparent binding energies are entirely appropriate, since they are then being applied in precisely the same way that they were derived. This was born out by the more recent example of cytidine deaminase ligands, where introduction of a particular hydroxyl also resulted in a seven orders of magnitude improvement in affinity. Observation of the crystal structure of the cytidine deaminase–ligand complex shows that there is a very similar network of interactions between the hydroxyl and both adenosine deaminase and cytidine deaminase. A more conservative estimate of the value of a charge-assisted hydrogen bond would be in the range of 16–$20\,kJ\,mol^{-1}$, based on the work of Fersht $et\,al.$ (1985). Page's estimate of 12–$14\,kJ\,mol^{-1}$ per CH_2 group, having been derived from observations on highly selective t-RNA synthetases, is probably also approaching the limit for an attractive interaction between non-polar groups.

The corresponding figures for charged groups, 18–$28\,kJ\,mol^{-1}$, are not based on examples where they are the primary determinants of specificity, and may be underestimates. An indication of this likelihood may be obtained using simple observations on the interactions of individual charged groups with appropriate enzymes. The phosphate ion, for example, binds alkaline phosphatase with a dissociation constant of $2.3 \times 10^{-6}\,M$, equivalent to a ΔG value of approximately $33\,kJ\,mol^{-1}$. Taking the most conservative estimate for the loss of rotational and translational entropy associated with this interaction, $12\,kJ\,mol^{-1}$ for a loosely bound complex, equation (2.4) then gives a lower estimate for binding of the phosphate ion of $45\,kJ\,mol^{-1}$. If the same value of ΔG_{t+r} is applied to the binding of oxalate ion to transcarboxylase, for which the dissociation constant is $1.8 \times 10^{-6}\,M$ (Northrop and Wood 1969) ($33\,kJ\,mol^{-1}$), equation (2.4) gives an apparent binding energy of $24\,kJ\,mol^{-1}$ per carboxylate group after allowance for a minimal conformational entropy loss of $3\,kJ\,mol^{-1}$.

2.6.2   How well does my ligand fit the receptor?

Summation of the average contributions of individual binding groups, including allowance for conformational, rotational and translational entropy terms as shown in equation (2.4), provides a simple back-of-the-envelope calculation of the strength of binding which might be expected for a ligand forming a typical interaction with a receptor. This figure, when compared to the observed affinity of the ligand for the target receptor, gives a direct indication of the relevance of the structure in 3D QSAR. If the observed binding is stronger than anticipated, it is reasonable to expect that the structure offers a reasonable fit to the receptor in a reasonably low energy conformation. If, on the other hand, the observed binding is significantly weaker than anticipated then it is likely that the ligand either matches its receptor less well than average, or binds to the receptor in a comparatively high energy conformation.

For this purpose, the optimal binding contributions determined from highly specific applications of the anchor principle are not appropriate, since the absence of detailed structural data means that the summation in equation (2.4) is necessarily done over all the functional groups in the ligand, regardless of whether or not they are directly involved in binding to the receptor. For those groups which make up the molecular framework, including most notably the sp^2 or sp^3 carbons, the average contribution should thus be much less than that derived from the anchor principle, while the contribution of substituents positioned to interact with corresponding receptor groups may be of similar magnitude.

Comparison with the other data in Table 2.1 suggests that the average values derived previously by Andrews *et al.* (1984) are a reasonable starting point for goodness of fit calculations. Clearly, they could be improved by adjusting the entropy terms to account for the extent to which rotational, translational and conformational entropy are lost in individual complexes, or even by employing a smaller entropy cost rather than $58.5 \, kJ \, mol^{-1}$ for ΔG_{t+r}. Either of these modifications would lead to a reduction in the size of the average functional group contributions, and this would be most significant for charged substituents.

Meanwhile, the two most extreme cases from the original set of 200 ligand–protein interactions studied by Andrews *et al.* (1984) offer simple examples of the application of the original 'average' numbers.

Substitution of these numbers into equation (2.4) for biotin suggested that it bound to the protein avidin almost $70 \, kJ \, mol^{-1}$ more tightly than anticipated on the basis of its constituent functional groups, implying an exceptional match to the structure of the protein. It has since been established that this is indeed the case, with polarization of the biotin molecule by the protein actually leading to an ionic interaction where a neutral hydrogen bonding interaction had been assumed.

At the opposite extreme is the case of methotrexate, for which equation (2.4) shows that the molecule binds to dihydrofolate reductase some $74 \, kJ \, mol^{-1}$ less tightly than anticipated, suggesting that despite its exceptional affinity for the enzyme the ligand does not offer a good overall fit to the active site of the enzyme. Again, the direct evidence of the crystal structure verifies this suggestion, with substantial parts of the structure, including one of the carboxylic acid groups, being exposed to solvent rather than utilized in binding to the enzyme.

2.6.3   Conclusion

It will be evident from the preceding discussion that the magnitudes of the intrinsic binding energies associated with different functional groups, or even types of interactions, are far from being precisely defined. The uncertainty in the numbers arises for two reasons.

First, the experimental data rarely provide any real degree of confidence that the observed change in binding energy actually reflects a single interaction between the target functional group and its binding partner in the receptor. Even in cases where there are structural data to show the binding interface with and without the additional functional group, as in the case of the phosphinate/phosphonamide inhibitor pairs described in Section 2.5.1, it is very difficult to predict the consequences of structural change on binding affinity. Binding affinity is a property of the state changes from the left-hand side to the right-hand side of equation (2.1), it is not attributable to the nature of the binding interface alone. It has become quite apparent that the task of predicting the state changes involved in ligand–receptor interactions is daunting. The medicinal chemist's traditional rigid receptor hypothesis is long since dead. Receptors have been shown to be capable of unpredictable conformational changes in response to different ligands, which may bring different ensembles of functional group interactions into play at the interface, further complicating the extraction of meaningful contributions (Davis and Teague 1999).

Second, the interpretation of the observed numbers invariably involves juggling differences between rather large entropy and enthalpy contributions in order to finally deduce the relatively small contribution due to the target binding group. The problem is akin to the legendary technique for weighing the ship's captain by weighing the ship before and after he comes aboard – except that in this case there is the additional complication of an unknown and variable number of stowaways!

The eventual solution to these uncertainties will require much more detailed analyses of structurally well-defined interactions, preferably including estimates of the extent to which each individual functional group is actually participating in the overall interaction (lengths and orientations of bonds, tightness of match between surfaces, states of ionization of binding groups, etc.) and the extent to which rotational, translational and conformational entropy have been lost in the process. With the increase in high-resolution structural details of intermolecular complexes and the rise of accurate calorimetric techniques (to independently calculate equilibrium constants, ΔH and ΔS) (Ladbury and Chowdhry 1996) improving our underlying knowledge, the goal of accurately predicting affinities may yet be achievable.

REFERENCES AND FURTHER READING

Ajay and Murcko, M.A. (1995) Computational methods to predict binding free energy in ligand–receptor complexes. *J. Med. Chem.*, **38**, 4953–4967.

Andrews, P.R., Craik, D.J. and Martin, J.L. (1984) Functional group contributions to drug–receptor interactions. *J. Med. Chem.*, **2**, 1648–1656.

Andrews, P. (1986) Functional groups, drug–receptor interactions and drug design. *Trends Pharmacol. Sci.*, **7**, 148–151.

Beddell, C.R., Goodford, P.J., Stammers, D.K. and Wootton, R. (1979) Species differences in the binding of compounds designed to fit a site of known structure in adult haemoglobin. *Br. J. Pharmacol.*, **65**, 535–543.

Ben-Tal, N., Sitkoff, D., Topol, I.A., Yang, A.-S., Burt, S.K. and Honig, B. (1997) Free energy of amide hydrogen bond formation in vacuum, in water, and in liquid alkane solution. *J. Phys. Chem. B.*, **101**, 450–457.

Bongrand, P. (1999) Ligand–receptor interactions. *Rep. Prog. Phs.*, **62**, 921–968.

Davis, A.M. and Teague, S.J. (1999) Hydrogen bonding, hydrophobic interactions, and the failure of the rigid receptor hypothesis. *Angew. Chem. Int. Ed.*, **38**, 736–749.

Dougherty, D.A. (1996) Cation-π-interactions in chemistry and biology: a new view of benzene, Phe, Tyr and Trp. *Science*, **271**, 163–168.

Epps, D.E., Cheney, J., Schostarez, H., Sawyer, T.K., Prairie, M., Krueger, W.C. and Mandel, F. (1990) Thermodynamics of the interaction of inhibitors with the binding site of recombinant human renin *J. Med. Chem.*, **33**, 2080–2086.

Fersht, A.R., Shi, J.-P., Knill-Jones, J., Lowe, D.M., Wilkinson, A.J., Blow, D.M. *et al.* (1985) Hydrogen bonding and biological specificity analysed by protein engineering. *Nature*, **314**, 235–238.

Finkelstein, A.V. and Janin, J. (1989) The price of lost freedom: entropy of bimolecular complex formation. *Protein Eng.*, **3**, 1–3.

Glusker, J.P. (1998) Directional aspects of intermolecular interactions. In *Design of Organic Solids*, edited by E. Weber, pp. 3–53. Berlin: Springer-Verlag.

Hunter, C.A. (1994) Meldola Lecture – the role of aromatic interactions in molecular recognition. *Chem. Soc. Rev.*, **23**, 101–109.

Jencks, W.P. (1981) On the attribution and additivity of binding energies. *Proc. Natl. Acad. Sci. USA*, **78**, 4046–4050.

Klotz, I.M. (1997) *Ligand–receptor energetics: a guide for the perplexed*, pp. 95–96. New York: John Wiley & Sons, Inc.

Kollman, P. (1993) Free energy calculations – applications to chemical and biochemical phenomena. *Chem. Rev.*, **93**, 2395–2417.

Ladbury, J.E. and Chowdhry, B.Z. (1996) Sensing the Heat: the application of isothermal titration calorimetry to thermodynamic studies of biomolecular interactions. *Chemistry & Biology*, **3**, 791–801.

McDonald, I.K. and Thornton, J.M. (1994) Satisfying hydrogen bonding potentials in proteins. *J. Mol. Biol.*, **238**, 777–793.

Morgan, B.P., Scholtz, J.M., Ballinger, M.D., Zipkin, I.D. and Bartlett, P.A. (1991) Differential binding-energy – a detailed evaluation of the influence of hydrogen-bonding and hydrophobic groups on the inhibition of thermolysin by phosphorus-containing inhibitors. *J. Am. Chem. Soc.*, **113**, 297–307.

Northrop, D.B. and Wood, H.G. (1969) Transcarboxylase VII. Exchange reactions and kinetics of oxalate inhibition. *J. Biol. Chem.*, **244**, 5820–5827.

Page, M.I. and Jencks, W.P. (1971) Entropic contributions to rate accelerations in enzymic and intramolecular reaction and the chelate effect. *Proc. Natl. Acad. Sci. USA*, **68**, 1678–1683.

Page, M.I. (1977) Entropy, binding energy and enzyme catalysis. *Angew. Chem. Int. Ed. Engl.*, **16**, 449–459.

Pang, Y.P. and Kollman, P.A. (1995) Applications of free energy derivatives to analog design. *Perspectives in Drug Discovery*, **3**, 106–122.

Searle, M.S. and Williams, D.H. (1992) The cost of conformational order: entropy changes in molecular associations. *J. Am. Chem. Soc.*, **114**, 10690–10697.

Wiley, R.A. and Rich, D.H. (1993) Peptidomimetics derived from natural-products. *Med. Res. Rev.*, **13**, 327–384.

Williams, D.H. and Bardsley, B. (1999) Estimating binding constants – the hydrophobic effect and cooperativity. *Perspectives in Drug Discovery and Design*, **17**, 43–59.

Williams, D.H., Cox, J.P.L., Doig, A.J., Gardner, M., Gerhard, U., Kaye, P.T., Lal, A.R., Nicholls, I.A., Salter, C.J. and Mitchell, R.C. (1991) Towards the semiquantitative estimation of binding constants. Guides for peptide–peptide binding in aqueous solution. *J. Am. Chem. Soc.*, **113**, 7020–7030.

Williams, D.H. and Westwell, M.S. (1998) Aspects of weak interactions. *Chem. Soc. Rev.*, **27**, 57–63.

Wolfenden, R. and Kati, W.M. (1991) Testing the limits of protein–legand binding discrimination with transition-state analog inhibitors. *Acc. Chem. Res.*, **24**, 209–215.

Chapter 3

Stereochemistry in drug design

Ian J. Kennedy and David E. Jane

3.1 INTRODUCTION

In the year 2000, the sales of chiral drugs reached $120 billion representing almost one-third of all drug sales world-wide (Figure 3.1), a fact which reinforces the importance of the link between chirality and drug design. In turn, this stems from the often overlooked reality that the biological targets for which these drugs are designed to interact with are themselves chiral. Therefore, dramatic differences are often witnessed in the action of one enantiomer over another in biological systems, ultimately in humans.

This raises the questions of why these drugs need to be chiral and how can such compounds be synthesized? In this chapter, we attempt to answer these questions by providing an overview of the rationale behind synthesizing asymmetric biologically active compounds and the methods that can be employed to obtain them. However, this is merely an introduction to this vast subject, individual points of

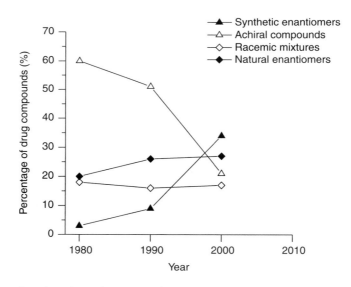

Figure 3.1 The sales of synthetic drugs as single enantiomers at the expense of achiral compounds.

which are described in more detail in the reference
chapter.

In summary, the first section gives an overview of tl
behind stereochemistry, merely intended as a brief revi
further information can be found in standard textbooks
ing on from this a rationale is presented as to why chiral
molecular recognition perspective and how they may be
this are several examples of how these methodologies l
synthesis of known drugs. The final section outlines analytical methods for the
assessment of the purity of chiral drugs.

3.2   WHAT ARE STEREOISOMERS?

There are a number of different types of isomerism that can be divided as
shown in Figure 3.2. Although both geometric and conformational isomers are
by definition classed as stereoisomers, optical isomers are probably the most
significant in terms of drug design and it is this type of isomerism that is
discussed in this chapter.

Such molecules that can possess optical activity are said to be chiral. Chirality is
simply a symmetry property of an object that describes its inability to be super-
imposed upon its mirror image i.e. it lacks reflectional symmetry. This generally
arises because of substitution around a tetrahedral carbon atom (the stereogenic
center) of four different groups, although other atoms such as nitrogen or phosphorous may also behave as stereogenic centers. The important point is that such
substitutions lead to the loss of symmetry and this is the prerequisite for a compound to be chiral. Such compounds can exist as two different stereoisomers, or
enantiomers, which are related as object to image through a reflectional plane. For
example, Figure 3.3 shows one of the simplest chiral molecules, lactic acid, produced by the body as a result of anaerobic respiration. It has a central stereogenic
center and no internal symmetry plane and thus can exist in one of two chiral
enantiomeric forms. However, propanoic acid possesses a symmetry plane down
the center of the molecule and so is achiral.

An important point concerning the enantiomers of a chiral molecule is that they
are identical except for two properties. First, they are chemically different only in

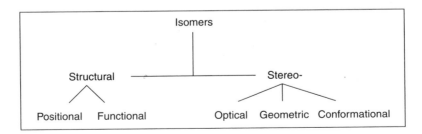

Figure 3.2 The different classes of isomerism. Stereoisomers are isomers that have the same
constitution but differ only in their 3D arrangement.

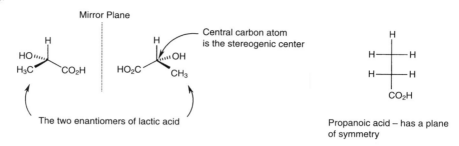

Figure 3.3 The two enantiomers of lactic acid are mirror images of each other. However, propanoic acid is achiral as it has a plane of symmetry through the center of the molecule.

the way that they react with other chiral molecules. This is a key attribute – the importance of which is discussed in more detail in the following sections. Second, their physical properties differ solely in the way in which they interact with plane polarized light, hence the term optical activity. All other properties such as melting point, solubility and spectroscopic data are identical.

The aforementioned differences in optical activity of chiral molecules can be simply explained by their lack of internal symmetry. When ordinary light is passed through a polarizer, the resultant light beam possesses electromagnetic waves that oscillate only in a single plane that is perpendicular to the direction of travel. If this light were to then pass through a solution containing a symmetrical molecule, collisions with the molecule in a particular orientation are canceled out by encounters with the mirror image molecular orientation. However, if this were to be repeated with a sample containing unequal amounts of enantiomers of a chiral compound then the plane of polarization will be altered. This is because there will be no 'canceling effect' and the net amount of rotation can then be measured. If a 50:50 (racemic) mixture of two enantiomers were to be examined, again there would be a net overall effect of zero rotation as each enantiomer would cancel out the rotation caused by the other.

The degree of rotation caused by a chiral molecule is easily measured using a polarimeter. If a molecule is seen to rotate the light anticlockwise it is labeled as *laevorotatory*, or if it is clockwise it is called *dextrorotatory*. The abbreviated labels (−) or L for laevo- and (+) or D for dextrorotatory are also used. Since this net rotation, termed $[\alpha]_D$ (or specific rotation), is an intrinsic property of an optically active molecule it can be used to quantify the amount or purity of a chiral molecule. This value is dependent on the wavelength of light used, the length of the sample tube through which the light is passed, temperature, solvent and sample concentration. The light source most often used for such determinations is that emitted by a sodium lamp at 589 nm (the so-called sodium D line).

The specific rotation at 20 °C can therefore be expressed as:

$$[\alpha]_D^{20} = \frac{\text{observed rotation (degrees)}}{\text{length of sample tube (dm)} \times \text{concentration (g/ml)}}$$

Optical purity can be defined as the ratio of the specific optical rotation of the enantiomeric mixture and the specific optical rotation of the pure enantiomer and is usually expressed as a percentage.

The observed optical rotation (D or L) was the earliest method of distinguishing between enantiomers, but this method gives no indication as to the actual spatial geometry of a molecule i.e. the configuration about the stereogenic centre. This was rectified by the introduction of the Fischer convention which labelled such centres as having either D or L configuration based on an arbitrary standard, (+)-glyceraldehyde. However, this system has now been superseded by the Cahn–Ingold–Prelog (or 'sequence rule') system which can be used to unambiguously assign any stereogenic center as possessing either (R) or (S) stereochemistry. This is deduced using a set of rules that assign priorities to the substituents attached to the stereogenic centre, the details of which are outside the scope of this review. A detailed discussion of these rules is available in any general organic chemistry textbook (e.g. Robinson 2000). Once the priorities of the substituents have been assigned, enantiomers are readily classified as being the (R) or (S) isomers. This is done by first viewing the molecule from the opposite group of lowest priority. If the remaining groups are seen to go from lowest to highest priority in a clockwise direction then the center is labeled as (R), and vice versa for (S). Lactic acid is again used as an example to demonstrate this (Figure 3.4).

Molecules such as lactic acid are relatively simple in that they only have one stereogenic center, but what are the implications if multiple stereogenic centers are present? As an example, the drug ephedrine has two stereogenic centers and thus there are four possible isomers (Figure 3.5). Since there can only be two possible enantiomers of a chiral compound then the relationship between these two pairs must be a

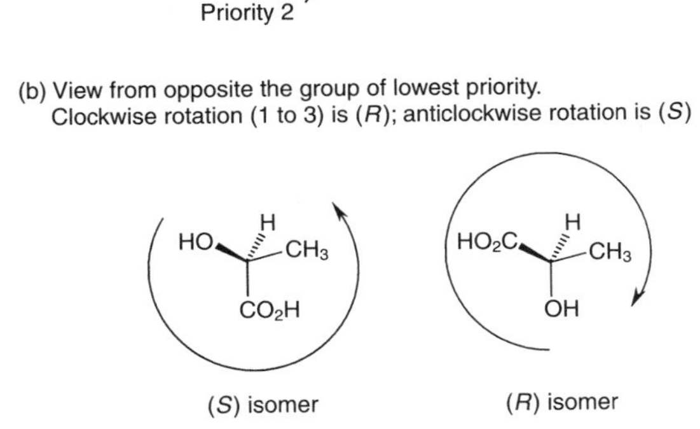

Figure 3.4 Procedure for assigning stereogenic centers as possessing either (R) or (S) configuration.

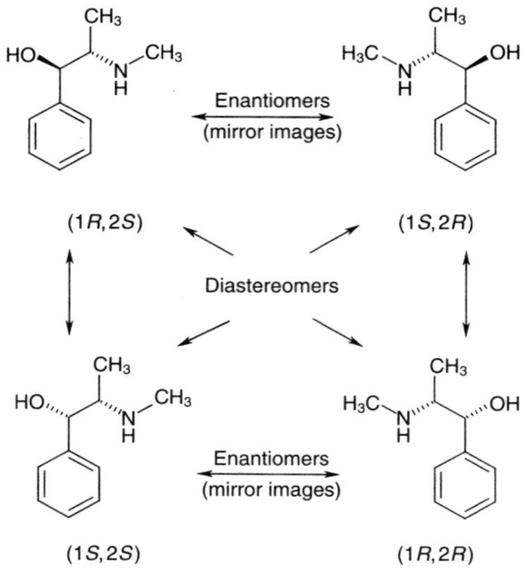

Figure 3.5 The relationship between enantiomers and diastereomers. The biologically active forms of ephedrine are those with the (1R, 2S) and (1S, 2S) configurations, which are diastereomers of each other.

non-mirror image one. Such stereoisomers that are non-superimposable, non-mirror images of each other are known as diastereomers.

Therefore, although enantiomers must have an opposite configuration at all stereogenic centers, diastereomers must be opposite at only some, but may be the same at the others. As previously described, two enantiomers of a racemate have identical chemical properties in an achiral environment. However, an extremely important property of diastereomers is that unlike enantiomers, they will (unless by coincidence) have non-identical physical and chemical properties such as boiling point, solubility and spectral properties. The potential applications of this are discussed in Sections 3.5.1 and 3.5.2.

As a general rule, the total number of isomers of any given molecule is also given by the rule:

Number of isomers $= 2^n$

where n is the total number of stereogenic centers.

So, as in ephedrine, a compound with two centers will have four isomers, three centers leads to eight isomers and so on. However, there are examples where this rule does not hold true because some isomers may be *meso* compounds. These can be described as isomers that contain stereogenic centers but are achiral due to the presence of a symmetry plane. This generally arises when the three groups attached to one stereogenic center are the same as those attached to another. All of this implies that a *meso* compound will be superimposable on its mirror image hence will be optically inactive. These principles are demonstrated well using

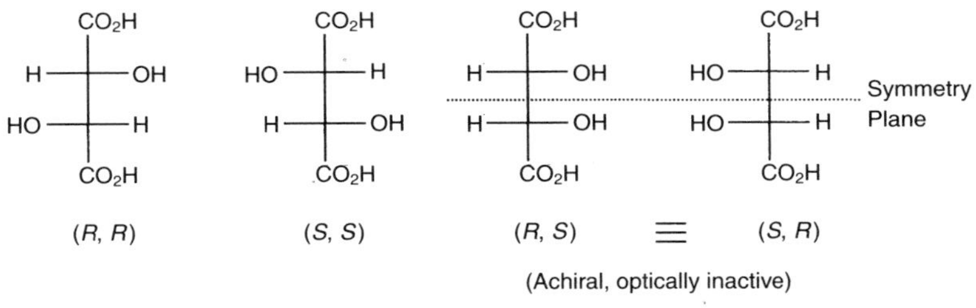

Figure 3.6 Tartaric acid has two stereogenic centers but only three stereoisomers.

tartaric acid. This compound has two stereogenic centers and so should have four isomers – two pairs of enantiomers. However, the (R, S) and (S, R) configurations are superimposable since they have a plane of symmetry. Therefore, tartaric acid has three isomers – a pair of enantiomers and a *meso* isomer (Figure 3.6).

The definition of optical purity discussed above has been largely superseded by two related terms enantiomeric excess (ee) and diastereomeric excess (de). Enantiomeric excess can be defined as the proportion of the major enantiomer less that of the minor enantiomer whereas de is defined as the proportion of the major diastereomer less that of the minor one. Both ee and de are usually expressed as percentages.

Should the only difference between enantiomers be their interaction with plane polarized light then their existence would be little more than academic. However, as described above stereochemistry has important implications in terms of biological activity. The origin and nature of these phenomena are described in the following section.

3.3 THE ORIGIN OF STEREOSPECIFICITY IN MOLECULAR RECOGNITION

In 1896, Emil Fischer proposed that the substrates of an enzyme must have a complementary shape to the active site, this theory being known as the lock and key hypothesis (Figure 3.7). This was the first attempt to explain the specificity of enzyme action. However, this theory was erroneous as it suggested that enzymes only have one optimal substrate and all others fit less well and therefore the catalyzed reaction is less efficient. This is not the case as some enzymes can catalyze reactions on a range of different substrates. In order to take this observation into account, Koshland later proposed that the enzyme is forced to change shape to some extent in order to take up the optimal shape to accommodate the binding of substrates to the active site. This induced fit model (Figure 3.8) explains why enzymes can accommodate a range of substrates. However, it is now thought that not only the enzyme can change shape, the substrate can also alter its shape to fix it in the optimal conformation for the reaction catalyzed by the enzyme.

Although the induced fit model was proposed for enzymes, it has also been proposed that it may also explain drug–receptor interactions. Receptors are made

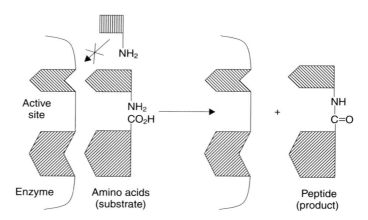

Figure 3.7 The lock and key hypothesis – the enzyme and substrate must have a complementary shape.

up of chiral building blocks and are themselves chiral and would therefore be expected to be enantioselective in their interactions with chiral drugs. In order to explain the stereoselective action of drugs on receptors, the three-point receptor theory was proposed (Figure 3.9). In this theory, only one enantiomer has the optimal spatial disposition of the three groups A, B and C to interact with the complementary sites on the receptor. The less active enantiomer binds less effectively with the receptor, as the groups on the ligand cannot align favorably with the corresponding sites on the receptor. This theory is successful in explaining stereoselectivity of drug action although it must be born in mind that there may be more than three interactions of a drug with a receptor. In addition, these interactions are not necessarily all ionic or hydrogen bonds; hydrophobic or steric interactions may also suffice.

The three-point receptor theory has been useful in understanding the mechanism of enzyme action and also in the rational design of inhibitors. An example of an

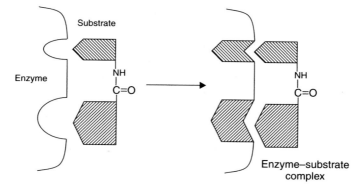

Figure 3.8 The induced fit model – the enzyme is forced to change shape to interact optimally with the substrate.

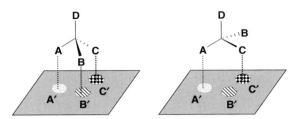

Figure 3.9 The three-point receptor theory.

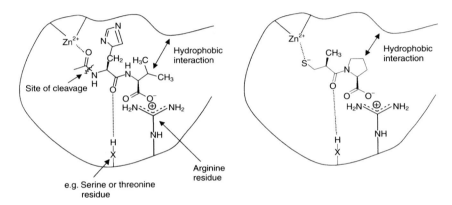

Figure 3.10 Left panel: Interaction of the terminal dipeptide sequence of angiotensin I with ACE showing site of peptide cleavage. Right panel: Note Captopril interacts with ACE in a similar fashion to angiotensin I.

inhibitor designed by such rational drug design is the angiotensin converting enzyme (ACE) inhibitor captopril, which is marketed as an antihypertensive drug. Captopril was developed by taking into account a model of the mechanism by which ACE converts angiotensin I into angiotensin II (Figure 3.10). It is worth noting that captopril has two stereogenic centers and despite this was developed and marketed as a single enantiomer. Only one of the four possible isomers of captopril can bind optimally with the active site (Figure 3.10) illustrating the usefulness of the three-point receptor theory (note, however, that captopril has four areas of contact with the active site).

The three-point receptor theory has also been used for understanding chromatographic resolution of mixtures of enantiomers on chiral stationary phases, which can be thought of as artificial receptors (see Section 3.5.2).

3.4 WHY IS STEREOCHEMISTRY IMPORTANT IN DRUG DESIGN?

The sale of single enantiomer drugs shot past the $120 billion mark in the year 2000 and is projected to increase further over the next few years. Thus, chiral drugs whether sold as racemates or as the active enantiomer are likely to dominate drug markets in the near future. There are a number of reasons for the growth of chiral drug sales. Pharmaceutical companies see it as a way of prolonging the patent life of their existing racemic drugs by patenting and then marketing the active enantiomer, thereby undercutting competition from generic drug sales (Agranat and Caner 1999). In addition, some companies see this switching from racemate to single active enantiomer as a way into the drug market. One such company, Sepracor synthesizes the individual enantiomers of racemic drugs that are already on the market. If the activity resides in a single enantiomer then Sepracor patents the drug and will then either licence the drug back to the original company or market the drug itself. There are problems associated with this approach, Sepracor obtained a patent claiming the use of (S)-fluoxetine (Prozac) and (R)-fluoxetine (Figure 3.11) for the treatment of migraine and depression, respectively. Eli Lilly, the company responsible for the initial discovery of Prozac had already determined that the individual enantiomers of fluoxetine had almost equal activity as serotonin reuptake inhibitors and did not patent the individual enantiomers. Eli Lilly therefore took out a licence on the Sepracor patent allowing them sole rights to market (R)-fluoxetine as an antidepressant. This was seen as a strategy for extending the fluoxetine program until 2015. However, Lilly have terminated the agreement with Sepracor as clinical data showed a statistically significant negative cardiac side effect of the (R)-enantiomer at the highest dose tested. The underlying reason for this is likey to involve the differences in rates of metabolism of the two enantiomers, which means that only 25% of the fluoxetine in the plasma is the (R)-enantiomer. Thus, higher doses of the (R)-enantiomer were needed in clinical trials to give an equivalent therapeutic effect. Another strategic reason may also have played a part in the decision as fluoxetine would be competing with a new generation of antidepressants with multiple modes of action rather than relying on only serotonin reuptake (Thayer 2000).

The Food and Drug Administration (FDA) strongly urges companies to evaluate both the racemates and the corresponding individual enantiomers as new drugs. Thus, even if a drug is to be sold as a racemate the individual enantiomers need to be evaluated which increases the cost and timescale of drug development. Increasingly, drug companies are developing single enantiomer drugs to avoid these unnecessary costs. This strategy has been aided by the considerable increase in the methodology available for the synthesis and the assessment of purity of chiral drugs.

However, these are not the only reasons for testing individual enantiomers of chiral drugs, lessons learned from mistakes made by marketing racemic drugs also

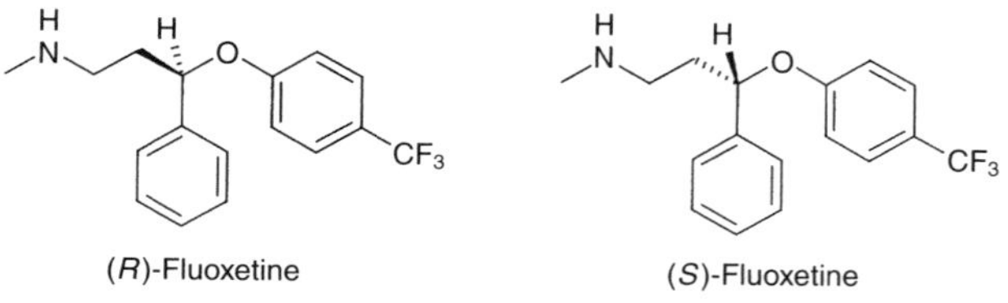

(R)-Fluoxetine   (S)-Fluoxetine

Figure 3.11 The structure of the serotonin reuptake inhibitor fluoxetine.

play a part such as in the tragic case of thalidomide (Figure 3.14). Racemic thalidomide was developed in the 1950s and was used as a sleeping pill and to treat morning sickness, but only outside the USA as FDA approval was not given. Unfortunately, the drug had serious side effects as it was found to be teratogenic causing foetal abnormalities. It was later discovered in tests with mice that the (S)-enantiomer possessed the teratogenic activity whilst the (R)-enantiomer possessed the sedative activity. However, subsequent studies using rabbits revealed that the enantiomers racemise under physiological conditions. Recently, thalidomide has hit the headlines again as the use of the racemate for treatment of leprosy has been approved by the FDA but only under the strictest of guidelines. It appears that thalidomide may also have therapeutic utility in the treatment of AIDS related disorders and tuberculosis.

The origin of the rising number of chiral drugs lies in the rational drug design process as medicinal chemists are now targeting receptors and enzymes, which are thought to be involved in the disease process. As these targets are themselves chiral, it is not surprising that the individual enantiomers of a drug may have differential activity. Indeed, Pfeiffer's rule states that 'the lower the effective dose of a drug the greater the difference in the pharmacological effect of the optical isomers'. This is simply stating that for drugs which potently interact with a receptor, it is unlikely that the individual enantiomers would both fit into the binding site. It should be noted that not only the pharmacodynamic aspects are important in the discussion of the activity of chiral drugs. Pharmacokinetics are also affected as the absorption and clearance of drugs involves interaction with enzymes and transport proteins. Thus, the individual enantiomers of a chiral drug may be metabolized by enzymes at different rates and may be transformed into different chemical entities. As a result of these considerations, it is very important that individual enantiomers of chiral drugs are tested in the clinic.

Ariëns (1986), a pioneer in the field of enantioselective drug actions, has proposed that the active enantiomer of a chiral drug be termed the eutomer whilst the less active enantiomer should be termed the distomer. The eudismic ratio (ER) is defined as the ratio of the activity of the eutomer to that of the distomer. The presence of the distomer in the racemic drug can have a number of consequences on the biological activity.

3.4.1   The distomer is inactive (high eudismic ratio)

In this case, the distomer is either inactive or displays no undesirable side effects. In the case of the antihypertensive agent (β-blocker) propranolol (Figure 3.12), the (S)-enantiomer is 130-fold more potent than the (R)-enantiomer as a β-adreno-ceptor antagonist (i.e. ER = 130). A number of other β-blockers based on this structure show high eudismic ratios. These drugs are therefore marketed as racemates as the distomer displays no side effects. Despite this, there would have been advantages in marketing the (S)-enantiomer if only to extend patent life. Some drugs show even greater enantioselectivity, dexetimide has 10 000-fold greater affinity for the muscarinic acetylcholine receptor than levetimide (Figure 3.12). The distomer in these cases has been termed isomeric ballast by Ariëns (1986) as at the very least marketing racemic drugs is wasteful of resources.

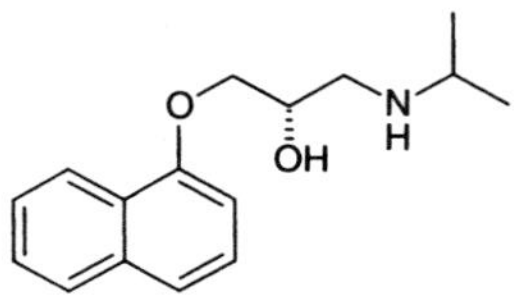

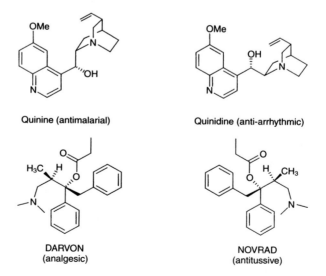

(*S*)-Propranolol (Eutomer, ER = 130) 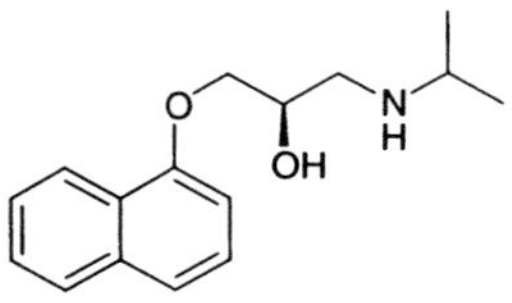   (*R*)-Propranolol (Distomer)

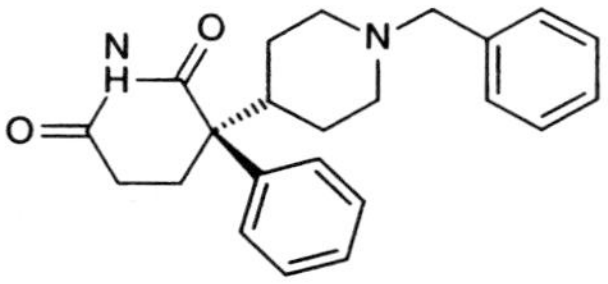

(*S*)-(+)-Dexetimide (Eutomer, ER = 10 000) 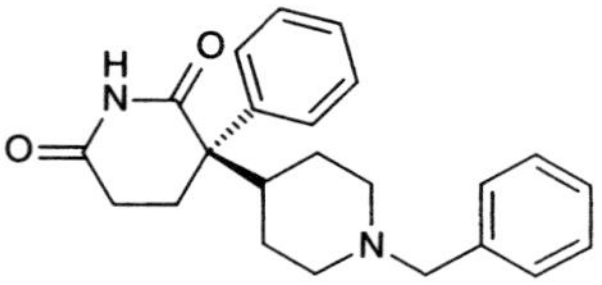   (*R*)-(−)-Levetimide (Distomer)

Figure 3.12 Examples of drugs where the distomer is weak/inactive.

3.4.2   Both enantiomers have independent therapeutic benefits

In some instances, both enantiomers of a drug may have different therapeutic value. The classical example of this behavior is quinine and quinidine (Figure 3.13). Quinine, which was originally obtained from the bark of cinchona trees was for centuries the only treatment for malaria. The first stereoselective synthesis of quinine has recently been published by Stork and co-workers (2001). Quinidine,

Quinine (antimalarial)   Quinidine (anti-arrhythmic)

DARVON
(analgesic)   NOVRAD
(antitussive)

Figure 3.13 Examples of drugs where both enantiomers possess therapeutic benefits.

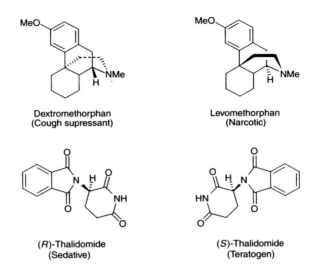

Figure 3.14 Examples of drugs where the distomer possesses harmful effects.

on the other hand, is used as a Class 1A anti-arrhythmic agent and acts by increasing action potential duration.

The drug dextropropoxyphene marketed by Eli Lilly has trade names reflecting the different activities of the enantiomers. Thus the (2R, 3S)-enantiomer, DARVON has analgesic properties whilst the (2S, 3R)-enantiomer NOVRAD (Figure 3.13) is an antitussive (prevents or relieves coughing).

3.4.3 Distomer possesses harmful effects

In some cases, it is known that the distomer produces harmful or undesirable side effects. Thus, dextromethorphan is used as a cough suppressant, whereas levomethorphan has antitussive properties it is also an opioid narcotic (Figure 3.14). The harmful teratogenic side effects of the (S)-enantiomer of thalidomide have already been discussed (Section 3.4).

3.4.4 The eutomer and the distomer have the opposite biological activity

It is sometimes observed that the enantiomers of a chiral drug may have opposite biological activity. One example of this is (−)-dobutamine, which is an agonist at α-adrenoceptors whereas (+)-dobutamine is an antagonist (Figure 3.15). However, (+)-dobutamine is ten-fold more potent than the (−)-isomer as a β_1-adrenoceptor agonist and is used to treat cardiogenic shock.

The individual enantiomers of the 1,4-dihydropyridine analog BayK8644 (Figure 3.15) have opposing effects on L-type calcium channels with the (S)-enantiomer being an activator and the (R)-enantiomer being an antagonist (see also Section 7.4.3).

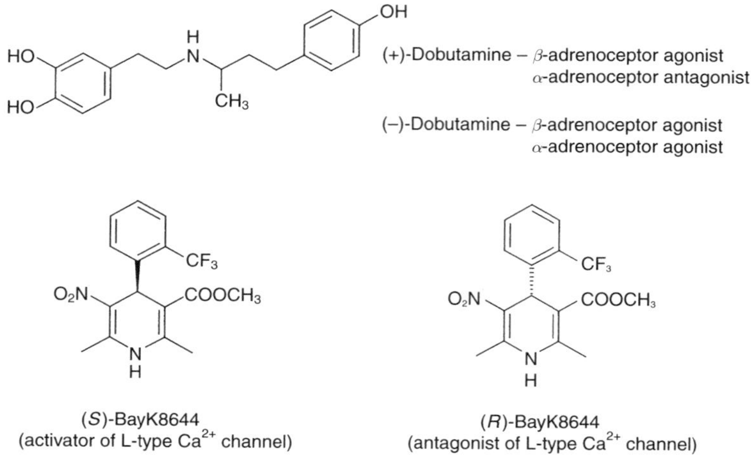

Figure 3.15 Examples of drugs where the eutomer and the distomer have the opposite biological activity.

3.4.5 The racemate has a therapeutic advantage over the individual enantiomers

Both enantiomers may contribute to the therapeutic effect though examples of chiral drugs exhibiting this phenomenon are quite rare. We have recently reported that racemic 3,4-dicarboxyphenylglycine (DCPG, Figure 3.16) displays a greater potency in preventing sound-induced seizures in an experimental model of generalized epilepsy seizures than either enantiomer alone (Moldrich *et al.* 2001). The (R)-enantiomer of DCPG has antagonist activity at the AMPA receptor subtype of ionotropic glutamate receptors whereas the (S)-enantiomer has agonist activity at the mGlu8 receptor subtype of metabotropic glutamate receptors (Thomas *et al.* 2001) (glutamate receptors; see also Section 9.3). Thus, combining an AMPA receptor antagonist with a mGlu8 receptor agonist leads to a potentiation of anti-epileptic activity. Interestingly, the racemate exhibited lower potency in the

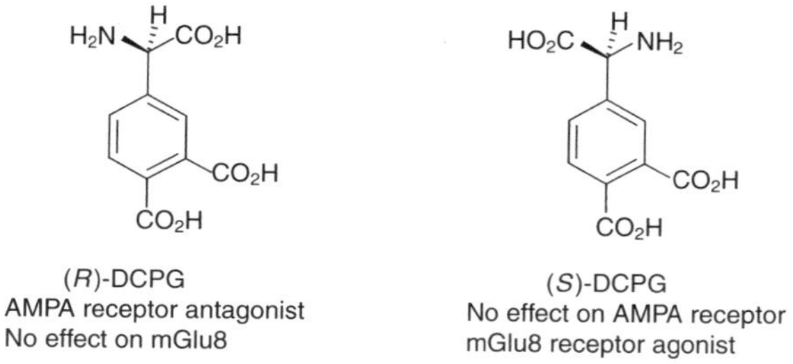

Figure 3.16 Both (R)- and (S)-3,4-DCPG have potential therapeutic value, the racemate, however, is more potent as an anti-epileptic agent.

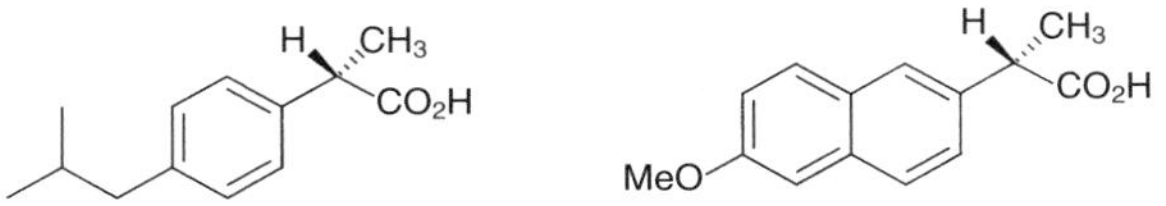

Figure 3.17 Examples of drugs where one enantiomer is converted into the other in the body.

rotarod test than the individual enantiomers suggesting that it did not impair motor performance beyond that experienced with either of the isomers alone.

3.4.6 One enantiomer converted into the other in the body

The inter-conversion of the enantiomers of thalidomide under physiological conditions has already been discussed. Another group of drugs which are known to exhibit this phenomenon are the α-arylpropionic acids, which are non-steroidal anti-inflammatory drugs (NSAIDs). These drugs are used to treat rheumatoid arthritis and as analgesics. It is known in the case of naproxen and ibuprofen (Figure 3.17) that the desired activity resides in the (S)-enantiomer while the (R)-enantiomer undergoes metabolic inversion to the (S)-enantiomer. Ostensibly, these drugs are safe to give in the racemic form as the distomer is converted to the eutomer in the body, however, it is known that in the course of the metabolism of the (R)-enantiomer, ibuprofen accumulates in fatty tissue in the body. The (S)-enantiomer is not metabolized in the same fashion and therefore marketing the biologically active (S)-enantiomer is advantageous.

Hopefully, these examples have persuaded the reader of the necessity of careful pharmacological testing of the individual enantiomers as well as the racemic mixture before marketing a chiral drug.

3.5 METHODS OF OBTAINING PURE STEREOISOMERS

Unfortunately, the preparation of pure stereoisomers is not trivial, arising from the fact that a reaction between two achiral starting materials, in an achiral environment, cannot generate a chiral product. This is essentially a description of the paradigm that chirality cannot just be created from nowhere. For example, the reaction between but-1-ene and hydrogen bromide (Figure 3.18) produces a compound containing a stereogenic center, so is it possible to generate a single enantiomer? The answer to this is no as the intermediate secondary carbocation contains a sp^2 hybridized carbon. It is therefore planar, has a plane of symmetry and is achiral.

As a result, subsequent attack by bromide ion can occur equally well from either the top or the bottom face. So, although the final product contains a stereogenic center, equal amounts of each isomer are produced leading to an achiral racemic mixture. So, how are pure chiral compounds obtained? Essentially, the answer to this is that there are three main methods: (1) resolution of racemates; (2) use

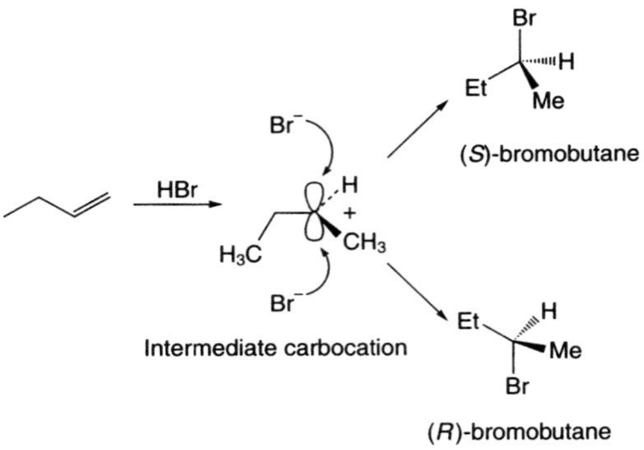

Figure 3.18 The reaction of achiral reagents in an achiral environment cannot produce an optically active product.

of naturally available chiral compounds (the chiral pool); or (3) stereoselective synthesis. These are described in more detail below, each of these methodologies being illustrated by examples taken from commercially available therapeutic agents.

3.5.1 Resolution of racemates by crystallization of diastereomers

Resolution is perhaps the oldest and most often used method of obtaining separation of a pair of enantiomers, and it is still widely used in the pharmaceutical industry for preparing optically active drugs. Although direct crystallizations of racemic mixtures can sometimes be performed in a chiral medium, the most common procedure utilizes the previously described principle that two diastereomers of a compound possess different chemical and physical properties. Of these, solubility disparities are widely used in order to produce differential crystallizations. The most common method of achieving this is to react a free carboxylic acid group of the racemate with a chiral base such as brucine, strychnine or basic amino acids such as lysine or arginine to produce diastereomeric salts (Figure 3.19). Other functional groups on the molecule such as bases, alcohols or aldehydes can also be used equally well. The resolving agents used have traditionally been derived from natural sources such as the alkaloid bases, but more recently advances have been made in the use of synthetic 'designer resolving agents'.

If the racemic mixture were reacted in this way with a pure optically active reagent then only two diastereomers are produced. These can then be crystallized and the initial precipitate should contain a higher proportion of one diastereomer (due to solubility differences), but usually this crystallization procedure needs to be repeated several times as the difference in solubility of the two isomers is rarely that pronounced. As the theoretical yield of this procedure is only 50% the racemization and recycling of the unwanted isomer is often performed in order to increase the economic viability of the procedure. This is

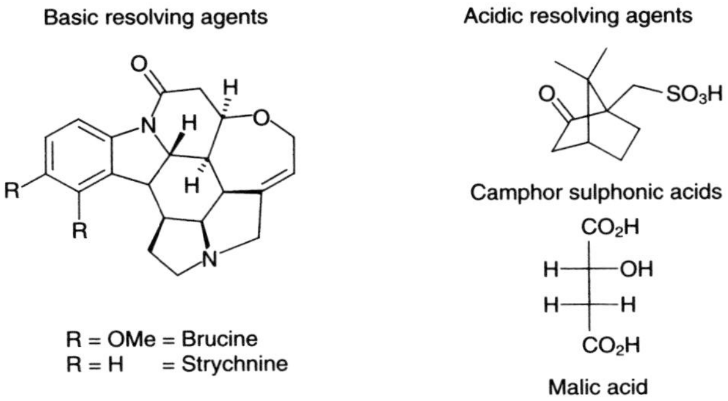

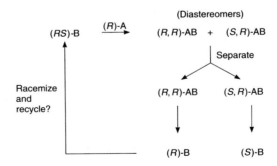

Basic resolving agents

R = OMe = Brucine
R = H = Strychnine

Acidic resolving agents

Camphor sulphonic acids

CO_2H
H——OH
H——H
CO_2H

Malic acid

Figure 3.19 Some commonly used resolving agents.

obviously of particular importance if this methodology is being used in large scale pharmaceutical production. Once the desired purity of the diastereomer has been achieved, the chiral auxiliary can then be removed to furnish the enantiomerically pure compound (Figure 3.20).

Although the predictability of success of such classical resolutions is not easy, a number of criteria for the choice of resolving agent have been proposed:

1   The asymmetric center should be in close proximity to the group used for salt formation.
2   The resultant salt should have a rigid structure.
3   Stronger acids and bases are preferential to weaker.
4   The resolving agent must be stable under the reaction conditions but be easily recovered after crystallization.

Despite this, the choice of which resolving agent to use often comes from trial and error experience. Overall, the disadvantages of this procedure are that it can be laborious and without recycling, it often results in a poor overall yield of the required diastereomer. There is also the requirement that the product needs to be

(Diastereomers)

(*RS*)-B —(*R*)-A→ (*R,R*)-AB + (*S,R*)-AB

Separate

(*R,R*)-AB   (*S,R*)-AB

(*R*)-B   (*S*)-B

Racemize and recycle?

Figure 3.20 Schematic procedure for resolution of a racemate by crystallization of its diastereomeric salt.

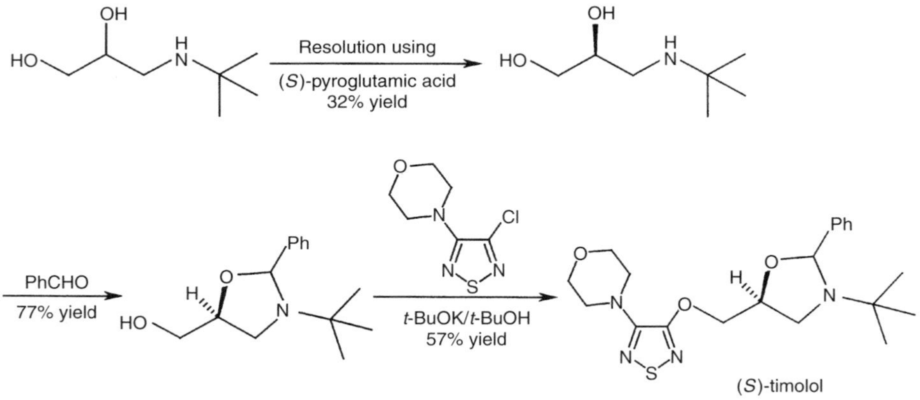

Figure 3.21 Synthesis of (S)-timolol using classical resolution.

a solid in order to be recrystallized! However, it is an inexpensive, well-established procedure, applicable to a variety of compounds on a large scale and requires no or little technical expertise or special equipment. There is also good availability and choice of chiral reactants from which to form the diastereomer. An example of the use of this technique can be found in the synthesis of (S)-timolol, a β-blocker antihypertensive drug (Figure 3.21).

3.5.2   Enantioselective chromatography

The preparative separation of the enantiomers of chiral drugs using chromatography is now an established procedure both in the pharmaceutical industry and in academic medicinal chemistry laboratories. Indeed, in some cases HPLC separation technology has been applied instead of synthesis or resolution to separate the individual enantiomers of chiral drugs, particularly at the development stage of drug discovery. New technology such as simulated moving bed (SMB) chromatography allows in some instances the resolution of chiral drugs up to 0.5–1.5 kg of racemate per kilogram of chiral stationary phase (CSP) per day. Separation of chiral drugs by chromatography relies on the formation of diastereomeric complexes. There are two main methods of accomplishing this either by precolumn derivatization using a chiral derivatizing agent followed by separation using conventional reversed-phase chromatography or separation using a column containing an immobilized CSP or via inclusion of a chiral mobile phase additive. There are a number of problems associated with precolumn derivatization, notwithstanding the inconvenience of having to perform a reaction before analysis. It is necessary to establish that the chiral derivatizing agent is enantiomerically pure and that racemization of either of the stereogenic centers of the diastereoisomer does not occur during the derivatization process. In addition, differential reaction rates of the sample with the derivatizing agent may lead to enantiomeric enrichment and racemization or enrichment may occur during the isolation and purification of the derivative. Addition of a chiral mobile phase additive (such as a cyclodextrin, or a (S)-proline copper complex) has met with success and has some advantages over CSPs such as the ability to use less expensive non-chiral columns. However, the direct separation of enantiomers using columns containing immobilized CSPs is usually the method of choice. Methodology for the resolution of chiral drugs on CSPs is now well developed and a number of different columns are commercially available. A brief overview of this methodology will be discussed. For a more detailed review see Francotte (2001).

3.5.2.1 Ligand-exchange

Chiral ligand-exchange chromatography relies on the covalent binding of an optically active ligand to the solid support. This type of separation is mainly used for the separation of amino acids using a CSP consisting of (S)-proline bound to the silica gel solid support. In order to separate racemic amino acids, copper (II) ions are first passed through the column to form a complex with the (S)-proline. The racemic mixture is then passed down the column and the (R)- and (S)-isomers displace one of the (S)-proline ligands from the copper complex resulting in the formation of transient diastereomeric complexes. These complexes formed with the two enantiomers of the amino acid of interest and immobilized (S)-proline have different stabilities resulting in one isomer of the amino acid being retained on the column for longer than the other.

3.5.2.2 Crown ethers

Chiral crown ethers have been immobilized on solid supports in order to affect the separation of both underivatized amino acids containing a primary amino group and chiral primary amines. The commercially available Crownpak column consists of a single enantiomer of a chiral dinaphthyl crown ether (Figure 3.23) immobilized on a stationary phase. Chiral separation using crown ether CSPs relies on the formation of a diastereomeric inclusion complex formed between the ammonium ion of the primary amino group and the oxygen atoms of the crown ether. In order to ensure protonation of the primary amino group separations are usually carried out in dilute acid solution such as aqueous perchloric acid. A preparative separation of the enantiomers of (RS)-3,4-DCPG (mentioned in Section 3.4.5) was obtained using the CR(+) column (see Figure 3.22 and Thomas *et al.* 2001).

For natural amino acids resolved on the Crownpak CR(+) column the D (or in most cases R) enantiomer is eluted before the L enantiomer. It has been claimed that the absolute configuration of an amino acid can be inferred from the elution order of the isomers from the CR(+) column. A CR(−) column which has the reverse enantioselectivity to the CR(+) column is also commercially available. One disadvantage of using this column is that mobile phases containing more than 15% methanol results in leaching of the chiral crown ether from the column and deterioration of CSP performance. Recently, a CSP bearing structural similarity to the crown ether found in the Crownpak column has been developed that has additional functionality allowing covalent immobilization on silica gel (Hyun *et al.* 2001).

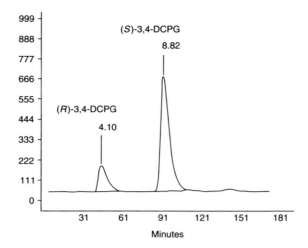

Figure 3.22 A mixture of (R)- and (S)-3,4-DCPG resolved on a Crownpak CR(+) column. Chromatography conditions: aqueous perchloric acid, pH 2, 20 °C, flow rate 0.4 ml/min. Detected at 230 nM.

3.5.2.3 *Pirkle columns*

These columns were mainly the result of the work of Pirkle and co-workers. There are two main types: (1) a π acceptor phase based mainly on N-(3,5-dinitrobenzoyl)-phenylglycine bonded via a linker to the silica (Figure 3.23); and (2) a π donor phase typically based on naphthylamino acid derivatives bonded to silica. The separation is achieved by the formation of a strong three-point interaction with only one enantiomer of a chiral drug. These interactions include the formation charge–transfer complexes, π–π bonding and steric effects. These types of column are commercially available and can be used for preparative separations. The main disadvantage of these columns is that they only separate aromatic compounds and therefore precolumn derivatization of the drug of interest may be necessary. Recently modified versions of these columns

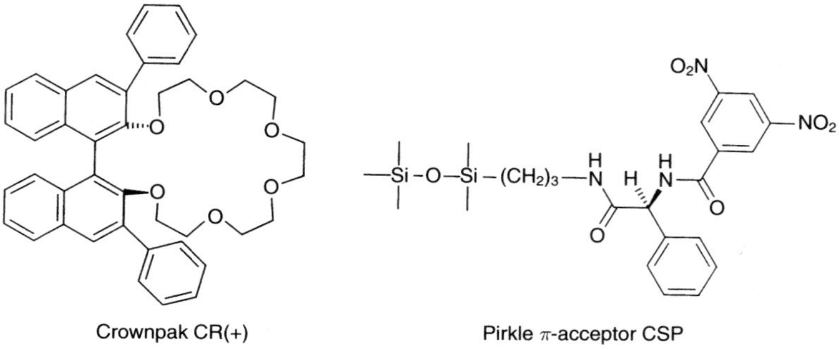

Crownpak CR(+)

Pirkle π-acceptor CSP

Figure 3.23 Examples of crown ether and Pirkle chiral stationary phases.

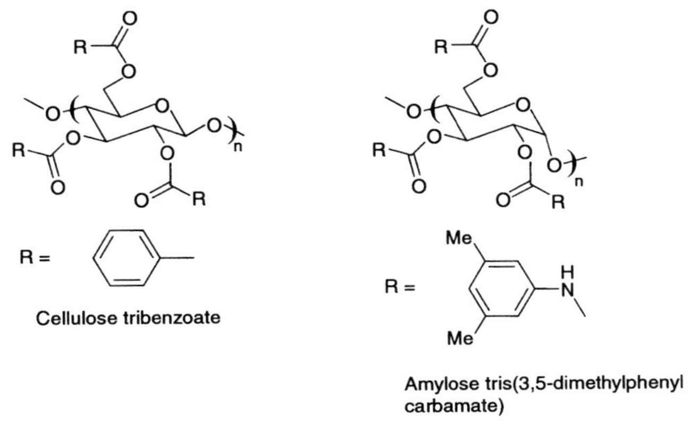

Figure 3.24 Examples of cellulose and amylose chiral stationary phases.

such as Whelk-O1 and α-Burke 1 have been used to separate β-blockers and NSAIDs.

3.5.2.4 *Cellulose and amylose phases*

A number of cellulose derivatives have been used as chiral stationary phases (e.g. cellulose tribenzoate marketed as Chiralcel OB). The amylose bonded phases are exemplified by amylose *tris*-(3,5-dimethylphenylcarbamate) marketed as Chiralpak AD (Figure 3.24). Both these types of column have been used to effect both analytical and preparative resolutions of a wide variety of chiral drugs. The current trend is to prepare immobilized polysaccharide-based stationary phases as these columns can be used with a wider variety of organic solvents in the mobile phase due to their low solubility in such solvents. This improves the resolution and also allows the use of more polar mobile phases thus increasing the solubility of the racemic drug (Francotte 2001).

3.5.2.5 *Miscellaneous phases*

Cyclodextrin based CSPs have also been used for both analytical and preparative separations. Cyclodextrins are cyclic oligosaccharides consisting of interlinked α-D-glucose units. The most commonly used cyclodextrins are comprised of 6, 7 or 8 glucose units, α-, β- and γ-cyclodextrin, respectively, arranged in a doughnut-shaped structure and differ in the size of the hydrophobic cavity and thus, the types of molecules that can be separated. Compounds can form inclusion complexes by binding inside the cavity and this forms the basis of the enantioselectivity.

Macrocyclic antibiotics such as vancomycin and teicoplanin have been incorporated into stationary phases. However, these phases are mostly used in analytical rather than preparative separations though separations of a few milligrams of material have been demonstrated. These phases have shown greatest applicability to the resolution of racemic amino acids.

material that resembles the skeleton of the target, the 'chiral group' is purposefully attached to the achiral substrate solely for the purpose of controlling the stereo-chemical outcome of subsequent reactions. The unit chosen is not an integral part of the target compound, but instead is removed once it has performed its function. Therefore, the three steps can be depicted as:

1   Appendage of the enantiomerically pure chiral auxiliary to the substrate;
2   Reaction with the achiral reagent producing two diastereomers with induction hopefully providing these in greatly unequal amounts; and
3   Removal of the auxiliary, avoiding conditions that may cause racemization.

The advantage of this methodology is that reaction of the chiral substrate (i.e. with auxiliary attached) produces a diastereomer. Therefore, even if a high level of induction in subsequent reactions is not produced the products can potentially still be separated to isolate the required material in good enantiomeric purity. But what is it that causes this induction to provide unequal amounts of diastereomers?

Virtually all reactions of this type can be explained in terms of kinetics. If the rate constant leading to the (R) product is different to that leading to the (S) product then these two isomers will be formed in different amounts and the enantiomeric ratio of products formed will reflect this. This rate constant is directly linked to the activation energy of the reaction by the Arrhenius equation so the greater the difference in activation energy to form the two isomers then the greater the selectivity. Conversely, if the two activation energies are the same then no selectivity is observed. This difference in activation energy can be explained by the fact that the transition states leading to the product are in themselves diastereo-meric and thus not equivalent and have different energies. As an example, the reaction between 4-methylhex-1-ene and hydrogen bromide, produces a chiral molecule containing a new stereogenic centre (Figure 3.26). This is because the carbocation intermediate has no symmetry plane and so attack by bromide ion from either the top or bottom faces is not equally favorable.

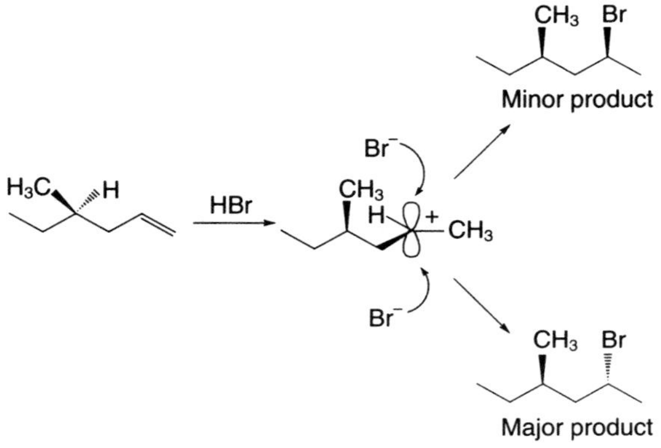

Figure 3.26 Preferential attack by bromide ion on the carbocation intermediate leads to dif-ferential formation of the two possible diastereomers.

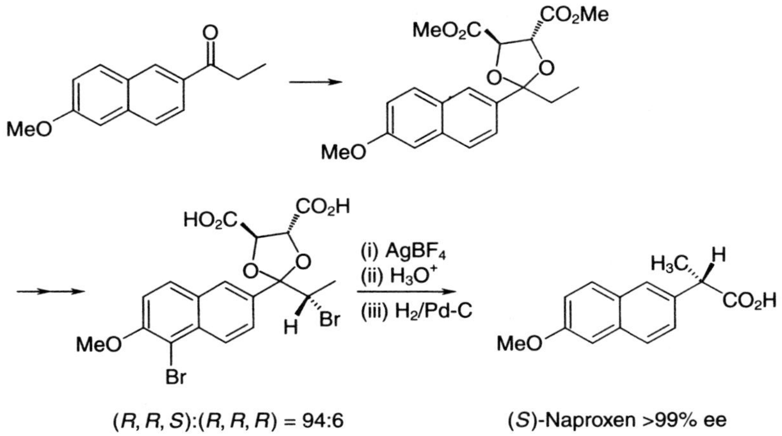

Figure 3.27 Synthesis of (S)-Naproxen using tartaric acid as a chiral auxiliary.

In this case, the non-equivalence is the result of steric interference, and this is generally the basis for first and second-generation asymmetric methods, although other factors such as chelation, hydrogen bonding and electrostatic interactions may also be important. A good example of this is the synthesis of the anti-inflammatory agent (S)-Naproxen. In this route, (2R, 3R)-tartaric acid is used as the chiral auxiliary which can be recovered in the penultimate step (Figure 3.27).

3.5.3.2.2 The use of chiral reagents and catalysts (third and fourth generation methodology)

The main disadvantage of using a chiral auxiliary is that additional steps are required in the synthesis for appendage and removal of the chiral group. However, if the chiral product is formed directly from an achiral starting material using a chiral reagent then this is avoided. An added advantage to this methodology over first and second generation methods is that the choice of starting material is now far wider as it now no longer needs to be derived from the chiral pool. However, although the number of chiral reagents is increasing, there are no comprehensive literature reviews covering the availability of chiral reagents for particular synthetic transformations. In order to overcome the additional problem of also requiring a stoichiometric amount of reagent, chiral catalysts have been developed. This is the most recent and perhaps pivotal area of asymmetric synthesis and essentially involves using a chiral catalyst to promote the reaction of an achiral starting material into a chiral product. By definition, the advantage is that only a small molar ratio of catalyst is required (often less than 0.05 equivalents being used), which can be recovered and reused.

One of the most widely exploited areas of catalytic asymmetric synthesis is hydrogenation using a chiral transition metal complex. Two important ligands in this area are (1) BINAP; and (2) DIPAMP, (Figure 3.28) which are often

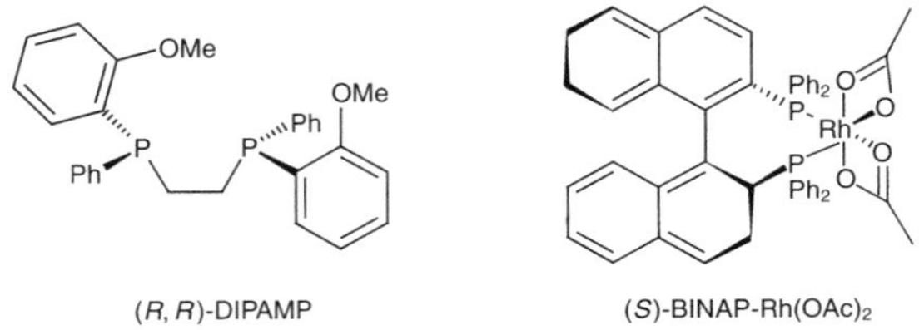

Figure 3.28 Two commonly utilized chiral catalysts for performing asymmetric hydrogenations. BINAP (right) is shown as its octahedral rhodium acetate complex.

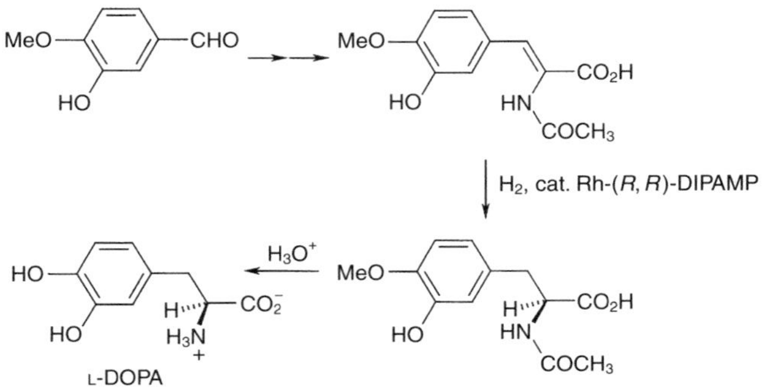

Figure 3.29 Synthesis of L-DOPA using asymmetric hydrogenation.

complexed to rhodium (II) or ruthenium (II) acetate. These are particularly effective because of the rigid structure of the complex, which is octahedral and can exist in two enantiomeric forms.

The DIPAMP is used in the industrial synthesis of (S)-3,4-dihydroxyphenylalanine (L-DOPA), an anti-Parkinson's agent (Figure 3.29). This compound is of particular interest as the actual active drug, dopamine, is the decarboxylated product of L-DOPA, but this cannot cross the blood–brain barrier to reach the target site. However, the prodrug DOPA can do this and after reaching the site of action it is only the L-isomer, which is stereoselectively decarboxylated by the enzyme DOPA decarboxylase. Therefore, it is essential to administer the prodrug in only the L-configuration in order to avoid a potentially dangerous build up of the D-isomer.

3.5.3.2.3   Use of enzymes and whole organisms

Enzymes are nature's chiral catalysts which are extremely versatile catalyzing almost every known chemical reaction. Common misconceptions about enzyme specificity following on from the Lock and Key hypothesis have hampered the development of the use of enzymes in enantioselective synthesis. This has been exacerbated due to the wrongly held view that aqueous conditions were needed for enzyme function and that only one enantiomer could be produced due to the stereospecificity of enzyme action. However, it is now generally agreed that enzymes can accommodate a variety of structurally diverse substrates and in some cases can be used under a wide variety of temperature, pressure and pH conditions. This being particularly applicable to the so-called extremophile class of enzyme isolated from microbes capable of surviving in extreme environments. Most enzymes can also carry out their function in organic solvents as long as they are not totally anhydrous.

Enzymes catalyzing a wide variety of chemical reactions are available for enantio-selective synthesis and thanks to the advent of molecular biological techniques, the choice of enzyme is not restricted to those found in nature. It is now a relatively straightforward process to manipulate enzyme structure using mutagenesis and recombinant technology allowing the stability, activity and substrate specificity of enzymes to be controlled. High throughput screening methods used in the discovery phase of drug development can be used to discover an appropriate enzyme for a particular chemical synthesis and also to adapt the enzyme to the reaction conditions.

One of the first decisions to make when considering an enantioselective synthesis using an enzyme is whether to use whole cells or a cell-free enzyme preparation. Cell-free enzyme preparations offer advantages in simplicity of use, as well as tolerance to harsh conditions such as the use of organic solvents but suffer from the disadvantage of being expensive and may also need additional co-factors to function correctly. On the other hand, whole cells are relatively cheap and all necessary co-factors are present but product isolation can be complex and side reactions may also occur due to the presence of other enzymes in the cells.

A comprehensive review of the use of enzymes in drug synthesis is beyond the scope of this chapter and therefore only selected examples are given. Readers are referred to more detailed reviews given in the reading list for further information (see Sheldon 1993; Roberts 1999; Schulze and Wubbolts 1999; McCoy 2001). Enzymes from all six major classes (see Table 3.1) have been used either in the production of chiral drugs or intermediates used in their synthesis.

The cardiovascular drug diltiazem (see Sections 7.3.3 and 7.5.3) is manufactured on a multihundred tonne scale from a chiral phenylglycidyl ester which is in turn produced via a lipase catalyzed resolution (Figure 3.30). Only the $(2S, 3R)$-isomer

Table 3.1 The classification of enzymes

Enzyme class	Examples of enzymes	Reactions catalyzed
Oxidoreductase	Dehydrogenases, oxidases, peroxidases	Oxidation/reduction reactions
Transferase	Aminotransferases	Group transfer reactions (e.g. methyl, acyl, phosphate)
Hydrolase	Lipases/esterases, proteases, amidopeptidases, acylases, hydantoinases	Hydrolysis (e.g. esters, amides, hydantoins)
Lyase	Decarboxylases, dehydratases, aldolases, oxynitrilases	Additions to, or formation of, C=C, C=O or C=N bonds
Isomerase	Racemases, epimerases	Structural and geometric rearrangements
Ligase	DNA ligase	Formation of C−C, C−N, C−O or C−S bonds

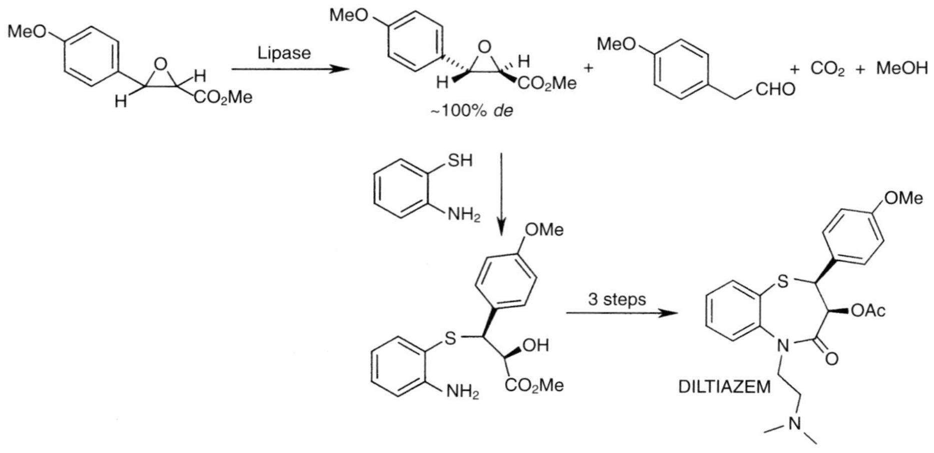

Figure 3.30 Route to diltiazem involving a lipase catalyzed resolution.

of the phenylglycidyl ester is hydrolyzed to the corresponding carboxylic acid which is unstable and decomposes to the corresponding phenylacetaldehyde.

Several antibiotics based on the penicillin or cephalosporin structure contain (R)-4-p-hydroxyphenylglycine as the acyl side-chain. This amino acid is produced on a multithousand tonne scale by dynamic kinetic resolution of the corresponding hydantoin (Figure 3.31). In resolutions of racemates using hydrolases, the maximum theoretical yield is 50% (one enantiomer is unaffected by the hydrolase). However, by allowing racemization to occur simultaneously the theoretical yield can be increased to 100%, this process being known as dynamic kinetic resolution. In the aforementioned hydantoin hydrolysis, racemization of the unchanged (S)-hydantoin is achieved either by carrying out the process at alkaline pH or by the inclusion of a hydantoin racemase.

Fermentation has also been used for the bulk preparation of a number of pharmaceutical and related compounds (for more details see Sheldon 1993). Fermentation is distinct from enzymatic transformations using whole cells as the

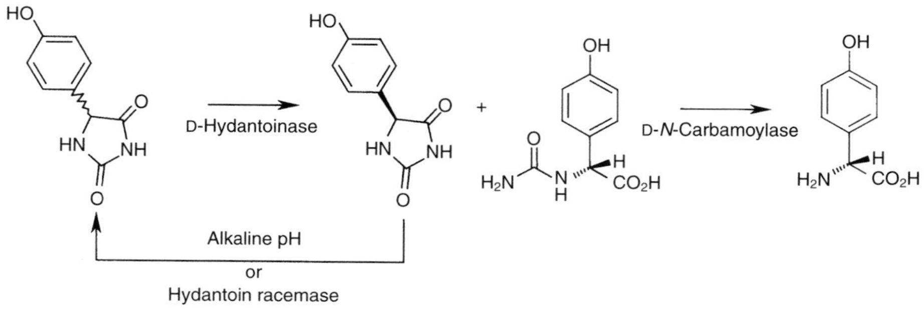

Figure 3.31 Industrial process for the production of (R)-p-hydroxyphenylglycine.

former involves the use of growing cells. In relation to pharmaceutical products, fermentation has been mainly used in the production of β-lactam antibiotics (cephalosporins and penicillins), steroid drugs (market value >\$1 billion), ephidrene, pseudoephidrine, and intermediates for the manufacture of β-blockers. Fermentation is the most cost-effective or in some cases the only way to produce complex chiral molecules such as cyclosporin (immunosuppressant agent), avermectins (anthelmintic agents) and vitamin B_{12}.

3.6 ANALYTICAL METHODS OF DETERMINING PURITY OF STEREOISOMERS

A number of methodologies are now available for the accurate assessment of enantiomeric purity, which are critical for all phases of the drug discovery process. In the drug development phase, it is vital to know the purity of individual enantiomers to understand the structure–activity relationships of drug candidates while in the pharmacokinetic phase, it is necessary to determine the levels of drug enantiomers in biological fluids. It should be a standard practice to use more than one analytical method to determine enantiomeric purity. Fortunately, a wide variety of analytical methods have been developed. One of the main methods of determining the purity of the individual enantiomers of chiral drugs concerns the use of HPLC using chiral stationary phases as discussed in Section 3.5.2. In this Section, some of the main alternative methods available for determining enantiomeric purity will be discussed.

3.6.1 Optical rotation

One of the oldest and most commonly used methods available for the assessment of enantiomeric purity involves measuring optical rotation using a polarimeter (for details of how this is measured see Section 3.2). The main advantage of this method is that it is quick and can be performed without the need for costly apparatus. However, there are problems associated with this method of purity assessment; care must be taken to remove chiral impurities from the sample and to ensure that it was isolated without accidental enantiomeric enrichment. This is particularly a problem with crystallization as enantiomers crystallize at different rates in a chiral medium (see Section 3.5.1). In the case of novel compounds, the maximum optical rotation of the pure enantiomer will not be known and in these cases pure samples of each enantiomer will be needed before using this form of purity assessment. When comparing optical rotations, it is essential to compare samples of the same concentration in the same solvent and to carry out the reading at the same temperature as used from the standard as all these factors can affect the sign and magnitude of the rotation. For water soluble compounds such as amino acids, optical rotation also depends on pH.

Empirical rules have been devised which allow the correlation of the sense of optical rotation with absolute configuration. However, these should be used with caution as closely related compounds with the same absolute configuration can rotate plane-polarized light in different directions. Thus, it is unlikely that such correlations will replace X-ray crystallography as the method of choice for determining absolute configuration.

3.6.2   NMR spectroscopy

Nuclear magnetic resonance (NMR) spectroscopy has been widely used to determine enantiomeric purity. Enantiomers cannot be distinguished by NMR spectroscopy and so this method relies on the formation of diastereoisomers by the addition of a chiral agent to the mixture of enantiomers. There are three main methods of forming diastereomeric mixtures, via a chiral derivatizing agent (CDA), a chiral lanthanide shift reagent or the use of a chiral solvent.

The formation of diastereomeric mixtures using a chiral derivatizing reagent suffers from the same disadvantages as highlighted in Section 3.5.2 covering precolumn derivatization of samples for HPLC analysis. Despite these limitations CDAs are still widely used. One CDA, α-methoxy-α-trifluoromethylphenylacetic acid (MTPA, Figure 3.32) developed by Mosher has been used to analyze enantiomeric purity of amino acids and α-hydroxy acids. Using ^{1}H NMR spectroscopy, the purity of the original enantiomer can be estimated by taking the ratio of the integral of the peaks due to the methoxy groups of the diastereoisomers formed via MTPA derivatization. The MTPA has the advantage over previously reported reagents such as O-methylmandelic acid (Figure 3.32) of being stable to racemization as it lacks an α-hydrogen atom. In addition, as MTPA contains a trifluoromethyl group, ^{19}F NMR spectroscopy can be used thus considerably simplifying the NMR spectrum.

A non-derivatizing method involves using a chiral lanthanide shift reagent which when complexed with the sample of interest shifts some of the signals in the NMR spectrum. As the lanthanide shift reagent is chiral, diastereomeric complexes are formed with the mixture of enantiomers in the analytical sample and these exhibit different shifts in the NMR spectrum. The europium shift reagents illustrated in Figure 3.32 have been used to analyze the purity of chiral compounds containing a wide range of functional groups such as alcohols, esters, ketones and sulphonamides.

Chiral solvating agents (CSAs) have been used to analyze the enantiomeric purity of a range of chiral compounds. This is illustrated by the use of 1-(9-anthryl)-2,2,2-trifluoroethanol to analyze chiral amines, alcohols, α-amino acid esters and lactones. This methodology involves the addition of 1–10 mol equivalents of the CSA to the bulk NMR solvent and relies on the formation of diastereomeric solvation complexes with the chiral analytical sample. The major drawback of this method is that there is

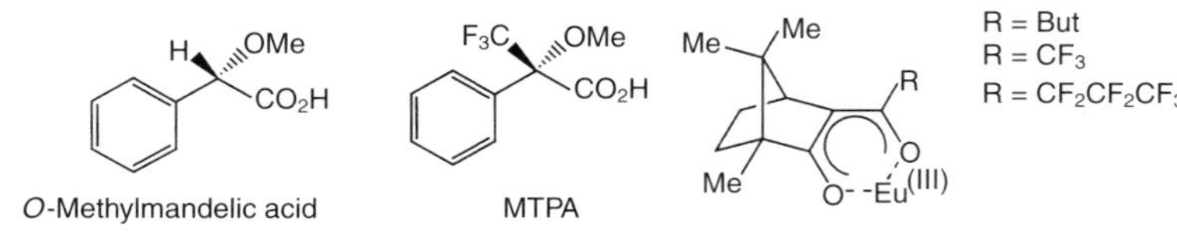

Figure 3.32 Examples of chiral reagents used for the determination of enantiomeric purity by NMR spectroscopy.

not one resolving agent that is applicable to all chiral compounds. The use of NMR for the analysis of the purity of chiral drugs is limited by the fact that non-polar solvents usually give optimal peak separations and this excludes the use of polar solvents such as DMSO, which are required to dissolve a number of polar pharmacologically active compounds. Analytical methods based on HPLC, GC and capillary electrophoresis are now used more often than those relying on NMR spectroscopy for determining enantiomeric purity of chiral drugs.

3.6.3 Gas chromatography

Chiral gas chromatography (GC) has emerged as an extremely efficient and sensitive method for the determination of the enantiomeric purity of chiral drugs (for a comprehensive review see Schurig 2001). In addition, it is now possible to effect preparative separations of volatile racemic compounds. The main limitation of this technique is that the sample needs to be readily vaporized without decomposition. However, there are a number of advantages to the use of chiral GC such as the ability to analyze multicomponent mixtures of enantiomers and to separate the enantiomers away from trace contaminants. It is possible to extend the detection of enantiomeric impurities down to the picogram level enabling the reliable determination of enantiomeric excess to levels >99.9%.

Chiral GC relies on the use of a CSP of high enantiomeric purity to effect resolution of mixtures of enantiomers. There are three main types of CSPs available for GC analysis:

1 Those using chiral amino acid derivatives, which resolve mixtures of enantiomers via the formation of diastereomeric complexes involving hydrogen bond interactions.
2 Phases including chiral metal complexes, which separate mixtures of enantiomers via the formation of diastereomeric metal complexes.
3 Phases including cyclodextrin derivatives, which separate mixtures of enantiomers via formation of inclusion complexes.

These phases are usually linked to polysiloxanes, which produces columns with enhanced thermal stability and separation efficiency.

In the case of the chiral inhalation anaesthetics enflurane (CHF_2OCF_2CHFCl), isoflurane and desflurane efficient separation on chiral GC, CSPs has allowed preparative scale resolution of the enantiomers which have been subsequently tested in biomedical trials. Using analogous methodology to that used in simulated moving bed (SMB) HPLC, the enantiomers of enflurane have been separated by enantioselective GC SMB on a large scale.

3.6.4 Capillary electrophoresis (CE)

A relatively new method of enantioseparation involves the use of capillary electromigration techniques, which have been developed over the past 15 years (for a review see Chankvetadze and Blaschke 2001). In common with chiral GC and HPLC, the origin of the enantioseparation lies in the non-covalent intermolecular interactions between the analyte and the chiral selector and is not based on electrophoretic mobility, as enantiomers possess the same charge densities. In HPLC, the CSP is usually chemically bonded to the silica gel, however, CE is usually carried out with bare silica capillaries. For this reason, the chiral selector is added to the electrolyte in order to form diastereomeric complexes with the analyte thereby effecting chiral discrimination.

In common with HPLC, a number of chiral selectors have been used to effect enantioseparation such as cyclodextrins, polysaccharides, macrocyclic antibiotics and proteins. In an elegant study, it has been shown that the enantiomers of N-derivatized amino acids such as (RS)-3,5-dinitrobenzoylleucine can be resolved in non-aqueous CE using t-butylcarbamoylquinine as a chiral selector. Conversely, t-butylcarbamoylquinine and t-butylcarbamoylquinidine can be separated using (R)- or (S)-3,5-dinitrobenzoylleucine as a chiral selector.

3.6.5 Mass spectrometry

A newly emerging technology for the rapid analysis of chiral drugs involves the use of mass spectroscopy (Tao *et al.* 2001; Jacoby 2001). Four main methods are available for mass spectrometry-based analysis of mixtures of enantiomers:

1   Generation of diastereomeric adducts using chiral reference compounds and chemical ionization, fast atom bombardment, or electrospray mass spectrometry. In this method, one enantiomer of the analyte is isotopically labeled so that the corresponding diastereomeric mixture can be mass resolved.
2   Using exchange reactions. A diastereomeric adduct typically generated from the chiral ligand and a chiral host such as a β-cyclodextrin is mass selected and allowed to exchange the chiral ligand with a neutral gas. Resolution is achieved as exchange rates vary with the chirality of the analyte incorporated into the adduct ion.
3   Collision-induced dissociation of diastereomeric adducts formed from the analyte and a chiral reference substance in a tandem mass spectrometry experiment.
4   Kinetic method using tandem mass spectrometry.

A recent report illustrating the application of the kinetic method describes the use of diastereomeric copper (II) complexes with a drug and a chiral reference compound (in this case (S)-amino acids) to analyze the enantiomeric purity of a range of chiral drugs (propranolol, DOPA, norepinephrine, ephedrine, isoproterenol and atenolol). Using electrospray mass spectroscopy these trimeric complex ions (three ligands – one of the analyte and two of the reference (S)-amino acid) are collisionally activated leading to loss of either a neutral reference or a neutral drug molecule. The ratio of these two competitive dissociation rates is then related via the kinetic method to the enantiomeric composition of the analyte. The advantage of this method over other previously described methods is that isotopic labeling is avoided and commercially available instruments can be used. In addition, the method is sensitive enough to allow analysis of mixtures with a few percent enantiomeric contamination (2–4% ee). Another advantage of using mass spectroscopy for analysis is that it can be coupled to other separation methods such as HPLC and GC.

FURTHER READING

Agranat, I. and Caner, H. (1999) Intellectual property and chirality of drugs. *Drug Discovery Today*, **4**, 313–321.

Aitken, R.A. and Kilenyi, S.N. (1994) *Asymmetric synthesis*, 1st edition. London: Chapman and Hall.

Ariëns, E.J. (1986) Chirality in bioactive agents and its pitfalls. *Trends Pharmacol. Sci.*, **7**, 200–205.

Chankvetadze, B. and Blaschke, G. (2001) Enantioseparations in capillary electromigration techniques: recent developments and future trends. *J. Chromatography A*, **906**, 309–363.

Francotte, E.R. (2001) Enantioselective chromatography as a powerful alternative for the preparation of drug enantiomers. *J. Chromatography A*, **906**, 379–397.

Hyun, H.H., Han, S.C., Lipshutz, B.H., Shin, Y.-J. and Welch, C.J. (2001) New chiral crown ether stationary phase for the liquid chromatographic resolution of α-amino acid enantiomers. *J. Chromatography A*, **910**, 359–365.

Jacoby, M. (2001) Fast separations for drugs. *Chemical & Engineering News*, **79** (21), 68–69.

McCoy, M. (2001) Making drugs with little bugs. *Chemical & Engineering News*, **79** (21), 37–43.

Moldrich, R.X., Beart, P.M., Jane, D.E., Chapman, A.G. and Meldrum, B.S. (2001) Anticonvulsant activity of 3,4-dicarboxyphenylglycines in DBA/2 mice. *Neuropharmacology*, **40**, 696–699.

Roberts, S.M. (1999) Preparative biotransformations. *J. Chem. Soc., Perkin Trans. 1*, 1–21.

Robinson, M.J.T. (2000) *Organic stereochemistry*. New York: Oxford University Press.

Schulte, M. and Strube, J. (2001) Preparative enantioseparation by simulated moving bed chromatography. *J. Chromatography A*, **906**, 399–416.

Schulze, B. and Wubbolts, M.G. (1999) Biocatalysts for industrial production of fine chemicals. *Current Opinion in Biotechnology*, **10**, 609–615.

Schurig, V. (2001) Separation of enantiomers by gas chromatography. *J. Chromatography A*, **906**, 275–299.

Sheldon, R.A. (1993) *Chirotechnology, industrial synthesis of optically active compounds*. New York: Marcel Decker.

Stork, G., Niu, D., Fujimoto, A., Koft, E.R., Balkovec, J.M., Tata, J.R. and Dake G.R. (2001) The first stereoselective total synthesis of quinine. *J. Am. Chem. Soc.*, **123**, 3239–3242.

Tao, W.A., Gozzo, F.C. and Cooks, R.G. (2001) Mass spectrometric quantitation of chiral drugs by the kinetic method. *Anal. Chem.*, **73**, 1692–1698.

Thayer, A. (2000) Eli Lilly pulls the plug on Prozac isomer drug. *Chemical & Engineering News*, **78** (40), 8.

Thomas, N.K., Wright, R.A., Howson, P.A., Kingston, A.E., Schoepp, D.D. and Jane, D.E. (2001) (S)-3,4-DCPG a potent and selective mGlu8a receptor agonist activates metabotropic glutamate receptors on primary afferent terminals in the neonatal rat spinal cord. *Neuropharmacology*, **40**, 311–318.

Triggle, D.J. (1997) Stereoselectivity of drug action. *Drug Discovery Today*, **2**, 138–147.

Chapter 4

Computer-aided development and use of three-dimensional pharmacophore models

Tommy Liljefors and Ingrid Pettersson

4.1 STRUCTURE- AND PHARMACOPHORE-BASED LIGAND DESIGN

The explosive development of computer technology and methodologies to calculate molecular properties have increasingly made it possible to use computer techniques to aid the drug discovery process. The use of computer techniques in this context is often called *computer-aided drug design (CADD)*, but since the development of a drug involves a large number of steps in addition to the development of a high-affinity ligand (bioavailability, toxicity and metabolism must also be taken into account as discussed in Chapter 1), a more appropriate name is *computer-aided ligand design (CALD)*.

If the 3D-structure of the target enzyme or receptor is available from X-ray crystallography, preferentially with a co-crystallized ligand so that the binding site and binding mode of the ligand is known, it is feasible to study the biomacromolecule–ligand complex in a direct way by interactive computer graphics techniques and computational chemistry. In this way, a detailed knowledge of the interactions between the ligand and the enzyme/receptor may be obtained. New candidate ligands may be 'docked' into the binding site in order to study if the new structure can interact with the receptor in an optimal way. This procedure is known as *structure-based ligand design*. An example of the use of this type of ligand design in the development of new high-affinity ligands for dihydrofolate reductase (DHFR) is discussed in Chapter 17.

It may seem straightforward to develop new ligands for known enzyme or receptor structures, but there are many difficult problems involved. For instance, conformational changes of the ligand and/or the biomacromolecule may be necessary for an optimal binding. In addition, conformational energies, multiple binding modes and differential solvation effects must be taken into account. However, much progress in this field have been made in recent years and several successful examples of the use of structure-based ligand design in a drug development process have been reported.

Many target receptors of high interest in connection with drug development, e.g. seven trans-membrane (7-TM) neurotransmitter receptors (see Chapter 6), are membrane-bound and all attempts to crystallize and determine the structure of these receptors by X-ray crystallography have so far been unsuccessful. In the absence of an experimentally determined 3D-structure for the receptor, ligand design may be performed by the use of a *pharmacophore model* based on the analysis and comparison of molecular properties and receptor binding data for known receptor ligands. In the present chapter, the development and use of 3D-pharmacophore models will be discussed.

In 3D-pharmacophore studies, the concept of *pharmacophore* is employed in an attempt to deduce the spatial relationships between those parts of the ligand which are essential for its binding to the receptor – the *3D-pharmacophore*. On the basis of this, a comparison of the molecular volumes of active and inactive compounds may additionally give information about the dimensions of the binding cavity. High-affinity ligands are characterized by being capable of assuming a conformation which positions those parts of the ligand which are crucial for the affinity in such a way that they are complementary to the 3D-arrangement of their binding partners (e.g. amino acid residues) in the binding cavity. An additional requirement for high affinity is that the ligand in this bioactive conformation does not display steric repulsions with the receptor.

A well-developed 3D-pharmacophore model, preferentially including informa-tion about the dimensions of the receptor binding cavity, may be employed to design new ligands which fit the model and/or to search databases for new compounds which are compatible with the model. It should be noted that a 3D-pharmacophore model in general does not yield quantitative predictions of receptor affinities. The main use of such models is restricted to the prediction of candidate ligands as active or inactive (high or low affinity). Such a classification may be fruitfully used in the selection of new molecules to be synthesized in a drug discovery project. However, 3D-pharmacophore models are starting points for the 3D-QSAR methodology (see Chapter 5) by which quantitative predictions may be made.

The development of a 3D-pharmacophore model and its use for ligand design is necessarily an iterative and multidisciplinary process. The initial model, based on known ligands, is used to design new compounds to test the model and the outcome of receptor binding studies of the new compounds is used to validate, refine (or discard) the model.

4.2 THE PHARMACOPHORE CONCEPT

Nineteenth century organic chemists developing organic dyes introduced the concept of *chromophore* for those parts of a molecule which are responsible for its color. In analogy, Paul Ehrlich in the early 1900s, introduced the term *pharmacophore* to describe those parts of a molecule which are responsible for its biological activity. Pharmacophore and pharmacophore elements are central concepts in medicinal chemistry. The idea behind these concepts comes from the common observation that variations of some parts of the molecular structure of a compound drastically influence the activity at a target receptor, whereas variations of other parts only cause minor activity changes. (In the following, the term receptor is used in a general sense for the biomacromolecular target and no distinction between enzymes and receptors is made).

A *pharmacophore element* is traditionally defined as an atom or a group of atoms (a functional group) common for active compounds with respect to a receptor and essential for the activity of the compounds. However, the concept of pharmacophore element may fruitfully be extended to include representations of interactions of functional groups with receptor sites as discussed in Section 4.4. The pharmacophore is a collection of pharmacophore elements and the concept of *3D-pharmacophore* may be used when the relative spatial positions of the pharmacophore elements are included in the analysis. Thus, a 3D-pharmacophore consists of a specific 3D-arrangement of pharmacophore elements. The pharmacophore concept has been used for a long time in medicinal chemistry in a topological sense (2D), however, the use of computer techniques has enormously facilitated the topographical (3D) use of the concept.

4.3 BASIC PRINCIPLES AND A STEP-BY-STEP PROCEDURE

The basic principles of the development of a 3D-pharmacophore model are illustrated in Figure 4.1. On the basis of conformational analysis of a set of active molecules with pharmacophore elements A, B and C, a conformation of each molecule is selected for which the pharmacophore elements of the molecules overlap in space as shown in the figure. The selected conformations are the putative bioactive conformations of the molecules and the overlapping pharmacophore elements and their spatial positions make up the 3D-pharmacophore. It is useful for the following discussion to separate the 3D-pharmacophore identification process into a number of discrete steps.

Step 1. A set of high-affinity ligands for the target receptor is collected and pharmacophore elements are selected. The molecules in the set should have as diverse structural frameworks as possible. Pharmacophore elements and their representations are discussed in Sections 4.4. In order to facilitate the next step in the process, the conformational analysis, the selected compounds should have as few torsional degrees of freedom as possible. The receptor binding data for the

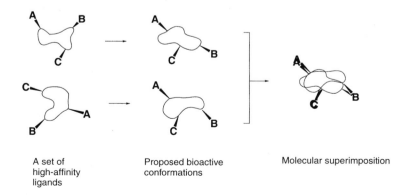

A set of high-affinity ligands

Proposed bioactive conformations

Molecular superimposition

Figure 4.1 The basic principles of 3D-pharmacophore identification.

selected compounds, preferably obtained by a radioligand binding assay, should be of high quality and preferably from the same laboratory.

Step 2. An exhaustive conformational analysis is performed for each compound in the set in order to identify low-energy conformations for each active molecule. Conformational properties and conformational analysis are discussed in Section 4.5.

Step 3. Molecular superimposition techniques are used to identify low-energy conformations of each molecule in the set, conformations for which the selected pharmacophore elements superimpose (see Section 4.6). The aim of this step is to identify the bioactive conformation of each molecule and a common 3D-pharmacophore for all high-affinity compounds.

Step 4. When a common 3D-pharmacophore for all high-affinity compounds have been identified, inactive or low-affinity compounds which fit the 3D-pharmacophore in a low-energy conformation may be used to explore the dimensions of the receptor cavity and to identify receptor-excluded and receptor-essential volumes. This is discussed in Section 4.7.

In addition, it may be necessary to take differential solvent properties into account in the interpretation of the affinity data and in the design of new compounds. This is discussed in Section 4.8.

4.4 PHARMACOPHORE ELEMENTS AND THEIR REPRESENTATIONS

The selection of pharmacophore elements is generally based on experimental observations about parts (atoms, functional groups) of a set of active molecules which are common for these molecules and essential for the activity. Pharmacophore elements used in the development of 3D-pharmacophore models are most often atoms or functional groups (or derived from atoms or functional groups) which may interact with receptor binding sites via hydrogen bonds, electrostatic forces or van der Waals forces (for a discussion of such interactions see Chapter 2). Thus, heteroatoms such as oxygens and nitrogens and polar functional groups such as carboxylic acids, amides and hydroxy groups are commonly found to be pharmacophore elements. Drug molecules frequently include aromatic ring systems. Since such ring systems may strongly interact with, for instance, aromatic side-chains of the receptor or hydrophobic receptor regions they are very often essential for the activity and therefore selected as pharmacophore elements.

Many potent dopamine D_2 receptor agonists are derived from the structure of dopamine itself (**4.1**). Thus, their structures often include an *ortho*-dihydroxy phenyl (catechol) moiety and a nitrogen atom as exemplified by (**4.2**). However, only the *meta*-hydroxy group is necessary for activity as shown by the active compound (**4.3**). Furthermore, it has been demonstrated that the catechol/phenol moiety may be bioisosterically replaced by, for instance, an indole ring (**4.4**) or a pyrazole ring (**4.5**). Considering these experimental observations, suitable pharmacophore elements for dopamine D_2 receptor agonists may include the

(4.1)   (4.2)   (4.3)

(4.4)   (4.5)

nitrogen atom corresponding to the one in (**4.1**), the aromatic ring and the *meta*-hydroxy group or its bioisosteric equivalent. A closer analysis of the structures suggests that it may be desirable to include the hydrogen bond donating and/or accepting properties of the hydroxy group in the pharmacophore. Similarly, explicit inclusion of the direction of the nitrogen atom-lone pair, or in the protonated case the N–H bond vectors, may extend the usefulness of the pharmacophore. Although, the pharmacophore concept originally was formulated in terms of atoms and functional groups it is often, as will be discussed in the next section, a great advantage to represent the functional group in terms of its possible interactions with the receptor.

4.4.1   Representation of pharmacophore elements as ligand points and site points

If we consider a hydroxy group as a pharmacophore element, the important properties of this functional group in connection with its binding to the receptor are its hydrogen bond donating and accepting properties. The hydroxy group pharmacophore element may be represented in various ways as shown in Figure 4.2.

The representation in Figure 4.2a does not specify any particular properties of the hydroxy group and a pharmacophore built on the selection of such a

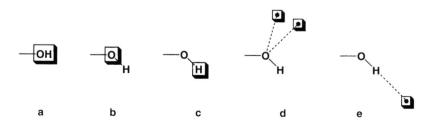

a   b   c   d   e

Figure 4.2 Various representations of a hydroxy group as a pharmacophore element.

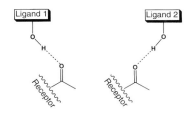

Figure 4.3 A hydroxy group may interact equally well with a carbonyl group in a ligand–receptor interaction without the requirement that the atoms of the hydroxy group in different ligands superimpose.

pharmacophore element merely requires that a hydroxy group is present at a particular location in 3D-space in all active compounds.

In Figures 4.2b,c, the hydrogen bond accepting and donating properties, respectively, are indirectly specified. The use of the oxygen or the hydrogen atom as a pharmacophore element (a *ligand point*) implies that the corresponding atoms should superimpose in space in all active compounds. However, this does not take into account that a hydroxy group of a set of ligands may bind equally well to the receptor, even if the atoms of the functional group in different ligands have different locations in space. For instance, as illustrated in Figure 4.3, the hydroxy group may bond hydrogen equally well to a carbonyl group of a receptor binding site without requiring that the hydroxy hydrogen atom or oxygen atom in all active compounds are located in the same positions in space.

The extension of the pharmacophore concept to include *site points* as shown in Figure 4.2d,e is a great advance in 3D-pharmacophore development. The dashed line between the site point and the ligand functional group represents a hydrogen bond interaction with a receptor site and the site point itself represents the interacting part of the receptor (e.g. an atom in an amino acid residue, see Section 4.4.2). Suitable site-points for some nitrogen and oxygen containing functional groups are shown in Figure 4.4. The site points for amines, ammonium groups and the imidazole group simulate possible hydrogen bonding interactions with

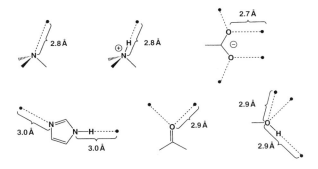

Figure 4.4 Site points for some oxygen and nitrogen containing functional groups.

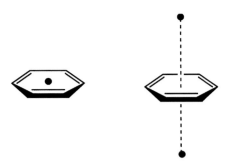

Figure 4.5 Ligand point and site points commonly used to represent a phenyl ring or other aromatic systems.

a receptor site. The site points are placed in the direction of the N–lone pair or N–H bond at typical hydrogen-bonding distances.

Depending on the structures and the structural diversity of the set of molecules to be analyzed, various combinations of site points and ligand points may be used. The use of the site point *and* the nitrogen atom as pharmacophore elements implies that not only the amino group as such is important, but that a specific direction of the interaction between the amine and the receptor is crucial for the activity. If *only* the site point is used and not the nitrogen atom, the implication is that the interaction with the receptor site represented by the site point may take place from different directions with different positions of the nitrogen atom.

An aromatic system such as a phenyl group is often represented by a ligand point positioned at the center of the aromatic ring (Figure 4.5). Specification of all carbon atoms in the ring will give such a ring an unrealistically large weight in a subsequent molecular least-squares superimposition (see Section 4.6). In some applications, it is useful to employ site points for an aromatic system located on the normal passing through the centroid of the aromatic system, above and below the ring plane (Figure 4.5). Such points may represent electrostatic and van der Waals interactions between the aromatic group and amino acid residues in the receptor binding site. They may also be used to enforce co-planarity of aromatic ring systems.

4.4.2   Comparison of site-points with experimentally observed ligand–protein interactions

Figure 4.6a shows the amino acid arginine including site points constructed according to the principles in Figure 4.4. These site points describe possible (optimal) hydrogen bond interactions between arginine and a receptor. The experimental structure of the complex between arginine and the amino acid transport protein LAO (lysine, arginine, ornithine-binding protein) is displayed in Figure 4.6b. On comparing the positions of the site-points in Figure 4.6a with the receptor atoms (including an oxygen of a water molecule) to which arginine is hydrogen bonded in the experimental structure (Figure 4.6b), it is clear that the site-points closely correspond to these hydrogen bonded receptor atoms. Only one out of the

(a)

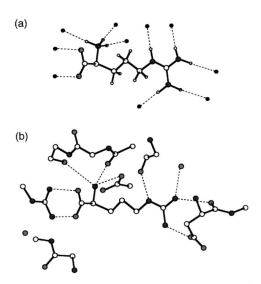

(b)

Figure 4.6 (a) The amino acid arginine with site points describing possible optimal hydrogen bonding interactions; and (b) arginine bound to the LAO transport protein.

ten site-points in Figure 4.6a does not correspond to a receptor atom in the experimental structure. (It may, however, correspond to a crystallographically unresolved water oxygen.) Other molecules may now be designed whose site points are able to overlap those of arginine. If this can be accomplished by a low-energy conformation of the designed molecule (see Section 4.5 for a discussion on conformational energies), it is predicted that the new molecule may bind to the protein in the same way as arginine.

4.4.3   Representation of pharmacophore elements by explicit molecular properties

As an alternative to (and extension of) the representations of pharmacophores elements by ligand points or site points, as described above, molecules may be analyzed in terms of ensembles of explicit molecular properties as hydrogen bond donors and acceptors, hydrophobic areas, charged groups etc. A computer-program which analyzes molecules in this way is CATALYST. Predefined properties are hydrogen-bond acceptor, hydrogen-bond donor, hydrophobic (aliphatic or aromatic), negative or positive charge, negatively or positively ionizable, and ring aromatic. In order to allow for variations in the geometry of the interaction between a molecule and its receptor, distance variation as well as angle variation is taken into account in this approach. For instance, a hydrogen bond acceptor is defined by a distance from the atom which accepts a hydrogen bond to the site which donates the hydrogen bond with an allowed variation at both ends. These

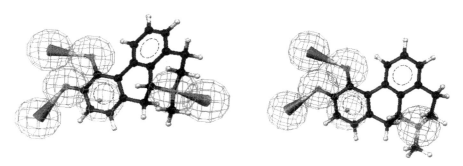

Figure 4.7 Two alternative pharmacophore models generated manually by using the program CATALYST.

allowed variations are defined by spheres and the optimal interaction is defined by the midpoint of the spheres.

CATALYST may be employed to generate a pharmacophore in a manual or in an automatic mode. Examples of *manually* generated pharmacophore models are shown in Figure 4.7. In the manual mode, a compound with a high biological activity in a proposed bioactive conformation is used and the user manually assign properties (pharmacophore elements) to the molecule. In this example, different properties proposed to be important for the dopaminergic activity of apomorphine have been assigned to the functional groups. As apomorphine is a very rigid molecule, the global energy minimum conformation is proposed to be the biological active one. In both alternatives in Figure 4.7, the hydroxyl groups are proposed to be hydrogen-bond donors (magenta colored spheres). In the Figure, it can be seen that there is a tolerance both at the start and end of the hydrogen bond. One of the aromatic rings has been assigned to be an essential hydrophobic group (blue sphere). Two different ways to treat the basic nitrogen are shown. To the left, the nitrogen is shown as a hydrogen bond acceptor (green spheres). To the right, the nitrogen atom is considered to be positively ionizable (red sphere). In order to add further constraints to the pharmacophore model, spheres representing volumes of steric repulsive interactions with the receptor (receptor essential volumes, see Section 4.7) may be added.

In order to generate a pharmacophore model by using CATALYST in an *automatic* mode (for an example, see Section 4.9.4), a set of compounds with measured biological activities is required. In the order of 20 compounds with activities covering 4–6 orders of magnitude is recommended for this approach. For each molecule, a set of conformations representing the available conformational space of the molecule is generated by the software. During the subsequent generation of the pharmacophore model, all conformations and relevant properties of the functional groups are being considered. The automatic procedure includes a QSAR calculation (for a discussion on QSAR, see Chapter 5). The software returns the ten best models in terms of fit of the compounds to the model and the ability of the model to account for the biological activities of the compounds.

Pharmacophore models generated by CATALYST either automatically or manually may be used in searching of large databases for new compounds which fit the model and which may be developed into new drugs (for an example, see Section 4.9.4). It should be noted, that in the databases used for such searching each compound is represented by a number of different conformations. This is necessary as it cannot be known in advance which (if any) conformation of a compound fits the pharmacophore model.

4.5   THE RECEPTOR-BOUND OR 'ACTIVE' CONFORMATION

4.5.1   Thermodynamic considerations

The great majority of drug molecules are flexible, which means that they through rotations about bonds and/or inversions about atomic centers may adopt a large number of conformations, giving the molecule a correspondingly large number of different 3D-shapes. In the context of the pharmacophore concept, this means that a ligand in general may exhibit a large number of possible spatial relationships between its pharmacophore elements. The pharmacophore hypothesis implies that for an active molecule, one of these conformations is optimally complementary to the receptor binding site and that the ligand, when bound to the receptor is characterized by a specific molecular conformation.

The single most important (and certainly most difficult) problem in 3D-pharmacophore identification is the identification of the *receptor-bound (bioactive) conformation*. If this can be accomplished, the spatial relationships of the pharmacophore elements in this conformation defines the 3D-pharmacophore (see Figure 4.1) and new candidate ligands may be tested to investigate if they fit this 3D-pharmacophore. Inactive molecules which fit the 3D-pharmacophore are of special interest since they may contain extra molecular volume which can be used for mapping of the dimensions of the receptor cavity (see Section 4.7).

The ligand–receptor interaction is characterized by the equilibrium (4.1), as illustrated in Figure 4.8.

$$\text{ligand} + \text{receptor} \overset{K}{\rightleftharpoons} \text{ligand}-\text{receptor complex} \tag{4.1}$$

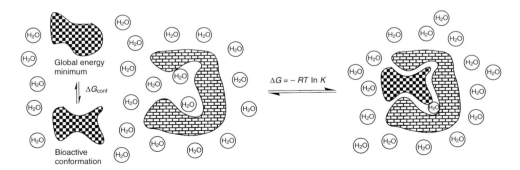

Figure 4.8 The equilibrium characterizing the ligand–receptor interaction.

The free energy difference ΔG is given by equation (4.2) where K is the equilibrium constant, R the gas constant $(8.314\,\mathrm{J\,K^{-1}mol^{-1}})$, T the absolute temperature in Kelvin (K_d is the dissociation constant).

$$\Delta G = -RT \ln K, \quad K_d = \frac{1}{K} \tag{4.2}$$

Neglecting for the moment conformational changes of the protein and the difference in solvation energy of the ligand–protein complex and the uncomplexed protein, the overall free energy of binding may be separated into three components as shown in equation (4.3).

$$\Delta G = \Delta G_{inter} + \Delta G_{conf} - \Delta G_{solv} \tag{4.3}$$

ΔG_{conf} is the free energy required for the ligand to adopt the bioactive conformation (the conformational energy penalty), ΔG_{inter} corresponds to the intermolecular interaction of this conformation with the receptor and ΔG_{solv} is the solvation free energy of the unbound ligand (these solvation effects are discussed in Section 4.8). In terms of the pharmacophore concept, ΔG_{inter} is due to binding interactions between the pharmacophore elements and the complementary binding sites of the receptor (e.g. amino acid residues and backbone atoms).

When ΔG_{conf} increases, equation (4.3) shows that ΔG becomes more positive and consequently, the equilibrium in equation (4.1) is shifted to the left, i.e. the affinity of the ligand decreases.

The factor of decrease in affinity (K_{conf}) corresponding to a conformational energy penalty (ΔG_{conf}) for the bioactive conformation may be calculated from equation (4.4) ($T = 310\,\mathrm{K}$).

$$\Delta G_{conf} = RT \ln K_{conf} = 5.9 \log K_{conf} \tag{4.4}$$

Thus, if the active conformation has a conformational energy penalty of $5.9\,\mathrm{kJ\,mol^{-1}}$ the decrease in the affinity is a factor of 10 due to this 'conformational effect'. For each additional $5.9\,\mathrm{kJ\,mol^{-1}}$ of conformational free energy, the affinity decreases by a further factor of 10.

An example of the relationship between conformational energy of the bioactive conformation and the affinity is shown in Figure 4.9. Compound (**4.6**) is a potent dopamine D_2 receptor agonist. The receptor-bound conformations of the related compounds (**4.6**)–(**4.9**) have been deduced by using (**4.9**) as a template and the conformational energies of the bioactive conformations have been calculated by molecular mechanics (see Section 4.5.3.1). These conformations are labeled

(**4.6**)   (**4.7**)   (**4.8**)   (**4.9**)

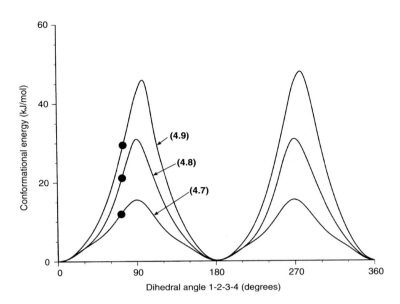

Figure 4.9 Calculated potential energy curves for rotation about the central bond in **(4.7)–(4.9)**. The bullets denote the deduced bioactive conformations of the compounds.

by bullets in Figure 4.9. The affinities as well as the agonist activities of **(4.7)–(4.9)** are significantly lower than that of **(4.6)**. Furthermore, the affinities and the agonist activities of **(4.7)–(4.9)** are in order **(4.7)**>**(4.8)**>**(4.9)**. These data are nicely accounted for by the calculated conformational energies of the bioactive conformations of **(4.7)–(4.9)** as shown in Figure 4.9. A higher conformational energy corresponds to a lower activity. Note that the deduced bioactive conformations of **(4.7)–(4.9)** are not energy minimum conformations.

4.5.2   The conformational energy of the bioactive conformation

As shown above by equations (4.3) and (4.4), the affinity of a ligand decreases when the conformational energy required to adopt the bioactive conformation (the conformational energy penalty) increases. Thus, a question of great practical importance in the development of 3D-pharmacophore models is how much above the global energy minimum we must go to be sure to include the bioactive conformation of a high-affinity ligand. In other words, which energy cut-off should we use in the conformational search for possible candidates for the bioactive conformation of a ligand? The conformational energies reguired for ligands to adopt their bioactive conformations have been calculated for a large number of experimentally determined ligand–protein complexes (Boström *et al.* 1998). It was found that for the great majority of ligand–protein complexes studied, the conformational energies for the bioactive conformations were calculated to be less

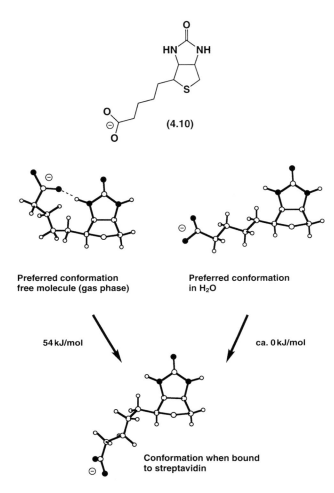

Figure 4.10 Calculated preferred conformations of biotin (**4.10**) in the gas phase and in aqueous solution and the bioactive conformation of (**4.10**) when it binds to streptavidin.

than 13 kJ mol^{-1}. Thus, the bioactive conformation of a high-affinity ligand most probably has a low conformational energy penalty (≤ 13 kJ mol^{-1}). It is important to note, that the conformational energy for the bioactive conformation must be calculated with reference to the internal energy of the ligand in *aqueous solution* (i.e. the energy of the ligand in aqueous solution excluding the solvation energy) (Boström *et al.* 1998). A conformational search performed for the 'free' ligand *in vacuo* may result in an unrealistically high calculated conformational energy for the bioactive conformation. An example of this is illustrated in Figure 4.10. Biotin (**4.10**) binds with very high affinity to the enzyme streptavidin. The experimentally observed bioactive conformation is shown in the figure. A conformational search *in vacuo* results in a preferred conformation with a strong hydrogen bond between the carboxylate group and the NH of the ureido group. The energy difference between the bioactive conformation and this global energy minimum conformation of the 'free' ligand is calculated to be very high, $54 \, kJ \, mol^{-1}$. Considering equation (4.4), such a high conformational energy penalty is clearly not compatible with the high affinity of (**4.10**). However, the global energy minimum conformation of (**4.10**) in aqueous solution (Figure 4.10) is similar to the observed bioactive conformation. In particular, the strong hydrogen bond displayed by the preferred conformation in gas phase is not present in the preferred conformation in aqueous phase. The internal energy difference between the bioactive conformation and the preferred conformation in aqueous solution is calculated to be essentially zero as expected from the high affinity of (**4.10**).

4.5.3 Conformational analysis

The bioactive conformation is not necessarily the lowest energy conformation of the molecule in solution, in the crystal or in the gas phase. (It may not even correspond to an energy minimum structure in any of these phases as shown by the example in the Section 4.5.2). Thus, experimental data on structures and conformational equilibria alone are of limited use in attempts to identify the bioactive conformation. A computational approach is required and the entire conformational space must be investigated.

There are two groups of methods which may be used for the calculation of conformational properties of molecules: (i) quantum chemical methods; and (ii) molecular mechanics or force field methods. In the quantum chemical methods (an approximation of) the Schrödinger equation is solved, treating the molecule as a collection of positively charged nuclei and negatively charged electrons moving under the influence of Coulombic potentials.

A hierarchy of quantum chemical methods at different levels of approximation are being used in computational chemistry. In the *ab initio* methods, all electrons are included in the calculations, whereas in the *semi-empirical methods* only the outer (valence) electrons are explicitly included in the calculations and many terms are not calculated but fitted to experimental data. Although several of these methods are being increasingly used in connection with problems in medicinal chemistry, the levels of theory necessary to yield reliable results are at the present time in general much too time-consuming to be of practical use for the extensive search of conformational space which is needed in connection with 3D-pharmacophore identification. These methods will thus not be considered here.

The other group of computational methods, molecular mechanics or force field methods, are well suited for extensive calculations on conformational properties of molecules of interest in medicinal chemistry and may also be used for calculations on biomacromolecules.

4.5.3.1 Molecular mechanics (force field) calculations

Molecular mechanics is a method for the calculation of molecular structures, conformational energies and other molecular properties using concepts from classical mechanics. A molecule is considered as a collection of atoms held together by classical forces. These forces are described by potential energy functions of structural features like bond lengths, bond angles, torsional (dihedral) angles, etc.

The energy (E) of the molecule is calculated as a sum of terms as in equation (4.5).

$$E = E_{\text{stretching}} + E_{\text{bending}} + E_{\text{torsion}} + E_{\text{van der Waals}} + E_{\text{electrostatic}}$$
$$+ E_{\text{hydrogen bond}} + \text{cross terms} \tag{4.5}$$

The first four terms in the sum are the energies due to deviations of bond lengths, bond angles, torsional angles and non-bonded distances, respectively, from their reference or 'ideal' values. $E_{\text{electrostatic}}$ gives the electrostatic attraction or repulsion between bond dipoles or partial atomic charges. Although a large part of the hydrogen bonding is included in the electrostatic energy component, many molecular mechanics methods include an additional hydrogen bonding term ($E_{\text{hydrogen bond}}$) to fine-tune the energies and geometries of a hydrogen bond interaction. More advanced force fields include cross terms such as stretch–bend, bend–bend, torsion–stretch etc. These terms are of importance for the accurate calculation of geometric properties of small rings (stretch–bend term) or for the calculation of vibrational frequencies (bend–bend term).

The energies are calculated using analytical potential energy functions similar to those used in classical mechanics. For a more comprehensive discussion on molecular mechanics see Burkert and Allinger (1982) in Further reading.

The molecular mechanics method calculates the energy as a function of the nuclear co-ordinates and energy minimization is an integral part of the method. A trial molecular geometry is constructed, most often by using computer graphics techniques, and the atoms are iteratively moved (without breaking bonds) using an energy minimization technique until the net forces on all atoms vanish and the total energy of the molecule reaches a minimum. The 3D-structure of the molecule corresponding to this energy minimum is one of the stable conformations of the molecule but *not necessarily* the most stable one (Figure 4.11). Since the energy minimization methods cannot move the molecule across energy barriers, the minimization of a trial molecule continues until the first *local energy minimum* is

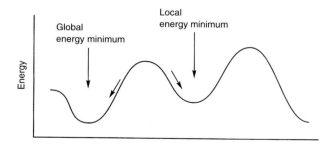

Figure 4.11 Energy minimization proceeds downhill to the nearest energy minimum.

found. Other local energy minima including the lowest energy one (the *global energy minimum*) may be found by repeating the calculation with another start geometry or more efficiently by the use of a conformational search method (see Section 4.5.3.2).

In general, the calculated results from a molecular mechanics calculation refer to the isolated molecule (*in vacuo*). However, the importance of including solvation in the conformational analysis was stressed in Section 4.5.2. Several methods are currently available by which solvent effects may be included in the calculation. In the present context, the most useful of these methods are the dielectric continuum methods (Cramer and Truhlar 1999).

4.5.3.2 *Conformational search methods*

As described in Section 4.5.3.1, the energy minimization procedure moves the molecule from the initial (trial) geometry to the *closest* local energy minimum. Many methods for conformational search have been devised but only the major ones, systematic search in torsional space and the random search methods, are described here. If well implemented, both methods are of similar efficiency and may be feasible for up to 10–15 rotatable bonds with current computer resources.

The systematic conformational search methodology is in principle simple and straightforward. New structures are generated using all combinations of torsional angle values at a preset resolution (angle increment) which gives a uniform grid search in torsional space. In the one-dimensional (one rotatable bond) or 2D (two rotatable bonds) cases, so-called *torsional driving* is feasible. Each torsional angle is incremented by a user defined value and the dihedral value is then kept fixed while the molecule is energy-minimized with respect to all other degrees of freedom. The result of a calculation using torsional driving is a potential energy curve or a potential energy (conformational) map which displays not only energy minima but also energy barriers and pathways for conformational interconversions. This type of calculations is very time consuming and is therefore seldom used for problems involving more than two rotatable bonds. Examples of potential energy curves calculated by the torsional driving method are shown in Figure 4.9 and in Section 4.9.2.

For three and more rotatable bonds, conformational search methods in general focus on finding energy minima. In random conformational search methods, random numbers are used to determine how many and which torsional angles to be incremented and by how much. A trial conformation generated in this way by the computer program is then energy minimized and the resulting conformation is compared with those already stored. If it is a new conformation, it is added to the storage. The procedure is repeated a large number of times and the completeness of the search may be estimated by how many times each stored conformation have been found. An advantage of this methodology is that it can be halted at any time and restarted and the results from repeated runs may be combined. For a thorough discussion on conformational search methods see Further reading (Leach 1991).

4.6   MOLECULAR SUPERIMPOSITION

4.6.1   Least-squares superimposition, flexible fitting and template forcing

A 3D-pharmacophore model is characterized by a particular 3D-arrangement of pharmacophore elements. Active (high affinity) ligands are able to assume a low-energy conformation in which the pharmacophore elements are positioned at closely similar relative positions in space as those of the 3D-pharmacophore model. During the development of a pharmacophore model, molecular super-imposition techniques are used to investigate similarities and differences between the accessible conformations of different molecules with respect to the spatial positions of their pharmacophore elements. When a 3D-pharmacophore model has been developed, molecular superimpositions are used to investigate if new molecules fit the model.

The most commonly used molecular superimposition method is the rigid-body *least-squares superimposition* of pharmacophore elements represented as ligand points or site points. The root mean square deviation (rms) between selected points in the test molecule and the corresponding points in the reference molecule is minimized by displacing and rotating the test molecule as a rigid body. The rms value of the resulting least-squares fit is given by equation (4.6).

$$\text{rms} = \sqrt{\left(\frac{\sum\limits_{i=1}^{N} R_i^2}{N}\right)} \qquad (4.6)$$

R_i in equation (4.6) is the distance between the ith pair of ligand or site points and N is the number of such pairs. The rms value is zero (Å) for a perfect fit and increases as the fit is decreased. For examples of superimpositions see Section 4.9.2.

It may not always be possible to obtain an optimal fit between two molecules in local energy conformations. Deviations of torsional angles from the values for a stable conformation of the molecule may be necessary for a good fit. Molecular superimposition algorithms often include possibilities to perform *flexible fitting* by automatic variations of the torsional angles of user defined rotatable bonds until an optimal fit between fitting points (pharmacophore elements) are found.

An alternative to the least-squares superimposition method is to connect the fitting points to be superimposed by an isotropic spring, which by the use of an energy minimization procedure forces the test molecule to be fitted to the reference molecule ('template forcing').

Molecular superimposition techniques have been developed in which molecular properties and fields are being fitted instead of ligand points and site points. The most interesting of these methods are based on the fact that in addition to shape complementarity, electronic complementarity is important for molecular recognition. That is, positively and negatively charged parts of the molecular surface should interact with oppositely charged parts in the receptor binding cavity. Thus, methods have been devised to identify a common charge pattern or even better a common pattern of electrostatic potentials on or just outside the molecular surface of low-energy conformations of a set of high-affinity ligands. (The electrostatic potential is the potential energy between a unitary positive charge placed at a position in space and the molecular charge distribution.)

4.6.2   The use of molecular superimposition techniques

The ultimate use of a 3D-pharmacophore model is for the design of new ligands. Molecular superimposition techniques are then indispensable tools for testing if newly designed ligands fit the model in low-energy conformations. Molecular superimpositions and their use are exemplified in Section 4.9.2. However, an equally important use of molecular superimposition techniques is to investigate if inactive (low affinity) compounds fit the model. If such a compound does not fit the model in any conformation, the obvious rationalization of its low affinity is its inability to present the pharmacophore elements in a correct way (see Section 4.3). If the compound fits the model but in a high-energy conformation, the equally straightforward rationalization of its lack of affinity is that the energy penalty for binding to the receptor is too high (see Section 4.5). However, if the inactive compound fits the model in a low-energy conformation, there are three possibilities to rationalize its inactivity: (i) the compound is too voluminous in some direction(s) causing steric repulsive interactions with the receptor (see Section 4.7); (ii) the compound has a very unfavorable free energy of solvation (see Section 4.8); or (iii) the electronic properties of the ligand are not complementary to the receptor binding site (see Section 4.6.1). If none of the cases is probable, the 3D-pharmacophore model is seriously in doubt and should be reconsidered. Thus, molecular superimposition studies may corroborate or discard a 3D-pharmacophore model. Testing of the 3D-pharmacophore model with all available high- and low-affinity ligands should be done before design of new molecules based on the model is attempted.

4.7   RECEPTOR-EXCLUDED AND RECEPTOR-ESSENTIAL VOLUMES

The volume of a molecule may be computed and graphically displayed in terms of the sum of atomic van der Waals radii. For a superimposed set of high-affinity ligands for the target receptor, the *combined volume* may be calculated as the union of the volumes for all the molecules in the set (Figure 4.12). This volume should be readily accomodated by the receptor and the combined volume gives an estimate of the lower bound of the receptor volume available for binding of ligands (the *receptor-excluded volume*). The volume occupied by the receptor is called the *receptor-essential volume* and is not available for ligand binding (Figure 4.12). The analysis of molecular volumes on the basis of a 3D-pharmacophore model may give valuable information about the dimensions of the receptor cavity. An inactive or low-affinity compound which fits the 3D-pharmacophore model in a low-energy conformation may have a van der Waals volume larger than the combined volume of

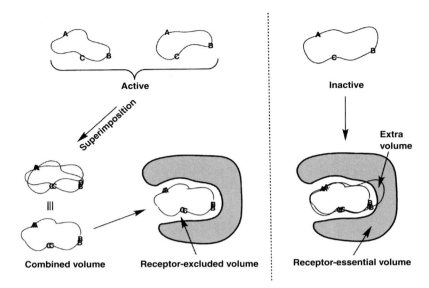

Figure 4.12 The *combined volume* gives an estimate of the lower-bound of receptor volume available for ligand binding (*receptor-excluded volume*). Inactive compounds may have an *extra volume* which overlaps the *receptor-essential volume* and thus causes steric repulsive interactions between the ligand and the receptor.

the high-affinity set of molecules (*extra volume*). For a valid 3D-pharmacophore model, the extra volume of the inactive compound indicates positions in space, where the ligand volume is in conflict with the receptor-essential volume (Figure 4.12). This information is extremely valuable in connection with design of new ligands based on a 3D-pharmacophore model as it provides knowledge about volumes in space where ligand fragments should not be present.

The potent $GABA_A$ receptor agonist muscimol ((**4.11**), Figure 4.13) displays an affinity for the $GABA_A$ receptor of 6 nM (IC_{50}, $^3H[GABA]$). The affinity of the 4-methyl analog (**4.12**) is drastically lower, 26 000 nM. An analysis of the molecular properties of (**4.11**) and (**4.12**) strongly indicates that the large decrease in the affinity of (**4.12**) compared to (**4.11**) is solely due to steric repulsive interactions between the methyl group in (**4.12**) and the receptor. In the superimposition of (**4.11**) and (**4.12**) in their deduced bioactive conformations shown in Figure 4.13, the 'extra volume' of the methyl group is displayed. Thus, in the design of new ligands for the $GABA_A$ receptor, care should be taken so that no parts of the ligands occupy this 'disallowed' volume in space.

4.8   SOLVATION EFFECTS

In Section 4.5.2, it was demonstrated that the conformational properties of a molecule may be strongly influenced by the solvent and that it is important to take

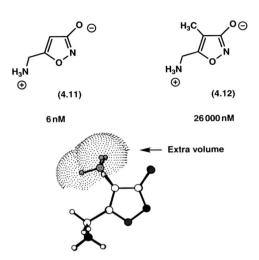

Figure 4.13 A superimposition of muscimol (**4.11**) and 4-methyl muscimol (**4.12**) illustrating the extra volume due to the 4-methyl group in (**4.12**).

solvation effects into account in the calculation of the conformational energy penalty of a bioactive conformation. In addition to its influence on the conformational properties, the aqueous environment in terms of the free energies of solvation (hydration) of the molecular species involved in the equilibrium in equation (4.1) and Figure 4.8 must also be taken into account. A larger stabilization of the ligand by the aqueous environment (i.e. a more negative free energy of hydration), shifts the equilibrium in Figure 4.8 to the left and the affinity for the receptor becomes lower.

As an example of this effect of the solvent, compound (**4.13**) binds to the enzyme thermolysin with a K_i-value of 9.1 nM. X-ray crystallography of the ligand–enzyme complex shows that the NH group indicated by an arrow interacts with a carbonyl oxygen of the enzyme binding site via a hydrogen bond. However, compound (**4.14**) binds equally well to the enzyme ($K_i = 10.6$ nM) in spite of the fact that the CH_2 group in (**4.14**), replacing the NH group in (**4.13**), cannot form a hydrogen bond to the enzyme. Computer simulations of the ligand–protein equilibrium show that (**4.14**) interacts less well with the enzyme than (**4.13**) by $10 \, \text{kJ mol}^{-1}$ ($\Delta\Delta G_{\text{inter}}$ in equation 4.3, Section 4.5.1). However, (**4.14**) is less well stabilized by

(**4.13**)

(**4.14**)

the solvent than (**4.13**) by $11 \, \text{kJ} \, \text{mol}^{-1}$ ($\Delta\Delta G_{solv}$). The net effect is that $\Delta\Delta G$ is close to zero and that (**4.13**) and (**4.14**) have essentially the same affinities for the enzyme (Merz Jr. and Kollman 1989).

In the development of 3D-pharmacophore models and in the design of new ligands based on such models, the free energies of hydration of the ligand must be taken into account. This may be done by only including compounds with similar free energies of solvation in the set on which the model is built. Otherwise such effects must be qualitatively estimated or explicitly calculated.

4.9   EXAMPLES OF 3D-PHARMACOPHORE MODELS AND THEIR USE

In this section, examples of development of 3D-pharmacophore models and their use are discussed. In addition to these examples, it should be noted that Chapter 11 includes a discussion on a pharmacophore model for the serotonin transporter.

4.9.1   Apomorphine congeners: conformational energies vs. agonist activities

An often used strategy in the structural elaboration of a lead compound is a simplification of the lead structure by ring-cleavage and/or deletion of rings. Compounds (**4.16**)–(**4.25**) are examples of such compounds, derived from the structure of the potent dopamine D_2 receptor agonist apomorphine (**4.15**).

Figure 4.14 displays a simple 3D-pharmacophore model for dopamine D_2 receptor agonists of the catechol type, based on three ligand points and a site point. Topologically (2D), compounds (**4.16**)–(**4.25**) all may display the same relative positions of the pharmacophore elements as (**4.15**). However, when

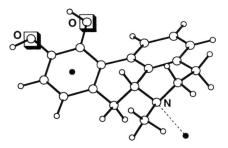

Figure 4.14 A 3D-pharmacophore model for dopamine D_2 agonists of the catechol type. The oxygen atoms, the center of the catechol ring and a site point 2.8 Å from the nitrogen atom in the direction of the nitrogen lone electron pair are selected as pharmacophore elements.

(**4.16**)–(**4.25**) are subjected to conformational analysis by molecular mechanics, it is found that most of the compounds require high conformational energies to fit the 3D-pharmacophore defined in Figure 4.14 (Pettersson and Liljefors 1987). Figure 4.15 displays the relationship between calculated conformational energies for the bioactive conformations of (**4.16**)–(**4.25**) and their obeserved agonist activities. The highly active compounds (**4.18**) and (**4.24**) have conformational energies of less

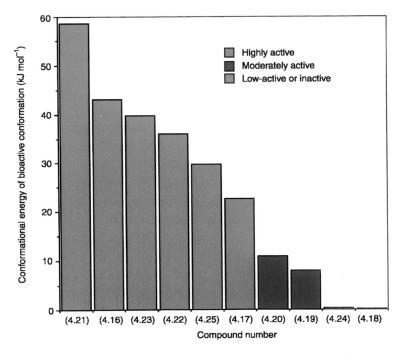

Figure 4.15 Calculated conformational energies of the deduced active conformations of compounds (**4.16**)–(**4.25**) vs. their dopamine receptor agonist activities.

than $2 \, \text{kJ} \, \text{mol}^{-1}$, whereas the moderately active compounds (**4.20**) and (**4.19**) display conformational energies of 8 and $11 \, \text{kJ} \, \text{mol}^{-1}$ respectively. All low active or inactive compounds have conformational energies in excess of $20 \, \text{kJ} \, \text{mol}^{-1}$. This clearly demonstrates that conformational energies must be taken into account in the design of new ligands from a template structure.

4.9.2   A 3D-pharmacophore model for dopamine D_2 receptor antagonists

(1*R*, 3*S*)-Tefludazine (**4.26**) and (*S*)-octoclothepin (*S*)-(**4.27**) are high-affinity dopamine D_2 receptor antagonists (Figure 4.16). On the basis of these compounds, a 3D-pharmacophore for D_2 receptor antagonists has been developed (Liljefors and Bøgesø 1988). The pharmacophore elements chosen are the centers of the aromatic rings, the nitrogen atoms encircled in Figure 4.16, and a site point in each molecule, $2.8 \, \text{Å}$ from the nitrogen atom in the direction of the nitrogen lone pair (Figure 4.16).

Based on exhaustive conformational analysis of the two compounds by molecular mechanics and molecular least-squares superimposition studies, the superimposition shown in Figure 4.17 was obtained (rms = $0.23 \, \text{Å}$). A closer inspection of this superimposition reveals that a simultaneous rotation in (**4.26**) and (*S*)-(**4.27**) about the C–N bond connecting the piperazine ring to the tricyclic ringsystem, preserves the excellent superimposition of the pharmacophore elements. However, such a simultaneous rotation generates an infinite number of possible 3D-pharmacophore candidates. It will be demonstrated below that calculated conformational energies may be used to select among these candidates.

Figure 4.18 displays calculated potential energy curves for different orientations of the piperazine rings in (**4.26**) and (*S*)-(**4.27**). The two curves are slightly displaced so that the pair of dihedral angles giving an optimal fit of the pharmacophore elements are placed directly above each other. The superimposition shown in Figure 4.17 corresponds to dihedral angles of $290°$ for (*S*)-(**4.27**) and $300°$ for (**4.26**).

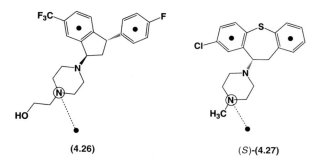

(4.26)   **(*S*)-(4.27)**

Figure 4.16 Pharmacophore elements used in the development of a 3D-pharmacophore model for dopamine D_2 receptor antagonists.

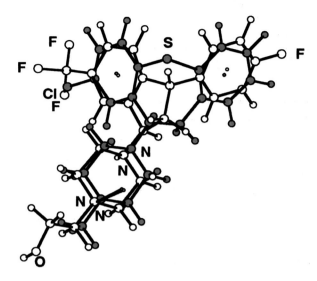

Figure 4.17 A least-squares molecular superimposition of compounds (**4.26**) (unfilled atoms) and (S)-(**4.27**) (green atoms). Note that the trifluoromethly group in (**4.26**) and the chloro substituent in (S)-(**4.27**) (the 'neuroleptic substituents') are very similarily positioned in space.

The potential energy curve for (**4.26**) displays several low-energy regions corresponding to possible receptor-bound conformations. However, the potential energy curve for (S)-(**4.27**) displays only a few such regions – only a small region with dihedral angles in the range of 260–315°, lies below 13 kJ mol^{-1} (see Section 4.5.2). Since the corresponding region in the potential energy curve of (**4.26**) (270–325°) has conformational energies well below 10 kJ mol^{-1}, the receptor-bound conformations for (**4.26**) and (S)-(**4.27**) are most probably to be found for dihedral angles in these regions. The conformations for (**4.26**) and (S)-(**4.27**) displayed in the superimposition in Figure 4.17 correspond to the lowest-energy conformations in these regions.

The enantiomers of (**4.27**) may be used to test the proposed receptor-bound conformation for (S)-(**4.27**) (Bøgesø *et al.* 1991). The conformational properties of (S)- and (R)-(**4.27**) are such that it is possible to find a conformation for (R)-(**4.27**) for which the pharmacophore elements superimpose extremely well with those of the proposed receptor-bound conformation of (S)-(**4.27**). This superimposition is shown in Figure 4.19. Note that in the superimposition, the two enantiomers have different conformations of their tricyclic ring systems.

The very high degree of similarity displayed by the two enantiomers in their proposed bioactive conformations (Figure 4.19) implies that energy contributions due to intermolecular interactions with receptor sites should be essentially the same for the enantiomers. $\Delta\Delta G$ should consequently be determined by the difference in conformational energies of the conformations shown in Figure 4.19, as discussed in Section 4.5.1. Experimentally, (S)-(**4.27**) binds stronger to the receptor than

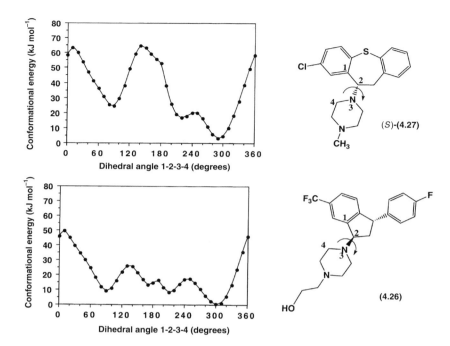

Figure 4.18 Potential energy curves calculated using molecular mechanics for the rotation about the C2–N3 bond in (**4.26**) and (S)-(**4.27**). Note that the global energy conformation for (S)-(**4.27**), (corresponding to a conformational energy of $0.0\,\mathrm{kJ\,mol^{-1}}$) is not included in the potential energy curve). The global energy conformation has another conformation of the tricyclic ring system.

(R)-(**4.27**) by $4.2\,\mathrm{kJ\,mol^{-1}}$. The conformational energy difference calculated by molecular mechanics is $5.8\,\mathrm{kJ\,mol^{-1}}$ in favor of (S)-(**4.27**). Since energy contributions due to desolvation, hydrophobicity, loss of entropy etc. are identical for enantiomers, the calculated energy may be directly compared with the experimental one. The very good agreement between calculated and experimental results strongly supports the proposed receptor-bound conformation for (S)-(**4.27**) (and thus for (**4.26**)). This analysis demonstrates that enantiomers having such conformational properties that pharmacophore elements are able to superimpose may be valuable tools in 3D-pharmacophore identification and validation.

A representation of the 3D-pharmacophore in terms of disconnected fragments derived from the superimposition in Figure 4.17 is shown in Figure 4.20.

4.9.3 3D-pharmacophore models for the design of selective 5-HT$_{2A}$ vs. D$_2$ receptor antagonists

On the basis of analyses of a large number of dopamine D$_2$ receptor antagonists and their receptor affinities, the basic pharmacophore model displayed in Figure 4.20 was extended to include further pharmacophore elements and, most importantly, receptor essential volumes (sterically disallowed regions). The final

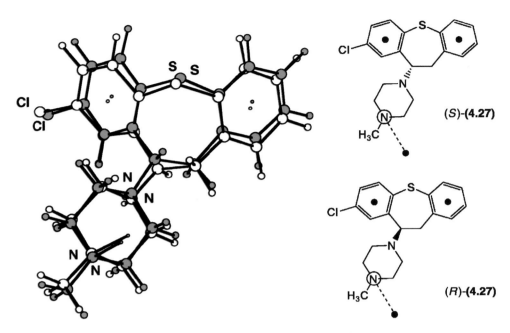

Figure 4.19 A molecular least-squares superimposition (rms = 0.28 Å) of (*S*)-(**4.27**) (green atoms) and (*R*)-(**4.27**) (unfilled atoms). The pharmacophore elements used in the superimposition are included in the structural formulas.

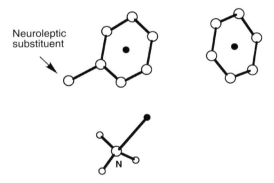

Figure 4.20 A representation of the basic 3D-pharmacophore model for dopamine D_2 receptor antagonists. The position of the 'neuroleptic substituent' which generally increases the affinity of the molecule for the dopamine D_2 receptor is included in the model.

model is displayed in Figure 4.21 (upper left part). The receptor essential volumes were identified by analyses of compounds with low affinity for the D_2 receptor as described in Section 4.7 and are represented by tetrahedrons in Figure 4.21. In order to study if differences in pharmacophoric features may be employed for the design of compounds selective for the serotonin 5-HT_{2A} receptor with respect to

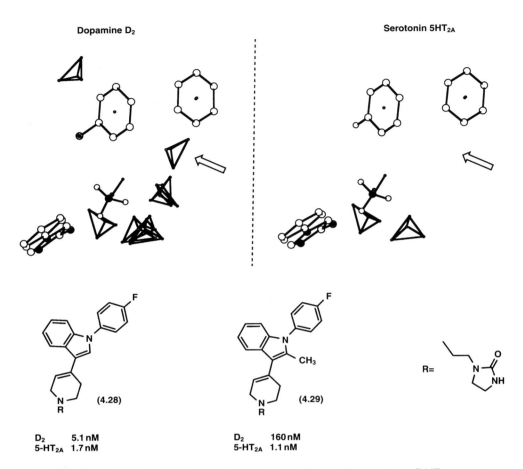

Dopamine D$_2$

Serotonin 5HT$_{2A}$

R=

(4.28)

(4.29)

| D$_2$ | 5.1 nM |
| 5-HT$_{2A}$ | 1.7 nM |

| D$_2$ | 160 nM |
| 5-HT$_{2A}$ | 1.1 nM |

Figure 4.21 3D-pharmacophore models for the dopamine D$_2$ and the serotonin 5-HT$_{2A}$ receptors. The tetrahedrons represent receptor essential volumes. The arrow points at one of the differences between the pharmacophore models. The effect of the indicated pharmacophore difference is illustrated for compounds (**4.28**) and (**4.29**). The D$_2$ and 5-HT$_{2A}$ affinity data are IC$_{50}$-values obtained by using [^{3}H]-spiroperidol and [^{3}H]-ketanserin, respectively, as radioligands.

the D$_2$ receptor, a 3D-pharmacophore model for 5-HT$_{2A}$ receptor antagonists was developed using the same methodology as described in Section 4.9.2 for D$_2$ receptor antagonists (Andersen *et al.* 1994). The final 3D-pharmacophore model for 5-HT$_{2A}$ antagonists is displayed in Figure 4.21 (upper right part). The two models are in many respects very similar. However, on comparing the receptor essential volumes in the two models, it is clear that the D$_2$ receptor causes steric repulsions between ligands and the receptor in a significantly larger number of volumes in space than the 5-HT$_{2A}$ receptor. One important difference is indicated by an arrow in Figure 4.21.

Compound (**4.28**) is a high affinity but essentially non-selective D_2 and 5-HT_{2A} receptor antagonist (Figure 4.21). This compound fits very well to both pharmacophore models in a low-energy conformation and there are no conflicts between (**4.28**) and the receptor essential volumes in either of the models. These findings are compatible with the high afffinity and non-selectivity of (**4.28**) .

Compound (**4.29**) can also be fitted to the two pharmacophore models in a low-energy conformation. However, the methyl group in (**4.29**) is in strong conflict with the sterically disallowed region indicated by an arrow in the D_2 pharmacophore model. This is reflected by its decreased affinity for the D_2 receptor (Figure 4.21). In contrast, the methyl group in (**4.29**) as may be predicted from the pharmacophore model does not have any effect on the affinity for the 5-HT_{2A} receptor. As a result, compound (**4.29**) displays selectivity for the 5-HT_{2A} receptor with respect to the D_2 receptor (by a factor of 145).

This example illustrates the importance of receptor essential volumes in the context of 3D-pharmacophore models and their usefulness for the design of new ligands. For further discussions on dopamine and serotonin receptor ligands, see Chapter 11.

4.9.4   A pharmacophore based database searching for new antimalarial drugs

Artemisinin (**4.30**), a naturally occurring compound isolated from the chinese plant *Artemisia annua* displays potent antimalarial activity. Since (**4.30**) is a quite complex molecule, structurally simpler 1,2,4-trioxanes have been synthesized and tested for antimalarial activity. Five structural classes of such analogs (**4.31**)–(**4.35**) have been used to develop a pharmacophore model for antimalarial activity with the aim of using the pharmacophore model for database searching for leads which may be developed into new antimalarial drugs (Grigorov *et al.* 1997).

On the basis of 23 compounds from the five structural classes of 1,2,4-trioxanes, pharmacophore models were developed by using the automatic pharmacophore generation capabilities of the CATALYST software (see Section 4.4.3). By using *in vitro* as well as *in vivo* data, two pharmacophore models corresponding to the

(**4.30**)   (**4.31**)   (**4.32**)

(**4.33**)   (**4.34**)   (**4.35**)

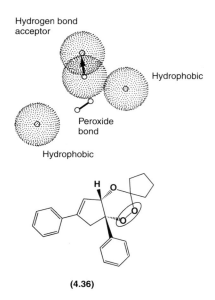

(4.36)

Figure 4.22 A schematic illustration of a CATALYST pharmacophore model used as a query for database searching.

(4.37)   **(4.38)   R=H**
                              (4.39)   R=OOH

two series of biological data were developed. The two models turned out to be very similar. A schematic illustration of the resulting *in vivo* pharmacophore model is shown in Figure 4.22. The model is made up by two hydrophobic pharmacophore elements corresponding to one of the phenyl groups and the cyclopentane ring system in (**4.36**), a representative of the compounds in the structural class (**4.34**). In addition, a hydrogen bond acceptor is included corresponding to the hydrogen accepting properties of the ether oxygen in (**4.36**). Finally, a peroxide moiety in an appropriate position was added to the pharmacophore model as this moiety is crucial for the antimalarial activity.

The pharmacophore was then used for searching the NCI (National Cancer Institute) database transferred by the CATALYST software into a multiconformational database (version 4.6 of the NCI database contains 98868 compounds). The database search resulted in four hits. Artemisinin (**4.30**) was one of the hits, the other three were (**4.37**)–(**4.39**). By using the QSAR capabilites of the

CATALYST software to estimate the activities of these compounds, compounds (**4.38**) and (**4.39**) were both predicted to be less active than artemisinin (**4.30**) by a factor of more than one hundred. However, compound (**4.37**) was predicted to have an antimalarial activity only ca. ten times lower than that of artemisinin which makes it an interesting lead for the development of new antimalarial drugs.

REFERENCES

Andersen, K., Liljefors, T., Gundertofte, K., Perregaard, J. and Bøgesø, K.P. (1994) Development of a receptor-interaction model for serotonin 5-HT$_2$ receptor antagonists. Prediction of selectivity with respect to dopamine D$_2$ receptors. *J. Med. Chem.*, **37**, 950–962.

Bøgesø, K.P., Liljefors, T., Arnt, J., Hyttel, J. and Pedersen, H. (1991) Octoclothepin Enantiomers. A reinvestigation of their biochemical and pharmacological activity in relation to a new model for dopamine D-2 receptor antagonists. *J. Med. Chem.*, **34**, 2023.

Grigorov, M., Weber, J., Tronchet, J.M.J., Jefford, C.W., Milhous, W.K. and Maric, D. (1997) A QSAR study of the antimalarial activity of some synthetic 1,2,4-trioxanes. *J. Chem. Inf. Comput. Sci.*, **37**, 124–130.

Liljefors, T. and Bøgesø, K.P. (1988) Conformational analysis and structural comparisons of 1R, 3S-(+)-, 1S, 3R-(−)-tefludazine, S-(+)-octoclothepin and (+)-dexclamol in relation to dopamine receptor antagonism and amine-uptake inhibition. *J. Med. Chem.*, **31**, 306–312.

Pettersson, I. and Liljefors, T. (1987) Structure–activity relationships for apomorphine congeners. Conformational energies vs. biological activities. *J. Computer-Aided Mol. Design*, **1**, 143–152.

FURTHER READING

Boström, J., Norrby, P.-O. and Liljefors, T. (1998) Conformational energy penalties of protein-bound ligands. *J. Computer-Aided Mol. Design*, **12**, 383–396.

Burkert, U. and Allinger, N. L. (1982) *Molecular Mechanics, ACS Monograph 177*. Washington D.C.: American Chemical Society.

Cramer, C.J. and Truhlar, D.G. (1995) Continuum solvation models: classical and quantum mechanics implementations. In *Reviews in Computational Chemistry*, Vol. 6, edited by K.B. Lipkowitz and D.B. Boyd, pp. 1–72. New York: VCH Publishers.

Cramer, C.J. and Truhlar, D.G. (1999) Implicit solvation models: equilibria, structure, spectra and dynamics. *Chem. Rev.*, **99**, 2161–2200.

Golender, V.E. and Vorpagel, E.R. (1993) Computer-assisted pharmacophore identification. In *3D QSAR in Drug Design. Theory Methods and Applications*, edited by H. Kubinyi, pp. 137–149. Leiden: Escom Science Publishers.

Güner, O.F. (ed.) (2000) *Pharmacophore Perception, Development, and Use in Drug Design*. La Jolla: International University Line.

Leach, A.R. (1991) A survey of methods for searching the conformational space of small and medium-sized molecules. In *Reviews in Computational Chemistry*, Vol. 2, edited by K.B. Lipkowitz and D.B. Boyd, pp. 1–55. New York: VCH Publishers.

Marshall, G.R. (1993) Binding site modeling of unknown receptors. In *3D QSAR in Drug Design. Theory, Methods and Applications*, edited by H. Kubinyi, pp. 80–116. Leiden: Escom Science Publishers.

Merz Jr., K.M. and Kollman, P.A. (1989) Free energy perturbation simulations of the inhibition of thermolysin. Prediction of the Free Energy of Binding of a New Inhibitor. *J. Med. Chem.*, **111**, 5649–5658.

Ripka, W.C. and Blaney J.M. (1991) Computer graphics and molecular modeling in the analysis of synthetic targets. In *Topics in Stereochemistry*, Vol. 20, edited by E.L. Eliel and S.H. Wilen, pp. 1–85. New York: J. Wiley & Sons.

Siebel, G.L. and Kollman, P.A. (1990) Molecular mechanics and the modeling of drug structures. In *Comprehensive Medicinal Chemistry*, Vol. 4, edited by C. Hansch, P.G. Sammes, J.B. Taylor and C.A. Ramsden, pp. 125–138. Oxford: Pergamon Press.

Sprague, P.W. and Hoffmann, R. (1997) CATALYST pharmacophore models and their utility as queries for searching 3D databases. In *Computer-Assisted Lead Finding and Optimization. Current Tools for Medicinal Chemistry*, edited by H. van der Waterbeemd, B. Testa and G. Folkers, pp. 225–240. Basel: Verlag Helvetica Chimica Acta.

Still, W.C., Tempczyk, A., Hawley, R.C. and Hendrickson, T. (1990) Semianalytical treatment of solvation for molecular mechanics and dynamics. *J. Amer. Chem. Soc.*, **112**, 6127–6129.

Wermuth, C.-G. and Langer, T. (1993) Pharmacophore identification. In *3D QSAR in Drug Design. Theory Methods and Applications*, edited by H. Kubinyi, pp. 117–136. Leiden: Escom Science Publishers.

Chapter 5

Quantitative structure–activity relationships and experimental design

Ulf Norinder and Thomas Högberg

5.1 INTRODUCTION

Pharmacophoric mapping is of great value in generating new chemical lead structures, especially when a limited number of compounds are available or when different chemical classes are used (see Chapter 4). A structural fit, reflected by the 3-D geometry of a structure in its active conformation is a necessary but not sufficient cause of activity, since electronic and hydrophobic forces between ligand and receptor are required for the response. An inherent limitation with pharmacophoric modeling techniques like the active analog approach is their inability to quantitatively describe the biological effect, i.e. one can usually only distinguish active from inactive compounds. In the process of optimizing a lead structure, it is necessary to utilize the information from quantitative activity data and from other structural properties in a more efficient way in order to predict more active congeners. Furthermore, quantitative structure–activity relationships (QSAR) can provide a great deal of information regarding the nature of ligand–target protein interactions. In series of homologous derivatives, various quantitative structure–activity analyses utilizing linear free energy relationships, multiple linear regression, and pattern recognition techniques have been applied. Furthermore, recent progress has been made in combining molecular modeling and statistical models, which allows for handling of non-congeneric series.

5.2 HANSCH ANALYSIS

5.2.1 Hydrophobic correlations

The biological activity can be regarded as a function of the physico-chemical and structural properties of the ligand. Already at the turn of the century, Meyer and Overton observed independently of each other that the anesthetic potency of simple organic molecules increases linearly with their oil/water partition coefficients (P). Four decades later Ferguson connected the narcotic activity and partition coefficients with thermodynamic principles. He stated that under equilibrium conditions, narcotic activity was correlated to the relative saturation of membranes by the gaseous narcotic substance. However, Hansch reasoned that too lipophilic molecules will partition into the first line of lipid membranes and be retained there.

Likewise, too hydrophilic molecules will not readily partition from the first aqueous compartment into the lipid of a membrane. Accordingly, Hansch and co-workers observed in the 1960s that the biological activity for several sets of congeners conformed with a parabolic dependence on lipophilicity ($\log P$) according to equation (5.1). Thus, an optimal $\log P$ value would correspond to the maximum probability of a compound to reach a receptor protein on a random walk between various lipophilic and hydrophilic compartments. The optimal lipophilic value, $\log P_o = a/2b$, is obtained from the derivative $d(\log 1/C)/d\log P$ being equal to zero. The biological activity is usually expressed as the logarithm of the inverse concentration or dose [$\log (1/C)$ or pC] which produces some standard response, e.g. $\log (1/IC_{50})$ or $\log (1/ED_{50})$.

$$\text{biological activity } \left(\log \frac{1}{C}\right) = a \log P - b(\log P)^2 + c \tag{5.1}$$

Phenomena involved in the transport of the ligand to its site of action and the hydrophobic interactions with the receptor are mainly determined by equation (5.1). For several classes of CNS active substances it has been found that the activity and thus the penetration over the blood–brain barrier (BBB) is optimal for $\log P_o$ (octanol) values in the range of 1.5–2.7, with a mean value of 2.1 (see also Section 5.4.5 for a more recent view). A linear dependence on $\log P$ might be expected up to a point where the hydrophobic region of the receptor is filled out and thereafter the activity decreases due to steric hindrance during the interaction of ligand and receptor. In several cases, the whole lipophilicity range may not have been investigated and, thus, only a linear dependence is revealed.

5.2.2 Multifactorial correlations

In order to take other types of molecular interactions into account, Hansch and Fujita included descriptors for steric, electronic and hydrophobic (= lipophilic) properties in the QSAR equation (5.2), which is based on the fact that the variables can be related to free energies in a linear free energy relationship (LFER). In the literature you will find the expressions parameter, descriptor or variable used with the same meaning.

$$\log\left(\frac{1}{C}\right) = a(\text{parameter}) + b(\text{electronic parameter})$$
$$+ c(\text{steric parameter}) + d(\text{other descriptor}) + e \tag{5.2}$$

where a, b, c, d and e are the regression coefficients determined by a least squares regression analysis (multiple linear regression, MLR), often referred to as a Hansch analysis. Different physico-chemical parameters have been used to describe the global properties of the molecule or the contribution from individual substituents. The most commonly used substituent parameters are shown in Table 5.1. These independent variables (parameters and descriptors) can be collinear, i.e. the same information is carried by the parameters, which will lead to false correlations. By including indicator variables, one can for example describe the presence or

Table 5.1 Physico-chemical parameters used in QSAR

Parameter	Symbol
Hydrophobic parameters	
Partition coefficient	$\log P$, CLOGP, Prolog P
Substituent constant	π
Hydrophobic fragmental constant	f, f'
Distribution coefficient	$\log D$
Apparent partition coefficient (fixed pH)	$\log P'$, $\log P_{app}$
Capacity factor in HPLC	$\log k$, $\log k_w$
Solubility parameter	δ
Electronic descriptors	
Hammett constants	$\sigma, \sigma^-, \sigma^+$
Taft's inductive (polar) constants	σ^*, σ_I
Swain and Lupton field parameter	$\Im$
Swain and Lupton resonance parameter	$\Re$
Ionization constant	pK_a, ΔpK_a
Chemical shifts (^{13}C and ^1H)	δ
Theoretical parameters	
Atomic net charge	q^σ, q^π
Superdelocalizability	S^N, S^E, S^R
Energy of highest occupied molecular orbital	E_{HOMO}
Energy of lowest unoccupied molecular orbital	E_{LUMO}
Electrostatic potentials	$V(r)$
Steric descriptors	
Taft's steric parameter	E_S, E^c
Molar volume	MV
Molecular weight	MW
Van der Waals radius	r
Van der Waals volume	V_W
Molar refractivity	MR
Parachor	P_r
STERIMOL parameters	$L, B_1, B_5 (B_2, B_3, B_4)$

absence of a certain substituent or other structural characteristics. In the ideal case, the biological data and physico-chemical parameters should be spread evenly and over a large range as will be discussed in the following Section 5.7 on experimental design.

The number of compounds (n) in the correlation must be considerably larger than the number of parameters used, i.e. four to six compounds (data points) per variable for medium-sized data sets in order to avoid chance correlations. In the PLS method described in Section 5.5, this is not a limitation even if redundant variables should be avoided. The correlation coefficient r, the relative measure of the quality of fit, should be around 0.9 for *in vitro* data, i.e. the explained variance r^2 should be over 80%, for acceptable regression equations. The standard deviation s, the absolute measure of the quality of fit, should not exceed the standard deviation in the biological data set too much. The regression coefficients (a, b, c, d etc.) should make sense from a physico-chemical standpoint (cf. ρ-values in physical organic chemistry) and be justified by confidence intervals at the 95% level (not shown in the following equations).

Importantly, the physico-chemical descriptors contain information that will give direct insight about properties essential for the transport to the site of action and for the interaction with the target protein required for the biological activity. Thus, one should select and statistically justify independent (low intercorrelation coefficients) variables, which describe different structural properties. In the analysis, one should aim for the simplest model to describe the data (principle of parsimony).

5.3 PHYSICO-CHEMICAL PROPERTIES

5.3.1 Electronic descriptors

The first and still most widely used electronic substituent parameter σ was developed by Hammett 1935 on the basis of ionization constants for benzoic acid derivatives. The Hammett equation (5.3) is expressed as

$$\rho\sigma = \log K_X - \log K_H \tag{5.3}$$

where K_H and K_X are the ionization constants for benzoic acid and a *para* or *meta* substituted derivative, respectively, and $\rho = 1$ for measurements in water at 25 °C. Positive σ values represent electron withdrawing properties ($X = CN, NO_2, CF_3$) and negative σ values electron donating properties ($X = NH_2, CH_3$).

A number of related Hammett parameters applicable for special circumstances, e.g. σ_p^-, σ_p^+, σ_m and σ_p, can provide mechanistic insight on the nature of the interaction if a considerably better correlation is obtained with a particular constant (cf. equation (5.18) below).

The inductive field (polar) component of the electronic substituent effect could be separated from the resonance part. Swain and Lupton described the Hammett σ constant as a linear combination of a resonance effect $\mathfrak{R}$ and a field effect $\mathfrak{F}$. These parameters are not position-dependent, which makes them useful and easy to handle in QSAR (cf. equation (5.20)). The Hammett constant σ is related to the $\mathfrak{F}$ and $\mathfrak{R}$ values as expressed in equation (5.4)

$$\sigma = f\mathfrak{F} + r\mathfrak{R} \tag{5.4}$$

where f and r are weighting factors.

5.3.2 Hydrophobic parameters

Analogous to the derivation of the Hammett constant, the substituent constant π for hydrophobic effect can be described by equation (5.5),

$$\pi = \log P_X - \log P_H \tag{5.5}$$

where P_X is the partition coefficient of a substituted derivative and P_H that of the parent compound. The distribution is measured between an organic solvent and water and the partition coefficient P is the ratio of the same solute in the two immiscible solvents. Octanol is the accepted standard system used and it has been justified as a suitable model for lipid constituents in biomembranes by the slightly amphiphilic nature introduced by the hydroxyl group in the long alkyl chain. The hydrogen bond donating and accepting properties facilitate the interaction with several types of solutes and octanol also dissolves an appreciable amount of water during equilibrium conditions. The partitioning to other solvent systems can be calculated by the Collander equation (5.6). This linear relationship between $\log P$ obtained in different systems makes it reasonable to apply one arbitrary standard system (octanol) even if limitations have been pointed out.

$$\log P_1 = a \log P_2 + c \tag{5.6}$$

A positive π corresponds to a lipophilic character and negative π to a hydrophilic character relative to hydrogen. In the case of ionizable solutes, $\log P$ for the non-ionized species can be determined from the distribution coefficient D, which is dependent on pH, by inclusion of the ionization constant(s) in the calculation (e.g. equations (5.7) and (5.8)). Partition through membranes is usually regarded to be associated with the non-ionized molecules.

$$\log D_{\text{acid}} = \log P - \log[1 + 10^{(\text{pH} - \text{pK}_a)}] \tag{5.7}$$

$$\log D_{\text{base}} = \log P - \log[1 + 10^{(\text{pK}_a - \text{pH})}] \tag{5.8}$$

However, the determination of partition coefficients by the classical shake flask technique is connected with several practical problems, e.g. disturbances from minor impurities, effects of ions in aqueous buffers, difficulties to analyze solutes in both phases especially for compounds with extreme $\log P$ values, necessity to work with very low concentrations of solute to diminish aggregation, and establishment of equilibrium conditions. These problems to determine $\log P$ values can largely be overcome by use of HPLC-derived hydrophobicity data. The HPLC methodology can also be applied to small and impure amounts of material and gives accurate data by frequent use of calibration standards. Furthermore, no quantitative methods for the determination of the solutes are required. The chromatographically derived values are not unique, but they can be converted into the familiar octanol/water partition coefficients. This makes HPLC the method of choice for experimental determination of $\log P$ values.

The slope a in equation (5.1) has been found to have values in the range from about 0.2 to 1.4. It has been argued that a-values of about unity implies complete desolvation and binding deep into a lipophilic pocket (cf. equations (5.13), (5.14), (5.17) and (5.25)), whereas a-values of about 0.5 reflects only partial desolvation and binding along the surface of a protein (cf. equations (5.12) and (5.15)). However, this view is under debate, since binding to a highly structured membrane reduces the freedom of an alkyl chain, which will diminish the slope a and the π values.

The additive properties of the π values make it possible to estimate $\log P$ of a new compound, either completely from tables or by combination of experimental values and tabulated data. For example, the $\log P$ value for xylene can be estimated with a high degree of accuracy from the $\log P$ values of benzene and toluene by the following simple calculation.

$$\pi_{Me} = \log P_{Ph-Me} - \log P_{Ph-H} = 2.69 - 2.13 = 0.56$$

$$\log P_{xylene} = \log P_{Ph-Me} + \pi_{Me} = 2.69 + 0.56 = 3.25 \text{ (Experimental 3.20)}$$

However, in several cases, especially for aliphatic compounds, large differences between observed $\log P$ values and partition coefficients calculated from π values are found. To overcome these limitations, Rekker introduced the concept of fragmental constants f, which are related to the π values according to equation (5.9). The fragmental constants, which were statistically derived from over thousand $\log P$ determinations, measure the absolute lipophilicity contribution of a given structural fragment i, which occurs a_i number of times in a structure. Interaction factors F were also introduced in order to correct for intramolecular electronic, steric or hydrogen bond interactions between fragments according to equation (5.10).

$$f_X = f_H + \pi_X \tag{5.9}$$
$$\log P = \Sigma a_i\, f_X + \Sigma F_i \tag{5.10}$$

The fragmental constant system has been modified by Leo and Hansch based on a small number of accurately determined $\log P$ values instead of the statistical approach used by Rekker. Based on this concept a computer program CLOGP was developed, which allows for more facile calculations of $\log P$ values.

5.3.3 Steric descriptors

The description of steric bulk of a substituent is difficult to assess, since the conformation may vary among the ligands in the test series as well as for the target protein. However, several parameters have been successfully applied. The steric effect has been described by Taft's steric parameter E_S, derived from acidic hydrolysis of esters (X-CH$_2$COOR). E_S is more negative for larger groups [t-Bu, CCl$_3$] and more positive for smaller groups (H, F, OH).

In order to better account for the shape of the substituents, Verloop has developed a set of parameters using the STERIMOL program based on CPK-models. The length parameter L and the four width parameters B_1, B_2, B_3, and B_4 which describe the dimensions of the group along fixed axes, were originally used. However, different possibilities may result for the B_2–B_4 parameters depending on the selection of B_1, which is not a very satisfactory situation. Because of this and also because of reported statistical chance correlations in the literature using the original STERIMOL parameters a new set of descriptors was developed by Verloop. These second generation parameters retained the STERIMOL length parameter L and the minimum width parameter B_1 but introduced a new width parameter B_5, which represents the largest width orthogonal to L but is independent of any angle between B_1 and B_5 (cf. equation (5.14)).

1   To determine the STERIMOL parameters one proceeds in the following manner: Determine the bond between the parent skeleton and the substituent and place that bond in the plane of the paper (or screen). Project the vdW surface of the substituent onto the same plane. Measure the length from the point of attachment (P) to the projected vdW surface along the bond of attachment. This value constitutes the STERIMOL parameter L.

2   Rotate the structure 90° to see the structure along the bond between the parent skeleton and the substituent. Project the vdW surface of the substituent onto the plane of the paper (or screen). Measure the shortest length as well as the longest length from the point of attachment (P) to the projected vdW surface. These two values constitute the STERIMOL parameters B_1 and B_5, respectively.

The definitions of the second generation STERIMOL parameters of L, B_1 and B_5 are shown in Figure 5.1. The parameters B_1 and B_5 are orthogonal to L as a consequence of the procedure described above. By using ratios of L/B_1 and B_5/B_1 one might get information on any directionality of importance for the receptor interaction.

Alternatively, the van der Waals radii and the molar volume $MV = MW/d$ have been used. The molar refractivity (MR) is related to the molar volume by the Lorentz–Lorenz equation (5.11).

$$MR = \left[\frac{(n^2 - 1)}{(n^2 + 2)}\right]\left(\frac{MW}{d}\right) \qquad (5.11)$$

where n is the refraction index, d is the density and MW is the molecular weight. Fragment values have been calculated since MR is an additive property of the molecule. A larger MR value for a substituent corresponds to a larger steric

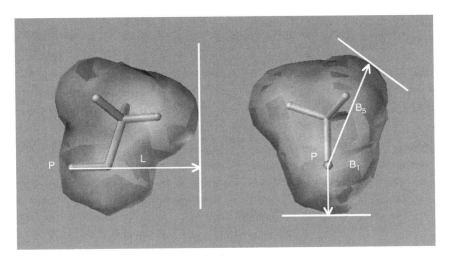

Figure 5.1 Definition of the second generation STERIMOL parameters used in QSAR work exemplified by a methoxy group substituent.

Table 5.2 Commonly used aromatic substituent parameters and principal properties (PP) calculated from the complete set of parameters by principal component analysis (Section 5.5)

Subst.	σ_m	σ_p	$\mathfrak{J}$	$\mathfrak{R}$	π	MR	L	B_1	B_5	PP_1	PP_2	PP_3
H	0.00	0.00	0.00	0.00	0.00	1.03	2.06	1.00	1.00	1.35	−3.00	−0.39
F	0.34	0.06	0.43	−0.34	0.14	0.92	2.65	1.35	1.35	2.38	−1.95	0.45
Cl	0.37	0.23	0.41	−0.15	0.71	6.03	3.52	1.80	1.80	2.22	−0.15	−0.57
Br	0.39	0.23	0.44	−0.17	0.86	8.88	3.82	1.95	1.95	2.08	0.38	−0.74
I	0.35	0.18	0.40	−0.19	1.12	13.94	4.23	2.15	2.15	1.49	1.00	−1.21
NO_2	0.71	0.78	0.67	0.16	−0.28	7.36	3.44	1.70	2.44	4.12	1.12	0.87
CH_3	−0.07	−0.17	−0.04	−0.13	0.56	5.65	2.87	1.52	2.04	0.25	−1.84	−1.36
CCH	0.21	0.23	0.19	0.05	0.40	9.55	4.66	1.60	1.60	1.30	−0.01	−0.60
$CHCH_2$	0.05	−0.02	0.07	−0.08	0.82	10.99	4.29	1.60	3.09	−0.09	−0.18	−0.65
C_2H_5	−0.07	−0.15	−0.05	−0.10	1.02	10.30	4.11	1.52	3.17	−0.71	−0.65	−0.90
C_3H_5	−0.07	−0.21	−0.03	−0.19	1.14	13.53	4.14	1.55	3.24	−1.02	−0.56	−0.83
C_3H_7	−0.07	−0.13	−0.06	−0.08	1.55	14.96	4.92	1.52	3.49	−1.35	0.15	−0.78
$CH(CH_3)_2$	−0.07	−0.15	−0.05	−0.10	1.53	14.98	4.11	1.90	3.17	−0.87	0.16	−1.89
C_4H_9	−0.08	−0.16	−0.06	−0.11	2.13	19.59	6.17	1.52	4.54	−2.43	1.22	−0.32
$CH_2CH(CH_3)_2$	−0.10	−0.20	−0.07	−0.13	1.98	19.62	4.92	1.52	4.45	−2.16	0.61	−0.55
$C(CH_3)_3$	−0.10	−0.20	−0.07	−0.13	1.98	19.62	4.11	2.60	3.17	−1.03	1.20	−3.70
C_5H_{11}	−0.08	−0.15	−0.06	−0.09	2.67	24.25	7.17	1.52	5.23	−3.22	2.21	−0.03
C_6H_5	0.06	−0.01	0.08	−0.08	1.96	25.36	6.28	1.71	3.11	−1.51	1.73	−0.64
C_6H_{11}	−0.15	−0.22	−0.13	−0.10	2.51	26.69	6.17	1.91	3.49	−2.68	1.67	−1.83
CF_3	0.43	0.54	0.38	0.19	0.88	5.02	3.30	1.99	2.61	2.83	1.00	−1.10
CN	0.56	0.66	0.51	0.19	−0.57	6.33	4.23	1.60	1.60	3.59	0.57	0.52
CHO	0.35	0.42	0.31	0.13	−0.65	6.88	3.53	1.60	2.36	2.51	−0.13	0.05
CH_2OH	0.00	0.00	0.00	0.00	−1.03	7.19	3.97	1.52	2.70	0.62	−1.22	−0.44
$COCH_3$	0.38	0.50	0.32	0.20	−0.55	11.18	4.06	1.60	3.13	2.13	0.73	0.42
COC_6H_5	0.34	0.43	0.30	0.16	1.05	30.33	5.81	1.60	5.98	−0.71	3.40	1.37
$CONH_2$	0.28	0.36	0.24	0.14	−1.49	9.81	4.06	1.50	3.07	1.90	−0.12	0.63
COOH	0.37	0.45	0.33	0.15	−0.32	6.93	3.91	1.60	2.66	2.36	0.28	0.17
$COOCH_3$	0.37	0.45	0.33	0.15	−0.01	12.87	4.73	1.64	3.36	1.60	1.21	0.42
$COOC_2H_5$	0.37	0.45	0.33	0.15	0.51	17.47	5.95	1.64	4.41	0.62	2.33	0.88
NH_2	−0.16	−0.66	0.02	−0.68	−1.23	5.42	2.78	1.35	1.97	−0.36	−3.85	−0.12
NCH_3	−0.30	−0.84	−0.11	−0.74	−0.47	10.33	3.53	1.35	3.08	−2.03	−3.29	−0.18
$N(CH_3)_2$	−0.15	−0.83	0.10	−0.92	0.18	15.55	3.53	1.35	3.08	−1.97	−2.76	0.46
NHC_4H_9	−0.34	−0.51	−0.28	−0.25	1.45	24.26	6.88	1.35	4.87	−4.18	0.46	−0.11
$N(C_2H_5)_2$	−0.23	−0.90	0.01	−0.91	1.18	24.85	4.83	1.35	4.39	−3.76	−1.37	0.66
NHC_6H_5	−0.12	−0.40	−0.02	−0.38	1.37	30.04	4.53	1.35	5.95	−3.30	0.53	0.82
$NHCOCH_3$	0.21	0.00	0.28	−0.26	−0.97	14.93	5.09	1.35	3.61	0.23	−0.27	1.54
$NHCONH_2$	−0.03	−0.24	0.04	−0.28	−1.30	13.72	5.06	1.35	3.61	−0.74	−1.11	0.84
OH	0.12	−0.37	0.29	−0.64	−0.67	2.85	2.74	1.35	1.93	0.96	−3.02	0.54
OCF_3	0.38	0.35	0.38	0.00	1.04	7.86	4.57	1.35	3.61	1.25	0.71	1.04
OCH_3	0.12	−0.27	0.26	−0.51	−0.02	7.87	3.98	1.35	3.07	0.06	−1.57	0.85
OC_2H_5	0.10	−0.24	0.22	−0.44	0.38	12.47	4.80	1.35	3.36	−0.57	−0.78	0.88
$OCH(CH_3)_2$	0.10	−0.25	0.22	−0.45	1.05	17.06	6.05	1.35	4.42	−1.62	0.37	1.31
OC_4H_9	0.10	−0.32	0.25	−0.55	1.55	21.66	6.86	1.35	4.79	−2.40	0.97	1.62
$OCH(CH_3)_2$	0.10	−0.45	0.30	−0.72	0.36	17.06	4.80	1.35	4.10	−1.33	−0.85	1.53
OC_6H_5	0.25	−0.03	0.34	−0.35	2.08	27.68	4.51	1.35	5.89	−1.64	1.63	1.74
SH	0.25	0.15	0.28	−0.11	0.39	9.22	3.47	1.70	2.33	1.47	−0.31	−0.48
SCF_3	0.40	0.50	0.35	0.18	1.44	13.81	4.89	1.70	3.94	1.16	2.11	0.17
SCH_3	0.15	0.00	0.20	−0.18	0.61	13.82	4.30	1.70	3.26	0.17	0.15	−0.28
SO_2NH_2	0.46	0.57	0.41	0.19	−1.82	12.28	4.02	2.04	3.05	3.04	1.08	−0.04

bulk and a greater tendency to interact via dispersion forces. A compilation of commonly used parameters for aromatic substituents is shown in Table 5.2.

5.3.4 Biological relevance

Recently, the relevance of several statistical correlations on enzyme inhibitors have been supported by computer modeling in cases where the solid-state structure of the enzymes have been determined (cf. equation (5.25)). For example, binding with substituents in certain positions correlated with hydrophobicity (π) whereas in other positions with molar refractivity (MR). The significance of the π terms in the correlation equations could be rationalized by van der Waals contacts with hydrophobic regions, where desolvation is the major driving force. On the other hand, correlations of substituents with MR appeared in polar regions of the protein where binding mainly involves dispersion forces. This means that it is possible not only to retrospectively correlate the data and predict more active congeners but also to gain mechanistic information on the nature of the interactions between the ligand/substrate and the receptor/enzyme.

5.4 APPLICATIONS OF HANSCH EQUATIONS

5.4.1 Hydrophobic and steric factors

A wide range of biological activities has been correlated with linear free energy-related parameters and a selection of examples will be given to show some of the information that can be obtained. For simple *in vitro* systems, e.g. enzyme inhibition data, simpler and more accurate relationships may be derived than for more complex biological systems, which involve a combination of transport, distribution and receptor-interaction phenomena.

Protein binding is a non-specific interaction to hydrophobic areas of serum proteins and linear relationships between $\log K$ (binding constant) and $\log P$ has indeed been found. Equation (5.12) shows the relationship for binding of sulfony-lurea derivatives to bovine serum albumin (BSA) and the small (0.33) regression coefficient indicates binding of an only partly desolvated compound.

$$\log K = 0.33 \log P + 0.24\ \mathrm{pK_a} + 1.48$$
$$n = 15, \quad r^2 = 0.90, \quad s = 0.090 \tag{5.12}$$

In concordance with the Meyer-Overton findings, the narcotic effect on tadpoles of a set of structurally diverse compounds was simply explained by the lipophilicity according to equation (5.13), which supports a non-specific interaction. In this case, the regression coefficient is close to unity, which is in line with a complete accumulation of the molecules in a lipophilic bioenvironment similar to that in octanol.

$$\log\left(\frac{1}{C}\right) = 0.94 \log P + 0.87$$
$$n = 51, \quad r^2 = 0.94 \tag{5.13}$$

(5.1)   **(5.2)**

The muscarinic effect of a series of *meta*-substituted benzyltrimethylammonium derivatives (**5.1**) investigated on isolated rat jejunum could be modeled by equation (5.14), which indicates binding of the *meta*-substituent X into a lipophilic pocket (large regression coefficient for the hydrophobic parameter π) of limited size (negative coefficient for the STERIMOL parameter B_5).

$$\log\left(\frac{1}{ED}\right) = 1.30\pi - 0.41\,B_5 + 5.68$$

$$n = 10, \quad r^2 = 0.90, \quad s = 0.186$$

(5.14)

The displacement of the benzodiazepine [^{3}H]flunitrazepam from bovine brain membranes of a series of quinolinones (**5.2**) was significantly correlated to steric and hydrophobic parameters, however for different positions, according to equation (5.15). The positive coefficient of Taft's steric constant for the *ortho*-positions ($E_S(2,6)$) might indicate a required co-planar arrangement of the phenyl ring during the receptor binding, which is abolished by too much bulk in these positions. However, lipophilic (and large) groups are favorable in other positions and the intermediate size of the π coefficient reflects a partial desolvation during the hydrophobic interaction of the *meta*-substituents ($\pi(3,5)$).

$$\log\left(\frac{1}{IC_{50}}\right) = 0.481\,E_S(2,6) + 0.606\pi(3,5) + 4.81$$

$$n = 20, \quad r^2 = 0.76, \quad s = 0.278$$

(5.15)

5.4.2   Influence of electronic and other factors

The *in vivo* activity of a series of 17 tricyclic antipsychotics (**5.3**) related to octoclothepin (X = Cl) have been correlated with the electronic and steric parameters of the X substituent according to equation (5.16).

$$\log\left(\frac{1}{ED_{50}}\right) = 0.698\,\sigma_p + 0.347\,E_S + 0.0458\,MV - 0.00059\,MV^2 + 0.297$$

$$n = 17, \quad r^2 = 0.93, \quad s = 0.128$$

(5.16)

An electron-withdrawing X group will enhance the activity as shown by the positive value of the coefficient for σ_p. The parabolic dependence on MV indicate that a too large X group could be detrimental for the activity by steric interference

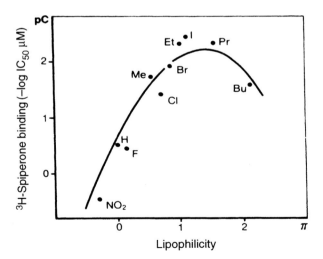

(5.3)   **(5.4)**

but smaller substituents interact favorably with the dopamine receptor, which is believed to mediate the antipsychotic activity. The latter aspect is also supported by the positive coefficient of E_S. In this case, the lipophilic parameters π and π^2 were not significantly involved.

The influence of the aromatic substituent X in a series of 12-mono-substituted potential antipsychotic salicylamides (**5.4**) on their ability to displace [³H]spiperone from the dopamine D_2 receptors *in vitro* has been investigated (Figure 5.2). The parabolic dependence on lipophilicity is clear from equation (5.17), which indicates that a limited size of the substituent X can be tolerated by the dopamine D_2 receptor since transportation effects should be negligible in this type of assay.

$$\log\left(\frac{1}{IC_{50}}\right) = 1.28\pi - 0.518\pi^2 - 0.692\sigma_{\mathrm{m}} + 1.495$$

$$n = 12, \quad r^2 = 0.94, \quad s = 0.399$$

(5.17)

The fungicidal activity against *Cladosporium cucumerinum* of a series of arylethyn-sulfones (**5.5**) could be explained by electronic, lipophilic and steric descriptors in

Figure 5.2 Relationship between the inhibition of [³H]spiperone binding and lipophilicity (π) of the 3-substituent (X) of 6-methoxysalicylamides (**5.4**). Reproduced with permission of the American Chemical Society.

equation (5.18). A favorable correlation was obtained with σ^-, which is based on ionization of substituted phenols in water and used for correlation of reactions having an electron-rich reaction center in conjugation with electron with drawing substituents. The correlation with this electronic substituent with a positive coefficient (ρ value) argues for a nucleophilic attack on the triple bond to be of importance for the biological action.

$$pC = 1.10\sigma^- + 0.84\pi - 0.07\pi^2 + 2.10\,E_S + 4.17$$
$$n = 25, \quad r^2 = 0.89, \quad s = 0.248 \tag{5.18}$$

5.4.3   Ionization constants

The acidity of the phenolic group in the antipsychotic 6-methoxysalicylamides (**5.6**) has been considered to be of importance for the biological activity. To better understand, the effects of the substituents on the acidity a number of models with steric and electronic descriptors were investigated. The most significant regression equation (5.19) was obtained with a σ parameter for the *ortho*-substituent X and the modified Taft parameter E^c for the *para*-substituent Y. The regression coefficient of σ_0 is in accordance with the well-known stabilization of anionic forms by electron withdrawing *ortho*-substituents. The steric effect induced by the *para*-substituent can be rationalized by the influence on the conformation of the methoxy substituent. A more perpendicular orientation of the methoxy group inflicted by a more bulky Y substituent could lead to a weakening of the $OH-O=C$ hydrogen bond, an effect which increases the acidity of the phenol.

$$pK_{a1} = -1.66\sigma_0 - 1.36\,E_p^c + 7.98$$
$$n = 9, \quad r^2 = 0.92, \quad s = 0.37 \tag{5.19}$$

5.4.4   Predictions from equations

A series of substituted benzamides (**5.7**) of the clebopride ($4 = NH_2, 5 = Cl, 6 = H$) type containing both phenols ($n = 12$) and non-phenols ($n = 10$) with substituents in the 3-, 4-, and 5-positions were treated in a Hansch analysis. The indicator variable I_{OH} is set to unity for phenols and zero for non-phenols (cf. example on PLS analysis of benzamides with pyrrolidine side chains in Section 5.5). The affinity for the [^{3}H]spiperone binding site could be modeled by a small number of substituents describing electronic properties, e.g. Swain and Lupton resonance parameters for the substituent in the 4-position ($\Re_4$) and the sum for the 3- and 5-substituents ($\Re_{(3+5)}$) as shown in equation (5.20).

(5.5)   (5.6)

$$\log\left(\frac{1}{IC_{50}}\right) = -1.75\,\Re_4 - 3.69\,\Re_{(3+5)} + 0.80\,I_{OH} + 0.04 \tag{5.20}$$

$$n = 22, \quad r^2 = 0.82, \quad s = 0.321, \quad F = 27.1$$

The equation (5.20) could be used to predict that compound (**5.8**) should have an IC_{50} value of 0.45 nM, i.e. ten-fold more active than the previous most potent member of the series. Synthesis and testing of this compound showed that the activity ($IC_{50} = 0.36$ nM) conformed with the predicted value to a degree we had not dare to expect. Figure 5.3 shows the new potent benzamide (**5.8**) included in the regression equation (5.21). Notably, the regression coefficients are virtually unchanged compared to equation (5.20), which is in accordance with the good prediction.

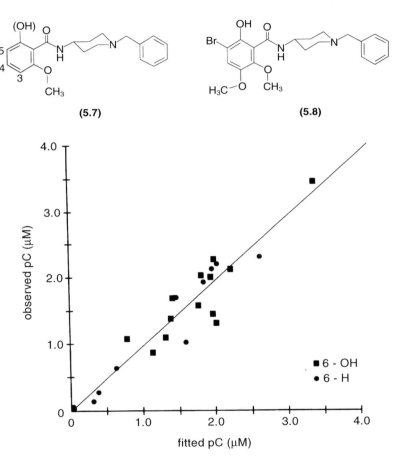

(**5.7**)   (**5.8**)

$\supset$und pC (log $1/IC_{50}$; µM)   values for [^{3}H]spiperone binding shown as a function of ata calculated according to the equation (5.21):

$$\log\left(\frac{1}{IC_{50}}\right) = -1.76\,\Re_4 - 3.75\,\Re_{(3+5)} + 0.81\,I_{OH} + 0.02 \tag{5.21}$$

$$n = 23, \quad r^2 = 0.87, \quad s = 0.313, \quad F = 41.8$$

It should be emphasized, however, that extrapolation outside the data set most often leads to large differences between predicted and found values, since the original model does not necessarily take the descriptors properly into account. In this case, we had included all the substituents used in the original test set, but the combinations of substituents were different in the predicted compound.

5.4.5   Blood–brain barrier penetration

As mentioned in Section 5.2.1, the optimal $\log P$ for penetration of the BBB is around 2.1 for a wide range of compounds. In a study aiming for centrally acting histamine H_2 antagonists, the physico-chemical properties of importance for the brain penetration was investigated in detail by Young and co-workers. A good correlation was found between the logarithms of the equilibrium brain/blood concentration ratios in the rat and the partition parameter $\Delta \log P$ (equation (5.22)) but not for $\log P$ in octanol (equation (5.23)).

$$\log\left(\frac{C_{\mathrm{brain}}}{C_{\mathrm{blood}}}\right) = -0.604\,\Delta \log P + 1.23$$
$$n = 6, \quad r^2 = 0.96, \quad s = 0.249$$
(5.22)

$$\log\left(\frac{C_{\mathrm{brain}}}{C_{\mathrm{blood}}}\right) = 0.150 \log P_{\mathrm{oct}} - 0.96$$
$$n = 6, \quad r^2 = 0.026, \quad s = 1.241$$
(5.23)

Seiler introduced the $\Delta \log P$ parameter, as the difference between the octanol/water and cyclohexane/water $\log P$ values, which is related to the overall hydrogen-bonding capacity of a compound by equation (5.24).

$$\Delta \log P = \log P_{\mathrm{oct}} - \log P_{\mathrm{cyh}} = \Sigma I_{\mathrm{H}} - 0.16$$
$$n = 195, \quad r^2 = 0.94, \quad s = 0.333$$
(5.24)

where I_{H} is the hydrogen-bonding ability for a given substituent. The larger the I_{H} value the more prone a substituent is to donate or accept a hydrogen bond, e.g. 2.60 for Ar–OH, 1.18 for Ar–NH_2, 0.45 for –NO_2, 0.31 for C=O, and 0.11 for ether –O–. Thus, the BBB penetration can be increased by lowering the overall hydrogen-bonding ability of a compound by, for example, encouraging intra-molecular hydrogen bonding, shielding with non-polar groups and by making less polar prodrugs. The principles could be utilized in the design of potent histamine H_2 antagonists, which readily cross the BBB, such as zolantidine (**5.9**) with a $\Delta \log P$ of 1.69 and a $\log P_{\mathrm{oct}}$ of 5.41.

5.4.6   Relations to molecular modeling

In a classical paper from the Hansch and Langridge groups (1982), the QSAR models for papain hydrolysis of phenyl hippurates (**5.10**) were compared with X-ray crystallography-based molecular modeling. Papain is a cystein protease

(5.9)   (5.10)

which hydrolyzes a number of esters, amides and peptides. A QSAR with the equation (5.25) was derived for a set of substituted phenyl hippurates.

$$\log\frac{1}{K_m} = 0.57\sigma + 1.03\pi'_3 + 0.61\ MR_4 + 3.80$$

$$n = 25, \quad r^2 = 0.82, \quad s = 0.208$$

(5.25)

where σ refers to substituents in any positions, MR_4 (scaled with 0.1 to be comparable with the other parameters) for the *para*-substituents and π'_3 indicates that only π for the most hydrophobic group in the *meta*-position is considered significant. The latter parameter makes mechanistic sense, since substituents that are hydrophobic ($\pi > 0$) partition into the enzyme, whereas those with negative values cause a rotation around the phenyl ring to place the less hydrophilic hydrogen onto the enzyme while the X-substituent is oriented into the aqueous phase. The term MR_4 cannot be replaced with π, which indicates that the *para*-substituent does not contact a lipophilic surface. On the other hand, the most lipophilic *meta*-substituent is making a hydrophobic interaction with complete desolvation as indicated by the correlation coefficient (1.03).

The solid-state structure has been determined for an enzyme–inhibitor complex between (benzyloxycarbonyl->L-phenylalanyl->L-alanylmethylene-papain, ZPA-papain), which allows for a proper orientation of the phenyl hippurates in the active site. The derived model was used to validate the QSAR equation (5.25) and indeed all terms could be shown to accommodate the modeling data. Thus, the 4-substituents collide with a highly polar amide moiety in Gln-142 and remain exposed to solvent. The hydrophobic *meta*-substituent is completely buried (desolvated) within a shallow hydrophobic pocket, whereas the other *meta*-position is oriented into the solvent as shown in Figure 5.4.

5.5 PATTERN RECOGNITION

5.5.1 PCR and PLS methods

In some cases where a structure–activity model is to be derived there are more variables, i.e. characteristics of the structures under investigation, than there are compounds. In such instances, traditional methods such as MLR (see previous Section 5.2) cannot be used since there are more unknown variables than available equations (one equation for each compound in the test set). This situation is especially true for the 3D-QSAR models (see Section 5.6) where the number of variables typically exceeds the number of compounds by a factor of a 100. Pattern

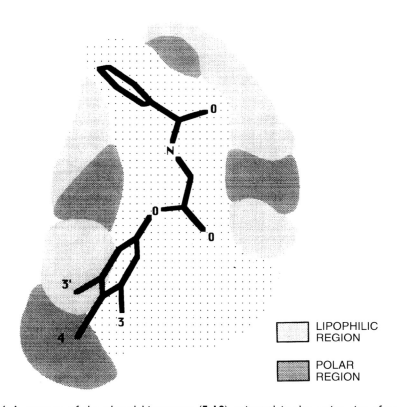

Figure 5.4 A cartoon of the phenyl hippurates (**5.10**) oriented in the active site of papain. The different shadings indicating hydrophobic and polar regions have been adopted by Magnus Jendbro according to the original modeling work by Hansch, Langridge and co-workers.

recognition methods, such as PLS (Partial least squares projections to latent structures), PCR (Principal component regression) and PCA (Principal component analysis), can be used to analyze these kinds of problems. All three methods contract (reduce) the original description of each molecule into a few descriptive dimensions, so-called principal components (PCs). Thus, these methods re-express the original matrix of data (X) for the compounds under investigation as a mean vector (X_m) plus the product of a score matrix T and a loading matrix P' (Figure 5.5). The scores, where each investigated compound has a computed set of score values, give the best summary of X and can be seen as the underlying factors of the studied system. Furthermore, the scores are, using the method described above, linear combinations of the original variables (equation (5.26)).

$$t_1 = C_1V_1 + C_2V_2 + C_3V_3 + \ldots + C_nV_n \tag{5.26}$$

where C_n are the weighting constants (loadings), V_n the original variables and t_1 is the first score value for a molecule (see Figure 5.5).

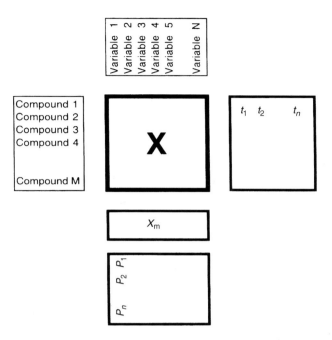

Figure 5.5 Schematic representation of the deconvolution of the structural descriptor matrix X into a score vector T ($t_1, t_2, \ldots, t_n$) and a loading vector P' ($P_1, P_2, \ldots, P_n$).

How are the principal components then calculated? Starting from the description of the investigated compounds (the mean centered data matrix X; see below for further explanation) the first PC is computed with the objective to explain as much information as possible in matrix X. This gives rise to the first score vector t_1 and the first row vector P'_1. The information contained in the first PC is then subtracted from the matrix X by subtracting the $t_1 P'_1$ matrix from X. A second PC with the same objective as that of the first PC, i.e. to explain as much information as possible in the new, updated matrix X is then calculated and so on for additional PCs. A mathematical consequence of the way the PCs are computed makes each PC orthogonal (independent) to all other PCs and that the first PC (PC1) contains the largest part of explained variance (information content) in the data. Subsequent PCs contain decreasingly smaller amounts of explained variance. It is desirable to first center the data matrix by subtracting the mean value of each column from the respective column (mean centering of the data matrix). Otherwise, the first PC will contain no interesting structural information but will instead represent a vector from origo to the point represented by the mean values.

How many components should then be calculated (extracted), i.e. used to describe the properties of the investigated compounds? Certainly one should only extract relevant information and stop when the amount of noise becomes too large in a calculated component. The term 'extracted' is mostly used in the literature instead of 'calculated', when dealing with PCs. A cross-validation (CV) procedure described by Wold (1979) is used to determine the stoppage point.

In CV, a portion of the data is left out, a PC is extracted and a model is created with the remaining data. The left out data are then predicted by the model. As long as the prediction of the left out data becomes better, the extracted component is judged to be significant and is kept in the model. When the prediction of the left out data does not improve any more, the extraction of components is stopped and the resulting model is based on the previously extracted significant components.

There is a fundamental difference between PLS and PCR in deriving the PCs. The PCR is composed of two steps. In the first step, a PCA is applied to the description of the structures (the X matrix; see Figure 5.5) and a relevant number of PCs are extracted. These PCs are then, in a second step, correlated against the biological activity using MLR. In PLS, a correlation between the chemical descriptors (variables) and biological activity (or other properties) is obtained where PLS uses the available biological information (biological activity) during the extraction of PCs. Thus, PLS tries to derive PCs that explain as much as possible of the biological information while PCR in the first step, the PCA, tries to explain as much as possible of the structural description of the molecules and then, in the second step, uses the derived PCs to derive a good model with respect to the measured activities. This means that the PCs from PLS and PCR differ from each other. Since PLS is targeted at explaining the activities this also means that PLS usually produces somewhat better QSARs compared with PCR. Some of the advantages of using PLS/PCR compared with multiple regression techniques are the following:

1   The number of compounds in the analysis can be significantly smaller than the number of variables used.
2   There are no collinearities between final variables since PLS/PCR is PC based, which means that addition of relevant variables will improve the relationship.
3   The original data set of chemical descriptor may contain 'missing data', i.e. a number of variables have not been assigned a value for some reason and are missing. The PLS/PCR tolerates a certain number of such data depending on the distribution in the data matrix X.

All evidence suggest that PLS gives at least as good relationships (predictions) as other linear regression techniques and sometimes much better.

5.5.2 Application of PLS

Partial least squares has been used by Norinder and Högberg to study the QSAR between the *in vitro* affinity to [^{3}H]spiperone binding sites of mono- and disubstituted benzamides (**5.11**) with a large number of physico-chemical descrip-

(5.11)

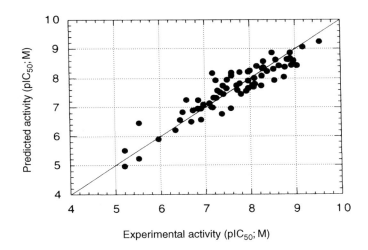

Figure 5.6 Plot of predicted vs. experimental [^{3}H]spiperone displacing activity (pIC$_{50}$; M) of substituted salicylamides (**5.11**). The QSAR was made with the PLS method as described in Section 5.5.

tors for size, lipophilicity and electronic characteristics. Each of the 3- and 5-substituents were described by the original physico-chemical parameters ($\sigma_m, \sigma_p, \Im, \Re, \pi, MR, L, B_1$ and B_5 in Table 5.1) and the corresponding squared values. Since only two choices exist for position $2(R_2 = H, OH)$ a so-called indicator variable (I_2) was used. This variable can assume two values; $I_2 = 0$ for $R_2 = H$ and $I_2 = 1$ for $R_2 = OH$. A similar indicator variable (I_S) was also used to represent the stereochemistry of the side chain (I_S; $R = -1$, $S = 1$, racemate $= 0$). In total, 38 variables were used to describe each compound.

The PLS analysis resulted in 4 PCs which explained 86% of the variance (information) in binding affinity (see Figure 5.6). The analysis pointed out the major importance of size, lipophilicity and electronic properties of the 3-substituent as well as a (*S*)-configuration of the side chain.

5.6 3D-QSAR METHODOLOGIES

5.6.1 Methods and strategy

Structure–activity relationships of traditional type, e.g. Hansch analysis or pattern recognition methods as discussed above, usually do not take the 3D structures of the investigated compounds into account in an explicit manner. Instead, they use substituent parameters and indicator variables to describe the structural variations.

Today it is well recognized that, at the molecular level, the interactions that produce an observed biological effect are usually non-covalent and that such steric and electrostatic interactions can account for many of the observed molecular properties. Extensions to the traditional QSAR approaches have been developed which explicitly uses the 3D geometry of the structures during the development of a QSAR model. These new technologies, commonly referred to as 3D-QSAR methodologies, include approaches such as the HASL method (Doweyko 1988), REMOTEDISC (Ghose *et al.* 1989) and GRID/GOLPE (Cruciani and Watson 1994). The presently most used technique, CoMFA (Comparative Molecular Field Analysis), was developed by Cramer and co-workers (Cramer *et al.* 1988).

The following steps have to be considered when trying to develop a 3D-QSAR model:

1   Identification of active conformation(s)
2   Alignment rule
3   3D-grid construction
4   Calculation of field values
5   Selection of training set compounds
6   PLS analysis
7   Interpretation of results (contour maps)
8   Predictions of new compounds.

One of the most fundamental problems when trying to develop a good and predictive 3D-QSAR model is the identification of the bioactive conformation(s) (cf. the detailed discussion in Chapter 4) of the investigated compounds and how to align them (steps 1 and 2). This becomes especially critical when one is dealing with a set of structurally diverse compounds. Considerable effort has been devoted to investigate and develop better protocols for alignment of compounds (see Norinder 1998 for a recent review). There are several available methods, such as SEAL, Catalyst and DISCO, by which atoms or molecular properties are super-imposed onto a reference compound or a set of reference compounds (Section 5.6.2). Fitting the interaction fields of the investigated compounds onto the corresponding fields of a reference compound (field fitting, see Section 5.6.3) as well as experimental geometries from X-ray crystallography (see Section 5.6.4) can also be used for alignment purposes. However, for flexible molecules there is usually not one unique 'best' way of identifying bioactive conformations and super-imposing the geometries. Attempts have been made to device iterative schemes where a number of conformations and alignments are investigated in order to find a self-consistent 3D-QSAR model. Examples of such programs are COMPASS (Jain *et al.* 1994) and TDQ (Norinder 1996). However, in the end the researcher must in most cases decide which superimpositioning scheme to use for the 3D-QSAR model. If a predictive model can be successfully be developed, then this may serve as an indication that the choice of alignment scheme was a reasonable one.

Once the choice of molecular alignments and conformations is made, then a 3D-grid box is spanned around the molecules under investigation. The box is filled with grid points (see Figure 5.7) with an internal distance of usually between 1 and 3 Å (step 3).

A probe atom with, in the cases used here as examples (see below), the van der Waals properties of a sp^3 carbon and a charge of $+1$ is placed at each grid point and two forces (interactions) related to steric and charge interactions are calculated for each molecule (step 4). Thus, all the computed values become a 'fingerprint' for each molecule. All values are stored in a large data matrix (see Figure 5.5) where each

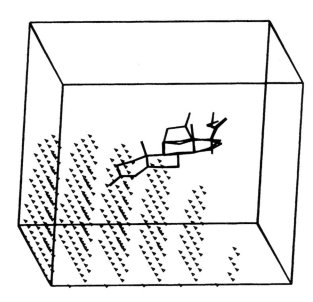

Figure 5.7 The 3D box, with partially depicted grid points, used in the 3D-QSAR example in Section 5.6. Steroids I and II are shown with hydrogens omitted for clarity.

row is related to a compound. Each of the two sets of calculated forces (steric and electrostatic, respectively) are usually referred to as a field. Thus, in this example we have a steric field and an electrostatic field. To delineate the relationship between biological activity and structural description, where the number of variables greatly exceeds the number of compounds, the method of PLS is used (step 6). Again, CV is used to judge the predictivity and statistical quality of the derived 3D-QSAR model by leaving a portion of the compounds out from the data set and building a model with the remaining compounds (see Section 5.5 for more details on CV). The results of a 3D-QSAR model are usually depicted as 3D contour maps. Each grid point in the box spanned around the molecules is associated with, in this case, two coefficients from the PLS analysis. One coefficient is related to the steric field and the other coefficient is related to the electrostatic field. Each of the two sets of coefficients are displayed as iso-contour maps (step 7). In most cases, it is not a trivial task to choose the appropriate iso-contour level in order to create a meaningful picture. The interpretation of contour maps are discussed in the following examples.

5.6.2 Application to steroids

Here the 3D-QSAR methodology will be exemplified by a data set of 30 steroids with affinities for human corticosteroid-binding globulins (CBG) where $\log(K)$ have been used as dependent variable which means that higher values indicate higher affinity for the receptor:

$$\log(K) = c_i E_{\text{steric}}(i) + c_j E_{\text{elec}}(j)$$

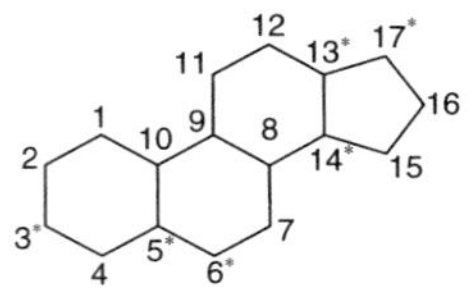

Figure 5.8 Steroid skeleton with atomic numbering system. Atoms indicated with an asterisk were used to superimpose steroids 2–30 in Figure 5.9 onto steroid 1.

where c_i and c_j are coefficients for grid points i and j, respectively, and E_{steric} and E_{elec} are the corresponding steric and electrostatic interaction energies.

This example is often used as a benchmark in 3D-QSAR investigations. Since all the compounds possess a common substructure, the steroid skeleton, the numbered atoms containing an asterisk in Figure 5.8 were used to superimpose compounds 2–30 onto compound 1 (see Figure 5.9).

Compounds 1–21 were used as training set (step 5) and the remaining steroids (22–30) were used as test set for which the affinities should be predicted by the derived 3D-QSAR model (step 8). A 3D-grid with an internal separation of $2.0\,\text{Å}$ between grid points was constructed based on the training set. Two fields (steric and electrostatic) were computed. Each steroid was defined by 1600 variables. A so-called leave-one-out CV scheme was used to determine the number of relevant PLS components. In a leave-one-out procedure one compound is held out and the remaining compounds are used to develop a model. The activity of the held-out compound is then predicted by the model. Then, all but the second molecule are used to generate a model that predicts the activity of the second molecule and so on. This procedure resulted in two significant PLS components. The Q^2 value was 0.791 for the training set and Q^2 is defined in equation (5.27).

$$Q^2 = 1.0 - \left\{ \frac{\Sigma(\text{Pred}_i - \text{Exp}_i)^2}{\Sigma(\text{Exp}_i - \text{Exp}_m)^2} \right\} \qquad (5.27)$$

where Pred_i and Exp_i are the predicted and experimental activity for the held-out compound i, respectively. Exp_m is the mean value of the experimental activities of all compounds and the summation in equation (5.27) runs over all compounds.

The R^2 value, where R^2 is defined analogous to Q^2, for the training set compounds was 0.901, and RMSE (root mean squared error) = 0.361. For the test set compounds 22–30, the RMSE was 0.471, which is a value indicating that the model has fair predictivity. The contours for the electrostatic interactions are here displayed as an iso-contour map depicting the 25% most influential areas (Figure 5.10).

How can these iso-contour maps (Figure 5.10) be interpreted and used for the development of new compounds? Let us examine the resulting negative electrostatic contour map (colored red) from the 3D-QSAR model based on steroids 1–21. The red region is mainly concentrated around (outside) the three position of the steroids. This location coincides very well with the keto moiety present in a large number of the steroids in the training set. Thus changing the electrostatic nature of this oxygen atom into something less negative or, to some extent, the direction of the oxygen atom, as in steroids 2, 3, 5, 9, 16, 17 and 18, will result in compounds with lower affinity. The steric iso-contour maps can be interpreted in a similar manner. Thus areas of positive steric regions (green), mainly centered around position 21 (the position at the end of the substituent on position 17) indicate that

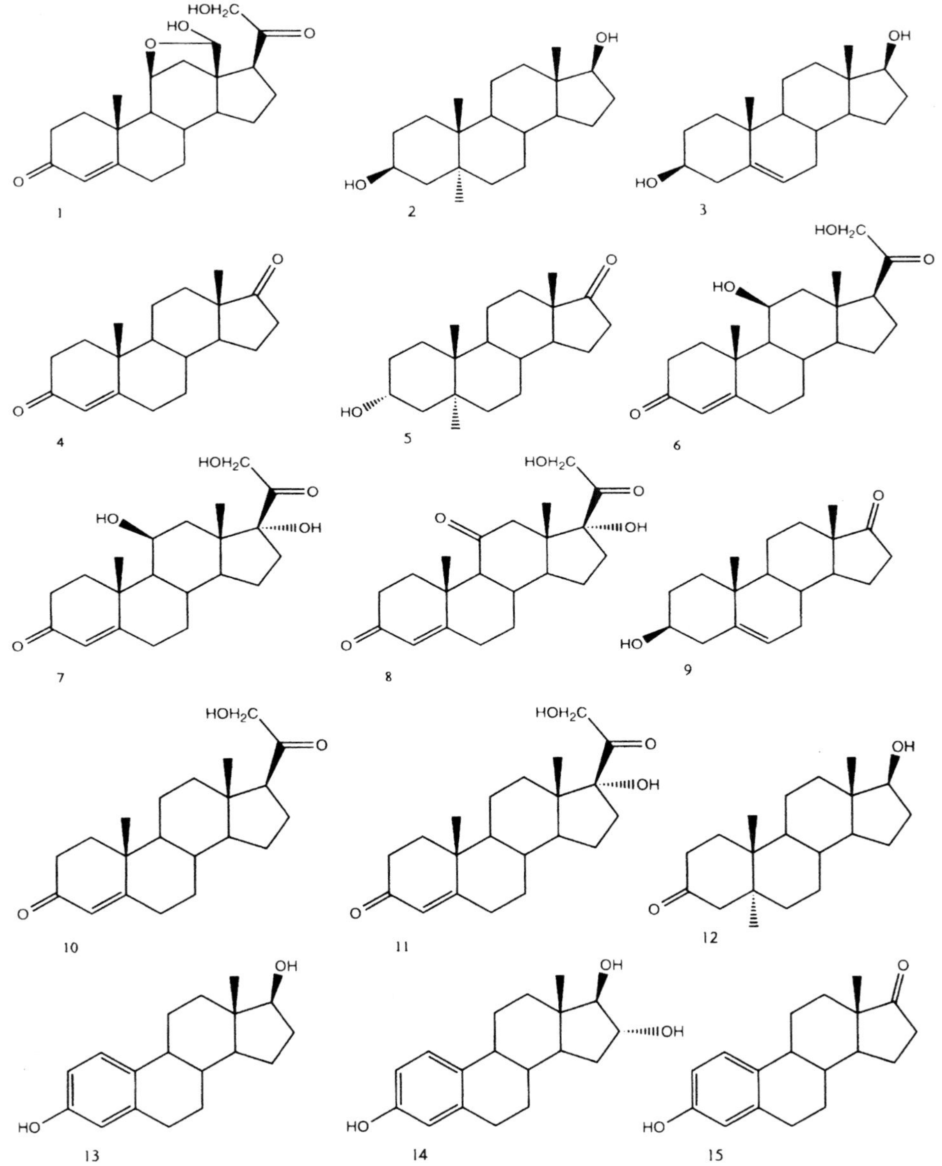

Figure 5.9 (Continued)

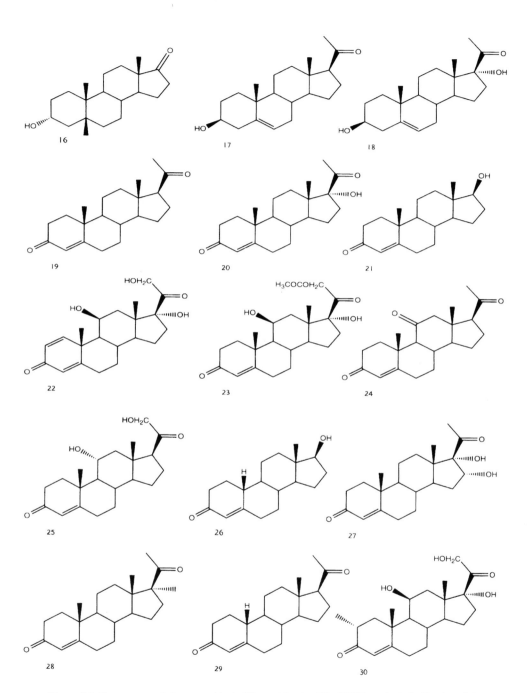

Figure 5.9 Structures of the steroids 1–30 used in the 3D-QSAR analysis in Section 5.6.

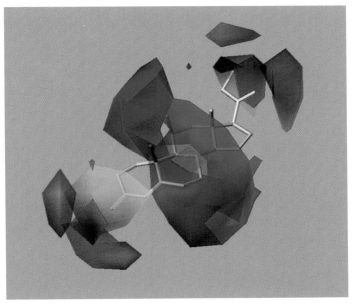

Figure 5.10 Contour map resulting from the 3D-QSAR analysis of steroids 1–21. The contours depict the 25% most influential areas (red and blue colors correspond to negative and positive electrostatic areas, respectively, while the yellow and green colors correspond to negative and positive steric areas). Steroids 1 and 11 are shown with hydrogens omitted for clarity.

it is favorable to have a substituent or substructure present close to these regions, e.g. steroids 6–8, 10–11 and 17–20.

5.6.3   Application to dopamine D₁ agonists

In the previous section, all compounds possessed a common substructure and the alignment procedure was not a problem. In this section, the investigated compounds are much more diverse (Figure 5.11) although they all contain two common elements that are of crucial importance for dopamine D_1 activity, namely an non-aromatic nitrogen atom and its electron lone-pair and an aromatic centre (Wilcox *et al.* 1998). With this knowledge at hand one may align the compounds in reasonable manner for a 3D-QSAR analysis. However, since we do not know the exact positions of the compounds, a field-fit method will be used here to construct the final alignments for the compounds in relation to a reference compound. The most potent compound is selected (in this case compound 6-Br-APB) as reference. The field-fit method operates in the following way. For each compound A:

1   The sum of the squared differences between the calculated interactions energies (steric and electrostatic) at each grid point for the investigated

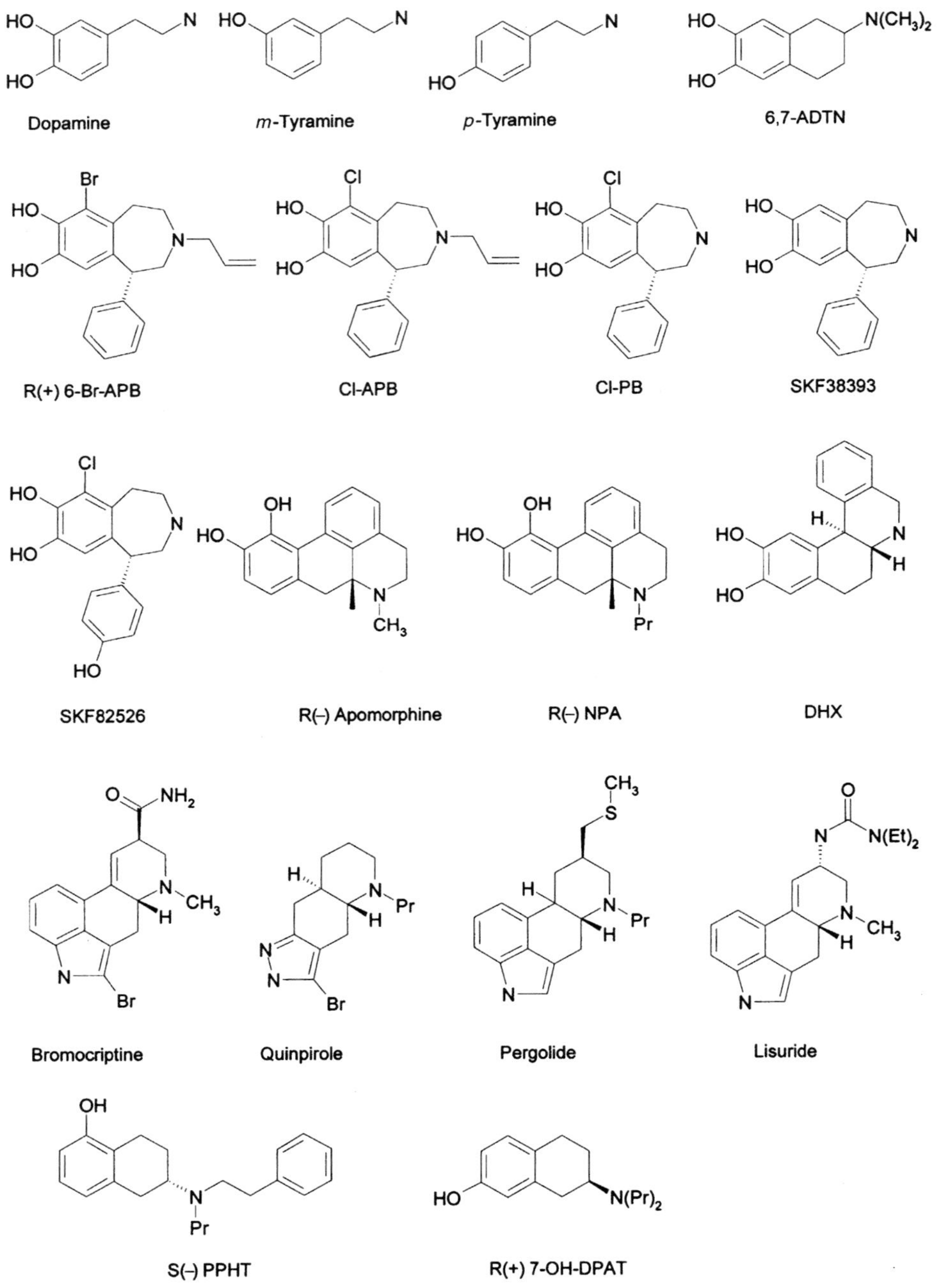

Figure 5.11 Structures of dopamine D$_1$ agonists.

compound and the corresponding values of the reference compound (in this case 6-Br-APB) are computed:

$$\text{Error}(A) = \sum_i (E_{\text{steric}}(i, \text{compound A}) - E_{\text{steric}}(i, \text{ref. compound}))^2$$
$$+ \sum_j (E_{\text{elec}}(j, \text{compound A}) - E_{\text{elec}}(j, \text{ref. compound}))^2$$

2   Compound A is then translated in the x, y and z directions of the co-ordinate system as well as rotated around the x-, y- and z-axis so that the computed error (Error(A)) is minimized.

3   The orientation of compound A corresponding to the smallest error is then used for the subsequent development of a 3D-QSAR model.

The training set of 12 compounds was selected using a field-based dissimilarity method. Thus, after the field-based alignment of the compounds, a PCA was performed on the two fields (steric and electrostatic) and 5 PCs were calculated. The 5-score values from the PCs of each compound were then used to select 12 compounds that were the farthest apart and, consequently, covered the field properties of the investigated data set most uniformly. The remaining 6-test set compounds were predicted with a RMSE value of 0.547, which implies that the derived model can predict new compounds with reasonable accuracy. The final 3D-QSAR model (4 PLS components) based on all 18 compounds had a good correlation ($Q^2 = 0.803, R^2 = 0.990, \text{RMSE} = 0.141$). In this example, the logarithm of the affinity to the D_1 receptor was used, i e. $- \log(K_i)$, which means that higher values indicate higher affinity to the receptor:

$$- \log(K_i) = c_i E_{\text{steric}}(i) + c_j E_{\text{elec}}(j)$$

Figure 5.12 shows the contour map of the model and indicates some interesting areas of importance. Negative electrostatic charge (colored red) in the region around the hydroxy groups, which can be attributed most certainly to hydrogen-bonding, favors high affinity. With respect to steric interactions, the area around the phenyl substituent of the 7-membered ring (colored green) is favorable with respect to steric bulk while the region around the non-aromatic nitrogen atom is not suited for placement of large substituents (yellow area).

5.6.4   Application to human rhinovirus

Sometimes uncertainties with respect to alignments of the ligands under investigation may be eliminated, or at least greatly reduced, with the existence of ligand/protein complexes. In this example of some antiviral compounds of human rhinovirus 14, there are complexes available from X-ray crystallography. Originally, Klebe and Abraham (1993) investigated this set of eight compounds using CoMFA.

The X-ray geometries of the ligands show that the four compounds (top set) with an 8 atom side-chain connecting the oxazole ring with the phenyl ring have opposite orientations compared with the four compounds (bottom set) with

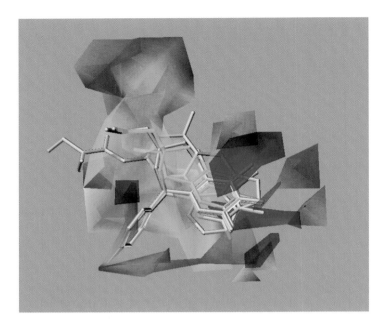

Figure 5.12 Contour map resulting from the 3D-QSAR analysis of the dopamine D_1 agonists. The contours depict the most influential areas (red and blue colors correspond to negative and positive electrostatic areas, respectively, while the yellow and green colors correspond to negative and positive steric areas). Compounds 6,7-ADTN, Cl-APB, Cl-PB, 6-Br-APB (bold structure), LISURIDE and SKF82526 are depicted.

a 6 atom side-chain connecting the corresponding rings (Figure 5.13). Without knowledge of the X-ray geometries of these compounds it is rather unlikely that the researcher would have suggested the X-ray orientation mode (Figure 5.14). Rather, the investigator would probably have tried to superimpose some 'obvious' pharmacophoric groups, such as the three rings present in all eight structures, or some maximum common substructure, such as the moiety consisting of the oxazoline ring and the pentyl phenyl ether group (Figure 5.15). In this example, we shall examine both choices of alignment and try to derive models for both orientations in order to see the consequences of our choices of alignment.

It is possible to derive a CoMFA model for the eight compounds based on the X-ray orientation mode (Figure 5.14) that have a $Q^2 = 0.515$ (leave-one-out validation, 3 PLS components) and an appreciable $R^2 = 0.997$. However, on the other hand, it is also possible to derive a corresponding model based on the maximum common substructure mode (Figure 5.15) of orientation: $Q^2 = 0.514$ (leave-one-out validation, 2 PLS components) and $R^2 = 0.976$. Furthermore, dividing the compounds into a training set and a test set each consisting of four compounds one can develop 2 CoMFA models that have quite reasonable predictive ability considering the very small training and test sets that we have available. The RMSE values for the test set are 1.260 and 1.280 for the X-ray and maximum common substructure orientation-mode, respectively. So, from this perspective, it

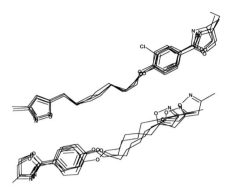

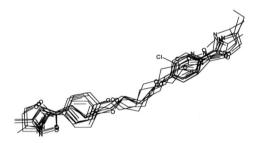

Figure 5.13 Structures of the human rhinovirus 14 antiviral compounds.

Figure 5.14 Superimpositioning of the human rhinovirus 14 antiviral compounds according to X-ray crystallography.

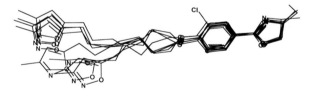

Figure 5.15 Superimpositioning of the human rhinovirus 14 antiviral compounds using atomistic substructure fitting.

would not have been possible either to distinguish between the two alternatives. Only further predictions of new compounds with failures and successes would, in the absence of the X-ray structure information, possibly give the researcher enough insight into the orientation problem to understand that the two series of compounds orient in opposite manners.

This example highlights that models can be developed with good statistical quality and predictive ability, but predict 'correct' observations from an 'incorrect' basis or understanding of the problem. Thus, it is important also to design experiments that challenges the models rather than confirms them.

5.6.5   Pros and cons

One advantage with 3D-QSAR studies is that the same protocol, i.e. steps 1–8 mentioned in Section 5.6.1, can be used for every new problem of interest. Also, the method can handle data sets to be investigated that contain structurally different compounds and predict new compounds of potential interest containing slightly different scaffolds than originally present among the training set compounds.

A limitation of the technique is that the models are only predictive in 3D space, which have been covered by substructures of sufficient variation. Thus, if in a certain position only a methyl-, ethyl-, and a propyl group have been present in the investigated structures, the 3D-QSAR model cannot make a reasonable prediction for the longer alkyl side chains such as butyl, pentyl and so on. A QSAR model based on some physico-chemical description, such as the 3D-dimensions of the side chain, can at least make a prediction for the latter group of substituents even though it represents an extrapolation. One interesting aspect of the contour maps of the derived 3D-QSAR models is their relationship to important drug–receptor interactions. Let us consider a case where the 3D-structure of the active site in a receptor is known. The compounds investigated in the study have been aligned by docking them into the active site. Each drug–receptor complex has then been brought into a common reference system by superimposing the receptor protein in each case onto each other. The compounds in their aligned orientations have then been taken out from the complex and used to derive a 3D-QSAR model. When the contour maps, which have the investigated compounds as reference, are overlaid on the drug–receptor complexes the spacial positioning of the most important parts of the contour maps may, in favorable cases, be located onto certain amino acid residues of the receptor protein. Then, this provides a description of the importance of various drug–receptor interactions. Thus, protein chemistry and biology, biotechnology, molecular modeling, conformational analysis, computational chemistry (to derive charges and other descriptors) and QSAR form a closely interlinked interdisciplinary entity in drug development.

5.7   EXPERIMENTAL DESIGN

5.7.1   Factorial design and principal properties

In order to be able to create a useful QSAR with good predictability, one wants the compounds included in the model (usually called the training set) to cover a large number of substituents and/or structural variation. However, at the same time it is desirable to keep the number of compounds to be synthesized and tested at a minimum. To obtain as much information as possible with a minimum of observations, one needs a protocol (experimental or statistical design) where the structures are varied in a carefully selected manner. Such protocols are found in the field of experimental design. There are several different types of protocols available but most often are factorial design schemes used due, in part, to the ease of evaluating these set-ups.

In a factorial design, each variable is assigned to a certain number of levels. A two level factorial design, which is most frequently used in chemistry, with four variables (a, b, c, d) involves 16 experiments (2^4). Each variable is designated a high level ($+$) and a low level ($-$) and the protocol is given in Table 5.3. The outcome of the 16 experiments may then be evaluated by some least squares method (like PLS).

Chemical substituents, however, are characterized by a large number of physico-chemical properties. To perform a complete two-level factorial or fractional factorial (reduced scheme) design using the original variables would involve too many compounds and be practically impossible. One method to circumvent this problem involves utilization of so called 'principal properties' (PPs), which are principal component derived variables (scores) from the original physico-chemical parameters. However, since the PPs are not continuous due to a limited number of substituents, it is not possible to construct a factorial design with exactly defined high and low levels. Instead, the substituents are classified according to the size and sign of their PPs. Table 5.2 shows the three first PPs of a number of aromatic substituents.

Practically, however, PPs are usually derived separately for each study since the objective is to span the chemical property space of the available substituents for the investigated compounds as effectively as possible. This will then, in turn, help to select compounds having a large variation in the mentioned physico-chemical property space. However, since different sets of substituents are used for different investigations and the purpose of each PCA is to explain as much information as possible with each PC the numerical values of the PPs may differ considerably between different PCAs (see Tables 5.2 and 5.4). Again, one must look upon these values (PPs) as guidance when selecting substituents having a large difference and variation in physico-chemical properties and pay less attention to the exact numerical values. The QSAR equations that are subsequently

Table 5.3 Experimental design protocol for a two level factorial design

#	a	b	c	d
1	+	+	+	+
2	−	+	+	+
3	+	−	+	+
4	−	−	+	+
5	+	+	−	+
6	−	+	−	+
7	+	−	−	+
8	−	−	−	+
9	+	+	+	−
10	−	+	+	−
11	+	−	+	−
12	−	−	+	−
13	+	+	−	−
14	−	+	−	−
15	+	−	−	−
16	−	−	−	−

derived from the selected compounds, the training set, are based on the original physico-chemical variables. However, an alternative approach is to use the PPs directly as variables in the QSAR model. In this case, all substituents must have the same framework. Thus, one must include all the substituents to be used both for the training set compounds as well as for those compounds that are to be predicted from the derived QSAR model in the PCA when one calculates the PPs, since the exact numerical values will be used in this case to derive the QSAR equation.

5.7.2 Applications of factorial design

An example of using PPs as design variables for some substituted benzamides (**5.11**) (the same compounds as used in Section 5.5) is given below. The number of different available 3- and 5-substituents were few (F, CN, NO_2, Cl, H, OH, NH_2, Me, OMe, I, Br, Et, n-Pr, n-Bu) in this retrospective study and the PPs derived for this subset are shown in Table 5.4.

The fractional factorial design protocol and the choice of substituents are listed in Table 5.5. The 16 selected compounds were then used to construct a model by which the activities of the remaining 54 benzamides were predicted using PLS.

Three significant components were extracted. They explained 89% of the variance in binding affinity. The model explained 61% of the variance of the biological data for the test set of 54 benzamides (**5.11**). Figure 5.16 shows a plot a calculated vs. experimental activities. The substituents R_3 and R_5 were described by a total of 38 variables, i.e. the parameters σ_m, σ_p, $\mathfrak{J}$, $\mathfrak{R}$, π, MR, L, B_1 and B_5 (cf. Table 5.1), the corresponding squared values and indicator values for R_2 and stereochemistry (*), in the same way as in the PLS analysis in Section 5.5. As can be seen in Figure 5.16, the small training set predicts the activity quite well and covers a large activity

Table 5.4 Design levels for the R_3- and R_5-substituents used in retrospective study of some benzamides (**5.11**)

Substituent	PP_1	PP_2	FDL^a
F	2.17	0.16	++
CN	0.79	2.51	
NO_2	0.56	2.94	
Cl	0.35	1.34	
H	2.46	−0.65	+−
OH	2.11	−1.46	
NH_2	1.92	−2.56	
Me	0.52	−0.62	
OMe	0.09	−1.29	
I	−1.34	1.65	−+
Br	−0.28	1.57	
Et	−1.30	−0.72	−−
n-Pr	−2.56	−0.69	
n-Bu	−4.38	−0.93	

Note
a FDL = factorial design levels.

Table 5.5 Experimental design protocol and selected substituents for the benzamides (**5.11**)[a]

#	R_3		R_5		R_2	R_3	R_5	R_2
	a	b	c	d	abcd			
1	+	+	+	+	+	Cl	Cl	OH
2	−	+	+	+	−	Br	OH	H
3	+	−	+	+	(−)	OMe	Cl	OH
4	−	−	+	+	+	Pr	Cl	OH
5	+	+	−	+	(−)	NO_2	Br	OH
6	−	+	−	+	(+)	Br	Br	H
7	+	−	−	+	+	Me	Br	OH
8	−	−	−	+	−	Et	Br	H
9	+	+	+	−	−	Br	OMe	H
10	−	+	+	−	(+)	I	OMe	H
11	+	−	+	−	(+)	Me	OMe	H
12	−	−	+	−	(−)	Pr	Me	OH
13	+	+	−	−	+	Cl	Pr	OH
14	−	+	−	−	(−)	Br	Et	OH
15	+	−	−	−	(−)	H	Et	OH
16	−	−	−	−	+	Et	Et	OH

Note
a   Parenthesis indicate a deviation from the protocol in selecting the substituent.

span which is quite frequently the consequence of the experimental design procedure. The model also predicts the remaining 54 benzamides in the test set reasonably well.

The second example is related to a set of β-adrenergic blockers analyzed by Norinder. The 101 compounds available are of the phenoxypropanolamine type (**5.12**) with a reasonable structural variation. Again a two-level PP fractional factorial design was applied and eight compounds were selected according to the design protocol (Table 5.8). Substituents R_1 and X were treated with indicator variables since only two choices existed in each case $\{R_1 = t\text{-Bu}(+1), i\text{-Pr}(-1);$ X = direct attached (-1), NH $(+1)\}$. Substituents R and R_2 were characterized by the following physico-chemical variables: R $= MR, L, B_1, B_5$; $R_2 = \mathfrak{F}, \mathfrak{R}, \pi, MR, L, B_1, B_5$. See Tables 5.6 and 5.7 for the calculated PPs of R- and R_2-substituents, respectively, using PCA on the original physico-chemical parameters.

The PLS analysis resulted in three significant components which explained 92% of the variance of the biological data in the training set (the eight compounds in Table 5.9). The model explained 67% of the variance of the biological data of the remaining 93 compounds. The model predicts compounds A–D (Table 5.9) to be interesting new structures with high activity.

If one uses all of the 101 available compounds to derive a model the same four compounds (A–D) are predicted by this model to possess high activity. Thus, not very much new information was added to the model by incorporating an additional 93 compounds, which is also indicated by the fact that the PLS regression coefficients were virtually the same for both models. This further proves the power of using experimental design to cover the available structural variation by a small number of compounds in a good manner.

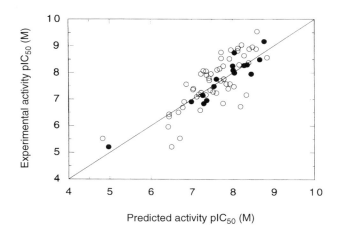

Figure 5.16 Plot of predicted vs. experimental [³H]spiperone displacing activity (pIC$_{50}$; M) of substituted salicylamides (**5.11**). The QSAR was made with the PLS method as described in Section 5.5. Solid and open circles represent the training set and test set compounds, respectively.

Table 5.6 Calculated score vectors for R-substituents in phenoxypropanolamine derivatives (**5.12**)

Substituent	PC_1	PC_2	FDL[a]
H	−4.06	−1.00	−−
$(CH_2)_2OCH_3$	−0.42	−0.73	
CH_2CHCH_2	−0.33	−0.36	
$(CH_2)_2CH_3$	−0.30	−0.23	
CH_3	−2.60	0.18	−+
CH_2CH_3	−1.24	−0.13	
$CH(CH_2)_2$	−0.95	−0.04	
$CH(CH_3)_2$	−0.52	0.98	
$(CH_2)_3CH_3$	1.02	−0.53	+−
$CH_2C_6H_5$	1.83	−0.46	
$(CH_2)_4CH_3$	2.15	−0.72	
$(CH_2)_5CH_3$	3.31	−0.93	
$CH_2CH(CH_3)_2$	0.45	2.99	++
C_6H_5	0.80	0.18	
$CH(CH_2)_4$	0.86	0.81	

Note
a   Designated factorial design levels.

Thus, using the predictive power of these models one can design compounds with the desired potency in a very efficient way, which is advantageous in the drug development phase. This also shows the usefulness of statistical design whereby structural variation is performed in an organized manner. These methods provide a broad basis for constructing a QSAR with good predictability, which makes it possible to keep the number of compounds to be synthesized and tested at a minimum.

Table 5.7 Calculated score vectors for R_2-substituents in phenoxypropanolamine derivatives (**5.12**)

Substituent	PC_1	PC_2	FDL^a
CH_2CHCH_2	−3.10	−0.92	− −
$(CH_2)_2CH_3$	−3.04	−0.76	
CH_2CH_3	−1.62	−1.09	
OCH_2CH_3	−1.20	−0.52	
SCH_3	−1.43	0.44	− +
I	−0.92	2.21	
$COCH_3$	0.00	1.28	
OCH_3	0.19	−0.79	+ −
CH_3	0.42	−1.52	
OH	2.46	−1.28	
H	2.58	−2.48	
Br	0.27	1.75	+ +
Cl	0.91	1.20	
NO_2	1.65	2.75	

Note
a Designated factorial design levels.

Table 5.8 Fractional factorial design protocol and choice of training set compounds of phenoxypropanolamine derivatives (**5.12**)

#	R			R_1^a	R_2		X^b	R	R_2
	a	b	c	abc	ab	bc		
1	+	+	+	+	+	(+)	$CH(CH_2)_4$	Cl
2	−	+	+	−	−	+	CH_2CH_3	CH_2CHCH_2
3	+	−	+	−	−	−	$(CH_2)_5CH_3$	CH_2CHCH_2
4	−	−	+	+	(+)	(−)	H	H
5	+	+	−	(−)	+	−	C_6H_5	Cl
6	−	+	−	+	−	−	$(CH_2)_2CH_3$	OCH_3
7	+	−	−	+	−	+	$(CH_2)_3CH_3$	CH_3
8	−	−	−	(−)	(+)	+	CH_2CHCH_2	CH_3

Parenthesis indicate a choice for the training set of a substituent which deviates from the protocol.
Notes
a R_1 has only two choices: $(+) = C(CH_3)_3$, $(−) = CH(CH_3)_2$.
b X has only two choices: $(+) = -NH-$, $(−) = (da)$.

Table 5.9 Predicted activities for compounds A–D of phenoxypropanolamine derivatives (**5.12**)

Compound	R	R_1	R_2	X	Pred. Act.
A	$(CH_2)_3CH_3$	$C(CH_3)_3$	I	NH	7.54
B	$(CH_2)_3CH_3$	$C(CH_3)_3$	Br	NH	7.42
C	$(CH_2)_3CH_3$	$C(CH_3)_3$	$(CH_2)_2CH_3$	NH	7.43
D	$(CH_2)_3CH_3$	$C(CH_3)_3$	Cl	NH	7.34

(5.12)

5.7.3   Combinatorial chemistry and experimental design

Nature manages to make large numbers of diverse compounds, e.g. proteins, from a limited number of building blocks. Combinatorial chemistry, mimicking this process, has evolved from producing large libraries of complex mixtures of oligomers to producing single drug-like molecules by parallel synthesis. Thus, it might be argued that combinatorial chemistry nowadays can eliminate synthetic capacity as a limitation in the lead finding and optimization once synthesis, isolation, analysis and data handling has effectively been automated. The number of possible endproducts increases rapidly with the number of building blocks and the number of positions varied which, in turn, effects resources like available physical space, time and money that all put limits to the size of a combinatorial library in practice (Figure 5.17).

A number of objectives may be envisaged for a combinatorial library:

1   Create a focused library of limited size with pure compounds for lead optimization.
2   Create a diverse library complementing already existing libraries in sparsely populated chemical space ('hole-filling').
3   Create a highly diverse general library, possibly as mixtures, for lead identification.

Experimental design can reinforce the utility and effectiveness of combinatorial chemistry to make it more than a 'numbers game'. The products obtained should have the properties needed for efficacy as well as for acceptable bioavailability and low toxicity. The reagents (building blocks) used should be available at reasonable costs and have the required reactivity for the specific chemistries. The following question comes to mind: Should one make the diversity selection in reagent chemical space or in the final product space (cf. Figure 5.17)? There are distinct advantages in diversity selection using the former set, namely, that, in most cases, the reagents are smaller compounds, both with respect to size and molecular weight, which permits easier, faster and more extensive characterization using quantum chemical calculations, should this be necessary. Besides, optimized diverse sets of reagents of different classes (Y_n, Z_m, etc.) can be utilized in reactions with several scaffolds (X) to produce many libraries, which makes the effectiveness even larger. Also, the combinatorial explosion is kept under control, i.e. there is no need for an explicit enumeration (creation) of all the compounds of the library, which simplifies the diversity analysis. Investigations have been performed that suggest that indeed it is possible to work in reagent (building block) chemical space without loosing diversity in product space.

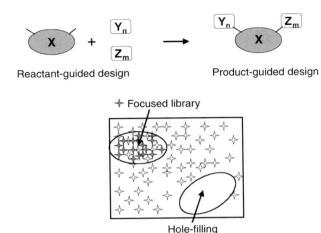

Figure 5.17 Combinatorial synthesis by reaction of scaffold X with reagents Y_n and Z_m to produce a library of n·m products by n + m reactions. Below is shown the product space with examples of a focused library and the need for hole-filling of the library.

Think of creating a library consisting of three building blocks A, B and C. Let us assume that we, at our disposal, have 50 different A:s, 100 different B:s and 75 different C:s. Evaluation in reagent space is rather trivial, but diversity selection in product space would involve calculating descriptors for $50 \times 100 \times 75 = 375\,000$ compounds. In many cases, the size of such a library would not permit us to perform adequate analysis using available software and techniques.

Thus, experimental design is as important as before considering the magnitude of compounds that potentially can be synthesized and tested by current high throughput techniques.

FURTHER READING

Box, G.E.P., Hunter, W.G. and Hunter, J.S. (1978) *Statistics for Experimenters*. New York: Wiley.

Cramer, R.D., Patterson, D.E. and Bunce, J.D. (1988) Comparative molecular field analysis (CoMFA). I. Effect of shape on binding of steroids to carrier proteins. *J. Am. Chem. Soc.*, **110**, 5959–5967.

Cruciani, G. and Watson, K.A. (1994) Comparative molecular field analysis using GRID force-field and GOLPE variable selection methods in a study of inhibitors of glycogen phosphorylase b. *J. Med. Chem.*, **37**, 2589–2601.

de Paulis, T., Hall, H., Kumar, Y., Rämsby, S., Ögren, S.O. and Högberg, T. (1990) Potential antipsychotic agents. 6. Synthesis and antidopaminergic properties of substituted N-(1-benzyl-4-piperidinyl)salicylamides and related compounds. QSAR based design of more active members. *Eur. J. Med. Chem.*, **25**, 507–517.

Dean, P.M. (1987) *Molecular foundations of drug–receptor interaction*. Cambridge: Cambridge University Press.

Doweyko, A.M. (1988) The hypothetical active site lattice. An approach to modelling sites from data on inhibitor molecules. *J. Med. Chem.*, **31**, 1396–1406.

Fauchére, J.L. (ed.) (1989) *QSAR: Quantitative Structure–Activity Relationships in Drug Design.* New York: Alan R. Liss.

Ghose, A., Crippen, G., Revankar, G., McKernan, P., Smee, D. and Robbins, R. (1989) Analysis of the in vitro activity of certain ribonucleosides against parainfluenza virus using a novel computer-aided molecular modeling procedure. *J. Med. Chem.*, **32**, 746–756.

Gupta, S.P. (1989) QSAR studies on drugs acting at the central nervous system. *Chem. Rev.*, **89**, 1765–1800.

Hansch, C. and Leo, A.J. (1979) *Substituent Constants for Correlation Analysis in Chemistry and Biology.* New York: Wiley.

Jain, A.N., Koile, K. and Chapman, D. (1994) Compass: Predicting biological activities from molecular surface properties. Performance comparisons on a steroid benchmark. *J. Med. Chem.*, **37**, 2315–2327.

Klebe, G. and Abraham, U. (1993) On the prediction of binding properties of drug molecules by comparative molecular field analysis. *J. Med. Chem.*, **36**, 70–80.

Kubinyi, H. (1993) QSAR: Hansch analysis and related approaches. In *Methods and Principles in Medicinal Chemistry*, edited by R. Mannhold., P. Krogsgaard-Larsen and H. Timmermann. Weinheim: VCH. This book provides an excellent overview of the different techniques in the field.

Kubinyi, H. (ed.) (1993) *3D QSAR in Drug Design. Theory, Methods and Applications.* Leiden: ESCOM Science Publishers.

Kubinyi, H. (ed.) (1998) *3D QSAR in Drug Design. Volume 2 Ligand–Protein Interactions and Molecular Similarity.* Dordrecht: Kluwer Academic Publishers.

Kubinyi, H. (ed.) (1998) *3D QSAR in Drug Design. Volume 3 Recent Advances.* Dordrecht: Kluwer Academic Publishers.

Linusson, A., Gottfries, J., Lindgren, F. and Wold, S. (2000) Statistical molecular design of building blocks for combinatorial chemistry. *J. Med. Chem.*, **43**, 1320–1328.

Nelson Smith, R., Hansch, C., Kim, K.H., Omiya, B., Fukumura, G., Dias Selassie, C., Jow, P.Y.C., Blaney, J.M. and Langridge, R. (1982) The use of crystallography, graphics, and quantitative structure–activity relationships in the analysis of the papain hydrolysis of X-phenyl hippurates. *Arch. Biochem. Biophys.*, **215**, 319–328.

Norinder, U. (1991) An experimental design based quantitative structure–activity relationship study on β-adrenergic blocking agents using PLS. *Drug. Des. Discov.*, **8**, 127–136.

Norinder, U. and Högberg, T. (1991) QSAR on substituted salicylamides using PLS with implementation of 3D-MEP descriptors. *Quant. Struct.-Act. Relat.*, **10**, 1–5.

Norinder, U. and Högberg, T. (1992) A quantitative structure–activity relationship for some dopamine D$_2$ antagonists of benzamide type. *Acta Pharm. Nord.*, **4**, 73–78.

Norinder, U. (1996) 3D-QSAR investigation of the tripos benchmark steroids and some protein-tyrosine kinase inhibitors of styrene type using the TDQ approach. *J. Chemometrics*, **10**, 533–545.

Norinder, U. (1998) Recent progress in CoMFA methodology and related techniques. *Perspec. Drug. Des. Dis.*, **12/14**, 25–39.

Perun, T.J. and Propst, C.L. (1989) *Computer-Aided Drug Design. Methods and Applications.* New York: Marcel Dekker.

Pliska, V., Testa, B. and van de Waterbeemd, H. (1996) Lipophilicity in drug action and toxicology. In *Methods and Principles in Medicinal Chemistry*, edited by R. Mannhold and H. Kubinyi. Weinheim: VCH.

Ramsden, C.A. (ed.) (1990) Quantitative drug design. In *Comprehensive Medicinal Chemistry*, Vol. 3, edited by C. Hansch, P. G. Sammes and J. B. Taylor. Oxford: Pergamon

Press. This book provides a full and critical account of all aspects of QSAR by experts in the field.

Tsai, R.-S., Carrupt, P.-A., Testa, B., Gaillard, P., El Tayar, N. and Högberg, T. (1993) Effects of solvation on the ionization and conformation of raclopride and other antidopaminergic 6-Methoxysalicylamides: insight into the pharmacophore. *J. Med. Chem.*, **36**, 196–204.

Wermuth, C.G. (ed.) (1993) *Trends in QSAR and Molecular Modeling 92*. Leiden: ESCOM Science Publishers.

Wilcox, R.E., Tseng, T., Brusniak, M.-Y. K., Ginsburg, B., Pearlman, R.S., Teeter, M., DuRand, Starr, C.S. and Neve, K.A. (1998) CoMFA-based prediction of agonist affinities at recombinant D1 vs. D2 dopamine receptors. *J. Med. Chem.*, **41**, 4385–4399.

Wold, S. (1979) Cross-validatory estimation of the number of components in factor and principal components models. *Technometrics*, **20**, 379–405.

Wold, S. and Dunn III, W.J. (1983) Multivariate quantitative structure–activity relationships (QSAR). Conditions for their applicability. *J. Chem. Inf. Comp. Sci.*, **23**, 6–13.

Young, R.C., Mitchell, R.C., Brown, T.H., Ganellin, C.R., Griffiths, R., Jones, M., Rana, K.K., Saunders, D., Smith, I.R., Sore, N.E. and Wilks, T.J. (1988) Development of a new physicochemical model for brain penetration and its application to the design of centrally acting H_2 receptor histamines antagonists. *J. Med. Chem.*, **31**, 656–671.

Chapter 6

Receptors: structure, function and pharmacology

Hans Bräuner-Osborne

6.1 INTRODUCTION

Communication between cells are mediated by compounds such as neurotransmitters and hormones which upon release will activate a receptor in the target cells. This communication is of pivotal importance for many physiological functions and dysfunction in cell communication pathways often have severe consequences. Many diseases are thus caused by dysfunction in the pathways and in these cases, drugs designed to act at the receptors have beneficial effects. Receptors are thus very important drug targets.

The definition of receptors is constantly debated, in particular as a consequence of the ever increasing knowledge of the many varying ways cells communicate. However, in general it is agreed that a receptor consist of one or more macromolecule(s) which upon binding of a signaling molecule will cause a cellular response. As will be exemplified in Chapters 9–11, the structural requirements for the signaling molecules are very specific. The receptor–ligand interaction has often been described by the 'lock and key' model. Likewise, the cellular responses mediated by the receptors are also very specific. Accordingly, receptors are classified by the signaling molecule, e.g. 'glutamate receptor', and by the signaling pathway. The latter is divided into four major superfamilies: (1) G-protein coupled receptors; (2) ligand-gated ion channels; (3) tyrosine kinase receptors; and (4) nuclear receptors. The structure and function of these families will be discussed in detail in this chapter.

The first receptors were cloned in the mid-eighties and since then hundreds of receptor genes have been identified. Based on the sequence of the human genome it is currently estimated that more than one thousand human receptors exist. Almost all receptors are heterogeneous, meaning that several receptor subtypes are activated by the same signaling molecule. One such example is the excitatory neurotransmitter glutamate for which 23 receptors have been cloned. As shown in Figure 6.1, the amino acid sequence of these receptors vary and the receptors form subgroups which, as will be discussed in Chapter 9, share pharmacology.

As can also be seen in Figure 6.1, the same signaling molecule can act on both G-protein coupled receptors and ligand-gated ion channels. One of the reasons for the heterogeneity is that it allows cells to be regulated in subtle ways. For example, whereas the fast synaptic action potential is initiated by glutamate receptors of the ligand-gated ion channel family, these receptors are by themselves regulated

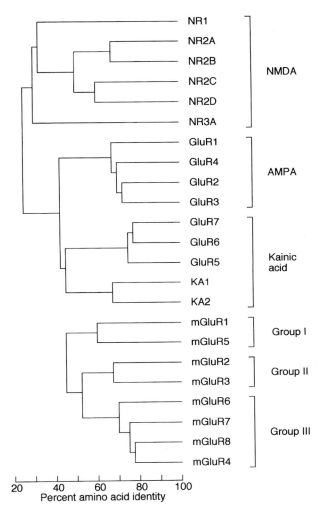

Figure 6.1 Phylogenetic tree showing the amino acid sequence identity between cloned mammalian glutamate receptors. The subgroups according to receptor pharmacology has been noted. The NMDA, AMPA, and kainic acid receptors belong to the superfamily of ligand-gated ion channels whereas the metabotropic glutamate receptors (mGluR1-8) belong to the superfamily of G-protein coupled receptors (Adapted from Bräuner-Osborne *et al.*, *J. Med. Chem.*, **43**, 2000, 2621).

by the slower and longer acting glutamate receptors from the G-protein coupled receptor family. The action on these two receptor families is actually shared by a number of other neurotransmitters such as GABA (Chapter 9), acetylcholine (Chapter 10) and serotonin (Chapter 11).

The receptor is activated upon release of the signaling molecule and it is evidently equally important to stop the signaling again. This is often achieved by transporters situated in the vicinity of the receptor which will remove the signaling molecule from the extracellular to the intracellular space, where it is either stored or degraded. Blockade of a transporter will cause an elevation of the extracellular concentration of the signaling molecule and thus lead to increased receptor activation, and transporters can thus be viewed as indirect receptor targets. However, in the strict sense, transporters are not receptors, but medicinal chemistry related to the two targets are very similar (Chapter 11). As a matter of fact, molecules acting on receptors, such as serotonin receptors, often also act on the transporters, such as serotonin transporters, which in some cases is desirable and in other cases not.

6.1.1   Synaptic processes and mechanisms

As exemplified above, receptors are located in a complex, integrated and highly interactive environment which can be further illustrated by the processes and mechanisms of synapses (Figure 6.2). The synapses are key elements in the inter-neuronal communication in the peripheral and the CNS. In the CNS, each neuron has been estimated to have synaptic contact with several thousand other neurones, making the structure and function of the CNS extremely complex.

Each neurotransmitter system operates through a characteristic set of synaptic processes and mechanisms (Figure 6.2), which are highly regulated and with distinct requirements for activation. In principle, each of these steps in the neurotransmission process is susceptible to specific pharmacological intervention. Synaptic functions may be facilitated by stimulation of the neurotransmitter biosynthesis, for example by administration of a biochemical precursor, or by inhibition of the metabolism/degradation pathway(s). There are several examples of therapeutically successful inhibitors of enzymes catalyzing intra- or extracellular metabolic processes. Similarly, it has been

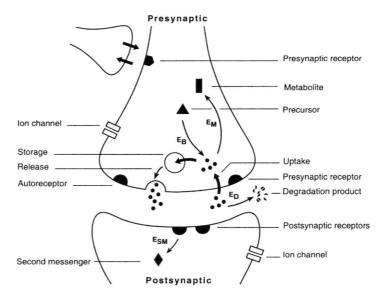

Figure 6.2 Generalized schematic illustration of processes and mechanisms associated with an axosomatic synapse in the CNS. E, enzymes; metabolic (E_M), biosynthetic (E_B), degradation (E_D), second messenger (E_{SM}); •, neurotransmitter.

shown in a number of cases that neurotransmitter function can be stimulated in a therapeutically beneficial manner via stimulation of neurotransmitter release or via inhibition of neuronal transport systems. It is possible that transport mechanisms in synaptic storage vesicles (Figure 6.2) also are potential sites for effective pharmacological intervention. Autoreceptors normally play a key role as a negative feedback mechanism regulating the release of certain neurotransmitters, making this class of presynaptic receptors therapeutically interesting.

Pharmacological stimulation or inhibition of the above mentioned synaptic mechanisms are, however, likely to affect the function of the entire neurotransmitter system. Activation of neurotransmitter receptors may, in principle, represent the most direct and selective approach to stimulation of a particular neurotransmitter system. Furthermore, activation of distinct subtypes of receptors operated by the neurotransmitter concerned may open up the prospect of highly selective pharmacological intervention. This principle may apply to pre- as well as post-synaptic receptors and also to ion channels associated with or independent of receptors (Figure 6.2) (see also Chapter 7).

Direct activation of receptors by full agonists may result in rapid receptor desensitization (insensitive to activation). Partial agonists are much less liable to induce receptor desensitization and may therefore be particularly interesting for neurotransmitter replacement therapies. Whereas desensitization may be a more or less pronounced problem associated with pharmacological or therapeutic use of receptor agonists, receptor antagonists, which in many cases have proved useful therapeutic agents, may inherently cause receptor supersensitivity. The presence of allosteric binding sites at certain receptor complexes, which may function as physiological modulatory mechanisms, offer unique prospects of selective and flexible pharmacological manipulation of the receptor complex concerned. Whilst some receptors are associated with ion channels, others are coupled to second messenger systems. Key steps in such enzyme-regulated multistep intracellular systems (Figure 6.2), which also include regulation of gene transcription by second messengers, represent targets for therapeutic interventions.

There is an urgent need for novel psycho-active drugs with specific actions. This demand is particularly pronounced in the field of neurologic disorders, where effective drugs in many cases are not yet available, even for symptomatic treatments. In terms of receptors, the heterogeneity offers opportunities to develop new ligands with increased receptor subtype selectivity and corresponding decrease of side effects. On the other hand, it simultaneously becomes a challenge to generate ligands with selectivity for one of many closely related targets.

6.2 RECEPTOR STRUCTURE AND FUNCTION

As mentioned in the previous section, receptors have been divided into four major superfamilies: (1) G-protein coupled receptors; (2) ligand-gated ion channels; (3) tyrosine kinase receptors; and (4) nuclear receptors. The three first receptor superfamilies are located in the cell membrane and the latter family is located intracellularly.

Our understanding of ligand–receptor interactions and receptor structure has increased dramatically during the last couple of years, not least due to the rapidly growing number of 3D-crystallographic structures that have been determined of either full receptors or isolated ligand binding domains. Thus today, structures of partial or full receptors of all four receptor superfamilies have been determined. Clearly, the information obtained from 3D-structures of ligand binding domains in the presence of ligands is very valuable for rational drug design. Likewise, knowledge of how the receptor functions can be used to e.g. design antagonists targeted to block mechanisms by which the receptor is activated (such as a conformational change).

6.2.1   G-protein coupled receptors

The G-protein coupled receptors (GPCRs) is the largest of the four superfamilies with some estimated 600 human receptor genes. A large fraction of these are taste and odor sensing receptors which are not of immediate interest for the pharmaceutical industry but are of interest, for e.g. fragrance manufactures. Nevertheless, it is estimated that 50% of all currently marketed drugs act on GPCRs and the superfamily thus remains a very important target for drug research. It is fascinating to note the very broad variety of signaling molecules which are able to act via this receptor superfamily, which, as already noted, include tastes and odors and for example light (photons), ions, monoamines, nucleotides, amino acids, peptides, proteins and pheromones.

The receptors are also referred to as 7TM receptors due to the seven α-helical transmembrane segments found in all GPCRs (Figure 6.3). The GPCRs have been further subdivided into family A, B and C based on their amino-acid sequence homology. Thus receptors within family A are closer related to each other than to receptors in family B and C etc. This grouping also coincides with the way ligands binds to the receptors. Thus, as illustrated in Figure 6.3, the endogenous signaling molecules bind to the transmembrane region of family A receptors (e.g. acetylcholine, histamine, dopamine and serotonin GPCRs, Chapters 10–11), to both the extracellular loops and amino-terminal domain of family B receptors (e.g. glucagon

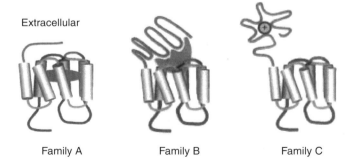

Extracellular

Family A   Family B   Family C

Figure 6.3 The three families of G-protein coupled receptors. All G-protein coupled receptors contain seven α-helical transmembrane segments and are thus also called 7TM receptors. Note the difference in agonist binding in the three families; family A receptors bind the agonist in the 7TM region, family B receptors bind the agonist in both the 7TM region and the extracellular amino-terminal domain, and family C receptors bind the agonist exclusively in the extracellular amino-terminal domain. (Adapted from Ji *et al.*, *J. Biol. Chem.*, **273**, 1998, 17299).

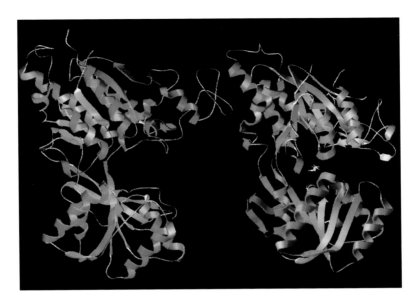

Figure 6.4 The structure of the amino-terminal domain of the metabotropic glutamate receptor subtype mGluR1 in the open inactive form (left) and the closed active form with glutamate bound in the cleft (right). The structures were generated using the program 'Swiss PDB viewer 3.5' with co-ordinates from Brookhaven Protein Data Base.

and secretin GPCRs) and exclusively to the extracellular amino-terminal domain of family C receptors (e.g. glutamate and GABA GPCRs, Chapter 9).

It is known that agonist binding to family A and presumably family B receptors cause a conformational change in the 7TM domain which is then relayed to the intracellular loops causing G-protein activation. It has yet to be fully elucidated how agonist binding to the amino-terminal domain of family C receptors is brought through the 7TM domains. The structure of the isolated amino-terminal domain of the glutamate GPCR subtype mGluR1 has recently been determined in the absence and presence of glutamate. As shown in Figure 6.4, the domain consist of two globular lobes forming an agonist-binding cleft which close upon agonist binding. The initial event in family C receptor activation is thus closure of the cleft which then induces a conformational change in the 7TM domain probably by direct interaction of the closed amino-terminal domain and the extra-cellular loops as illustrated in Figure 6.13.

As already eluted to above, the intracellular loops of GPCRs interact with G-proteins. The G-proteins are trimeric and consist of G_α, G_β and G_γ subunits (Figure 6.5). Receptor activation will cause an interaction of the receptor with the trimeric $G_{\alpha\beta\gamma}$-protein, catalyzing an exchange of GDP for GTP in the G_α subunit whereupon the G-protein disassociate into activated G_α and $G_{\beta\gamma}$ subunits. Both of these will then activate effector molecules such as adenylate cyclase and potassium channels (Figure 6.5). 27 G_α, 5 G_β and 13 G_γ subunits have been identified in humans and like the receptors they form groups based on the amino acid homology and the

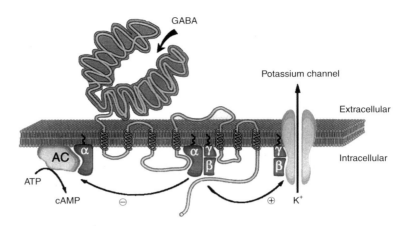

Figure 6.5 Cartoon of the family C receptor subtype GABA$_B$R1 interacting with an intracellular trimeric G-protein consisting of α-, β- and γ-subunits. Receptor activation will catalyze an exchange of GDP for GTP in the α-subunit which leads to activation and separation of the α- and $\beta\gamma$-subunits. Both of these will modulate downstream effectors such as inhibition of adenylate cyclase (AC) by the α-subunit and activation of potassium channels. (Adapted from Bettler *et al.*, *Curr. Opin. Neurobiol.*, **8**, 1998, 345).

effectors they interact with. For example, the G_α proteins have been divided into the $G_{\alpha i}$ class (inhibits adenylate cyclase), the $G_{\alpha s}$ class (stimulates adenylate cyclase), the $G_{\alpha q}$ class (stimulates phospholipase C) and the $G_{\alpha 12}$ class (function not fully elucidated). The GPCRs are classified as to which class of G_α proteins they mainly interact with. Thus, the GABA$_B$ receptor shown in Figure 6.5 would be termed a $G_{\alpha i}$ coupled receptor. Given that receptors prefer a given subset of G-proteins which again preferentiall interact with a given subset of effector proteins, each of which are differentially expressed in cell types, it is clear that the response of the same receptor might not be exactly the same in all cells. For example, the GABA$_B$ receptor shown in Figure 6.5 will inhibit adenylate cyclase and potassium channels in some cells but only inhibit adenylate cyclase in others where the potassium channel is not expressed. This will of course lead to different cellular effects in the two cell types which exemplifies the dynamic complexity of GPCR function and pharmacology.

6.2.2 Ligand-gated ion channel receptors

Ligand-gated ion channels can both be excitatory (e.g. ionotropic glutamate receptors and nicotinic acetylcholine receptors) or inhibitory (e.g. glycine and GABA$_A$ receptors) by conduction of Na^+/Ca^{2+} or Cl^- ions which will hypo- or hyperpolarize the cell, respectively (see Chapter 7 for further details). The nicotinic acetylcholine receptor, at the nerve-muscle synapse, is the best understood ligand-gated ion channel which upon acetylcholine binding allow as many as 10 000 potassium and sodium ions per millisecond to pass through the channel. As shown in Figure 6.6, the receptor consist of two acetylcholine binding α_1 subunits and three other subunits (β_1, γ and δ) which form a pentameric pore in the cell membrane.

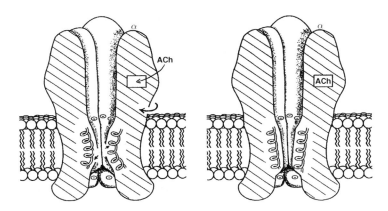

Figure 6.6 Cartoon based on the actual 3D-structure of the neuromuscular nicotinic acetylcholine receptor which belong to the superfamily of ligand gated ion channels.
The receptor consists of five subunits (two α-, one β-, one γ- and one δ-subunit).
The receptor is shown in the inactive form where the ion channel pore is closed by
five α-helices with kinks pointed toward the channel pore (left). Agonist binding to the α-
subunits cause a conformational change relayed to the pore lining α-helices
which rotate and thereby open the channel (right). (Adapted from Unwin, *J. Struc.
Biol.*, **121**, 1998, 181).

A low-resolution 3D-structure of the nicotinic acetylcholine receptor has been
determined in the absence and presence of acetylcholine (Figure 6.6). The pore
itself is lined with five α-helices, one from each of the five receptor subunits, which
have a kink in the middle of the membrane spanning part. This bend is the gate
of the receptor, which in the closed state points toward the channel. Agonist
binding to the extracellular part of the α-subunits induces local conformational
changes which are then relayed to the three additional subunits and ultimately
leads to rotation of the pore-lining α-helices whereby the channels opens.

Nicotinic acetylcholine receptors are also present in the central nervous system.
In humans, these receptors consist of at least one of five different acetylcholine
binding α-subunits (α_2–α_6) and at least one of three different β-subunits (β_2–β_4).
The number of subunit combinations forming functional receptors is thus stagger-
ing high, but in reality only certain combinations are present. Furthermore, even
fewer combinations such as the $\alpha_4\beta_2$ receptor, has therapeutic interest. Finally, a
homopentameric α_7-subunit receptor has been identified in humans which has
also been of significant therapeutic interest. Other ligand-gated ion channels also
consist of four or five homo- or heteromeric subunits.

High-resolution 3D structures of the isolated ligand binding domain of the
ionotropic glutamate receptor subunit GluR2 (Figure 6.1) has been determined.
As shown in Figure 6.7, the overall structure and function of this domain show
a striking resemblance with the domain from the mGluR1 receptor (Figure 6.4).
Thus, the agonist binding cleft of both GluR2 and mGluR1 close around
the agonist upon binding, which in the case of GluR2 is relayed to the membrane spanning part of the receptor causing an opening of the channel pore
(Figure 6.7).

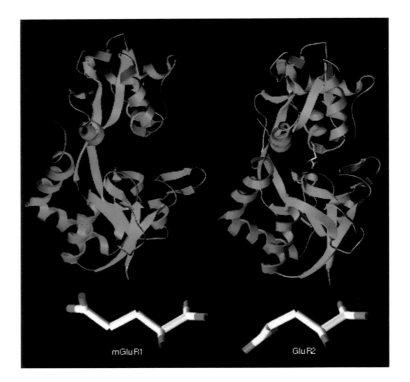

Figure 6.7 Structure of the agonist binding domain of the ionotropic glutamate receptor subtype GluR2 which belong to the superfamily of ligand gated ion channels. The domain is shown in the open inactive form (upper left) and the closed active form with glutamate bound in the cleft (upper right). Note the similarity in the overall structure of the agonist binding domain of GluR2 and mGluR1 (compare with Figure 6.4). The difference in conformation of glutamate bound to mGluR1 and GluR2 are also shown. The structures were generated using the program 'Swiss PDB viewer 3.5' with co-ordinates from Brookhaven Protein Data Base.

The conformation of glutamate bound to GluR2 and mGluR1 is quite different as illustrated in Figure 6.7. Such information is very valuable in the design of glutamate receptor subtype selective compounds which is discussed in further detail in Chapter 9.

6.2.3   Tyrosine kinase receptors

The tyrosine kinase receptors (TKR) have a large extracellular agonist binding domain, one transmembrane segment and an intracellular domain. The receptors can be divided into two groups: (1) those that contain the tyrosine kinase as an integral part of the intracellular domain; and (2) those that are associated with a Janus kinase (JAK). Examples of the former group are the insulin receptor family, the fibroblast growth factor (FGF) receptor family and examples of the latter are the cytokine receptor family such as the erythropoietin (EPO) receptor and the thrombopoietin (TPO) receptor. However, both groups share the same mechanism of activation: Upon agonist binding two intracellular kinases are brought together which will initiate autophosphorylation of tyrosine residues of the intracellular tyrosine kinase domain (Figure 6.8). This will attract other proteins (e.g. Shc/Grb2/Sos and STAT for the two receptor groups, respectively) which are also phosphorylated and this will initiate protein cascades which will ultimately lead to regulation of transcriptional factors (e.g. Elk-1, Figure 6.8) and thus regulation of genes involved in e.g. cell proliferation and differentiation. As described for the G-protein coupled receptors, all the proteins in the intracellular activation cascades are heterogeneous leading to individual responses (i.e. regulation of different subset of genes) in individual cell types.

Some of the receptors exist as monomers in the absence of agonist whereas other exist as covalently linked dimers (the insulin receptor family) or non-covalently linked dimers. In case of the monomers, the agonist will bring the two receptor subunits together by binding to both subunits simultaneously and thereby initiate

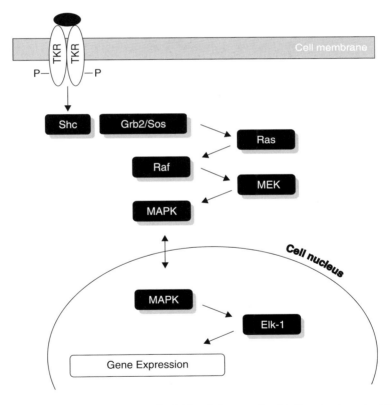

Figure 6.8 Cartoon of a protein cascade initiated by agonist binding to two tyrosine kinase receptors (TKR) causing autophosphorylation of the dimerized intracellular receptor domains. This cause activation of a cascade of intracellular proteins (abbreviated Shc, Grb2/Sos, Ras, Raf, MEK and MAPK), which ultimately leads to activation of transcription factors (e.g. Elk-1) and thus regulation of gene expression. (Adapted from Campbell *et al.*, *Oncogene*, **17**, 1998, 1395).

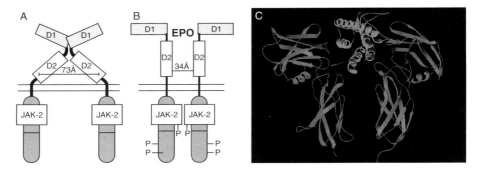

Figure 6.9 Cartoon of the activation mechanism of the EPO receptor which belong to the JAK/STAT receptor class of the superfamily of TKR: (A) The receptor is dimerized in the inactive conformation by interaction of amino acids which are similar to those involved in binding of EPO and the intracellular JAK kinases are kept too far apart to initiate autophosphorylation; (B) binding of EPO to the dimer interface tilts the structure and brings the JAK kinases in close proximity which initiates the autophosphorylation; and (C) the actual structure of EPO (in cyan) bound to the extracellular receptor domains of the EPO receptor (in green). (Adapted from Wilson *et al.*, *Curr. Opin. Struc. Biol.*, **9**, 1998, 696. The structure was generated using the program 'Swiss PDB viewer 3.5' with co-ordinates from Brookhaven Protein Data Base).

the autophosphorylation. In case of the preformed inactive dimers, agonist binding will cause a conformational change in the receptor, which brings the two intracellular kinases together and thus initiate the autophosphorylation. The best understood example in this regard is the EPO receptor of which the 3D-structure of the extracellular agonist binding domain has been determined in the absence and presence of EPO (Figure 6.9). In the absence of EPO, the domain is a dimer in which the ends are too far apart for the JAK's to reach each other. The EPO binds to the same amino acids on the receptor that forms the dimer interface and thereby tilts the two receptor subunits. This brings the JAK's close together and initiate the autophosphorylation (Figure 6.9).

6.2.4   Nuclear receptors

Nuclear receptors are cellular proteins and are thus not embedded in the membrane like the previously described receptors. In contrast to the membrane bound receptors, they bind small lipophilic hormones and function as ligand modulated transcription factors. The nuclear receptors have been classified according to the type of hormone they bind. Thereby, receptors have been divided into those which bind steroids (glucocorticoids, progestestins, mineralocorticoid androgens and estrogens) and steroid derivatives (vitamin D_3), non-steroids (thyroid hormone, retinoids, prostaglandins), and orphan receptors for which the physiological agonist has yet to be discovered. The receptor family is relatively small (~ 70 subtypes) of which the majority actually still belongs to the group of orphan receptors.

The nuclear receptors consist of a ligand binding domain and a DNA binding domain. Upon activation, the two receptors dimerize, as homo- or heterodimers, and bind to specific recognition sites on the DNA. Co-activators will then associate with the dimeric receptor and initiate transcription of the target gene(s). Each receptor recognize specific DNA sequences, also known as the hormone response elements, which are located upstream of the genes that are regulated.

A 3D high-resolution structures of both ligand and DNA binding domains have been determined. In drug research the main focus has been on the structures of the ligand binding domains which for several receptors have been determined in absence and presence of ligands. One such example is shown in Figure 6.10 which illustrate the mechanism of agonism and antagonism of the superfamily of nuclear receptors. The ligand binding site is a hydrophobic pocket in the center of the protein which in the absence of ligand is partially filled with hydrophobic residues from α-helix H11. Upon agonist binding, H11 is displaced by the agonist and α-helix H12 folds back over the binding pocket. The co-activators binds to and recognize residues in α-helices H3, H4 and H12, and agonist binding thus reposition H12 such that the co-activator binding motif is generated. This also explains how some antagonists work at the molecular level. The antagonist BMS614 is larger than the physiological hormone and thus pushes H12 away from the ligand binding pocket. In this way, H12 now occupies the space between H3 and H4 and thus prevent the co-activator from binding (Figure 6.10).

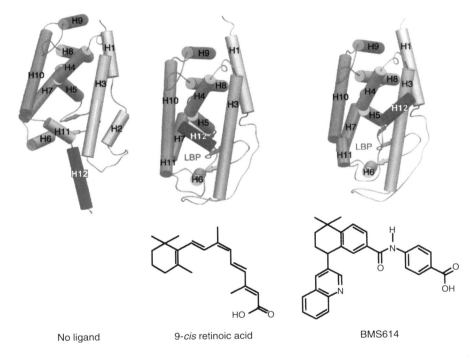

No ligand   9-*cis* retinoic acid   BMS614

Figure 6.10 Structures of nuclear retinoic acid receptors in the absence of ligand (left), binding the agonist 9-*cis* retinoic acid (middle) or the antagonist BMS614 (right) in the ligand binding pocket (LBP). Note the difference in location of α-helix H12 which is the key player in the activation mechanism (see text for further details). (From Bourguet *et al.*, *Trends Pharmacol. Sci.*, **21**, 2000, 381).

6.3   RECEPTOR PHARMACOLOGY

6.3.1   Recombinant vs. *in situ* assays

The last decade has had a profound impact on how receptor pharmacology is performed. As mentioned in the introduction, receptor cloning was initiated in the mid-eighties and today the majority of receptors have been cloned. Thus, it is now possible to determine the effect of ligands on individual receptor subtypes expressed in recombinant systems rather than a mixture of receptors in e.g. an organ. This is very useful given that receptor selectivity is a major goal in terms of decreasing side effects of drugs and development of useful pharmacological tools which can be used to elucidate the physiological function of individual receptor subtypes. Furthermore, recombinant assay systems allow one to assay cloned human receptors which is otherwise often not possible to obtain. Although most receptors are more than 95% identical between humans and rodents, there have been cases of drugs developed for rats rather than for humans due to the fact that the compounds were active on the rat receptor but not on the human receptor due to the small differences in primary amino acid sequence.

It should be noted that the use of organ and whole animal pharmacology is still required. As previously noted, the cellular effects of receptor activation depends on the intracellular contents of the proteins involved in e.g. the signaling cascades. These effects can only be determined when the receptor is situated in its natural environment rather than in a recombinant system. In most situations, both recombinant and *in situ* assays are thus used to fully evaluate the pharmacological profile of new ligands. Furthermore, once a compound with the desired selectivity profile has been identified in the recombinant assays, it is important to confirm that this compound has the predicted physiological effects in e.g. primary non-recombinant cell lines which express the receptor, in organs and/or in whole animals.

6.3.2   Binding vs. functional assays

Binding assays used to be the preferred choice of method for pharmacological evaluation which was mainly due to the ease of these assays compared to functional assays which generally required more steps than binding assays. However, several factors have changed this perception: (1) biotechnological functional assays have evolved profoundly and have decreased the number of assay steps and increased the throughput; (2) functional assay equipment has been automated; (3) ligand binding requires a high-affinity ligand which for many targets identified in genome projects simply does not exist; (4) binding assays are unable to discriminate between agonists and antagonists; and (5) binding assays will only identify compounds binding to the same site as the radioactively labeled tracer.

The Fluorometric Imaging Plate Reader (FLIPR^{TM}) illustrates this development towards functional assays. Cells transfected with a receptor coupled to increase in intracellular calcium levels (e.g. a $G_{\alpha q}$ coupled GPCR or a Ca^{2+} permeable ligand-gated ion channel) are loaded with the dye Fluo-3 which in itself is not fluorescent. However, as shown in Figure 6.11, the dye becomes fluorescent when exposed to Ca^{2+} in the cell in a concentration dependent manner. In this manner, ligand

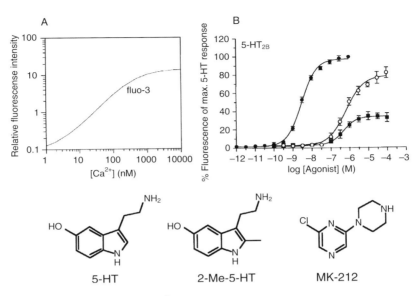

Figure 6.11 (A) Relation between Ca^{2+} concentration and relative fluorescence intensity of the fluorescent probe fluo-3. (B) The 5-HT$_{2B}$ receptor subtype belong to the superfamily of G-protein coupled receptors and are coupled to increase in inositol phosphates and intracellular Ca^{2+}. Cells expressing 5-HT$_{2B}$ receptors were loaded with fluo-3 and the fluorescence was determined upon exposure to the endogenous agonist 5-HT and the partial agonists 2-Me-5-HT and MK-212 on a FLIPR^{TM}. (Adapted from Jerman *et al.*, *Eur. J. Pharmacol.*, **414**, 2001, 23).

concentration–response curves can be generated on the FLIPR^{TM} very fast as it reads all wells of a 384-well tissue culture plate simultaneously. Many other functional assays along these lines have been developed in recent years.

6.3.3 Partial and full agonists

Agonists are characterized by two pharmacological parameters, potency and maximal response. The most common way of describing the potency is by measurement of the agonist concentration which elicit 50% of the compounds own maximal response (the EC$_{50}$ value). The maximal response is commonly described as per cent of the maximal response of the endogenous agonist. The maximal response is also often described as efficacy or intrinsic activity which were defined by Stephenson and Ariëns, respectively. Compounds, such as 2-Me-5-HT and MK-212 in Figure 6.11, which show a lower maximal response than the endogenous agonist 5-HT are termed partial agonists. The parameters potency and maximal response are independent of each other and on the same receptor it is thus possible to have e.g. a highly potent partial agonist and a low potent full agonist. Both parameters are important for drug research, and it is thus desirable to have a pharmacological assay system which is able to determine both the potency and maximal response of the tested ligands.

6.3.4   Antagonists

Antagonists do not activate the receptors but block the activity elicited by agonists and accordingly they are only characterized by the parameter affinity. The most common way of characterization of antagonists is by competition with an agonist (functional assay) or a radioactively labeled ligand (binding assay). In both cases, the antagonist concentration is increased and the agonist or radioligand, which are being displaced, are held at a constant concentration. It is then possible to determine the concentration of antagonist which inhibits the response/binding to 50% (the IC_{50} value). The IC_{50} value can then be transformed to affinity (K) by the Cheng–Prusoff equation.

Functional assay:

$$K = \frac{IC_{50}}{\left(1 + \frac{[\text{Agonist}]}{EC_{50}}\right)} \tag{6.1}$$

where [Agonist] is the agonist concentration and EC_{50} is for the agonist in the particular assay.

Binding assay:

$$K = \frac{IC_{50}}{\left(1 + \frac{[\text{Radioligand}]}{K_D}\right)} \tag{6.2}$$

Where [Radioligand] is the radioligand concentration and K_D is the affinity of the radioligand.

It is important to observe that the Cheng–Prusoff equation is only valid for competitive antagonists.

The Schild analysis is often used to determine whether an antagonist is competitive or non-competitive. In the Schild analysis, the antagonist concentration is kept constant while the agonist concentration is varied. For a competitive antagonist, this will cause a rightward parallel shift of the concentration–response curves without a reduction of the maximal response (Figure 6.12A). The degree of rightshifting is determined as the dose ratio (DR), which is the concentration of agonist giving a particular response in the presence of antagonist divided by the concentration of agonist that gives the same response in the absence of antagonist. Typically one will choose the EC_{50} values to calculate the DR. In the Schild analysis, the log $(DR - 1)$ is depicted as a function of the antagonist concentration (Figure 6.12B). When the slope of the curve equals 1 it is a sign of competitive antagonism and the affinity can then be determined by the intercept of the abscissa. When the slope is significantly different from 1 or the curve is not linear it is a sign of non-competitive antagonism which invalidates the Schild analysis.

As shown in the example in Figure 6.12, five concentration–response curves are generated to obtain one antagonist affinity determination and it can thus be seen that the Schild analysis is rather work intensive compared to e.g. the transformation by the Cheng–Prusoff equation where one inhibition curve generates one antagonist affinity determination. However, the latter cannot be used to determine whether an antagonist is competitive or non-competitive which is the advantage of the Schild analysis.

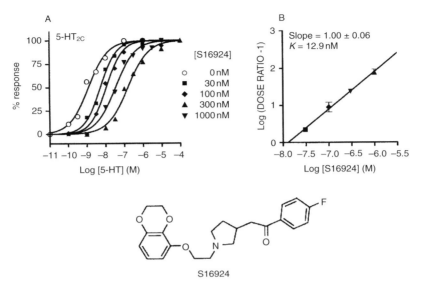

Figure 6.12 Schild analysis of the competitive antagonist S16924 on cells expressing the 5-HT$_{2C}$ receptor. (A) Concentration–response curves of the agonist 5-HT were generated in the presence of varying concentrations of S16924. Note the parallel right shift of the curves and the same level of maximum response; and (B) dose ratios are calculated and plotted as a function of the constant antagonist concentration generating a straight line with a slope of 1.00 ± 0.06. These results and the observations from (A) are in agreement with a competitive interaction and the antagonist affinity can thus be determined by the intercept of the abscissa; $K = 12.9$ nM. (Adapted from Cussac *et al.*, *Naunyn Schiedbergs Arch. Phamacol.*, **361**, 2000, 549).

When testing a series of structurally related antagonists one would thus often determine the nature of antagonism with the Schild analysis for a couple of representative compounds. If these are competitive antagonists, it would then be reasonable to assume that all compounds in the series are competitive and thus determine the affinity by use of the less work intensive Cheng–Prusoff equation.

6.3.5 Allosteric modulators

Allosteric modulators can both be stimulative or inhibitory (non-competitive antagonists) and typically these compounds bind outside the endogenous agonist binding site. This class of compounds modulate the effect of agonist and accordingly they show no activity in the absence of agonist. Well-known examples are the benzodiazepines which enhance the effect of GABA on GABA$_A$ receptors and PCP which inhibit the effect of glutamate on NMDA receptors (Chapter 9).

As noted in Section 6.3.4, the Schild analysis is very useful to discriminate between competitive and non-competitive antagonists, and an example of the latter is shown in Figure 6.13. The ligand CPCCOEt is a selective antagonist at the mGluR1 receptor, and the Schild analysis clearly demonstrate that the antagonism is non-competitive due to the depression of the maximal response (compare Figure 6.12A and 6.13).

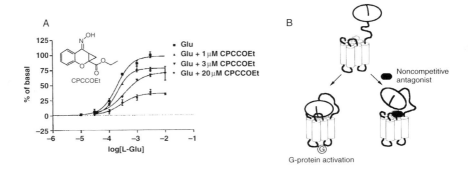

Figure 6.13 Schild analysis of the non-competitive antagonist CPCCOEt on cells expressing the metabotropic glutamate receptor subtype mGluR1: (A) Concentration–response curves of the agonist glutamate (Glu) were generated in the presence of varying concentrations of CPCCOEt. In contrast to the Schild analysis shown in Figure 6.12, a clear depression of the maximal response is seen with increasing antagonist concentrations. This shows that the antagonist is non-competitive; and (B) cartoon showing the interaction between the closed glutamate bound amino terminal domain of mGluR1and the seven transmembrane domain (lower left). Receptor mutagenesis studies have shown that CPCCOEt binds to the 7TM domain of mGluR1 and thus act by obstructing the intramolecular agonist-induced interaction (lower right). (Adapted from Litschig *et al., Mol. Pharmacol.,* **55**, 1999, 453 and Bräuner-Osborne *et al., J. Med. Chem.,* **43**, 2000, 2621).

As noted previously, glutamate binds to the large extracellular amino-terminal domain whereas CPCCOEt has been shown to bind to the extracellular part of the 7TM domain (Figure 6.13B). CPCCOEt thus blocks the intramolecular communication between the amino-terminal domain and the 7TM domain.

FURTHER READING

Bourguet, W., Germain, P. and Gronemeyer, H. (2000) Nuclear receptor ligand-binding domains: three-dimensional structures, molecular interactions and pharmacological implications. *Trends Pharmacol. Sci.,* **21**, 381–388.

Bräuner-Osborne, H., Egebjerg, J., Nielsen, E.Ø., Madsen, U. and Krogsgaard-Larsen, P. (2000) Ligands for glutamate receptors: design and therapeutic prospects. *J. Med. Chem.,* **43**, 2609–2645.

Egea, P.F., Klaholz, B.P. and Moras, D. (2000) Ligand–protein interactions in nuclear receptors of hormones. *FEBS Lett.,* **476**, 62–67.

Ji, T.H., Grossmann, M. and Ji, I. (1998) G-protein-coupled receptors. I. Diversity of receptor–ligand interactions. *J. Biol. Chem.,* **273**, 17299–17302.

Kenakin, T.P. (1997) *Pharmacologic analysis of drug–receptor interaction,* 3rd edition. London: Lippincott Williams & Wilkins.

Schlessinger, J. (2000) Cell signalling by receptor tyrosine kinases. *Cell,* **103**, 211–225.

Unwin, N. (1998) The nicotinic acetylcholine receptor of the *Torpedo* electric ray. *J. Struct. Biol.,* **121**, 181–190.

Wilson, I.A. and Jolliffe, L.K. (1999) The structure, organization, activation and plasticity of the erythropoietin receptor. *Curr. Opin. Struct. Biol.,* **9**, 696–704.

Chapter 7

Ion channels: structure, function and pharmacology

David J. Triggle

7.1 INTRODUCTION

7.1.1 Ion channels and cellular function

'*The grave's a fine and private place*', wrote the Elizabethan poet Andrew Marvel, but the cell is not. Ions moving through the ion channels of the cell's membranes are both an integral component of the music of life and a constant reminder of the cellular traffic that defines cellular excitability. Ion channels serve as one of the mechanisms through which cells respond to informational inputs. Under physiological conditions ion channels permit the orderly movement of ions across cellular membranes – both plasma membranes and the membranes of cellular organelles. Under pathological conditions ion channels generate disorderly ionic traffic and cellular death.

7.1.2 Ion channels as membrane effectors

Excitable cells respond to a variety of informational inputs, chemical and physical, including neurotransmitters, hormones, pheromones, heat, light and pressure. These informational inputs are coupled to cellular response through transduction systems that include enzyme activation, substrate internalization and ion channel opening and closing (Figure 7.1). Ion channels are one class of biological effectors. They function to permeate ions, including the physiological cations Na^+, K^+, Ca^{2+} and Mg^{2+} and the anion Cl^-, in response to diverse cell stimuli. The resultant ionic current may itself be the end consequence as in the maintenance of membrane potential or the discharge of potential in electric fish. More commonly, the ion current is coupled to other events, including the alteration of cellular sensitivity to other stimuli and the major generic processes of excitation–contraction coupling and stimulus–secretion coupling. In the latter examples, there is a dual function for calcium since it both carries current and serves as a cellular messenger coupling cell excitation to the calcium-dependent events of contraction and secretion.

The cell maintains a highly asymmetric distribution of ions across its membranes. Na^+, Ca^{2+} and Cl^- are maintained at low intracellular levels and K^+ at high intracellular level relative to the extracellular environment. Maintenance of this asymmetric distribution depends upon the selective permeability of cell membranes and the work of ionic pumps including Na^+, K^+-ATPase and Ca^{2+}-ATPase

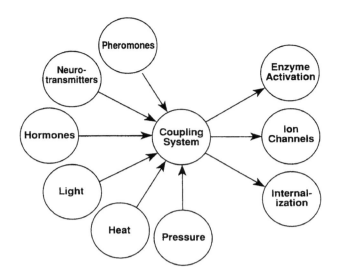

Figure 7.1 Ion channels as one of several mechanisms by which informational inputs are translated through intermediate coupling devices into cellular responses.

that maintain ionic gradients in the face of constant leakage and to restore these gradients subsequent to dissipation by channel activating stimuli.

The lipid bilayer of the cell is essentially impermeable to ions and ion channels (or an equivalent function) are therefore necessary components of cellular membranes and likely arose relatively early during cellular evolution. Uncontrolled movements of ions represent toxic or lethal stimuli and ion channels are, therefore, regulated species. The processes of channel regulation of opening and closing are thus critical to any understanding of the physiologic and pharmacologic control of channel activity.

7.1.3   Ion channels and ion distribution

The relationship between ion concentrations, membrane potential and ion chemical and electrical gradients is depicted in Figure 7.2. At a typical resting cellular potential of 70 mV (by convention negative interior) both electrical and concentration gradients combine to provide a net inward driving force for Na^+ entry of 120 mV. When the membrane potential is maintained at the equilibrium potential for Na^+ (positive interior) the inwardly directed concentration gradient is exactly balanced by the outwardly directed electrical gradient and there is no net movement of Na^+ ions. A representative comparison of the equilibrium potentials for Na^+, K^+, Ca^{2+} and Cl^- is presented in Table 7.1. Quite generally, the opening of Na^+ and Ca^{2+} channels will dissipate membrane potential – depolarize – to mediate cellular excitation. In contrast, opening of K^+ or Cl^- channels will maintain or elevate membrane potential – hyperpolarize – to mediate inhibitory responses. Conversely, the closing of K^+ or Cl^- channels will be disinhibitory in nature leading to cell excitation and the blockade of Na^+ or Ca^{2+} channels will prevent

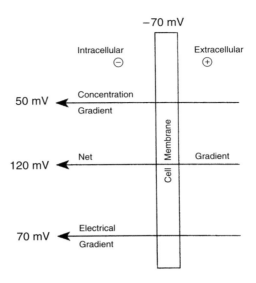

Figure 7.2 Ion movements across a cell membrane are determined by the net product of the concentration gradient and the electrical gradient. In the example where the net membrane potential is −70 mV both concentration and electrical gradients favor Na$^+$ entry into the cell. If the membrane potential is set at the equilibrium potential for Na$^+$, ~ +50 mV, then these gradients will balance and there will be no net movement of Na$^+$.

Table 7.1 Ionic concentrations and equilibrium potentials in excitable cells

Ion	[X]$_{ext}$ mM	[X]$_{int}$ mM	Equilibrium potential mV (approximate)
Na$^+$	145	12	+70
K$^+$	4	155	−90
Ca^{2+}	1.5	<10^{-4}	>+120
Cl$^-$	123	4	−90

depolarization and thus mediate inhibitory responses. When two or more ion channels open or close together the resultant membrane potential, and response, will represent the sum of these events.

There are very important implications to this elementary analysis of ion movements for the actions of drugs on ion channels. Drugs that open Na$^+$ or Ca^{2+} channels will tend to depolarize cells and to be excitatory in nature while drugs that open K$^+$ or Cl$^-$ channels will hyperpolarize cells and be inhibitory in nature. A similar, but opposing relationship, will apply to antagonists at these channels (Figure 7.3). However, the control of ion channels must not be viewed in isolation or as one channel at a time, but rather should be seen as linked events whereby channels are multiply involved in the control of cellular function. Thus, the influx of Ca^{2+} through Ca^{2+} channels – an excitatory event – can lead to the activation of Ca^{2+}-dependent K$^+$ channels – an inhibitory event. This is depicted in Figure 7.4

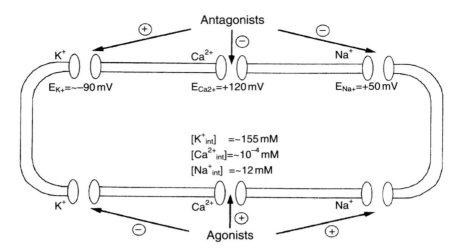

Figure 7.3 The equilibrium potentials for Na^+, K^+ and Ca^{2+} and the effects of drugs that open or close selectively these channels (see text for additional details). $(+)$ indicates excitatory event and $(-)$ indicates an inhibitory event.

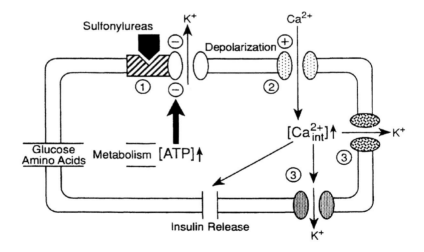

Figure 7.4 Ion channels frequently function in co-operation or sequentially. In this insulin-secreting β-cell of the pancreas ATP derived from metabolic input blocks K^+_{ATP} channels (1) thus depolarizing the cell. This K^+ channel is the target for the hypoglycemic sulfonylurea antidiabetic drugs that block the channel at a specific receptor site. Depolarization activates Ca^{2+} channels (2) that causes an influx of Ca^{2+} into the cell to stimulate the release of insulin. The elevation of intracellular Ca^{2+} also activates Ca^{2+}-dependent K^+ channels (3) that open to restore membrane potential. Thus, the net balance of electrical activity in the cell will be determined by the combined activities of the three types of ion channels.

where in an insulin-secreting pancreatic β-cell, there exist both ATP-sensitive K^+ channels and voltage-gated Ca^{2+} channels. When the ATP levels are elevated in response to rising glucose or amino acid concentrations post-feeding the K^+ channel closes: the resultant depolarization activates the voltage-gated Ca^{2+} channel and the resultant Ca^{2+} influx promotes insulin release. Subsequently, the activation of Ca^{2+}-sensitive K^+ channels serves to repolarize the cell.

7.1.4 Activation and inactivation of ion channels

The schematized depiction of impulse conduction in a nerve fiber indicates the association between different ionic processes and the different behavior of distinct ion channels (Figure 7.5). The depolarization of a nerve axon by a step depolarization results in the rapid activation of Na^+ channels to permit a fast inward and depolarizing current that is carried virtually exclusively by Na^+ ions and a later outward and repolarizing current carried by K^+ ions. Two important differential properties of ion channels are illustrated in Figure 7.5. Channels may open rapidly or slowly and they may stay open in response to a constant stimulus or they may open and close in a relatively transient manner. Thus, the rates and properties of activation and inactivation are important characteristics of ion channels and these differential properties are increasingly being linked to specific components of channel molecular structure. Figure 7.5 also illustrates the principle of the voltage clamp procedure whereby the application of a specific voltage step or 'clamp' permits the magnitudes, directions and kinetics of ion currents to be measured. This may be achieved at the macroscopic level where large number of channels

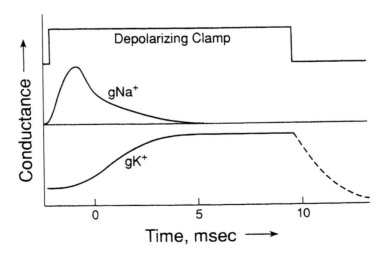

Figure 7.5 Schematic representation of Na^+ and K^+ conductance changes during the period of maintained depolarization ('depolarizing clamp'). The Na^+ conductance (gNa^+) activates and inactivates rapidly and the K^+(gK^+) conductance activates less rapidly and does not inactivate over the period of the clamp depicted.

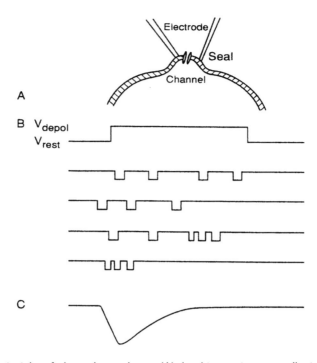

Figure 7.6 The principle of the voltage clamp: (A) In this version a small piece of membrane containing a single ion channel is clamped between two electrodes; (B) The opening and closing of single channels is observed as an all-or-none stochastic event and the sum of these events is depicted under (C).

are studied simultaneously (tissue or whole cell), with a few channels and even with single ion channels in patch-clamp techniques that study small patches of native or reconstituted membranes (Figure 7.6).

7.2   STRUCTURE AND FUNCTION OF ION CHANNELS

7.2.1   Ion channels as efficient and regulated species

Ion channels are discriminating cellular entities. Ion channels translocate ions on the basis of ion type – cations vs. anions – on the basis of ion charge – monovalent vs. divalent – and on the basis of ion size – Na^+ vs. K^+. Channels permeate ions very efficiently at rates $>10^7$ ion/sec, that approach diffusion-controlled limits. Enzymes and carriers operate generally at orders of magnitude lower efficiency. To charge a membrane of capacity $1\,\mu F/cm^2$ by $100\,mV$ requires the transfer of some 6000 ions per square micrometer and with a channel of conductance $20\,pS$ this can be accomplished in $0.5\,sec$. Because of this efficiency ion channels are frequently relatively minor components of excitable cells. Channels

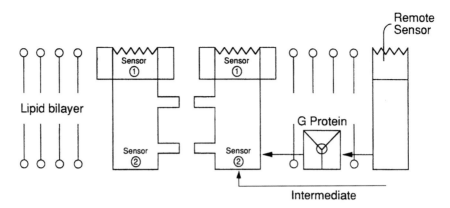

Figure 7.7 The fundamental architecture of ion channels depicting sensors (integral and remote), gates in the channel pore and both G protein and cytoplasmic routes for messenger modulation of the channel.

are also regulated species, regulated most frequently by changes in chemical or electrical potential, and hence must possess a certain minimal organization structure (Figure 7.7). It is helpful to regard ion channels through an analogy to allosteric enzymes, functioning to accelerate ion transit across an essentially impermeable membrane barrier, through changes in chemical or electrical potential recognized at sites distal to the channel pore itself.

7.2.2   The structure of ion channels

The structure of Figure 7.7 includes sensors that function as the regulatory components ('allosteric sites') and that are responsive to chemical or physical stimuli, gates that open and close in response to these stimuli, a pore through which ions pass and a 'selectivity filter' that confers upon the channel its ionic selectivity. In principle, the ionic selectivity of a channel may be mediated through two very different mechanisms. The channel may discriminate on the basis of ionic size through 'molecular sieving' or may discriminate through a process of selective ionic binding with components of the channel pore. There is increasing evidence that the latter is the dominant mechanism and that ions do bind with channel components during transit and, moreover, that ion channels have multiple ion binding sites and that multiple occupancy of these sites facilitates ion transit. The 2D representation of an ion channel depicted in Figure 7.7 was derived from indirect evidence obtained during a century of biophysical, largely electrophysiological, investigations. The essential validity of this model has now been confirmed through a direct structure determination of a K^+ channel (Figure 7.8). Although this is a structure of a bacterial ion channel and one that is gated by changes in pH, rather than voltage or chemical transmitters, there is general agreement that the underlying molecular details are generally applicable to other ion channels.

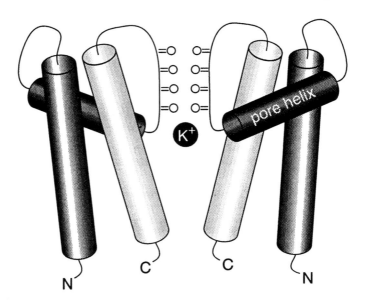

Figure 7.8 Schematic representation of two of the four subunits that make up the functional bacterial K^+ channel. The 'selectivity filter' comprises the aligned carbonyl residues and the pore helices (two are shown) project a dipole field that lowers the energy barrier for K^+ ion entry into the pore of the channel. One K^+ ion is shown in the pore region.

7.2.3   Families of ion channels

Structural studies indicate that there are at least two major families of ion channels. This structural classification into the voltage-gated and ligand-gated families parallels the functional classification established from biophysical and pharmacologic studies. The primary sequences and subunit organization of a large number of channels are now available and with the determination of the 3D-structure of a K^+ channel (Figure 7.8) there is a good foundation upon which to analyze drug–channel interactions.

Each of these major channel families is internally homologous, but both families share fundamental structural and topological similarities. This common structural plan consists of an approximately symmetric disposition of homologous subunits or domains surrounding a central pore. Ligand-gated channels are composed of a set of subunits which, though substantially homologous, bear individually specialized functions including the receptor and regulatory drug binding sites. Thus, the typical ligand-gated ion channel is a heteromeric expression of these subunits – typically a pentameric arrangement as in the nicotinic acetylcholine receptor-channel of skeletal muscle – $\alpha_2\beta\gamma\delta$ – where the α-subunits bear the acetylcholine binding sites. However, homomeric expression does occur as in neuronal nicotinic receptors that can be made up of α- and β-subunits or exclusively of α-subunits. Each of the five homologous subunits of the acetylcholine receptor ion channel has four transmembrane helices and the five subunits are arranged around a central transmembrane pore that is lined with the polar residues of the M2 helices. Concentrations of negative charge are to be found at the top and the bottom of the channel.

Voltage-gated channels for Na^+ and Ca^{2+} are also of subunit organization, but the principal channel functions are associated with a large subunit of approximately 200 kDA and which is made up of four homologous domains – I–IV. This major subunit carries the drug binding sites and makes up the architecture of the channel pore. This subunit is associated with other subunits that can regulate both the expression of the channel and its functional properties (Figure 7.9). Each of the domains of the voltage-gated Na^+ and Ca^{2+} channels is composed of six transmembrane helices and the pore is composed up of residues between S5 and S6. Helix S4 contains a sequence of positively charged residues and these confer voltage-sensing upon the channel. In contrast, the voltage-gated K^+ channel is comprised of a smaller peptide that is homologous to one of the domains of the Na^+ or Ca^{2+} channels: a functional K^+ channel is formed as tetrameric association of these individual subunits. The smaller size of the K^+ channel suggests that it may be ancestral to the Na^+ and Ca^{2+} channels and, consistent with this argument, there are more variations on the structure of the K^+ channel including those with six transmembrane helices – voltage-gated, Ca^{2+}-activated and HERG (human ether-a-go-go related gene) channels, the latter contributing to important human cardiac arrhythmias. K^+ channels with two transmembrane helices include the inwardly rectifying channel family that includes K^+_{ATP} channels.

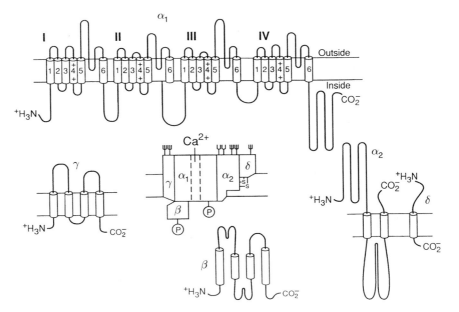

Figure 7.9 Schematic arrangement of the subunits that comprise the voltage-gated Ca^{2+} channel and their organization. The α_1 subunit is the major structural and functional component and bears the permeation machinery and the principal drug binding sites. The cytosolic β-subunit is of particular importance in facilitating the expression of the α_1 subunit and for modifying its gating properties upon activation. Channel diversity arises from the presence of distinct α, β, γ and δ subtypes.

Quite generally, ion channels show remarkable conservation across species – from *Drosophila* to man. This serves as eloquent testimony to the cellular importance of ion channels and to the fitness of design once achieved.

7.2.4   Structure–function correlations

Increasingly, knowledge of the sequences of the channels, their subunit organizations and, most recently, their 3D structures makes it possible to assign specific structural motifs to defined functions, including the sites of drug action and aberrant function as in 'ion channel diseases'. A detailed exposition of these findings lies outside the scope of this chapter, but some illustrative examples may be illustrative of the advances that are being made.

The GABA-gated Cl⁻ channel is a heteromeric organization of homologous subunits. The pentameric association is derived dominantly from the α-, β-and γ-subunits and the opening of this channel by GABA which leads to inhibitory responses is potentiated by benzodiazepines; this action is the basis for their therapeutic effectiveness as sedatives, anxiolytics, muscle relaxants and antiepileptics (Chapter 9). The benzodiazepines bind to a regulatory site located between the α- and γ-subunits. Depending upon the type of α-subunit, α_1–α_6, the GABA receptor may be sensitive or insensitive to benzodiazepines. Only the α_1, α_2, α_3 and α_5 subunits confer sensitivity to benzodiazepines in the GABA receptor channel. These subunits all contain histidine at position 101 and its replacement by arginine abolishes benzodiazepine sensitivity. Furthermore, selective replacement of histidine by arginine in only the α_1-subunit abolishes the sedating effects of benzodiazepines, but leaves the anxiolytic actions unchanged.

The nicotinic acetylcholine receptor channel is a pentameric association of subunits with the α-subunit bearing the acetylcholine receptor site. The pore of the channel is formed from the lining of the M2 helices and is comprised of polar residues with non-polar leucine side chains intruding into the pore at rest ('closed gate'). During activation by acetylcholine the M2 helices twist, rotating away the leucine residues and replacing them with smaller polar residues, and permit ions to flow through the channel pore (Figure 7.10).

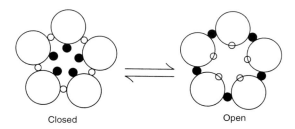

Closed   Open

Figure 7.10 The opening of the nicotinic acetylcholine receptor channel complex subsequent to binding of two molecules of acetylcholine to the α-subunits. Twisting of the M2 helices rotates the non-polar leucine residues (dark circles) away from the pore and replaces them with smaller polar residues (open circles) that permits ion flow through the pore.

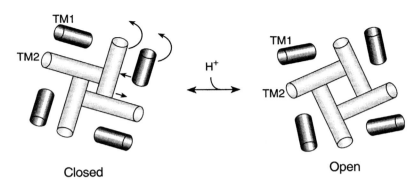

Figure 7.11 The transition between the closed and open states of the bacterial K^+ channel that is activated by a change in pH. Anticlockwise rotation of the MI and M2 helices opens the channel to K^+ ions.

Voltage-gated ion channels present a similar transmembrane profile, but have six transmembrane helices designated S1 to S6 (Figure 7.9). The S4 helix has a common sequence in all voltage-gated channels being composed of positively charged lysine or arginine residues separated by two non-polar residues. Each helix thus carries five or six positive charges and serves as the voltage sensor for the channel. As the membrane depolarizes, this helix unscrews by breaking and remaking hydrogen bonds to adjacent helices and thus effectively transfers one gating charge. Progressive replacement of these positive charges by neutral residues shifts the voltage-dependence of the channel activation process. Other components of the sequence can be identified with other functions. The intracellular sequence linking domains II and IV of the Na^+ channel is critical to channel inactivation. Although the primary biophysical and pharmacological properties for Na^+ and Ca^{2+} channels are carried within the major α-subunit, other subunits notably the β-subunits play major roles. In the voltage-gated Ca^{2+} channel, the β-subunit interacts specifically with the α-subunit in the cytoplasmic loop between domains I and II.

Finally, the actual direct determination of the structure of a K^+ channel (Figure 7.8) permits explanation of the channel activation mechanisms for voltage-gated ion channels. In the model of Figure 7.11, a counter-clockwise rotation of the two transmembrane domains of each subunit of the tetrameric complex leads to pore opening.

7.3   THE CLASSIFICATION OF ION CHANNELS

7.3.1   Criteria for ion channel classification

Ion channels may be classified according to a variety of criteria. The nature of the permeant ion serves as one scheme to designate Cl^-, Na^+, K^+ and Ca^{2+} channels. Although appropriately descriptive this classification is extremely broad, since it is now clear that multiple classes of channels exist for single ions. Additionally, few channels are totally selective for a single ion and ionic selectivity can be altered, sometimes dramatically so, by differing experimental conditions. Channels may be classified according to the nature of the regulatory signal – as potential-dependent channels, activated by changes in membrane potential or as ligand-gated channels, activated by interaction with specific physiological chemical signals. Most recently, mechanically-dependent channels, activated by changes in cellular pressure or tension, have been described: these are important in hair cells of the ear and in cells, such as cardiac cells, where changes in pressure occur during contraction.

The differentiation of voltage-gated and ligand-gated channels (Table 7.2) has been of particular value and has been confirmed by structural studies (Section 7.2.3). The former class responds primarily to changes in membrane potential over defined ranges of electrical activity, and the latter to changes in chemical potential through drug–receptor interactions. Ligand-gated channels may have the chemical sensor as an integral component of the channel or as a remote component (Figure 7.12). Thus in Figure 7.12a which represents the nicotinic acetylcholine receptor–channel complex (and proteins of the same family) the channel and receptor functions are clearly part of the same heteromeric protein assembly, whereas in Figures 7.12b and c, they are clearly quite separate. An example of the latter process is the activation of voltage-gated cardiac Ca^{2+} channels through interaction of norepinephrine at the β-adrenoceptor. The activating ligand is actually an intermediate soluble second messenger, c-AMP.

The distinction at the molecular level between voltage- and ligand-gated ion channels is, however, less than absolute. All channels exhibit sensitivity to endogenous or exogenous chemical species, both naturally occurring and synthetic, and potential-dependent channels are well recognized to exhibit remarkable chemical sensitivity and ligand-gated channels are not insensitive to changes in membrane potential. The basis for channel activation by a signal lies in an understanding that the ion channel is a stochastic molecular device that opens and closes in a probabilistic manner:

$$I = N_f P_o i$$

where I is the total current through the channel, N_f is the total number of functional ion channels, P_o is the opening probability and i is the unitary current. Changes in chemical or electrical potential can increase or decrease P_o or N_f (or both) and thus change the total current through the channel.

Table 7.2 Summary of channel classes

Voltage-gated	Ligand-gated	Mechano-gated	pH
Na^+	GABA	Various ions	K^+
K^+	Glycine		
Ca^{2+}	n-AchR		
	c-AMP		
	Purines		
	Glutamate		

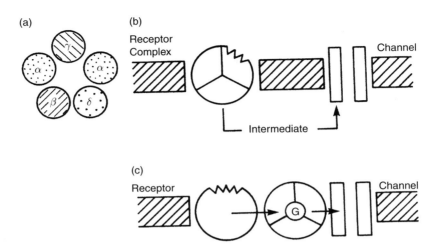

Figure 7.12 Schematic arrangements of ligand-gated ion channels depicting: (a) An oligomeric association of subunits which contain both the channel machinery and the drug receptor; (b) a separate assembly where the drug binding site and the channel machinery are linked through an intermediate (soluble) messenger; and (c) a separate assembly where the drug binding site and the channel machinery are coupled through an intermediate guanine nucleotide (G) binding protein.

7.3.2   Ion channel classification by electrophysiologic criteria

Channels are also classified according to their electrophysiologic characteristics – conductance (current carried) and kinetics and completeness of activation and inactivation. Such distinctions can be seen clearly in the currents of Figure 7.5 where the Na^+ current activates rapidly and inactivates rapidly and the K^+ current activates slowly and does not inactivate during the time course of the trace.

7.3.3   Ion channel classification by drug action

Ion channels may also be classified according to the drugs with which they interact. This classification is obviously in place for ligand-gated channels such as the nicotinic acetylcholine receptor or the GABA and glycine receptors, but it is also applicable to voltage-gated channels that demonstrate a remarkable degree of sensitivity to chemical ligands. Thus, the Na^+ and K^+ currents of Figure 7.5 are sensitive to tetrodotoxin (**7.1**) and tetraethylammonium (**7.2**) that serve as inhibitors of Na^+ and K^+ channels, respectively (Figure 7.13). The actions of tetrodotoxin (**7.1**), a toxin from the puffer fish, underlies its lethal effects and the occasional fatalities from individuals who dine on this delicacy. The 1,4-dihydropyridine nifedipine (**7.3**) (Figure 7.13) blocks voltage-gated Ca^{2+} channels and these actions underlie its clinical cardiovascular uses.

Naturally occurring toxins and synthetic chemicals continue to be of major utility in both the classification of ion channels and in the generation of therapeutic agents.

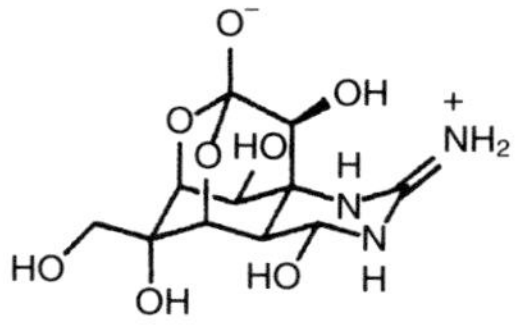

Figure 7.13 Drugs that interact with ion channels: tetrodotoxin (7.1) at Na⁺ channels and tetraethylammonium (7.2) at K⁺ channels. Nifedipine (7.3), verapamil (7.4) and diltiazem (7.5) are the first generation Ca^{2+} channel anatagonists. These drugs interact potently and selectively with the L-type voltage-gated Ca^{2+} channel.

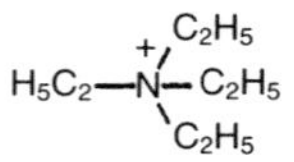

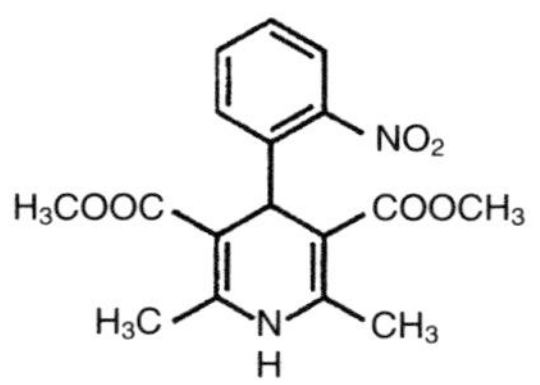

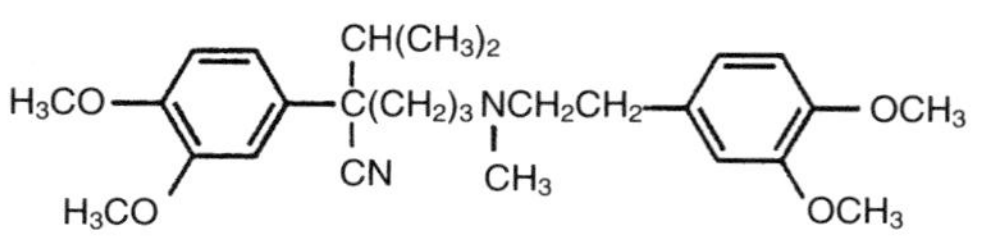

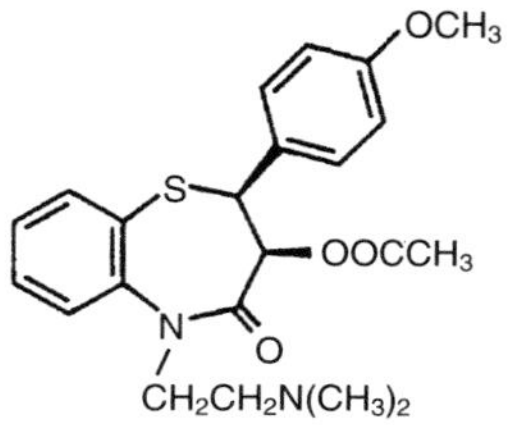

Thus, lidocaine, procaine and related agents owe their local anesthetic and antiarrhythmic properties to their selective interactions with Na⁺ channels. Similarly, the heterogeneous group of agents depicted in the lower portion of Figure 7.13, including the 1,4-dihydropyridine nifedipine (7.3), the phenylalkylamine verapamil (7.4) and the benzothiazepinone diltiazem (7.5) are all used as molecular tools with which to classify Ca^{2+} channels and as major cardiovascular drugs (Table 7.3).

In practice, all of these properties of ion channels – ion selectivity, electrophysiological properties, pharmacological sensitivity, and location – are used to classify ion channels. This is illustrated in Table 7.4 for voltage-gated Ca^{2+} channels and in Table 7.5 for K⁺ channels, a particularly diverse group. The application of molecular biologic techniques has added a particularly fundamental base – classification according to sequence. Collectively, these techniques have

Table 7.3 Therapeutic uses of Ca^{2+} channel antagonists

Uses	Verapamil	Nifedipine	Diltiazem
Angina pectoris	+++	++	+++
PSVT	+++	−	++
Atrial fibrillation and flutter	++	−	++
Hypertension	++	+++	++
Hypertrophic cardiomyopathy	+	−	−
Raynaud's disease	++	++	++

Notes
+++, most common use; ++, common use; +, less common use; −, not indicated.

Table 7.4 Classification of voltage-gated Ca^{2+} channels

Nomenclature	Channel class				
	T	L	N	P/Q	R
Sequence, CaV	3.1–3.3	1.1–1.3	2.2	2.1	2.3
Current	I_T	I_L	I_N	$I_{P/Q}$	I_R
Conductance, pS	5–10	25	20	10–20	–
Activation threshold	low	high	high	high	high
Inactivation rate	fast	slow	moderate	rapid	–
Permeation	$Ba^{2+} > Ca^{2+}$	$Ba^{2+} > Ca^{2+}$	$Ba^{2+} > Ca^{2+}$	$Ba^{2+} > Ca^{2+}$	$Ba^{2+} = Ca^{2+}$
Function and location	Cardiac SA node, neurons, rep. spiking, spike activity	E-coupling in muscle cells, neurons	------------------neurons only------------------ neurotransmitter release		
Pharmacology blockers	mibefradil flunarizine kurotoxin	nifedipine verapamil diltiazem	ω-CTXGVIA	ω-AGAIVA	–
Agonist		BayK8644			
Subunit composition (α subunits only)	$\alpha_1 G$, $\alpha_1 H$, $\alpha_1 I$	$\alpha_1 S$, $\alpha_1 C$, $\alpha_1 D$, $\alpha_1 F$	$\alpha_1 B$	$\alpha_1 A$	$\alpha_1 E$

Table 7.5 Classification of K^+ channels

Class	Type	Pharmacology	Properties
Voltage-gated			
K_V	delayed rectifier (delayed outward)	TEA, 4-AP PCP, 9-AA	Delayed activation; slow inactivating
K_{VR}	rapid delayed rectifier	dofetilide, sotalol quinidine, tedisamil	rapidly activating component of cardiac current
K_{VS}	slow delayed rectifier		very slow activating component of cardiac current
K_A	transient outward current	4-AP, quinidine PCP, dendrotoxin	activated by hyperpolarization following depolarization
K_{IR}	inward rectifier	TEA, gaboon Viper venom	channel conductance highest when hyperpolarized
Calcium-activated			
BK_{Ca}	high-conductance (maxi-K)	TEA, charybdotoxin noxius toxin, iberatoxin	activated by Ca^{2+}_{int}
IK_{Ca}	intermediate-conductance	TEA, quinine, charybdotoxin	activated by Ca^{2+}_{int}
SK_{Ca}	small conductance	quinine, mepacrine, Apamin, leiurotoxin I	activated by Ca^{2+}_{int}
Receptor-coupled			
K_M	muscarinic-inactivated K^+ channel	W.7	slow to activate at negative potentials, nn-inactivating
Other			
K_{ATP}	ATP-sensitive K^+ channel	glibenclamide, tolbutamide pinacidil, nicorandil	inhibited by $[ATP_{int}]$

revealed that ion channels fall into a limited number of families and that within each family substantial homology exists. Additionally, it is clear that ion channels of apparently fundamentally different characteristics exhibit considerable similarities in their proposed membrane topologies. One of the most important questions now in active resolution is that of relating ion channel structure and function and of generating mechanisms for channel opening and closing processes.

7.4 ION CHANNELS AS PHARMACOLOGICAL RECEPTORS

7.4.1 Receptor properties of ion channels

The pharmacological properties of ion channels indicate that they may be considered as pharmacological receptors with the following overall properties:

1 Channels should exist as homologous protein families.
2 Channels should posses specific drug binding sites which exhibit defined structure–activity relationships, including stereoselectivity, for interacting ligands.
3 Both activator and antagonist drugs should exist.
4 Channels should be regulated by drug and hormone action and by pathological states.
5 Channels should contribute to specific molecular disease states by virtue of aberrant expression or mutated channel structure.

These expectations have been fully realized for many ion channels, including the voltage-gated Ca^{2+} channels where drug interactions have been studied with particular intensity. However, ion channels also exhibit a number of specific and distinctive properties of ligand interaction.

7.4.2 State-dependent interactions of ion channels

Ion channels exist in a number of states or families of states where, quite generally, they are resting and activatable, open and permeant and, in the case of voltage-gate channels, inactivated following the activation process (Figure 7.14). Each of these states represents a different channel conformation and, in principle, a different conformation of, or access pathway to the drug binding site. In the scheme of Figure 7.14, a drug may exhibit higher affinity for the inactivated state of the channel and will thus serve as an antagonist. In contrast, an agent may stabilize the open state of a channel and thus serve as a channel activator or agonist. Alternative pathways of drug access to a binding site may exist. A hydrophilic drug with preferential affinity for the inactivated state may access its binding site through the open state of the channel (pathway A, Figure 7.14), whereas a hydrophobic species that partitions extensively into the membrane may access the site through the lipid bilayer pathway of the membrane (pathway B, Figure 7.14). Similar considerations dictate the pathways through which these drugs leave their binding sites. According to this 'modulated receptor' hypothesis:

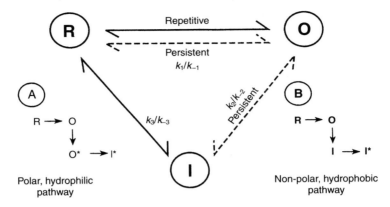

Figure 7.14 The 'modulated receptor' mechanism of drug action at ion channels. Drugs may bind to or access preferentially receptors in the channel in the resting, open or inactivated states of the channel. Each of the states can have a different affinity for a drug. The equilibrium between the channel states will be determined by the physiologic, pathologic or experimental conditions prevailing and hence the apparent drug affinity will vary according to this equilibrium. Repetitive depolarization defines a frequency-dependent process and persistent depolarization defines a voltage-dependent process as in cardiac and vascular smooth muscle, respectively, and thus the action of the Ca^{2+} channel antagonists (see text for further details).

1 Different channel states have different affinities for drugs.
2 Drugs may exhibit quantitatively and qualitatively different structure–activity relationships for different channel states.
3 Drugs stabilize different channel states.
4 Drugs alter the kinetics of channel state inter-conversion.

These considerations apply both to voltage-gated and ligand-gated ion channels and examples of drugs that exhibit such state-dependent interactions are readily available for both channel classes. In a simple two-state model where two states of the channel, A and B, have dissociation constants K_A and K_B for a drug, then K_{app}, the observed dissociation constant, will be given by:

$$K_{app} = \frac{1}{\left[\dfrac{h}{K_A}\right] + \left[1 - \dfrac{h}{K_B}\right]}$$

where h is the fraction of the channel in state A and $1 - h$ is the fraction in state B.

These state-dependent interactions are illustrated in a number of ways. The local anesthetic lidocaine demonstrates enhanced affinity by a factor of several hundred-fold for the depolarized (inactivated) state of the Na^+ channel (Figure 7.15). Access to and from binding sites associated with the ion channel will also control drug–receptor interactions. Interaction of local anesthetics with Na^+ channels reveals a clear dependency of potency upon stimulation frequency. This frequency-dependent property is consistent with a process whereby drug binding requires

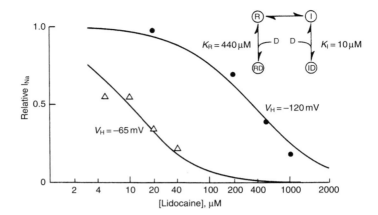

Figure 7.15 The voltage-dependent binding of lidocaine at the Na$^+$ channel. Dose–response curves for lidocaine inhibition of the Na$^+$ current (I_{Na^+}) are measured at holding potentials of -120 mV (when the channels are essentially all in the resting R state) and at -65 mV when the channels are in the inactivated I state. (Reproduced with permission from Bean, Cohen and Tsien, *J. Gen. Physiol.*, **8**, 1983, 613–642).

channel opening, whereas drug dissociation can occur during stimulus-free intervals. Thus, with increasing frequency of stimulation – increased channel opening – drug progressively accumulates at drug binding sites to produce greater block. With a decrease in frequency, channel block decreases correspondingly. Such state-dependent interactions define the anti-arrhythmic actions of a number of drugs.

Quaternary ammonium ions block K$^+$ channels and reveal further complexities in channel–drug interaction schemes (Figure 7.16). Quaternary ammonium ions applied intracellularly to excitable cells will enter and block the channel only

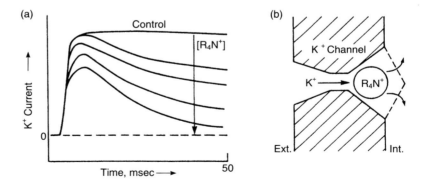

Figure 7.16 (a) Time-dependent blockade of K$^+$ current by quaternary ammonium ion. The extent of block is dependent upon time and progressively increases with increasing duration of channel open time. This indicates that the drug accesses its binding site *only* when the channel is open; (b) schematic representation of a quaternary ammoniumion being trapped in the pore after channel closure. K$^+$ ion movement and channel opening serve to displace the blocker.

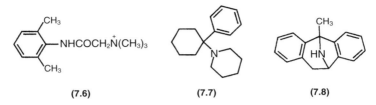

(7.6)   (7.7)   (7.8)

Figure 7.17 Structural formulae of drugs that show selective interaction with the open state of the Na$^+$ channel [QX-222 (**7.6**)] or the ligand-gated NMDA channel [PCP (**7.7**) and MK-801 (**7.8**)].

during the open state. The channel may close with drug trapped at the binding site from which it cannot escape until the channel is reopened.

Similarly, drugs that function as non-competitive antagonists in ligand-gated channels may interact at sites associated with the channel rather than the receptor component of the receptor-channel complex (Figure 7.17). The quaternary ammonium local anesthetic QX 222 (**7.6**) interacts preferentially with the open state of the channel, and at the *N*-methyl-D-aspartate class of excitatory amino acid receptors the agents phencyclidine (**7.7**) and MK-801 (**7.8**) also bind with highest affinity to the open channel state (see Chapter 9).

These state-dependent aspects of drug interactions are important from at least three perspectives. They are important in the determination of the selectivity of drug action. The voltage- and frequency-dependent actions of local anesthetics define their utility as Class 1 anti-arrhythmic agents, whereby the very efficacy of the drug is enhanced by the pathological condition and minimized by the physiologic condition. The state-dependent interactions also serve as valuable molecular probes of channel structure and function by revealing subtleties of interactions and access pathways. Finally, these interactions are important to the determination and analysis of structure–activity relationships of drugs active at ion channels.

7.4.3 Structure–activity relationships and state-dependent interactions

The interpretation of structure–activity relations for channel-active drugs is complex since it may depend significantly upon the choice of experimental conditions. These conditions may best be controlled through electrophysiologic studies. These may not generate large data bases, but they can establish the fundamental mode of interaction of lead compounds. Accordingly, comparisons of drug activities obtained under different conditions or in different preparations must be interpreted with caution. Differences in activity may indicate the existence of channel subtypes, but may be equally consistent with the existence of state-dependent interactions. The comparisons of pharmacologic and radioligand binding activities in a series of 1,4-dihydropyridine Ca^{2+} channel antagonists depicted in Figure 7.18 is illustrative of this issue. Clearly, the higher pharmacologic activity of this series in smooth muscle relative to cardiac muscle may be consistent with different channel

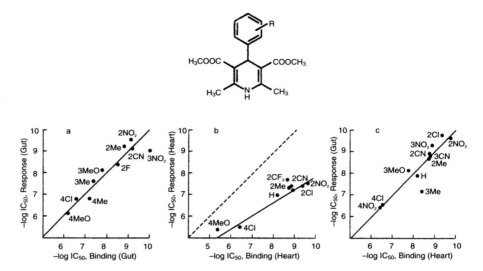

Figure 7.18 Comparison of the binding and pharmacologic affinities of a series of 1,4-dihydro-pyridines in smooth and cardiac muscle. The 1,4-dihydropyridines are all analogs of nifedipine (7.3) with the indicated phenyl ring substituents. Binding and pharmacologic affinities were measured in (a) intestinal smooth muscle, and (b) cardiac muscle. A comparison of the binding affinities in the two preparations is depicted in panel (c). The filled line represents the line of best fit and the dashed line 1:1 equivalence.

subtypes and there is evidence for this (Section 7.5.3). However, the equal binding affinities of the same compounds obtained from depolarized membrane preparations are also consistent with the existence of voltage-dependent binding as defining the different structure–function relationships. Binding affinity increases with increasing and maintained depolarization: this will be the situation with smooth muscle where maintained depolarization is the stimulus mode, rather than the repetitive depolarization observed for cardiac muscle.

A further example from the 1,4-dihydropyridine series, derives from the enantiomeric pair of Figure 7.19. In this series, the S- and R-enantiomers show activator and antagonist properties respectively. However, if the S-enantiomer interacts with the voltage-gated Ca^{2+} channel in the depolarized state it shows

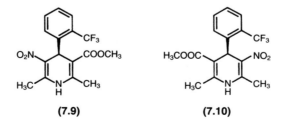

Figure 7.19 The enantiomers of a 1,4-dihydropyridine that show activator, (S)-BayK8644 (7.9), and antagonist, (R)-BayK8644 (7.10), properties.

antagonist activity. Thus, state–dependent interactions may generate both quantitative and qualitative changes in structure–activity relationships for drugs active at ion channels.

7.5 DRUGS ACTING AT SPECIFIC ION CHANNELS

7.5.1 Multiple sites for drug action

A principal feature of ion channels and drug action is the presence of multiple, discrete sites of action. These sites or receptors are frequently linked one to the other and to the functional machinery of the channel by complex allosteric interactions. Thus, binding of a drug to one channel receptor site may alter not only the ion permeation characteristics but may also simultaneously alter the interactions of drugs at other, but allosterically, linked receptor sites. These interactions render complex the interpretation of the actions of drugs at ion channels. Useful examples of this complexity are provided by drugs that act at voltage-gated Na^+, Ca^{2+} and K^+ channels and at the K_{ATP}^+ and NMDA receptors as examples of ligand-gated ion channels.

7.5.2 Drugs acting at Na^+ channels

At least nine major classes of drugs interact at the Na^+ channel at discrete receptors where they mediate distinct responses (Table 7.6). The guanidinium toxins, tetrodotoxin and saxitoxin, are generally assumed to block the permeation pathway of the channel. However, structure–activity relationships in these molecules are extremely limited, principally because of their complex synthetic chemistry. However, both the guanidinium group and the hydroxyl functions do appear necessary for activity. The other structural classes of Na^+ channel drugs exhibit more complex interactions with their interaction properties being profoundly state-dependent. Veratridine (**7.12**) and the lipid-soluble alkaloid toxins (Figure 7.20)

Table 7.6 Drug interactions at voltage-gated Na^+ channels

Site	Toxin or drug	Activity
1	Tetrodotoxin, saxitoxin	block activation
2	Batrachotoxin, veratridine grayanotoxin	persistent activation
3	α-Scorpion toxins sea anemone II toxin	block activation persistent activation
4	β-Scorpion toxins	shift voltage-dependence
5	Brevetoxins	repetitive firing
6	δ-Conotoxins	block inactivation
7	DDT, pyrethroids	block activation shift voltage-dependence
8	Coral toxin	block activation
9	Local anesthetics anticonvulsants	block activation

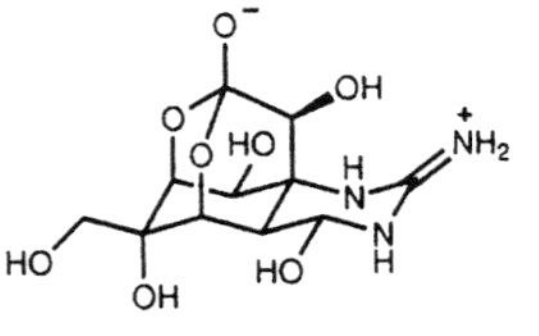

Figure 7.20 Structural formulae of toxins that interact at the Na^+ channel. Tetrodotoxin (7.1), batrachotoxin (7.11), veratridine (7.12) and grayanotoxin (7.13).

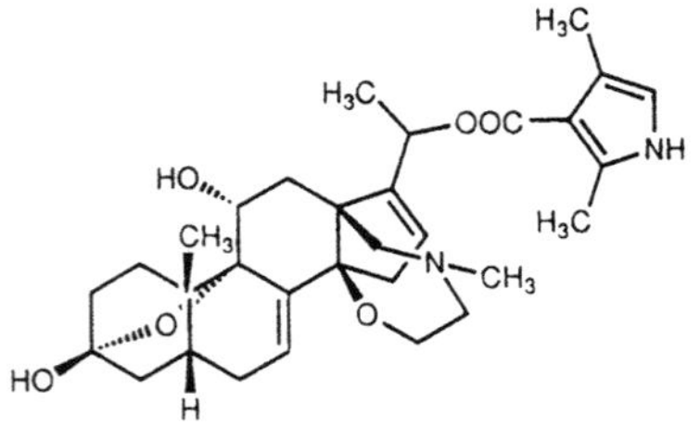

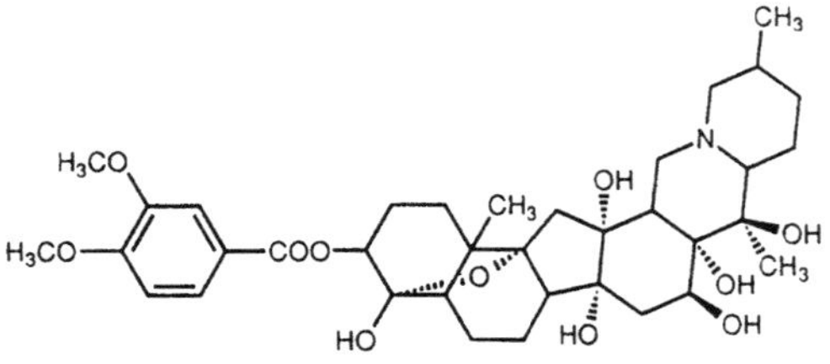

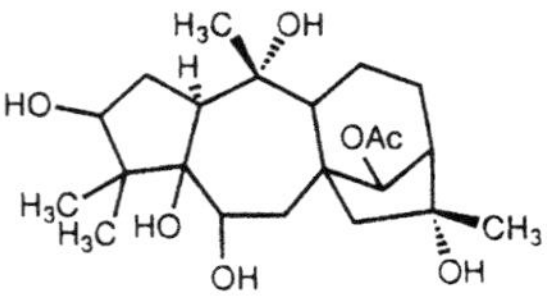

have the common property of activating the Na^+ channels and maintaining their open state. Although, consistent with their very different chemical structures, these agents do not interact at identical binding sites, they do share and the net consequence of their interaction to produce a state of persistent activation of the Na^+ channel. This activation occurs through an allosteric stabilization of the channel open state. Accordingly, drug-bound channels are activatable at membrane potentials far more negative than unmodified channels: the action of the drug is effectively to shift the voltage-activation curve for the Na^+ channel leftward to more negative membrane potentials.

A variety of peptide toxins also interact at Na^+ channels and are derived from scorpions, sea anemones and fish hunting cone snails of the *Conus* genus. These polypeptide toxins all contain several disulfide bridges that serve to maintain a relatively rigid structure. The toxins from sea anemones and scorpions are small proteins of 45–50 and 60–70 residues, respectively, while the conotoxins (Figure 7.21) are significantly smaller in size with some 20 residues. Although they are all disulfide-bridged entities they appear to interact in different ways. The conotoxins act in a manner similar to tetrodotoxin (7.1) and saxitoxin, whereas the sea anemone and scorpion toxins have more complex modes of interaction that appear to involve shifts of the channel activation curves to more negative membrane potentials in a manner similar to that of veratridine (7.12).

Other examples of drugs that interact at Na^+ channels include the pyrethroid insecticides, analogs of the pyrethroid neurotoxins isolable from *Chrysanthemums*. These agents (Figure 7.22) also interact allosterically with the channel and bind

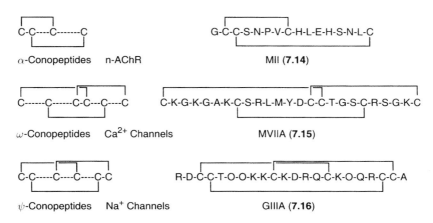

Figure 7.21 Structural formulae of representative examples of the conotoxin (derived from cone snails) series of peptide toxins. The α-, ω- and ψ-conopeptides are illustrated by general formulae with specification of cysteine disulfide bridges and one example from each group (7.14–7.16) with the amino acid sequence given by one-letter abbreviations.

preferentially to the open state causing a persistent channel activation: this underlies their neurotoxic properties. Local anesthetics, including lidocaine and procaine, also interact with the Na$^+$ channel and this forms the basis for their anesthetic actions and for their anti-arrhythmic properties.

Currently, therapeutic attention at the Na$^+$ channel is directed to the search for new anticonvulsants, neuroprotective agents and analgesia. The principal compounds available are the anticonvulsants phenytoin (7.21) and carbamazepine (7.22), lamotrigine (7.23) for neuropathic pain and riluzole (7.24) for the neurodegeneration observed in amyotrophic lateral sclerosis (Figure 7.23).

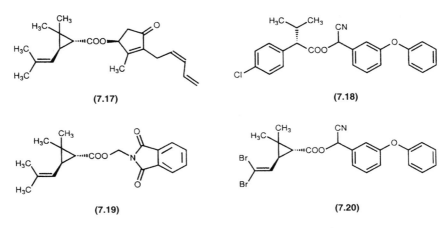

Figure 7.22 Pyrethrins (7.17–7.20) active at the Na$^+$ channel.

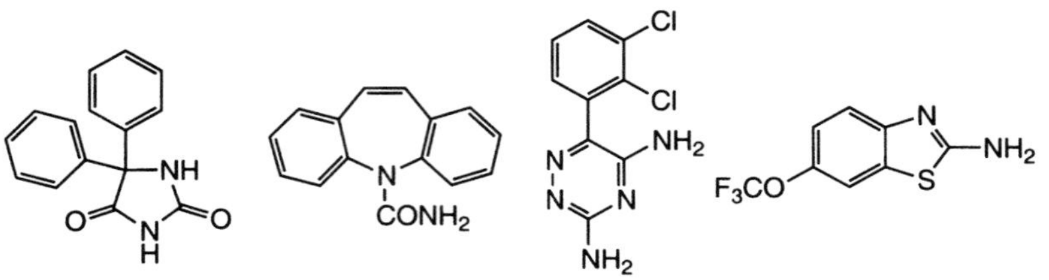

(7.21)   **(7.22)**   **(7.23)**   **(7.24)**

Figure 7.23 Clinically useful Na$^+$ channel antagonists. Phenytoin (**7.21**), carbamazepine (**7.22**), lamotrigine (**7.23**) and riluzole (**7.24**).

7.5.3   Drugs acting at Ca^{2+} channels

In contrast to the situation with K$^+$ channels, the pharmacology of the voltage-gated Ca^{2+} channels has been dominated by synthetic agents of the 1,4-dihydropyridine, benzothiazepinone and phenylalkylamine classes (Figure 7.13). These agents have served simultaneously as major therapeutic agents for cardiovascular diseases (Table 7.3) including hypertension and angina, and as molecular tools with which to analyze channel structure and function. The structures depicted in Figure 7.13 are inhibitors of Ca^{2+} influx through one particular class of Ca^{2+} channel – the L-type channel that functionally dominates the cardiovascular system – but there is considerable interest in drugs that may selectively modulate other classes of Ca^{2+} channels (Table 7.4) since such drugs may have prominent effects in neuronal and other disorders. Some drugs that act on these channel types are depicted in Figure 7.24.

The drugs of Figure 7.13 interact at separate and discrete sites on the L-type channel as shown in Figure 7.25 which demonstrates schematically the arrangement of these sites and the allosteric linkages that exist. The drug–receptor interactions depicted all show state-dependent properties with preferential drug interaction at the open and/or the inactivated states of the channel. Thus, depolarizing conditions that favor the formation of these states enhances the activity of these agents. However, verapamil (**7.4**) and diltiazem (**7.5**), are protonated species at physiological pH, exhibit frequency-dependent interactions, whereas the neutral nifedipine (**7.3**) exhibits voltage-dependent interactions. This difference in mechanism may reflect hydrophilic and hydrophobic access pathways for these drugs and may also underlie their different therapeutic applications with verapamil being an effective Class IV anti-arrhythmic agent and nifedipine (and all other 1,4-dihydropyridines) lacking such properties.

Consistent with their different chemical classes and their interaction at discrete receptor sites there is a separate structure–activity relationship that exists for each of the chemical classes. That for the 1,4-dihydropyridines has been particularly well described and is of interest since both activator and antagonist drugs exist. The overall structure–activity relationship is depicted in Figure 7.26. In a QSAR approach the activity of nifedipine analogs bearing substituents in the 4-phenyl ring could be described by:

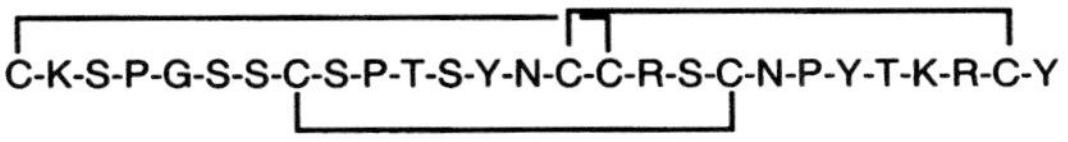

C-K-S-P-G-S-S-C-S-P-T-S-Y-N-C-C-R-S-C-N-P-Y-T-K-R-C-Y

(7.25)

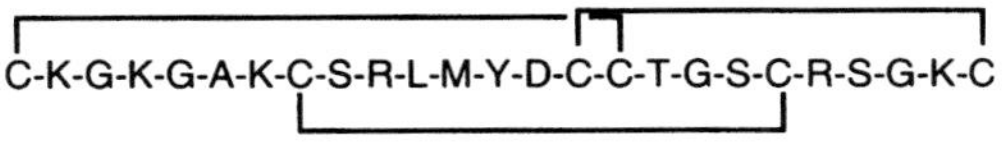

C-K-G-K-G-A-K-C-S-R-L-M-Y-D-C-C-T-G-S-C-R-S-G-K-C

(7.15)

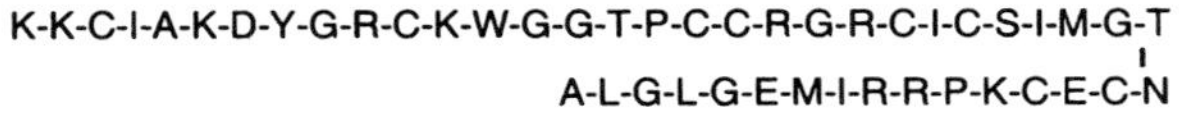

K-K-C-I-A-K-D-Y-G-R-C-K-W-G-G-T-P-C-C-R-G-R-C-I-C-S-I-M-G-T
A-L-G-L-G-E-M-I-R-R-P-K-C-E-C-N

(7.26)

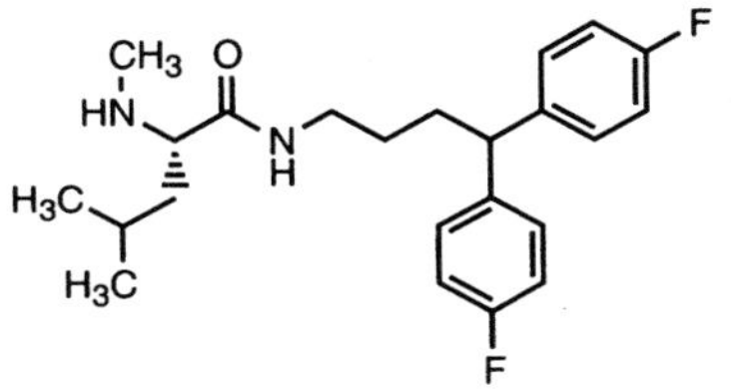

(7.27)

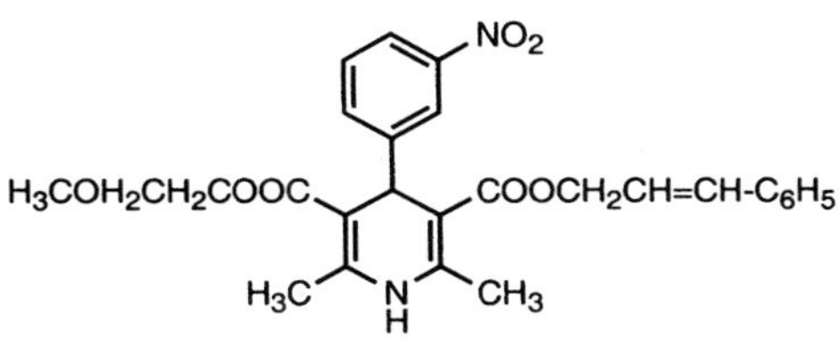

(7.28)

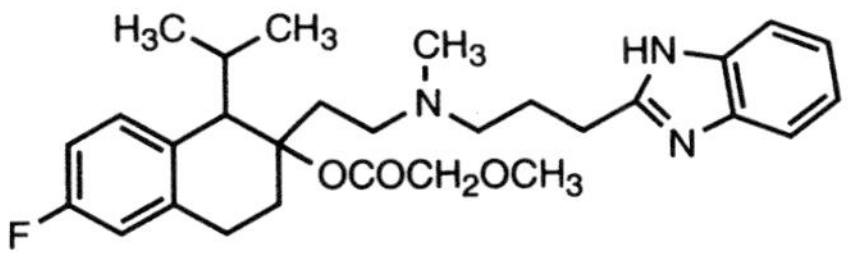

(7.29)

Figure 7.24 Drugs that interact with non-L-type voltage-gated Ca^{2+} channels. ω-Conotoxin GVIA (**7.25**, N-type channels); ω-Conotoxin MVIIA (**7.15**, N-type channels); ω-Agatoxin IVA (**7.26**, P-type channels), **7.27** (N-type channels), cilnidipine (**7.28**, N-type channels) and mibefradil (**7.29**, T-type channels).

$$\log 1/IC_{50} = 0.62\pi + 1.96\delta m - 0.44L_{\text{meta}} - 3.26B_{1\text{para}} - 1.51L_{\text{meta}'} + 14.23$$

$$n = 46, \quad r = 0.90, \quad s = 0.67, \quad F = 33.93$$

where δm is the electronic parameter, π a hydrophobicity index, and L and B_1 are steric parameters. The stereochemical requirements for interaction at the 1,4-dihydropyridine receptor have been examined in considerable detail through the synthesis of rigid analogs, the determination of solid state and solution conformations, and the application of computational techniques. There is general agreement that optimum activity of the 1,4-dihydropyridines requires a flattened boat conformation for the 1,4-dihydropyridine ring and a pseudoaxial phenyl ring oriented orthogonally to the 1,4-dihydropyridine ring with the aryl substituents

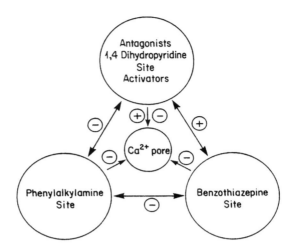

Figure 7.25 Representation of three primary pharmacologic receptors at the voltage-gated Ca^{2+} channel depicting their linkage to the permeation and gating machinery of the L-type channel and the allosteric linkages between these discrete receptors (+, positive allosteric interaction; −, negative allosteric interaction).

oriented away (antiperiplanar) from the 1,4-dihydropyridine ring (Figure 7.26). Additionally, there is an interesting stereochemical discrimination of pharmacological activity where, in appropriately substituted 1,4-dihydropyridines, there is activator activity in the *S*-enantiomer and antagonist activity in the *R*-enantiomer

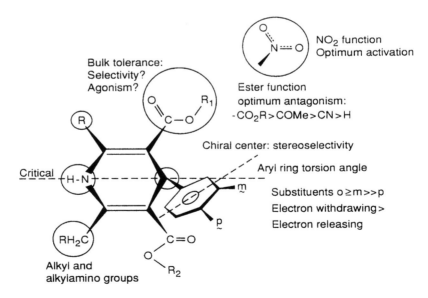

Figure 7.26 The structure–activity relationship for 1,4-dihydropyridine antagonists and activators at the L-type voltage-gated Ca^{2+} channel.

(Figure 7.19). Furthermore, because the interactions of the 1,4-dihydropyridines with their receptor site are voltage-dependent the *S*-enantiomer can transition from activator to antagonist as the membrane potential becomes progressively less polarized.

The 1,4-dihydropyridines also provide a series of second generation drugs, including nimodipine (**7.30**), nitrendipine (**7.31**), nicardipine (**7.32**), amlodipine (**7.33**), felodipine (**7.34**) and isradipine (**7.35**) (Figure 7.27). These agents have greater vascular selectivity than the parent 1,4-dihydropyridine, and this originates, in part, from their greater degree of voltage-dependence of interaction.

Molecular biology studies have defined both the location of the 1,4-dihydropyridine, benzothiazepinone and phenylalkylamine binding sites in the major $\alpha 1$ subunit of the L-type Ca^{2+} channel and the residues that are involved in binding the drugs. The 1,4-dihydropyridine binding site is located on the IIS5, the IIS6 and the IVS6 domains with critical contributions from tyrosine-1152 (IIIS6), isoleucine-1156 (IIIS6), methionine-1161 (IIS6) and asparagine-1472 (IVS6). A schematic arrangement of the binding sites at the α_1 subunit of the L-type Ca^{2+} channel is sketched in (Figure 7.28).

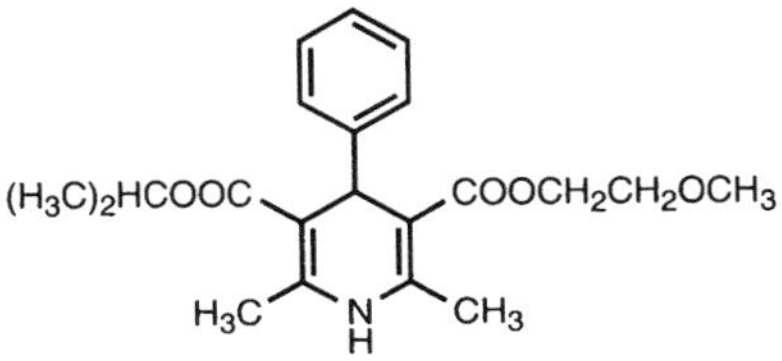

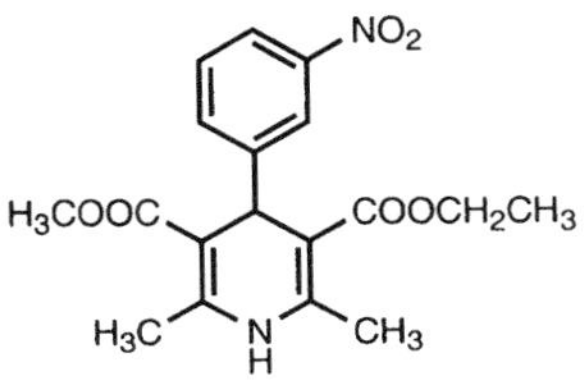

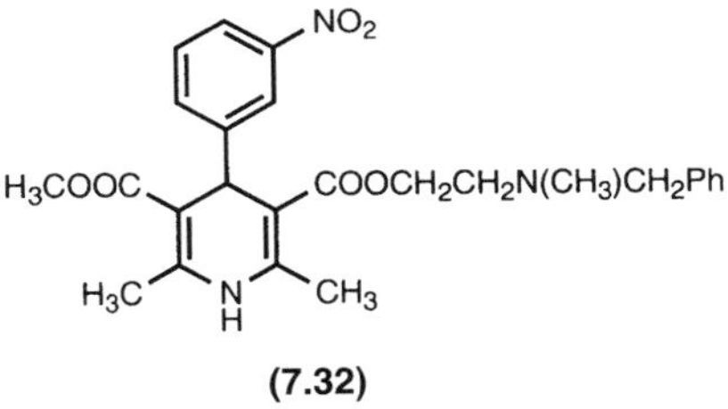

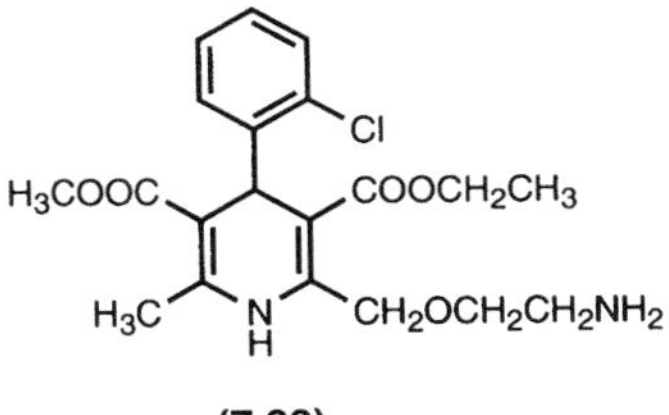

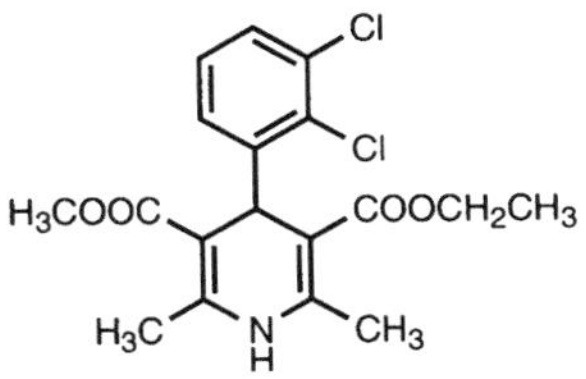

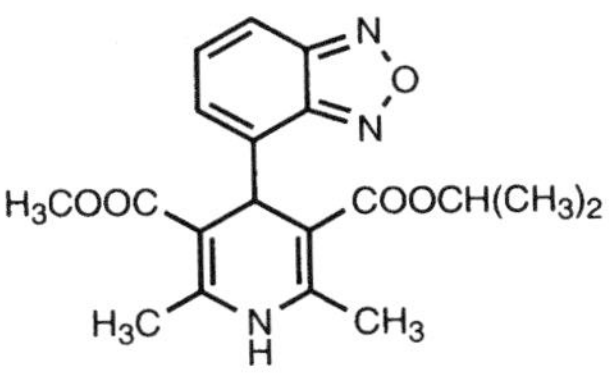

Figure 7.27 Structural formulae of second generation 1,4-dihydropyridines: Nimodipine (**7.30**), Nitrendipine (**7.31**), Nicardipine (**7.32**), Amlodipine (**7.33**), Felodipine (**7.34**) and Isradipine (**7.35**).

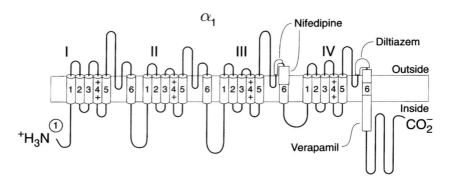

Figure 7.28 The α_1 subunit of the L-type voltage-gated Ca^{2+} channel showing the location of the principal binding sites for the antagonists nifedipine (**7.3**), verapamil (**7.4**) and diltiazem (**7.5**).

7.5.4   Drugs acting at K^+ channels

K^+ channels constitute a remarkably diverse molecular group of excitable proteins and their pharmacology is correspondingly diverse (Table 7.5). Quaternary ammonium ions, including tetraethylammonium, are channel blockers acting through pore mechanisms but are not very discriminating with respect to channel type. The specific pharmacology of the voltage-gated channels (K_V) is dominated by toxins from scorpions including agitoxin, charybdotoxin and kaliotoxin that block the channel pore as well as by toxins from sea anemone, snails of the *Conus* genus and from spiders including tarantulas. The scorpion toxins are globular miniproteins that share a common scaffold with 29–39 amino acid residues and three or four disulfide bridges with a common motif – G26-K27-C28-M/I29-N/G30-X31-K32-C33-(n)34-C35 where (n) represents a charged residue. The lysine residue at position 27 (K27) appears to be of critical significance and it is suggested that it may 'plug' the pore acting as a surrogate K^+ ion.

From a clinical perspective the ATP-sensitive K^+ channels are of particular importance. These were first recognized in the heart, but are now known to be of widespread distribution and to exist as several major subtypes. They serve to couple the cell metabolic state to membrane potential: with an increase in the cellular ATP levels the channel is blocked and membrane potential decreases. The structure of the channel is a subunit organization consisting of an inward rectifier channel K_{ir} with an sulfonylurea receptor (SUR) subunit that interacts with the synthetic sulfonylurea hypoglycemic agents. The sulfonylurea receptor family are large transmembrane proteins that contain 15 transmembrane sequences and two large cytoplasmic loops (Figure 7.29). The sulfonylurea receptors are members of the ABC transporter superfamily of proteins, which also includes the cystic fibrosis transmembrane regulator gene product. It is the combination of K_{ir} and SUR as an octameric complex that constitutes the active K^+ATP channel: expression of either subunit alone does not generate channel activity. This channel is the location for the hypoglycemic sulfonylureas (Figure 7.30), including the first- and second generation tolbutamide (**7.36**) and glibenclamide (**7.37**) that function

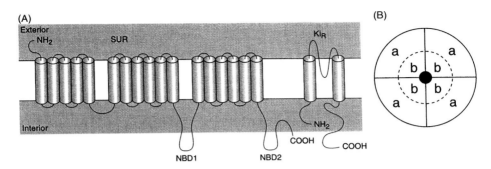

Figure 7.29 (A) The linear sequence of the SUR and its association with the K_{ir} channel subunit; and (B) a functional K_{ATP}^+ channel is an octamer consisting of four channel subunits (b) and four SUR subunits (a).

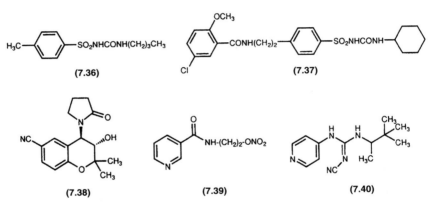

Figure 7.30 Drugs active at the K_{ATP}^+ channel (see also Figure 7.4). Antagonists: tolbutamide (**7.36**) and glibenclamide (**7.37**). Activators: cromakalim (**7.38**), nicorandil (**7.39**) and pinacidil (**7.40**).

as antagonists, as well as the K^+ channel activators including cromakalim (**7.38**), nicorandil (**7.39**) and pinacidil (**7.40**). The K^+ channel activators continue to attract attention because of their potential as selective cardiovascular (hypertension, angina), non-cardiovascular (asthma, urinary incontinence) and central nervous system (anticonvulsant, antineurodegenerative) therapeutic roles.

7.6 ION CHANNELS AND DISEASES

As benefits, their status as a class of pharmacological receptors ion channels are associated with defined molecular diseases that arise from specific mutations in channel proteins and that are associated with aberrant function or altered expression. A very partial list of such diseases and mutations is presented in Table 7.7.

Hyperkalemic periodic paralysis is a dominant mutation of the α-subunit of the skeletal muscle voltage-gated Na^+ channel. Mutations in this subunit are associated with a group of diseases referred collectively to 'potassium-aggravated myotonias'. Enhanced serum K^+ brought on by exercise or K^+-rich foods brings about a non-life-threatening muscle paralysis.

Long QT syndrome is a cardiac disease associated with arrhythmias and sudden death. It can arise from mutations in either voltage-gated Na^+ or K^+ channels. A severe form of the disease associated with Na^+ channels arises from a three amino acid deletion in the cytoplasmic loop between domains III and IV of the α-subunit. This produces a non-inactivating current and increases the QT interval of the electrocardiogram. The most common form of the disease is associated with mutations in the K^+ channel. The LQT syndrome has become an area of considerable importance to drug development since drugs that can induce such behavior either directly or by interfering with the P450 drug metabolism system are obviously to be avoided prior to clinical introduction. A number of drugs, including the antihistamines terfenadine and astemizole, the gastric motility agent cisapride and the antihypertensive agent mibefradil, have all been withdrawn from clinical use because of this occurrence.

In persistent hyperinsulinaemia there is an unregulated secretion of insulin with consequent profound hypoglycemia. The disease can arise from mutations in either the SUR or the K_{ir} subunits and activity of the channel is lost leading to a persistent depolarization of the cell and insulin release.

A number of molecular diseases are associated with defects in voltage-gated Ca^{2+} channels. Murine muscular dysgenesis involves a lack of excitation–contraction coupling in skeletal muscle with an absence of functional α_1-subunits: the protein is truncated at the C-terminal and expression of this aberrant protein is reduced. Familial hemiplegic migraine is associated a migraine aura and involves paralysis of one-half of the body during an attack. Several mutations within the α_1-subunit have been associated with this disease.

Cystic fibrosis is the most common molecular disease associated with the Caucasian population and involves defects in the epithelial Cl^- channel with

Table 7.7 Ion channel diseases

Channel	Disease
Voltage-gated Na^+	Hyperkalemic periodic paralysis
	Long QT syndrome
	Generalized epilepsy with fever
Voltage-gated K^+	Episodic ataxia
	Long QT syndrome
Inward rectifier $K^+(K_{ATP}^+)$	Familial persistent hyperinsulineamia
	Hypoglycemia of infancy
Voltage-gated Ca^{2+}	Muscular dysgenesis (murine)
	Hypokalemic periodic paralysis
	Familial hemiplegic migraine
Chloride channels, CFTR	Cystic fibrosis

associated defects in the excretion of NaCl (high salt concentration in the sweat), pathological abnormalities in the lung, intestine and male reproductive system. Although some 400 separate mutations have been described in the cystic fibrosis transmembrane regulator, the most common defect arises from a single amino acid deletion, phenylalanine, at position 508.

7.7   ION CHANNELS AS LETHAL SPECIES

The focus on ion channels thus far has been on ion channels as integral and endogenous protein species. However, there are exogenous proteins that when incorporated into the cell membrane form ion channels and these can serve as lethal species by disrupting ion and solute flow. There are some 40 families of pore- and channel-forming proteins and peptides, including a number of bacterial toxins. This toxin family includes diphtheria, botulinum, tetanus, α-hemolysin and insecticidal δ-toxins. Many species produce amphiathic, bioactive and pore-forming peptides. Frogs generate the magainins that serve virucidal, bactericidal and fungicidal actions thus serving to defend frogs against infections. Melittin, a 26 amino acid peptide, is produced by bees and defensins, 35–95 residues, are produced by mammals and have anti-infective functions. Such agents are likely to be of value in the search for new antibiotics.

7.8   FUTURE DEVELOPMENTS

Ion channels continue to represent both a major challenge and a major opportunity to the discipline of medicinal chemistry. They are a major challenge because of the complex kinetic interconversions that are integral to channel function, because of the multiplicity of subtypes and because determination of structure–function relationships of drug action has been more difficult than with other classes of receptors. The opportunities arise because these difficulties are being approached at the very time that molecular biology is making available detailed information about the structure and function of ion channels, including 3D structure. Ion channels, of course, serve as major integrating loci of cells where many different signals are integrated to modulate the health and welfare of the cell. Ion channel drugs are important to human therapy and are likely to become increasingly so in the twenty-first century.

FURTHER READING

Alexander, S.P.H. and Peters, J.A. (eds.) (2000) Receptor and ion channel nomenclature supplement. *Trends Pharmacol. Sci. Suppl.*

Anger, T., Madge, D.J., Mulla, M. and Riddall, D. (2001) Medicinal chemistry of neuronal voltage-gated sodium channel blockers. *J. Med. Chem.*, **44**, 115–137.

Ashcroft, F.M. (2000) *Ion Channels and Disease*. London and San Diego: Academic Press.

Endo, M., Kurachi, Y. and Mishina, M. (eds.) (1999) *Pharmacology of Ionic Channel Function. Activators and Inhibitors*. Berlin and Heidelberg: Springer.

Gura, T. (2001) Innate immunity: ancient system gets new respect. *Science*, **291**: 2068–2071.

Hille, B. (1992) *Ionic Channels in Excitable Membranes*, 2nd edition. Sinauer Associates, Sunderland, MA.

Hofmann, F., Lacinova, L. and Klugbauer, N. (1999) Voltage-dependent calcium channels: from structure to function. *Rev. Biochem. Physiol.*, **139**, 33–88.

Mulvaney, A.W., Spencer, C.I., Culliford, S., Borg, J.J., Davies, S.G. and Kazlowski, R.Z. (2000) Cardiac chloride channels: physiology, pharmacology and aproaches for identifying novel modulators of activity. *Drug Discovery Today*, **5**, 492–505.

Narahashi, T (2000) Neuroreceptors and ion channels as the basis for drug action: past, present and future. *J. Pharmacol. Exp. Therap.*, **294**, 1–26.

Rudy, B. and Seeburg, P. (eds.) (1999) Molecular and functional diversity of ion channels and receptors. *Ann. New York Acad. Sci.*, **868**.

Saier, M.H., Jr. (2000) Families of proteins forming transmembrane channels. *J. Membrane Biol.* **175**, 165–180.

Triggle, D. J. (1990) Drugs acting on ion channels. In *Comprehensive Medicinal Chemistry*, Vol. 3, edited by C. Hansch, J.C. Emmett, P.D. Kennewell, C.A. Ramsden, P.G. Sammes and J.B. Taylor, pp. 647–899. Oxford, UK: Pergamon Press.

Watling, K.J. (ed.) (2001) *The RBI Handbook of Receptor Classification and Signal Transduction*. RBI, Natick, Maine.

Chapter 8

Radiotracers: synthesis and use in imaging

Christer Halldin and Thomas Högberg

8.1 INTRODUCTION

Molecules labeled with radioactive isotopes (radionuclides) have been used extensively to study transformations and distributions of endogenous compounds and pharmaceuticals, since it allows for detection of very low levels of materials. Thus, it is a useful technique to track transformed compounds with a common origin without the need for development of specific analytical methods for each of the constituents. Recently, this field has entered a new area with the development of techniques to measure and display radioactivity in 3D by computerized tomography.

The chapter illustrates the synthesis of radioactive compounds. It is divided in sections depending upon the half-life of the radionuclides used, since this will have a profound influence on the synthetic strategy. It is not a comprehensive treatment, but it will give the reader some insight into this special discipline of organic chemistry. The second part of the chapter illustrates the use of different types of imaging.

Compounds radiolabeled with long-lived radionuclides such as ^{14}C, ^{3}H and ^{125}I are commonly used in *in vitro* imaging autoradiographic studies. Several imaging techniques are available for the *in vivo* visualization of morphology or biochemical processes in the human body, i.e. X-ray CT (Computed Tomography), MRI (Magnetic Resonance Imaging), SPECT (Single Photon Emission Computed Tomography) and PET (Positron Emission Tomography). X-ray CT provides anatomical information based on the differential absorption of X-rays by tissue. The MRI uses magnetic and radiofrequency fields to afford anatomical information based on the proton relaxation properties and proton density of tissue. The SPECT is used to visualize and measure the relative concentration of radioactivity in tissue after injection of compounds labeled with a relatively short-lived single photon emitting radionuclide such as ^{123}I. The PET has been widely used to visualize and quantify different biochemical processes such as metabolic processes and receptor densities. The PET technique utilizes radiotracers labeled with relatively short-lived positron emitting radionuclides such as ^{18}F or ^{76}Br or ultrashort-lived radionuclides such as ^{11}C, ^{13}N and ^{15}O. With this technique, minute amounts of radiotracers can be used due to the very high specific radioactivity obtainable by the short-lived radionuclides.

Biochemical changes can be determined by PET and SPECT in order to monitor pathological conditions in living humans even before any anatomical defects occur.

This has a great diagnostic value and gives new information about disease states and their potential therapeutic treatments. Radiolabeling of endogenous compounds such as glucose, amino acids and acetate have been used in studies on metabolism and synthesis of various human tissues such as tumor, cardiac and brain tissue. Receptor selective radioligands which display a high affinity for the receptor and a minimal metabolic degradation are used to probe receptor status. Imaging of CNS receptors in the human brain is a rapidly expanding area which previously was restricted to postmortem binding studies. While both PET and SPECT can detect radiotracer distribution, the SPECT technique is more readily available than PET. The development of a new generation of SPECT cameras, coincidence positron imaging using a gamma camera should significantly increase PET utilization. The PET requires a cyclotron to generate the radionuclides in close connection to the radiochemistry laboratory and the PET camera. However, the PET technique offers several advantages such as the ability to measure the concentration of the tracer quantitatively, a greater sensitivity, a higher resolution and chemically more diverse radiotracers.

8.2   NUCLEAR CHEMISTRY

An array of precursors and compounds labeled with the long-lived radionuclides ^{14}C, ^3H and ^{125}I are commercially available. These radiolabeled compounds have been used for a long time in biochemical and pharmaceutical research, e.g. metabolic, receptor binding and autoradiographic studies. The SPECT uses γ-emitting radionuclides such as ^{123}I, ^{99m}Tc, ^{67}Ga and ^{111}In. The former radionuclide is commercially available and can be produced by the $^{121}Sb(\alpha,2n)^{123}I$ reaction (Table 8.1), i.e. by bombardment of α-particles on a target containing the stable isotope ^{121}Sb to produce the radionuclide ^{123}I and two neutrons. Iodine-123 has a half-life of 13 h and can easily be incorporated with a sufficient level of

Table 8.1 Preparation and some physical properties of commonly used radionuclides

Nuclide	Half-life	Reaction[a]	Mode of decay	Maximum specific radioactivity (Ci/mmol)
^{15}O	2 min	$^{14}N(d,n)^{15}O$	β^+ (100%)	9.1×10^7
^{11}C	20 min	$^{14}N(p,\alpha)^{11}C$	β^+ (100%)	9.2×10^6
^{13}N	10 min	$^{16}O(p,\alpha)^{13}N$	β^+ (100%)	1.9×10^7
^{18}F	110 min	$^{18}O(p,n)^{18}F$	β^+ (97%)	1.7×10^6
^{76}Br	16 h	$^5As(d,n)^{76}Br$	β^+ (57%)	1.9×10^5
^{99m}Tc	6 h	$^{99}Mo(generator)^{99m}Tc$	γ (89%)	–
^{123}I	13 h	$^{121}Sb(\alpha,2n)^{123}I$	E.C. (100%)	2.4×10^5
^{125}I	60 days	$^{124}Xe(n,\gamma)^{125}I$	E.C. (100%)	2.2×10^3
^3H	12 years	$^6Li(n,\alpha)^3H$	β^- (100%)	29
^{14}C	5730 years	$^{14}N(n,p)^{14}C$	β^- (100%)	6.2×10^{-2}

Notes
a   The nuclear reactions indicate the target isotope and the bombarding particle, e.g. $^{14}N(d,n)^{15}O$: nitrogen-14 produce, upon bombardment with one deuteron, oxygen-15 and eject a neutron. d = deuteron; n = neutron; p = proton; α = alpha particle.

radioactivity into several types of organic molecules such as receptor radioligands. The transportation of ^{123}I from the cyclotron to the laboratory/hospital should be rapid and the experimental logistics effective. Compounds labeled with the short-lived PET radionuclides ^{18}F and ^{76}Br (half-lives 110 min and 16 h) and the ultrashort-lived ^{11}C, ^{13}N and ^{15}O (half-lives 20, 10 and 2 min) are not commercially available and must be prepared in the vicinity of a cyclotron, even if ^{76}Br potentially should be able to handle in a similar fashion as ^{123}I.

In a PET facility, the cyclotron, the radiochemistry laboratory and the PET camera constitute the three main operative units. Today, most centers employing PET are using low or medium energy sized cyclotrons to produce one or more of the positron-emitting radionuclides: ^{11}C, ^{13}N, ^{15}O and ^{18}F. The ultrashort half-lives of ^{11}C, ^{13}N and ^{15}O, implies that they must be produced immediately prior to use by an adjacent cyclotron. They are formed by means of nuclear reactions that occur on bombardment of target mediums with charged particles (Table 8.1). The production of ^{11}CO$_2$ is demonstrated in Figure 8.1 as an example of this special type of chemistry. The irradiated materials can be either in a solid, liquid or gaseous state. Radiochemical yields are dependent on factors including target shape, design of target foil and efficiency of target cooling. The amount of radioactivity that can be obtained is regulated by the energy of the accelerated particles and the beam current imposed on target.

Labeling of a compound without affecting its biochemical properties is possible by exchange of stable atoms present in the parent molecule. For instance, carbon-12 (^{12}C) or oxygen-16 (^{16}O) is replaced with the corresponding positron emitting radionuclides ^{11}C or ^{15}O. The small kinetic isotope effect that may occur is considered negligible for most applications. The ultrashort half-lives of especially ^{11}C or ^{15}O make them advantageous for sequential investigations with short time intervals in the same individual (animal or human), thereby allowing the subject to be its own control. The use of radionuclides with relatively longer half-lives such as ^{18}F or ^{76}Br provides an opportunity to follow the radioactivity from the radiolabeled compound for a longer period of time, but leads to use of analogs rather than that of natural compounds.

The specific radioactivity is defined as the ratio of radioactivity per mole of the labeled compound with a maximum specific radioactivity inversely related to the physical half-lives of the radionuclide. The maximum theoretically possible specific radioactivity for ^{11}C is 10^7 Ci/mmol (Table 8.1), but due to the difficulties of completely eliminating external sources of ^{12}C this high specific radioactivity is never obtained. A specific radioactivity higher than 1000 Ci/mmol (37 GBq/μmol), is sufficient for most of the radioligands in use in PET investigations of receptors. In addition, when highly potent radioligands are used an even higher specific radioactivity should be used to avoid mass effect on the receptor.

8.3   LONG-LIVED RADIONUCLIDES

Access to ^{14}C-, ^{3}H- or ^{125}I-labeled precursors or common compounds for biological work can in most cases be obtained from commercial sources. This is especially the case for ^{14}C- and ^{3}H-labeled materials with the longest half-life. The simpler the structure

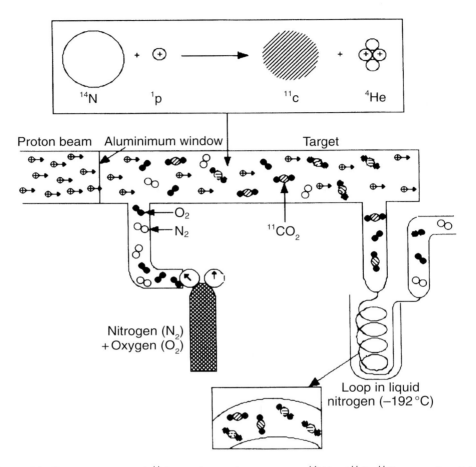

Figure 8.1 The production of ^{11}C via the nuclear reaction $^{14}N(p,\alpha)^{11}C$. ^{11}C is produced by proton bombardment of N_2 which is reacting with trace amounts of O_2 to give $^{11}CO_2$. The prepared $^{11}CO_2$ is trapped in a loop cooled with liquid nitrogen until further use.

the lower the price, i.e. in many situations it is preferable to make the target structure via a lengthy sequence from very simple compounds. For example, $[^{14}C]CH_3I$, $[^{14}C]BaCO_3$, $[^{14}C]KCN$, $[^3H]H_2$ and $[^3H]CH_3I$ are commonly used sources for the introduction of these long-lived radionuclides. Some representative examples of the synthesis of labeled compounds will be given to show what the effect of considerations such as price, availability and half-life will have on the synthetic strategy.

8.3.1 ^{14}C-labeled compounds

Studies of metabolism and disposition of drugs in animals are preferably made with ^{14}C-labeled derivatives in order to avoid exchange of labile tritium for hydrogens *in vivo* (cf. Section 8.3.2), which is a common problem with tritium-labeling, and to give more easily identified metabolites. However, synthetic limitations or the low obtainable specific radioactivity may necessitate other labeling protocols especially with tritium as discussed in 8.3.2. Depending upon the structure, the radiolabel should be introduced in the part of the structure that will provide most of the expected metabolites in radioactive form. One should for example avoid synthetically attractive choices like methylation of a heteroatom (e.g. N-^{14}CH$_3$), which is likely to be lost via P450 mediated α-oxidation to form radioactive formaldehyde instead of the radioactive desmethyl metabolite needed for the identification work.

NNC 756 (**8.8**) is a potent dopamine D$_1$ receptor ligand, which was needed in radiolabeled form for studies on the distribution and metabolic fate. The obvious way to label the nitrogen with ^{14}CH$_3$ was not used for reasons outlined above. Instead, the label was introduced in the ring via a six step sequence shown in Scheme 8.1. The radioactive precursor (**8.1**) was made with tetrafluoroborate as counteranion and reacted with 7-benzofurancarbaldehyde to produce the epoxide (**8.2**), which was reacted with N-methyl-3-chloro-4-methoxyphenethylamine. Opening of the epoxide produced two compounds (**8.3**) and (**8.4**) in a ratio of 9:1, with the desired isomer (**8.3**) in excess. Separation by reversed-phase chromatography and acid catalyzed ring closure with sulphuric acid in trifluoroacetic acid of (**8.3**) gave (**8.5**), which was resolved as dibenzoyl-D-tartrate (DBDT) salt to yield (**8.6**). Demethylation with boron tribromide gave optically pure (**8.7**). Finally, the hydrogenation over Rh/C gave [^{14}C]NNC 756 ([^{14}C]**8.8**) with a specific radioactivity of 24 mCi/mmol and an enantiomeric purity of >97%.

8.3.2 ^{3}H-labeled compounds

Tritium is the most commonly used radionuclide for radiolabeling in biology and medicine. Often the introduction of tritium is made at a late stage in the sequence via exchange or synthetic techniques, which are associated with certain limitations:

1   Exchange reactions with tritiated water or acetic acid (CH$_3$COOT) under acid, base or metal-catalyzed conditions often produce compounds with a low-specific radioactivity;

2   hydrogenation reactions are restricted by the availability of multiple C–C bond precursors and the required chemoselectivity in the reactions (e.g. interference from reactions with other multiple bonds and halogens);

3   hydrogenolysis of aryl-halogen derivatives (especially Ar-I and Ar-Br) has similar selectivity problems as hydrogenation;

4   methylation reactions require a desmethyl precursor and an applicable structure; and

5   hydride reductions are limited by the availability and quality of commercial hydride reagents, i.e. [^{3}H]NaBH$_3$ has often a lower specific activity than theoretically possible.

Since the frequent loss of tritium as tritated water renders the data more difficult to interpret, non-specific equilibration and exchange of labile hydrogens for tritium is less suitable when the tracer will be used for *in vivo* work. Besides, the degree of labeling with tritium in the different positions is usually not known, which can be of importance in studies where metabolic transformations may occur

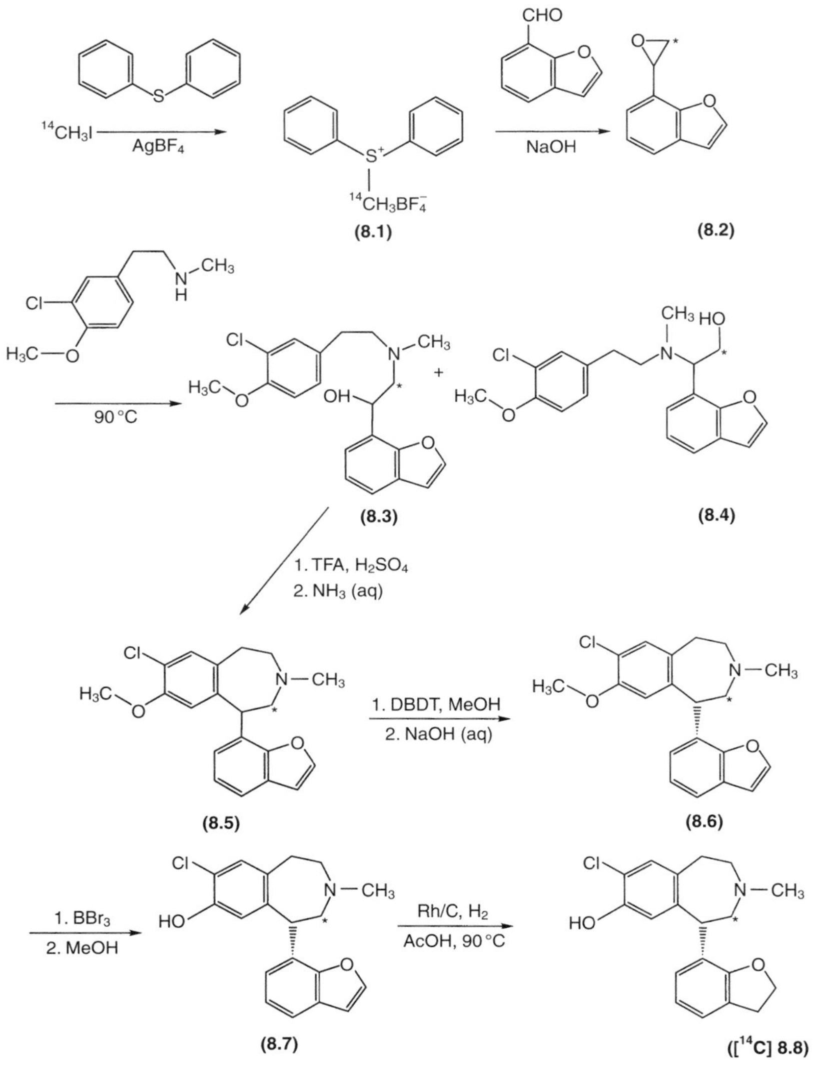

Scheme 8.1

(cf. Section 8.3.1). The development of transition metal catalyzed exchange reactions with tritium gas in which heteroatoms (oxygen and nitrogen) in the target structure can co-ordinate to the metal and promote insertion of tritium in a C–H bond offers a possibility to introduce tritium in positions that are not equally prone to uncatalyzed loss of tritium.

Reduction of olefins will lead to a well-defined regiochemistry even if the stereochemistry could be characterized to a lesser degree. The choice of catalyst will have a large effect on the obtained specific radioactivity, since hydrogen adsorbed on many

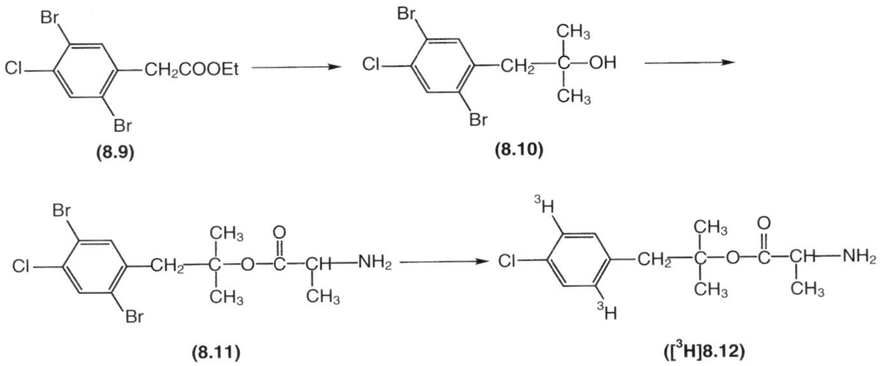

Scheme 8.2

catalysts will equilibrate with tritium if the reaction is too slow. Alternatively, hydrogenolysis of halogen derivatives can be applied to ascertain a well defined labeling. Many studies of receptor binding, especially at low-affinity binding sites, require high degree of specific radioactivity which translates into two tritium atoms per molecule.

Alaproclate (**8.12**) was developed as a selective synaptic serotonin uptake inhibitor. It also possessed affinity for other unknown receptor sites which prompted the preparation of a derivative with two tritium atoms in positions resistant to metabolic attack (Scheme 8.2). The 2,5-dibromo-4-chlorophenylacetate ester (**8.9**), prepared from 4-chlorotoluene, was subjected to a Grignard reaction with methyl magnesium iodide to give (**8.10**). The alanine ester (**8.11**) was obtained by acylation of (**8.10**) with 2-bromopropionyl bromide followed by amination. After optimization of the conditions, the two bromine atoms could selectively be hydrogenolyzed with tritium gas over Pd/C as catalyst in DMF and one equivalent triethylamine. The positions of the tritium atoms in ([³H]**8.12**) can be established by ³H-NMR, which shows *ortho* and *meta* ¹H–³H couplings in a fully coupled spectrum and the expected *para* substitution of the tritium atoms as two uncoupled peaks of equal intensity in a proton decoupled spectrum.

The glucocorticosteroid budesonide (**8.13**) is used in the treatment of asthma, rhinitis and inflammatory bowel diseases. It has been made in tritiated form by an efficient reductive and oxidative sequence (Scheme 8.3). Thus, hydrogenation with tritium gas of budesonide gives the corresponding 1,2-ditritio derivative (**8.14**). The following oxidation provides [³H]budesonide containing different levels of tritium in the 1- and 2-positions. In the case of (**8.14**), the hydrogens in the α-position are labile due to the possibility of enolization, which will lead to loss of tritium, in contrast to ([³H]**8.13**) which is not subject to a facile tritium-hydrogen exchange.

8.3.3   ¹²⁵I-labeled compounds

In order to obtain higher specific radioactivity, than is possible with ³H, the radionuclide ¹²⁵I can be used in applicable cases, which is especially advantageous for

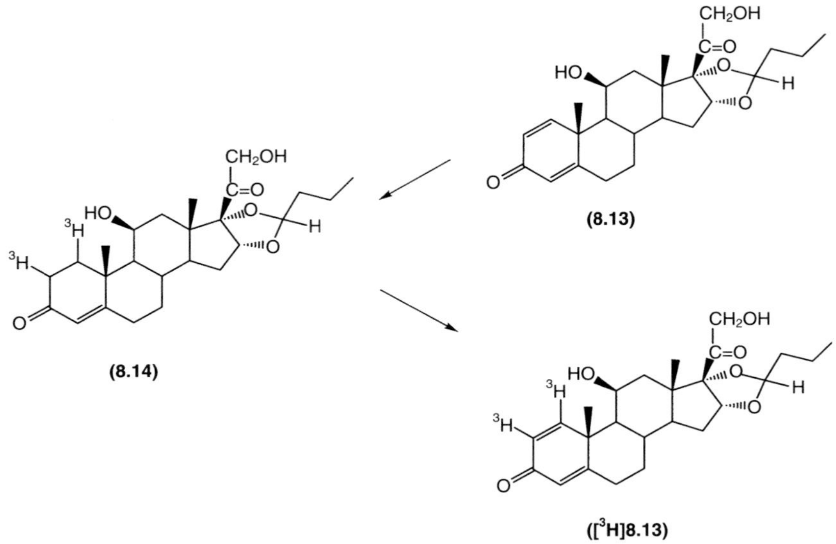

Scheme 8.3

autoradiographic studies. The gamma emitting radionuclide ^{125}I has a half-life of 60 days which enables work during a reasonable time span. Tritium ligands can be made with a specific radioactivity up to 29 Ci/mmol per tritium, compared to 2200 Ci/mmol for ^{125}I-labeled ligands. One reason for the high specific radioactivity of ^{125}I is that the preparation is carrier-free with no dilution of stable iodine. For the development of ^{123}I-labeled radioligands for SPECT (see Sections 8.4.1 and 8.6.2), the use of ^{125}I-labeled radioligands provides essential initial information about the binding properties of the ligand *in vitro* and *in vivo* in animals.

It is common to make non-specific labeling of proteins with this radionuclide. Several types of radioligands for use in receptor binding studies have been designed with ^{125}I substituents. The synthetic work with iodine is, however, more demanding with respect to safety aspects than synthesis with tritium.

NCQ 298 (**8.18**) is a highly selective and potent ligand, developed in our laboratories, for labeling of dopamine D$_2$ receptors. The regiospecific synthesis of [^{125}I]NCQ 298 ([^{125}I]**8.18**) from the dimethoxy compound (**8.15**) is shown in Scheme 8.4. The desiodo compound (**8.17**) is made by *ortho*-lithiation of the benzamide to produce the doubly chelated intermediate (**8.16**), which is reacted with tributyl borate and oxidized with hydrogen peroxide. Carrier-free ^{125}I was oxidized by chloramine-T in dilute hydrochloric acid and reacted with (**8.17**) to produce the radioligand ([^{125}I]**8.18**) in high radiochemical yield and purity. Notably, the direct halogenation reaction proceeds with full regiocontrol.

On the other hand, if the 2,3-dimethoxybenzamide (**8.15**) is iodinated or brominated (see Section 8.4.2) a mixture of halogenated isomers will be formed. In order to achieve a regioselective introduction, one can for example use the *ipso*-directing effect of silicon or use a halogen-metal exchange reaction by starting

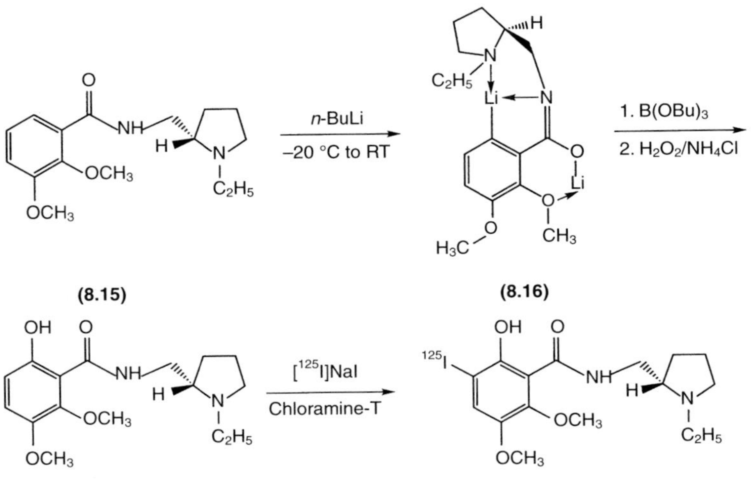

(8.15)   (8.16)

(8.17)   ([^{125}I]8.18)

Scheme 8.4

with the corresponding trialkyltin-derivative (**8.22**), as exemplified in Scheme 8.6 in the synthesis of [^{76}Br]FLB 457.

8.4 SHORT-LIVED RADIONUCLIDES

8.4.1 ^{123}I- and ^{99m}Tc-labeled compounds

The most widely used gamma emitting radionuclides in SPECT are ^{99m}Tc and ^{123}I. A number of successful ligands labeled with ^{123}I for SPECT imaging of various receptors have been developed during the past 10 years. Introduction of ^{123}I is usually carried out in a similar way as for ^{125}I, i.e. by electrophilic substitution of an electron-rich aromatic ring by reaction with [^{123}I]NaI in the presence of oxidation agents such as chloramine-T or peracetic acid.

An example of preparation of a ^{123}I SPECT tracer is given by the cocaine analogs [^{123}I]β-CIT ([^{123}I]**8.19**) (Scheme 8.5), which has been used for examination of Parkinson's disease as demonstrated in Section 8.6.2. The introduction of iodine-123 in the phenyl ring, which is not electron-rich enough to permit an efficient direct oxidative iodination analogous to the one used in the synthesis of ([^{125}I]**8.18**), requires a different strategy. Thus, a trimethyltin precursor (**8.20**) was made by a palladium catalyzed reaction using hexamethylditin in the presence of palladium-tetrakis-triphenylphosphine of the parent iodo compound (**8.19**) as shown in Scheme 8.5. This reaction is an efficient chemoselective way (note the ester and tertiary amine functions) to set up the molecule for a mild iodostannylation reaction. The trimethyltin precursor (**8.20**) is treated with no-carrier-added

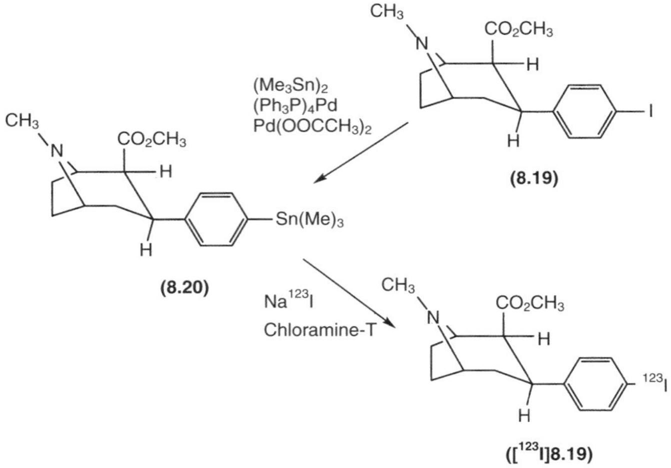

Scheme 8.5

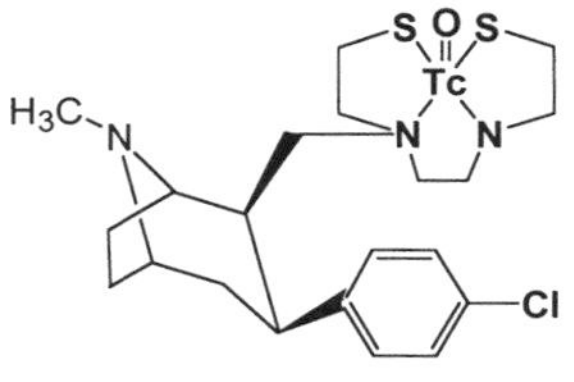

([^{99m}Tc]8.21)

(no dilution with stable iodine) [^{123}I]NaI to form [^{123}I]β-CIT ([^{123}I]**8.19**) with high specific radioactivity (usually >12000 Ci/mmol). When using this labeling method careful purification of the trimethyltin precursor must be performed to ensure a precursor which is free from unlabeled (^{127}I)β-CIT. Presence of carrier β-CIT will reduce the specific radioactivity of the final product and may also result in undesired pharmacological effects for the patient. The advantages of the iodostannylation method are a rapid reaction, high yield, mild radioiodination conditions and a regiospecific incorporation of the iodine. Alternatively, one can use a Cu(I) assisted reaction starting from the corresponding bromo precursor or a method based on direct iodination of the desiodo precursor at oxidative conditions. An advantage with the latter method is facile access to the precursor and elimination of the risk for unlabeled β-CIT in the final solution. Disadvantages are, however, that the direct iodination is not regiospecific, requires heating and results in lower yields. The nuclide ^{99m}Tc is often chelated to the molecule, which can be a suitable tagging technique for studies of e.g. formulations of pharmaceuticals or vascular perfusion (e.g. [^{99m}Tc]hexamethylpropyleneamine oxime) ([^{99m}Tc]

HMPAO). Imaging of dopamine transporters in human with ^{99m}Tc labeled TRODAT–1([^{99m}Tc]**8.21**), a tropane analog, has recently been performed.

8.4.2 ^{76}Br-labeled compounds

The positron emitting radionuclide ^{76}Br has a half-life of 16 h, which makes it possible to follow the radioligand distribution for more than 24 h, if the biological half-life of the compound is long enough. However, the limited access to ^{76}Br and the relatively high doses of radiation to target organs, when ^{76}Br is injected into the body, are disadvantages compared to other PET radionuclides with shorter half-lives. Several substituted benzamides and salicylamides developed at the Astra laboratories have high affinity and selectivity for central dopamine D$_2$ receptors. These properties and a low level of non-specific binding are reasons for their suitability as radioligands for PET.

One recently developed ligand, FLB 457 (**8.23**) has an extremely high affinity for the dopamine D$_2$ receptors, which makes it possible to also study regions containing low densities of receptors outside the striatum. This ligand has also been prepared in carbon-11 labeled form by a reaction analogous to the one described for raclopride ([^{11}C]**8.41**) in Section 8.5.1. Scheme 8.6 shows the preparation of the bromine-76 labeled benzamide FLB 457 ([^{76}Br]**8.23**) as well as the corresponding salicylamide FLB 463 ([^{76}Br]**8.24**). In the former case, a bromostannylation reaction of the tributyltin derivative (**8.22**) is required in order to establish full regiocontrol, whereas the bromination of (**8.17**) provides only one regioisomer (cf. the synthesis of the corresponding iodo derivative ([^{125}I]**8.18**)).

8.4.3 ^{18}F-labeled compounds

Compared to ^{11}C, the half-life of 110 min of ^{18}F allows for a relatively long synthesis and transportation of the radiotracer over moderate distances as well as studies

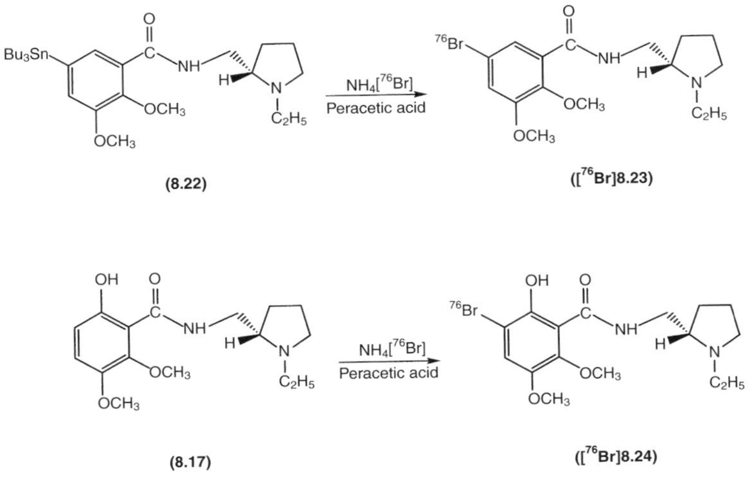

(8.22)　　　　　　　　　　　　　　([^{76}Br]8.23)

(8.17)　　　　　　　　　　　　　　([^{76}Br]8.24)

Scheme 8.6

([¹⁸F]8.25)

of relatively slow biological processes. The labeling of radiotracers with radioactive halogen nuclides usually implies synthesis of analogs rather than of the natural molecules. However, the small size of fluorine makes it possible to replace a hydrogen in many cases without distorting the properties. Accordingly, ^{18}F is a widely used tag in PET of naturally occurring molecules and therapeutic agents. However, the unique electronic properties of fluorine may lead to compounds with deviating properties, which must be investigated prior to the use. For example, a profound influence on the pK_a of amines substituted with fluorine in α- or β-position has been shown to affect the binding affinities of ligands. There are also possibilities to take advantage of the slightly altered properties inflicted by fluorine incorporation in the design of the tracer, e.g. in the most extensively used tracer 2-[^{18}F]fluoro-2-deoxyglucose ([^{18}F]FDG) ([^{18}F]8.25). [^{18}F]FDG has been widely used in metabolic studies of the brain and the heart. After intravenous administration, [^{18}F]FDG is phosphorylated to FDG-6-phosphate mediated by hexokinase. Because FDG-6-phosphate is not a substrate for glycolysis and does not undergo further metabolism, it remains trapped in the cell over the course of several hours. [^{18}F]FDG is usually prepared from [^{18}F]fluoride which can be produced from ^{18}O(p,n)^{18}F using H$_2$^{18}O as target (Table 8.1). [^{18}F]Fluoride can be separated by an anion-exchange column and allowed to react with 1,3,4,6-tetra-O-acetyl-2-O-trifluoromethanesulphonyl-β-D-mannopyranose in the presence of an aminopolyether such as Kryptofix[2.2.2] to enhance the nucleophilicity of fluoride to yield [^{18}F]FDG in about 50% total yield.

Another example of fluorine labeling is the preparation of [^{18}F]NCQ 115 ([^{18}F]8.30) (Scheme 8.7) which is a selective dopamine D$_2$ receptor antagonist. Notably, the affinity of this N-benzyl pyrrolidine (8.30) for the receptor resides in the opposite stereoisomer compared to the other mentioned benzamides with N-ethyl pyrrolidine side chains, e.g. (8.18), (8.23) and (8.24). NCQ 115 has a fluorine in a synthetically accessible position in the parent compound and was therefore suggested as a potential ^{18}F-labeled radioligand for PET. [^{18}F]4-Fluorobenzyl iodide (8.28) was prepared in a 3-step synthesis from potassium [^{18}F]fluoride. The first critical step relies upon a nucleophilic displacement of the quaternary anilinium group which proceeds with regiocontrol due to the influence of the electron-withdrawing aldehyde para-substituent. The nucleophilicity of the fluoride ion is enhanced by using the aminopolyether cryptand Kryptofix[2.2.2] to complex the potassium counterion. N-4-Fluorobenzylation of the corresponding secondary

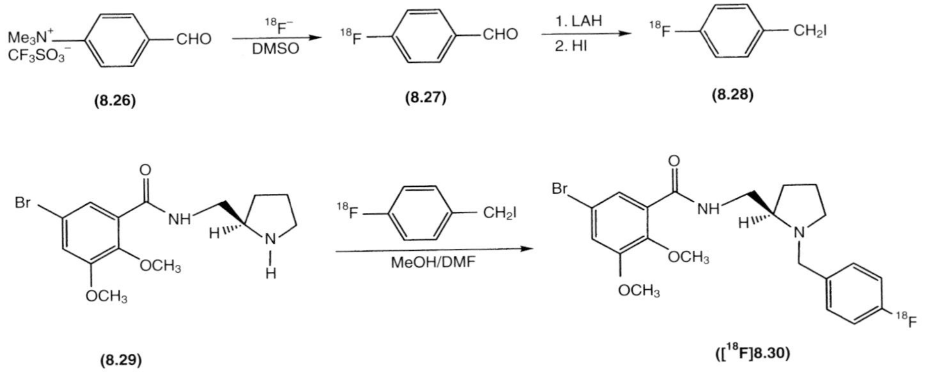

Scheme 8.7

pyrrolidine precursor (**8.29**) was performed giving ([^{18}F]**8.30**) with a total synthesis time of 90 min including purification with semi-preparative HPLC (Scheme 8.7).

8.5 ULTRASHORT-LIVED RADIONUCLIDES

In the preparation of compounds labeled with radionuclides such as ^{11}C, ^{13}N or ^{15}O (half-lives 20, 10 and 2 min) a series of requirements related to the ultrashort half-life of the radionuclide must be considered. When optimizing the radio-chemical yield of a reaction, influence of conventional parameters such as sub-strate and reagent concentrations, temperature, pH and solvent compositions are considered. However, the most critical parameter in the synthesis of these ultra-short-lived tracers is time. Even if a reaction is completed within two half-lives of the radionuclide, it may be favorable to stop the reaction earlier since the radioactivity decay has also to be considered (Figure 8.2).

8.5.1 ^{11}C-labeled compounds

The radioactivity must be introduced by readily accessible radiolabeled precursors. Examples of ^{11}C-labeled precursors that can either be produced directly in the target or obtained via rapid on-line reactions starting from ^{11}CO$_2$ are shown in Scheme 8.8. The most widely used labeled ^{11}C-labeled precursor today is [^{11}C]methyl iodide. Recently, a more reactive precursor [^{11}C]methyl triflate was shown to give higher yields in the synthesis of some commonly used PET radioligands.

The labeling reactions must occur rapidly and in high yields. The complete procedure, from the production of the labeled precursor to the delivery of the purified labeled compound should not exceed more than three half-lives of the radionuclide. A typical total synthesis time for a ^{11}C-labeled radioligand including purification is 30 min. The principal strategy is to introduce the labeled precursor as late as possible, followed by none or just a few additional reactions before the final purification. In addition, handling of high levels of radioactivity on a routine

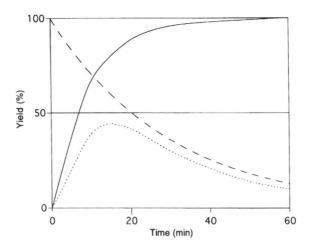

Figure 8.2 The radiochemical yield of a hypothetical ^{11}C-reaction as a function of time (dotted line). Dashed line: the decay curve of the radionuclide. Solid line: the chemical yield of the reaction.

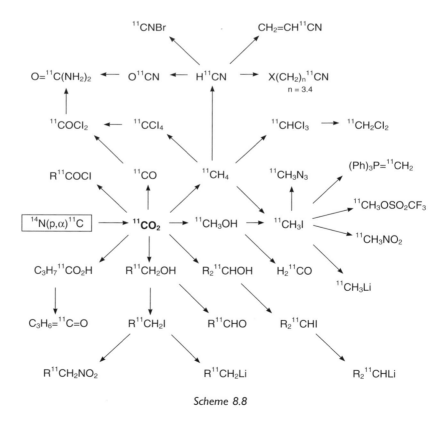

Scheme 8.8

basis requires an automated/remote-controlled experimental set-up installed in a lead-shielded hot-cell to ensure maximal radiation protection. On-line and one-pot reactions shorten the total synthesis time and reduce radioactivity losses.

The stoichiometry of a radiolabeling reaction differs from that of an ordinary chemical synthesis. The amount of the radionuclide produced in the cyclotron is in the nanomolar range. With such small amounts, all other substrates or reactants used are necessarily in large excess. This condition will favor a fast incorporation of the labeled precursor. However, because of the small amounts of the labeled precursor a general problem is that even small amounts of impurities might disturb the reaction. The various steps for the synthesis and PET-application of a radiotracer are presented in Figure 8.3. Efficient PET investigations require an

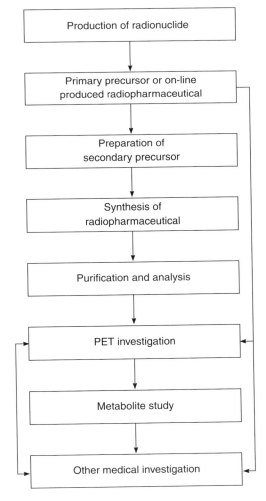

Figure 8.3 Various steps involved before and during medical investigations using positron-emitting radionuclides.

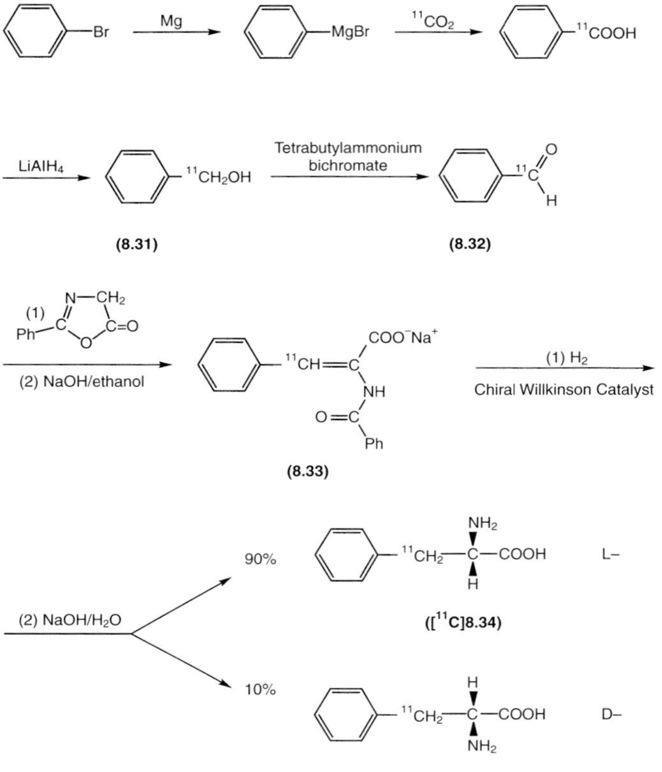

Scheme 8.9

unusually high degree of interdisciplinary collaboration and co-ordination set in a very tight time frame. Thus, PET centers have been established to optimize all steps in this sequence of events and to be cost-effective units. At the end of 1994, the number of PET research centers has reached more than 120 compared to only about 30 centers 10 years ago.

An example of a multi-step synthesis that can be performed with ^{11}C is the seven-step synthesis of optically enriched L-[3-^{11}C]phenylalanine ([^{11}C]8.34) from [^{11}C] carbon dioxide via [^{11}C]benzaldehyde (8.32) (Scheme 8.9). The labeled benzaldehyde was prepared by a selective oxidation of [^{11}C]benzylalcohol (8.31). The three steps from [^{11}C]CO_2 to (8.32) were accomplished within 5 min. [^{11}C]Benzaldehyde was condensed with a 2-phenyl-5-oxazolone to give the [α-^{11}C]-4-benzylidene-2-phenyl-5-oxazolone which was opened by sodium hydroxide in ethanol to give the amide protected α-aminocinnamic acid (8.33). Asymmetric catalytical hydrogenation was performed using a chiral Wilkinson catalyst to obtain the L-form of the amino acid ([^{11}C]8.34) in 80% e.e. The total synthesis time for this seven-step synthesis was 50 min including HPLC purification.

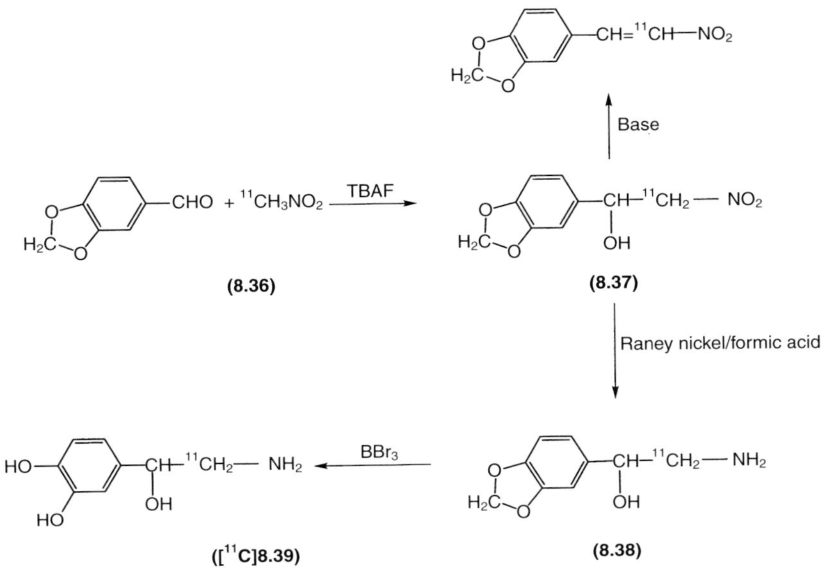

Scheme 8.10

Many analogs of norepinephrine have been radiolabeled for investigation of presynaptic binding sites of the heart. In order to investigate the sympathetic nerve terminal and the noradrenaline metabolism it may be of advantage to use the endogenous transmitter norepinephrine itself and not an analog. A synthetic approach has been developed for the preparation of racemic [^{11}C]norepinephrine ([^{11}C]**8.39**) starting from [^{11}C]nitromethane (**8.36**) (Scheme 8.10). In the first step, piperonal is reacted with [^{11}C]nitromethane with the mild base tetrabutylammonium fluoride (TBAF) as catalyst to give 80–90% of the initial condensation product (**8.37**). Usual bases employed in Knovenagel reactions, such as sodium hydroxide or secondary amines, lead to the nitrostyrene derivative after dehydration of (**8.37**). Reduction of the nitro group is accomplished with Raney nickel/formic acid to give (**8.38**), which is deprotected with boron tribromide.

The salicylamide [^{11}C]raclopride ([^{11}C]**8.41**) is the most extensively used PET radioligand for the quantitative examination of dopamine D$_2$ receptors in striatum by PET. Both enantiomers, [^{11}C]raclopride ([^{11}C]**8.41**) and the inactive isomer C[^{11}C]**8.43**), have been labeled with ^{11}C by O-methylation with [^{11}C]methyl iodide from the corresponding desmethyl precursors (Scheme 8.11). Both enantiomerically pure precursors were obtained by resolving 2-aminomethyl-1-ethylpyrrolidine by fractional crystallization of the ditartrates. The enantiomeric excess of both enantiomers was over 99.8% according to gas chromatographic analysis of the diastereomeric O-methylmandelic amides. Coupling of the resolved pyrrolidine amines with 3,5-dichloro-2,6-dimethoxybenzoyl chloride followed by bisdemethylation gave the enantiomerically pure and symmetrical precursors

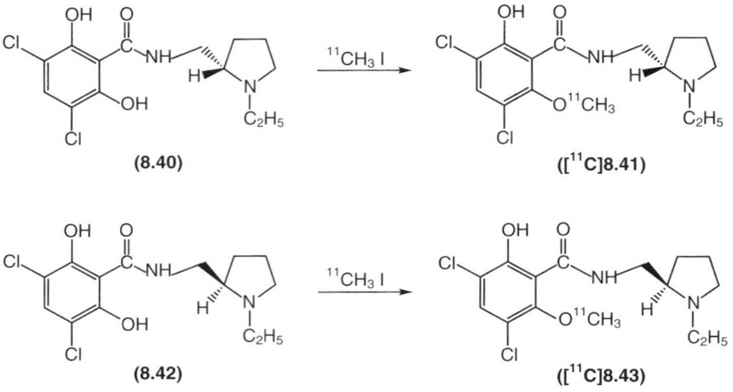

Scheme 8.11

(8.40) and (8.42). The *O*-methylation with [^{11}C]methyl iodide was performed by use of 5 M NaOH as the base in dimethylsulphoxide (DMSO) (Scheme 8.11).

8.5.2 ^{13}N-labeled compounds

The half-life of 10 min of ^{13}N limits the reaction time available and gives an unusual challenge for the development of synthesis methods and strategy for its incorporation into suitable PET tracers. Both synthetic and enzymatic approaches have been applied to the preparation of ^{13}N labeled radiotracers. Nitrogen-13 can be produced by the ^{16}O(p,α)^{13}N reaction. [^{13}N]NH$_3$ is a blood flow tracer, which can be produced by reduction of [^{13}N]nitrate and nitrite in the presence of a mixture of NaOH and TiCl$_3$, with a radiochemical purity greater than 99%. An alternative method is the deuteron irradiation of methane from which [^{13}N] ammonia is collected in an acidic water solution.

A number of enzymatically synthesized L-[^{13}N]amino acids, such as alanine, leucine, aspartic acid, valine, tyrosine and phenylalanine, have been reported. The general reaction used is glumatic acid dehydrogenase catalyzed formation of L-[^{13}N]amino acids from [^{13}N]NH$_3$ and an α-keto acid. Alternatively, [^{13}N]glutamic acid is synthesized and the ^{13}N amino group is transferred to an α-keto acid in a transaminase reaction catalyzed by glutamate–pyruvate or glutamate–oxaloacetate transferase. A variety of ^{13}N-labeled tracers has thus been synthesized, but the half-life limits the number of tracers used routinely today.

8.5.3 ^{15}O-labeled compounds

Preparation of oxygen-15 tracers for PET provides the ultimate challenge in organic synthesis due to the ultrashort half-life of 2 min. Despite the short half-life of ^{15}O the following tracers are used routinely worldwide today:

1    $[^{15}O]O_2$ is produced by the $^{14}N(d,n)^{15}O$ or $^{15}N(p,n)^{15}O$ reaction. $[^{15}O]O_2$ has been used to determine blood flow, oxygen extraction fraction and oxygen metabolism after administration to patients by inhalation.

2    $[^{15}O]CO_2$ is produced by passing $[^{15}O]O_2$ over activated charcoal heated at $400\,^{\circ}C$ to $600\,^{\circ}C$.

3    $[^{15}O]H_2O$ is prepared by bubbling $[^{15}O]CO_2$ into water or by direct action of $[^{15}O]O_2$ with hydrogen. Cerebral blood flow is measured routinely with $[^{15}O]H_2O$.

4    $[^{15}O]$butanol, a new tracer for blood flow, is produced by the reaction between tri-n-butyl borane and $[^{15}O]O_2$. The yield is high, and more than $100\,mCi$ of $[^{15}O]$butanol can be prepared with intervals of $10\,min$.

8.6   IMAGING TECHNIQUES

8.6.1   Autoradiography

The use of radioligands in autoradiographic imaging studies of small animals can give valuable information on distribution, density and kinetics. Slices of the human post-mortem brain can also be incubated with radioligands in order to map the distribution of different receptors. For autoradiography the brain is cryosectioned using a cryomicrotome into $100\,\mu m$ whole hemisphere sections. The tissue sections are transferred to glass plates, put into specially designed incubation chambers and incubated with radiolabeled compounds. The sections are then put into X-ray cassettes together with beta radiation sensitive film for exposure, 4 days for ^{125}I labeled compounds and 4 weeks for ^{3}H-labeled compounds. The films are developed and fixed using conventional techniques. The autoradiograms can be analyzed using computerized densitometry and with a high resolution video camera. Also ^{11}C- and ^{18}F-labeled compounds can be used with exposure times of only 1–4 h. Because of the differences in the range of the radiation, higher resolution is obtained with radioligands labeled with ^{3}H ($0.0072\,mm$ in H_2O) and ^{125}I than with ^{11}C ($4.12\,mm$ in H_2O) or ^{18}F.

An example of an autoradiogram of a whole hemisphere section of a human brain post mortem is given in Figure 8.4. It illustrates the binding of the highly selective and potent serotonin 5-HT$_{1A}$ receptor radioligand $[^{3}H]$WAY-100635. The image of the whole hemisphere demonstrates a high uptake of radioactivity in the hippocampus, raphe nuclei and neocortex regions known to have a high density of serotonin 5-HT$_{1A}$ receptors.

8.6.2   SPECT

The most common SPECT systems consists of a gamma camera with one or three NaI detector heads mounted on a gantry, an on-line computer for acquisition and processing of data, and a display system. The detector head rotates around the axis of the patient at small angle increments (3°–10°) for 180° or 360° angular sampling. The data are collected at each angular position and normally stored in the computer for later reconstruction of the images of the planes of interest.

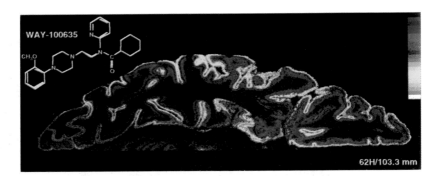

Figure 8.4 [³H]WAY-100635 binding to serotonin 5-HT$_{1A}$ receptors in a post-mortem human brain using whole hemisphere autoradiography. The figure was kindly provided by Dr Håkan Hall, Karolinska Institutet, Sweden.

Multi-head gamma cameras collect data in several projections simultaneously and reduce the time of imaging. The best SPECT cameras of today have a resolution of 5–6 mm.

The SPECT radiopharmaceuticals are used for detecting radioactivity in the whole body. For brain imaging, there exists a large number of tracers for monitoring blood–brain barrier transport, cerebral perfusion, receptor binding and binding to monoclonal antibodies. A perfusion tracer which is widely used for detection of a number of diseases is [^{99m}Tc]hexamethylpropyleneamine oxime ([^{99m}Tc]HMPAO, [^{99m}Tc]**8.21**).

The SPECT tracer [^{123}I]β-CIT ([^{123}I]**8.19**) is an analog to cocaine with a high affinity for the dopamine transporter ($K_d = 0.11$ nM). This recently developed radioligand has proven to be useful for studies of Parkinson's disease. Figure 8.5 shows a 52-year-old control subject (upper images) and a 55-year-old patient with Parkinson's disease (lower images). The patient had recieved no medication before this study. A reduced uptake of [^{123}I]β-CIT was demonstrated in the Parkinson's patient in a brain region normally having a high density of dopamine transporters (localized by arrows). This finding is of high diagnostic value in the examination of Parkinson's patients.

8.6.3 PET

The influence of the biological system on the radioligand *in vivo* cannot easily be simulated *in vitro*. Several conditions such as protein binding in plasma and the extracellular fluids, radioligand metabolism and ligand transport across the blood–brain barrier cannot be explored *in vitro*. By use of imaging techniques such as PET, *in vivo* visualization of biochemical processes can be performed in the human body.

While SPECT is more readily available than PET, the PET technique offers advantages such as the ability to measure the concentration of the tracer quantiatively, a greater sensitivity, a higher resolution and more diverse types of

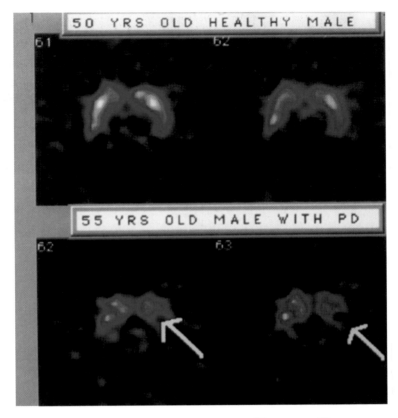

Figure 8.5 SPECT images taken 21 h after injection of $[^{123}I]\beta$-CIT ($[^{123}I]$**8.19**) in a healthy male (top) and a patient with Parkinson's disease (bottom). The images demonstrate highly reduced uptake in the patient with Parkinson's disease (arrow). The figure was kindly provided by Dr Jyrki Kuikka, Kuopio University Hospital, Finland.

radiotracers. The use of short-lived radionuclides and PET gives a low radiation dose to the subject. In addition, repeated investigations can be performed within short-time intervals.

The principles of the PET technique is demonstrated in Figure 8.6. Positron emitting radionuclides disintegrate and emit positrons (positively charged electrons, β^+), that interact with the corresponding antiparticle, an electron (β^-) after traveling in tissue for 1–2 mm. The mass of the two particles is converted to gamma (γ) radiation (annihilation) and two 511 keV photons are emitted simultaneously in opposite directions. The rays emitted are detected externally by a ring of scintillation detectors placed around the subject. The two γ-signals have to be registered by two coincidence coupled detectors within a time window to be counted as originating from the same disintegration. The last generation of PET-systems is used for data acquisition and image reconstruction of 47 slices in the 3D mode with a spatial resolution of 3–4 mm where 2 mm is the maximum theoretical resolution.

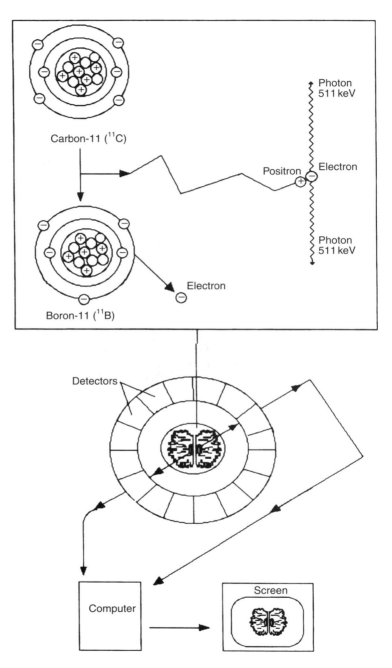

Figure 8.6 The positron-emitting radionuclide ^{11}C decays to form a positron, which annihilates with an electron. The resulting gamma energy, two photons traveling in opposite directions, can be detected externally by a ring of scintillation detectors placed around the subject in the PET camera.

Several PET radiopharmaceuticals are today used as standard tools for investigations of various disease states and control of treatment effects with drugs. The following examples can be mentioned:

1   2-[^{18}F]fluoro-2-deoxyglucose ([^{18}F]FDG, ([^{18}F]**8.25**) is the most frequently used tracer. It measures the glucose metabolism in tumors, heart and especially brain in various disease conditions.
2   [1-^{11}C]acetate, which enters the Krebs tricarboxylic acid cycle at the last possible step by binding to coenzyme-A, can be used as a tracer to reflect the oxygen consumption in the heart. It is prepared from methylmagnesium bromide and [^{11}C]CO$_2$.
3   [^{13}N]ammonia is a precursor that can be incorporated into biomolecules. However, it is a readily diffusible tracer and it enters tissues and metabolic processes, which will reflect the regional blood flow.
4   L-[^{11}C]methionine reflects the amino acid utilization, i.e. transport, protein synthesis, transmethylation and other metabolic processes. It can be easily prepared from the sulfide anion of L-homocysteine and [^{11}C]CH$_3$I.
5   n-[^{15}O]butanol and [^{15}O]H$_2$O are used to study blood flow in the brain and other organs. The partition coefficient of n-[^{15}O]butanol is 1.0, which is an advantage compared to [^{15}O]H$_2$O.
6   [^{11}C]raclopride ([^{11}C]**8.41**) is a selective antagonist for the dopamine D$_2$ receptors that has been used to measure the receptor occupancy in patients treated with different antipsychotics. The preparation is shown in Scheme 8.11.
7   [carbonyl-^{11}C]WAY-100635 is a selective antagonist for the serotonin 5-HT$_{1A}$ receptors which is used to measure receptor density in diseases such as depression, schizophrenia and epilepsy.

Besides [^{11}C]raclopride ([^{11}C]**8.41**) and [carbonyl-^{11}C]WAY-100635, a large number of receptor radioligands have been developed during the past 10 years. Selective radioligands are prepared and widely used in PET for visualization of dopamine, benzodiazepine, muscarinic and serotonin receptors.

Several PET radioligands have been developed for the presynaptic norepinephrine uptake system in the heart. Most of them are, however, analogs labeled with either ^{18}F or ^{76}Br. Recently, the endogenous compound itself, [^{11}C]norepinephrine ([^{11}C]**8.39**), has been synthesized and evaluated in the monkey with PET. Figure 8.7 shows two PET experiments in the monkey heart. The first experiment is a control study (left). In the second pretreatment experiment (right), the selective norepinephrine uptake inhibitor desipramine was given 30 min before injection of [^{11}C]norepinephrine. The results demonstrate that a major part of the radioactivity visualized by PET results from neuronal uptake of racemic ([^{11}C]**8.39**) in the monkey heart.

The preparation and PET examination of radiolabeled stereoisomers are important in radioligand development. Stereospecificity has been demonstrated for drug binding to plasma proteins to a moderate degree. Active transport across membranes is also stereospecific, whereas passive diffusion is primarily related to lipophilicity, which is identical for enantiomers. Stereospecificity is a basic criterion for specific binding to a receptor, an enzyme or a transport mechanism. The active enantiomer (sometimes called eutomer) with specific binding should have a higher

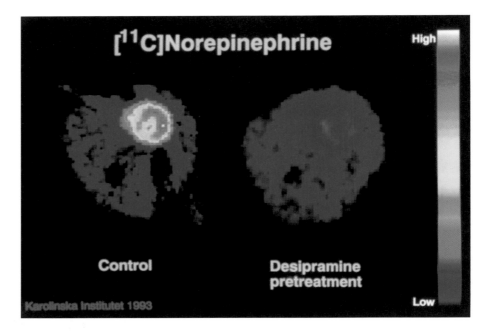

Figure 8.7 PET images showing distribution of radioactivity in the chest of a monkey after injection of [^{11}C]norepinephrine ([^{11}C]**8.39**) in a control experiment (left) and a pretreatment experiment with desipramine (right). The figure was kindly provided by Dr Lars Farde, Karolinska Institutet, Sweden.

accumulation in a target region *in vivo* than the inactive enantiomer (distomer). Comparative PET studies with enantiomers have been suggested as a method to differentiate specific from non-specific binding, which is the key problem in quantitative determination of receptor binding. The usefulness of this method has been demonstrated by PET for several enantiomeric pairs and is exemplified here with the dopamine D_2 receptor antagonist [^{11}C]raclopride ([^{11}C]**8.41**) and its inactive enantiomer ([^{11}C]**8.43**).

Enantiomers have identical physicochemical properties, such as partion coefficient, in a symmetrical environment. In general, if there is no involvement of chiral transport processes across the blood–brain barrier, then the identical partition coefficient of the enantiomers will result in an identical distribution ratio (radioactivity in brain/radioactivity in plasma). Accordingly, it may be possible in PET studies to use the measured brain radioactivity after the injection of an inactive enantiomer as an estimate of the background concentration of radioactivity obtained after the injection of an active enantiomer (Figure 8.8). In radioligand binding experiments *in vitro*, the background level is reduced by simply washing away the free radioligand before the radioactivity is measured. This cannot be accomplished in *in vivo* experiments with PET, because the free radioligand concentration adds to the non-specific binding and increases the background.

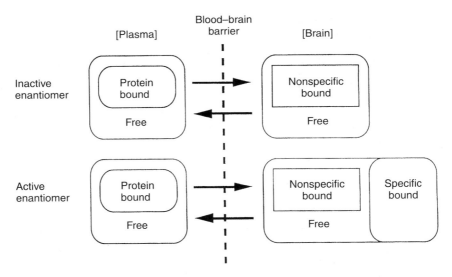

Figure 8.8 Compartments for the distribution of enantiomers.

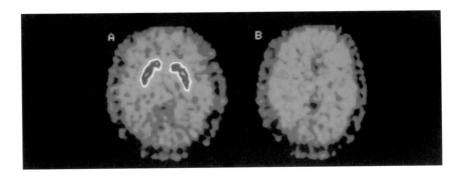

Figure 8.9 PET images showing distribution of radioactivity in the brain after injection of [^{11}C]raclopride ([^{11}C]**8.41**) (A) and the inactive enantiomer ([^{11}C]**8.43**) (B). The figure was kindly provided by Dr Lars Farde, Karolinska Institutet, Sweden.

After the injection of ([^{11}C]**8.41**), there was a high accumulation of radioactivity in the dopamine-rich basal ganglia, whereas the concentration of radioactivity in any other regions could not be differentiated reliably from the background level (Figure 8.9). After the injection of ([^{11}C]**8.43**), there was no such accumulation of radioactivity. Thus, the binding of [^{11}C]**8.41** is stereoselective.

It is generally assumed that the antipsychotic effect of neuroleptic drugs is mediated by blockade of dopamine receptors. By the use of this *in vivo* technique, it is possible to relate clinical drug effects to receptor binding data obtained in the same living subjects. New information of relevance for the identification of tentative target regions for the antipsychotic drug effect may be found by a regional examination of radioligand binding *in vivo* in the human brain.

FURTHER READING

Aquilonius, S.-M., Eckernäs, S.-Å. and Gillberg, P.-G. (1983) Large section cryomicrotomy in human neuroanatomy and neurochemistry. In *Brain Microdissection Techniques*, edited by A.C. Cuello, pp. 155–170. New York: Wiley.

Bengtsson, S., Gawell, L., Högberg, T. and Sahlberg, C. (1985) Synthesis and ^{3}H NMR of ^{3}H alaproclate of high specific activity. *J. Labelled Compd. Radiopharm.*, **22**, 427–435.

Coenen, H.H. (1986) Radiohalogenation methods: an overview. In *Progress in Radiopharmacy*, edited by P.H. Cox, S.J. Mather, C.B. Sampson and C.R. Lazarus, pp. 196–220. Dordrecht: Kluwer Academic Publishers.

Coenen, H.H., Moerlein, S.M. and Stöcklin, G. (1983) No-carrier-added radiolabelling methods with heavy halogens. *Radiochemica Acta*, **34**, 47–68.

Farde, L., Hall, H., Ehrin, E. and Sedvall, G. (1986) Quantitative analysis of dopamine D_2 receptor binding in the living human brain by positron emission tomography. *Science*, **231**, 258–261.

Farde, L., Halldin, C., Någren, K., Suhara, T., Karlsson, P., Schoeps, K.-O., Swahn, C.-G. and Bone, D. (1994) PET shows high specific [^{11}C]norepinephrine binding in the primate heart. *Eur. J. Nucl. Med.*, **21**, 345–347.

Farde, L., Pauli, S., Hall, H., Eriksson, L., Halldin, C., Högberg, T., Nilsson, L., Sjögren, I. and Stone-Elander, S. (1988) Stereoselective binding of [^{11}C]raclopride in living human brain – a search for extrastriatal central D_2-dopamine receptors by PET. *Psychopharmacology*, **94**, 471–478.

Fleming, J.S., Goatman, K.A., Julyan, P.J., Boivin, C.M., Wilson, M.J., Barber, R.W., Bird, N.J. and Fryer T.D. (2000) A comparison of performance of three gamma camera systems for positron emission tomography. *Nucl. Med. Commun.*, **21**, 1095–1102.

Foged, C., Hansen, L. and Halldin, C. (1993) ^{14}C-Labelling of NNC 756, a new dopamine D_1 antagonist. *J. Labelled Compd. Radiopharm.*, **33**, 747–757.

Fowler, J.S. and Wolf, A. (1986) Positron emitter-labelled compounds: priorities and problems. In *Positron Emission Tomography and Autoradiography: Principles and Applications for the Brain and Heart*, edited by M. Phelps, J. Mazziotta and H. Schelbert, pp. 391–450. New York: Raven Press.

Hall, H., Högberg, T., Halldin, C., Köhler, C., Ström, P., Ross, S.B., Larsson, S.A. and Farde, L. (1991) NCQ 298, A new selective iodinated salicylamide ligand for the labelling of dopamine D_2 receptors. *Psychopharmacology*, **103**, 6–18.

Hall, H., Lundkvist, C., Halldin, C., Farde, L., Pike, V.W., McCarron, J.A., Fletcher, A., Cliffe, I.A., Barf, T. and Sedvall, G. (1997) Autoradiographic localization of 5-HT1A receptors in the post-mortem human brain using [^{3}H]WAY-100635 and [^{11}C]WAY-100635. *Brain Research*, **745**, 96–108.

Hall, H., Sedvall, G., Magnusson, O., Kopp, J., Halldin, C. and Farde, L. (1994) Distribution of D_1- and D_2-dopamine receptors, dopamine and its metabolites in the human brain. *Neuropsychopharmacology*, **11**, 245–256.

Halldin, C. (1991) Radioligands for dopamine receptor PET studies: benzamides and ligands for dopamine D_1-receptors. In *Brain Dopaminergic Systems: Imaging with Positron Tomography*, edited by J.C. Baron, D. Comar, L. Farde, J.L. Martinot and B. Mazoyer, pp. 23–38. Dordrecht: Kluwer Academic Publishers.

Halldin, C. (1995) Dopamine receptor radioligands. *Med. Chem. Res.*, **5**, 127–149.

Halldin, C., Farde, L., Högberg, T., Hall, H., Ström, P., Ohlberger, A. and Solin, O. (1991) A comparative PET-studies of five carbon-11 or fluorine-18 labelled salicylamides. Preparation and *in vitro* dopamine D_2 receptor binding. *Nucl. Med. Biol.*, **18**, 871–881.

Halldin, C., Högberg, T. and Farde, L. (1994) Fluorine-18 labelled NCQ 115, a selective dopamine D_2 receptor ligand. Preparation and positron emission tomography. *Nucl. Med. Biol.*, **21**, 627–631.

Halldin, C. and Långström, B. (1985) Asymmetric synthesis of L-[3-^{11}C]phenylalanine using chiral hydrogenation catalysts. *Int. J. Appl. Radiat. Isot.*, **35**, 945–948.

Halldin, C. and Nilsson, S.-O. (1992) Carbon-11 radiopharmaceuticals – radiopharmacy aspects. In *Progress in Radiopharmacy*, edited by P.A. Schubiger and G. Westera, pp. 115–129. Dordrecht: Kluwer Academic Publishers.

Halldin, C., Suhara, T., Farde, L. and Sedvall, G. (1995) Preparation and examination of labelled stereoisomers *in vivo* by PET. In *Chemist's Views of Imaging Centers*, edited by A.M. Emran, pp. 497–511. New York: Plenum.

Högberg, T. (1993) The development of dopamine D$_2$-receptor selective antagonists. *Drug Design and Discovery*, **9**, 333–357.

Högberg, T., Ström, P., Hall, H., Köhler, C., Halldin, C. and Farde, L. (1990) Synthesis of [^{123}I], [^{125}I]- and unlabelled (S)-3-iodo-5,6-dimethoxy-*N*-((1-ethyl-2-pyrrolidinyl) methyl) salicylamide (NCQ 298), selective ligands for the study of dopamine D$_2$ receptors. *Acta Pharm. Nord.*, **1**, 53–60.

Kuikka, J., Bergström, K., Vanninen, E., Laulumaa, V., Hartikainen, P. and Länsimies, E. (1993) Initial experience with single-photon emission tomography using iodine-123 labelled 2β-carbomethoxy-3β-(4-iodophenyl)tropane in human brain. *Eur. J. Nucl. Med.*, **20**, 783–786.

Kung, H.F. (1990) Radiopharmaceuticals for CNS receptor imaging with SPECT. *Nucl. Med. Biol.*, **17**, 85–92.

Kung, H.F., Kim, H.-J., Kung, M.-P., Meegalla, S.K., Plössl, K. and Lee, H.-K. (1996) Imaging of dopamine transporters in humans with technetium-99m TRODAT-1. *Eur. J. Nucl. Med.*, **23**, 1527–1530.

Långström, B., Antoni, G., Gullberg, P., Halldin, C., Malmorg, P., Någren, K., Rimland, A. and Svärd, H. (1987) Synthesis of L- and D-[methyl-^{11}C]methionine. *J. Nucl. Med.*, **28**, 1037–1040.

Loch, C., Halldin, C., Bottleander, M., Swahn, C.-G., Moresco, R.-M., Maziere, M., Farde, L. and Maziere, B. (1994) Preparation and evaluation of [^{76}Br]FLB 457, [^{76}Br]FLB 463 and [^{76}Br]NCQ 115, three selective benzamides for mapping dopamine D$_2$ receptors with PET. *J. Labelled Compd. Radiopharm.*, **35**, 437–438.

Maziere, B. and Delforge, J. (1994) Contribution of positron emission tomography to pharmacokinetic studies. In *Pharmacokinetics of Drugs*, edited by P.G. Welling and L.P. Balant, pp. 455–480. New York: Springer-Verlag.

Maziere, B., Coenen, H.H., Halldin, C., Någren, K. and Pike, V.W. (1992) PET radioligands for dopamine receptors and re-uptake sites: chemistry and biochemistry. *Nucl. Med. Biol.*, **19**, 497–512.

Någren, K., Schoeps, K.-O., Halldin, C., Swahn, C.-G. and Farde, L. (1994) Selective synthesis of racemic 1-^{11}C-labelled norepinephrine, octopamine and phenethylamine and *in vivo* study of [1-^{11}C]norepinephrine in the heart with PET. *Appl. Radiat. Isot.*, **45**, 515–521.

Pike, V.W., Halldin, C. and Wikström, H. (2000) Radioligands for the study of brain 5-HT1A receptors *in vivo*. *Progr. Med. Chem.*, **38**, 189–247.

Saha, G.B. (1993) *Physics and Radiobiology of Nuclear Medicine*, 1st edition. New York: Springer-Verlag.

Saha, G.B., MacIntyre, W.J. and Raymundo, T.G. (1994) Radiopharmaceuticals for brain imaging. *Seminars in Nuclear Medicine*, **24**, 324–349.

Stöcklin, G. (1992) Tracers for metabolic imaging of brain and heart. Radiochemistry and radiopharmacology. *Eur. J. Nucl. Med.*, **19**, 527–551.

Stöcklin, G. and Pike, V.W. (eds) (1993) *Radiopharmaceuticals for Positron Emission Tomography. Methodological Aspects.* Dordrecht: Kluwer Academic Publishers.

Chapter 9

Excitatory and inhibitory amino acid receptor ligands

Ulf Madsen and Bente Frølund

9.1 THERAPEUTIC PROSPECTS FOR EXCITATORY AND INHIBITORY AMINO ACIDS

γ-Aminobutyric acid (GABA) and (S)-glutamic acid (Glu) are the major inhibitory and excitatory neurotransmitters, respectively, in the CNS. The balance between the activity of the two are of utmost importance for CNS functions, and dysfunctions of either of the two can be related to various neurologic disorders in the CNS.

9.1.1 Neurodegenerative diseases

In relation to the development of a number of neurodegenerative diseases, hypoactivity of GABA and/or hyperactivity of Glu neuronal functions seem to be involved. Neurodegenerative disorders such as epilepsy, Huntington's chorea, Parkinson's disease, AIDS dementia and amyotrophic lateral sclerosis are examples of progressive diseases, where compounds interacting with the GABAergic and/or glutamatergic receptor systems may be of therapeutic value. Analysis of brain tissue samples from sites near seizure foci in epileptic patients or from animal models of epilepsy have revealed severe impairment of the GABAergic system. Reduction in the level of the GABA-synthesizing enzyme, Glu decarboxylase (GAD) (Figure 9.2) has been reported as well as reduction in the number of and/or efficiency of GABA transporters in models of epilepsy. Pharmacological studies have shown compounds enhancing GABA levels to be anticonvulsive and compounds with the reverse action to be convulsive. Similar studies using Glu receptor active compounds have shown the opposite effects in animal seizure models, convulsive action of agonists and anticonvulsive action of antagonists.

The primary causes of such neurodegenerative diseases are far from being fully elucidated. Several factors may play important roles, including genetic factors, free radicals and autoimmune mechanisms. Studies in recent years have, however, been focused on the role of Glu in the processes causing neurone injury and, ultimately, death. The view that hyperactivity of Glu neurones is an important causative factor in neurodegenerative processes is supported by *in vitro* and *in vivo* studies in a variety of model systems.

Focus has also been put on the function of GABA. The neurodegenerative process probably depends on the balance between excitatory and inhibitory mechanisms. Thus, inhibition of central glutamatergic activity represent one therapeutic strategy, whereas enhancement of central GABAergic activity represents another. Such strategies may, at least, slow down the progress of these very severe chronic disorders, and/or be used as symptomatic treatment, correcting the level of neuronal GABA and/or Glu activity. The question is whether such interventions can be performed without unwanted side effects. A general activation of inhibitory amino acid receptors or a general blockade of excitatory amino acid receptors may cause severe adverse effects due to the many physiological functions of these receptors. Development of selective agents interacting with specific subtypes of receptors involved in the neurodegenerative processes may be a possible therapeutic strategy.

9.1.2   CNS ischemia

Extensive neurodegeneration can also be observed in the brain after ischemic insults such as stroke or cardiac arrest. The neurodegeneration is, at least in part, caused by an excessive efflux of Glu, which is closely related to a compromised energy supply. Similarly, elevated extracellular levels of GABA are observed after ischemic insults. Data from experimental models of stroke shows that stimulation of GABA functions results in neuroprotection and suggests an increase of GABA activity to be a therapeutic approach. Stimulation of GABAergic activity should in any event, decrease glutamatergic activity. An immediate treatment with Glu antagonists may also be of beneficial value, and the concern towards side effects will be less strict for a short-term treatment compared to chronic administration. In numerous animal models of focal and global ischemia, various Glu receptor antagonists have shown promising neuroprotective properties, and several Glu antagonists have been subjected to clinical trials. In spite of effective blockade of Glu neurotoxicity, these compounds have all been withdrawn due to serious unwanted effects. However, different types of Glu antagonists are still being tested, in the search for candidates with fewer or no side effects.

9.1.3   Alzheimer's disease

In Alzheimer's disease an especially complicated neuropathological pattern is observed. Brain tissue from Alzheimer patients is characterized by extensive degeneration of especially cholinergic neurones. The prominent symptoms of Alzheimer patients are cognitive impairment and memory deficits, and a progressive, inevitable fatal, neurodegeneration. Hyperactivity of Glu neurones are believed to be involved in the development of the disease. However, neurodegeneration of Glu neurones are also observed at a certain stage of the disease.

The cause for this degeneration is not known, but the concomitant reduction of Glu neuronal function may be part of the learning and memory deficits observed in Alzheimer patients. The dual role of Glu neurones, involving both hypo- and hyperactivity, is illustrated in Figure 9.1. A Glu antagonist, capable of preventing the neurotoxicity due to Glu hyperactivity (Figure 9.1B), may simultaneously aggravate the hypoactivity observed at other Glu synapses (Figure 9.1C). On the other hand, a Glu agonist, administered in order to restore activity in the latter situation, may enhance the neurotoxicity observed in the hyperactivity situation.

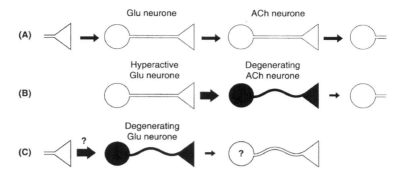

Figure 9.1 Schematic illustration of the interaction between a glutamatergic (Glu) and a cholinergic (ACh) neurone; (A) normal condition; (B) hyperactive; and (C) hypoactive Glu neurones, the two latter representing situations in Alzheimer's disease.

A possible therapeutic solution, at least in theory, may be the use of a partial agonist (see Section 6.3.3). A partial Glu agonist with an appropriately balanced agonist/antagonist profile may partially block the hyperactivity in certain brain areas, whereas in areas of hypoactivity a certain level of activity may be maintained due to the intrinsic activity, although reduced, of the partial agonist itself. It is not known whether such a strategy can be exploited therapeutically, but it does focus pharmacological attention on partial agonists (see Section 9.3.2.4).

9.1.4 Other neurologic disorders

The GABAergic compounds, notably benzodiazepines (see Section 9.2.5.3) have been successfully used for treatment of anxiety. Recent animal studies have also shown inhibitors of Glu activity to be anxiolytic. However, clinical application of Glu antagonists for this indication will require development of compounds with very limited or no side effects.

Increasing evidence from animal studies support the proposal that GABA as well as Glu receptors are involved in pain transmission and the plasticity which accompanies sensitization to pain. Thus, enhancement of GABA activity or inhibition of Glu activity may be used in the treatment of chronic pain.

Finally, abnormal inhibitory and/or excitatory amino acid neurotransmission seems to play a role in schizophrenia. Apart from the well-established imbalance observed for dopaminergic and cholinergic neurotransmission, there has been some controversy as to whether hypo- or hyperactivity at GABA and Glu receptors are implicated in the neurologic pattern of schizophrenia. Activation of the GABAergic system produce psychotomimetic effects in normal human beings and stimulate the psychotic symptoms in schizophrenic patients, and drug abuse of a Glu antagonist (PCP, see Section 9.3.1.3) has caused schizophrenic symptoms. These observations have been interpreted as indicative of GABA hyper- and Glu hypoactivity, respectively, to be part of schizophrenia. However, recent contradictory results seem to indicate that Glu hyperactivity is involved, and clinical trials are going on with both an antagonist as well as with a positive modulator of AMPA receptors.

9.2   GABA: INHIBITORY NEUROTRANSMITTER

The role of the neutral amino acid GABA (**9.1**) as the major inhibitory neurotransmitter in the CNS is fully established. Furthermore, GABA is involved in the regulation of a variety of physiological mechanisms in the periphery. GABA is present in high concentrations in many brain regions and the majority of central neurones are sensitive to GABA and receive synaptic input from GABAergic neurones. The major role of the GABAergic neurotransmitter system is to balance neuronal excitability. Imbalance due to impaired operation of the GABA-mediated inhibitory synapses may be an important factor in several neurologic disorders as described in Section 9.1. These aspects have focused interest on the various processes and mechanisms associated with GABA-mediated neurotransmission in the CNS as potential targets for clinically useful drugs.

9.2.1   Therapeutic targets

The GABAergic neurotransmitter system involves a number of synaptic processes and mechanisms, which have been studied pharmacologically and constitute potential therapeutic targets. GABA is formed in the presynaptic nerve terminals

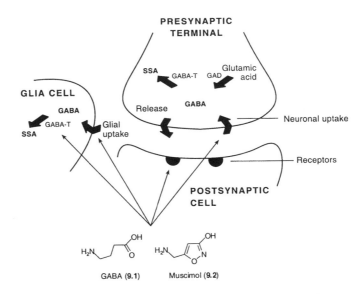

GABA (**9.1**)   Muscimol (**9.2**)

Figure 9.2 Schematic illustration of the biochemical pathways, transport mechanisms, and receptors at a GABA-operated axo-somatic synapse. GAD: (S)-glutamic acid decarboxylase; GABA-T: GABA:2-oxoglutarate aminotransferase; SSA: succinic acid semi-aldehyde. The interactions with various GABA synaptic mechanisms of GABA and the heterocyclic GABA analog muscimol (**9.2**), is indicated.

and released into the synaptic cleft, where it activates the postsynaptic GABA receptors (Figure 9.2). This activation causes an opening of the chloride channels, resulting in hyperpolarization of the nerve membrane potential. GABA is taken up by presynaptic nerve terminals and glial cells, and subsequently, it is enzymatically metabolized to form succinic acid semialdehyde (SSA).

Many drugs with effects in the brain, such as anxiolytics, anticonvulsants, myorelaxants, sedatives and general anaesthetics have been shown to interact with the GABA neurotransmitter system. Possible targets of action of these drugs include direct GABA receptor agonism/antagonism, allosteric modulation of the GABA receptors or interference with GABA reuptake or metabolism.

9.2.2   The GABA molecule

The structural requirements for activation of the different targets in the GABA neurotransmitter system have been extensively studied using GABA as a lead compound.

The GABA molecule has a very high degree of flexibility and there is strong evidence supporting the view that GABA adopts dissimilar active conformations at different synaptic recognition sites. Thus, pharmacological studies of GABA analogs with restricted conformations may lead to compounds with selective actions. Synthesis and structure–activity studies of GABA analogs, in which the conformational and electronic parameters have been systematically changed, have shed much light on the molecular pharmacology of the GABA synaptic mechanisms.

Muscimol (**9.2**), a constituent of the mushroom *Amanita muscaria*, is a very potent GABA$_A$ (see Section 9.2.5 for receptor classification) agonist but muscimol is also an inhibitor of neuronal and glial GABA uptake and a substrate for the GABA-metabolizing enzyme GABA transaminase (GABA-T) (Figure 9.2). Muscimol has been used as a lead for the design of different classes of GABA analogs, and systematic variation of the molecular structure of muscimol in order to separate the multiple affinities of this compound, has provided a number of specific GABA$_A$ receptor agonists and GABA uptake inhibitors (Figure 9.3). Conversion of muscimol into THIP (**9.3**) and the isomeric compound THPO (**9.4**) effectively separated GABA$_A$ receptor and GABA uptake affinity; THIP proved to be a specific GABA$_A$ agonist, whereas THPO is a GABA uptake inhibitor. Further development led to the monoheterocyclic compounds isonipecotic acid (**9.5**), isoguvacine (**9.6**), nipecotic acid (**9.7**) and guvacine (**9.8**), where **9.5** and **9.6** were shown to be specific GABA$_A$ agonists and **9.7** and **9.8** GABA uptake inhibitors (Figure 9.3).

The degree of stereoselectivity of the GABA transport mechanisms has been compared with that of the GABA$_A$ receptor binding sites using the *S*- and *R*-forms of chiral GABA analogs as test compounds (Figure 9.4). The *S*- and *R*-forms of the flexible GABA analog 4-aminopentanoic acid (**9.9**) are equally effective at GABA$_A$ receptor sites, and both interact with the neuronal as well as the glial GABA uptake systems. Conformational restriction of the C2-C3 bonds of the enantiomers of 4-aminopentanoic acid as in (*S*)- and (*R*)-*trans*-4-amino-2-pentenoic acid (**9.10**) has quite dramatic effects on the pharmacological profiles. Thus, the *S*-form of this

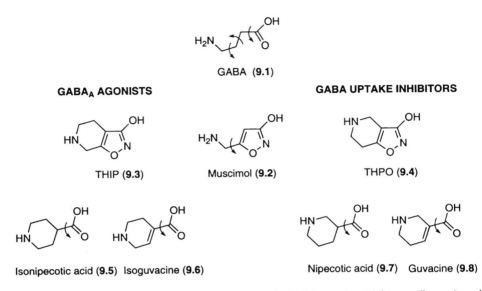

GABA (9.1)

GABA_A AGONISTS

GABA UPTAKE INHIBITORS

THIP (9.3)   Muscimol (9.2)   THPO (9.4)

Isonipecotic acid (9.5) Isoguvacine (9.6)   Nipecotic acid (9.7) Guvacine (9.8)

Figure 9.3 Structures of some GABA_A agonists and GABA uptake inhibitors illustrating the structural requirements for activation of GABA_A receptors and for inhibition of GABA uptake.

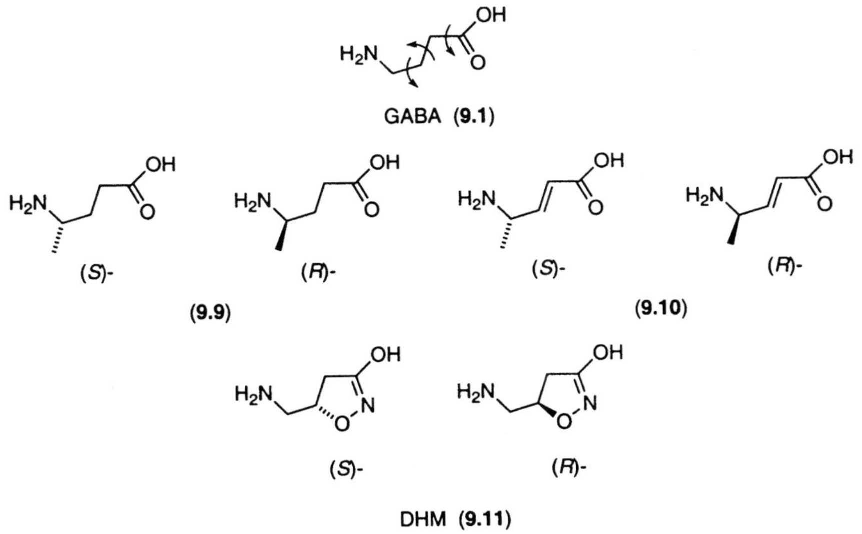

GABA (9.1)

(S)-   (R)-   (S)-   (R)-

(9.9)   (9.10)

(S)-   (R)-

DHM (9.11)

Figure 9.4 Structures of S- and R-forms of GABA analogs.

conformationally restricted GABA analog specifically binds to and activates GABA_A receptors, whereas its *R*-isomer interacts with neuronal and glial GABA uptake systems without showing detectable affinity for GABA_A receptor sites. These results show that the degree of stereoselectivity of GABA synaptic mechanisms depends on the conformational mobility of the chiral GABA analog tested. Thus, enantiomers of semi-rigid, chiral GABA analogs show markedly different pharmacological profiles.

Studies on chiral analogs of muscimol have supported these structure–activity relationships. Thus, the S-form of dihydromuscimol (DHM, **9.11**) is an extremely potent and highly selective GABA$_A$ agonist and (R)-DHM is a selective inhibitor of GABA uptake.

9.2.3   GABA biosynthesis and metabolism

The biochemical pathways underlying the synthesis and catabolism of GABA, have largely been mapped out and the key enzymes are identified and characterized. The main pathway for GABA synthesis is decarboxylation of Glu catalyzed by GAD which uses pyridoxal-5'-phosphate (PLP) as a cofactor (Figure 9.2). GABA is released via a specific release system into the synaptic cleft by depolarization of the presynaptic neurone. The initial step of the degradation of GABA is transformation into SSA. This transamination step, which is catalyzed by the PLP-dependent GABA-T, takes place within presynaptic GABA terminals as well as in surrounding glia cells (Figure 9.2). Extracellular enzymatic degradation does not seem to play any role in the inactivation of GABA.

The crystal structure of GABA-T has recently been reported, which undoubtedly will assist the development of new inhibitors on a more rational basis. The compounds discussed in the following section have all, however, been developed prior to the determination of the crystal structure of the enzyme.

9.2.3.1   Inhibitors of GABA metabolism

A number of mechanism-based inactivators of GABA-T has been developed and has been shown to work *in vitro* and *in vivo*. These compounds are typically analogs of GABA, containing appropriate functional groups at C4 of the GABA backbone. The functional group are converted by GABA-T into electrophiles, which react with nucleophilic groups at or near the active site of the enzyme and thereby inactivate the enzyme irreversibly. Although GABA-T, like other PLP-dependent enzymes, does not show strict stereospecificity with respect to inactivation by mechanism-based inactivators, such inhibitors do react with the enzyme in a stereoselective manner. Thus, the S-forms of the GABA-T inhibitors 4-amino-5-hexenoic acid (Vigabatrin) (**9.12**), 4-amino-5-hexynoic acid (**9.13**) and the fluoromethyl derivative (**9.14**) are more active as GABA-T inactivators than the respective R-isomers (Figure 9.5). These observations are in good agreement with results obtained from modeling studies of the inhibitors using the reported crystal structure of the enzyme. Selective inactivation of GABA-T using Vigabatrin is successfully applied in treatment of epilepsy. In this regard, it is interesting and fortunate that the active S-isomer of Vigabatrin is actively taken up by the neuronal as well as the glial transport mechanisms, whereas the R-isomer is not transported.

A number of conformationally rigid analogs of Vigabatrin and 4-amino-5-halopentanoic acid has recently been developed. The saturated 5-fluoro analog **9.16** exhibit inactivation of GABA-T similar to, although not as potent

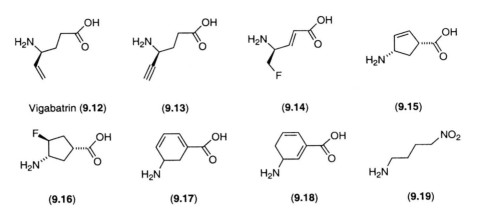

Figure 9.5 Structures of some GABA-T inhibitors, compound **9.15** being inactive.

as, the corresponding open-chain analogs. This is in contrast to the unsaturated conformationally constrained Vigabatrin analog **9.15**, which does not inactivate GABA-T. Gabaculine (**9.17**), a naturally occurring neurotoxin isolated from *Streptomyces toyacaensis* and isogabaculine (**9.18**) are potent irreversible inactivators of GABA-T. In contrast to Vigabatrin (**9.12**), the cyclic analogs of GABA do not alkylate the enzyme. As a result of enzymatic processing by GABA-T these compounds are converted into aromatic pyridoxamine-5-phosphate adducts, which do not desorb from the active site of the enzyme. 4-Nitro-1-butanamine (**9.19**) is a GABA-T inhibitor, in which the weakly acidic nitromethylene group participates in the inactivation of the enzyme (see Scheme 9.2).

The mechanism for inactivation of GABA-T by Vigabatrin (**9.12**) is outlined in Scheme 9.1. As shown, a Schiff base (**9.20**) is formed between the co-factor PLP and the terminal amino group from a lysine residue. Transamination with **9.12** generates a new iminium ion **9.21**, which undergoes rate-determining enzyme-catalyzed deprotonation to give the iminium ion **9.23** after reprotonation. In analogy with transamination reaction on GABA, **9.23** could be hydrolyzed to give the SSA analog **9.25** and pyridoxamine-5-phosphate **9.24**. However, **9.23** is a Michael acceptor electrophile, which undergoes conjugate addition by an active-site nucleophile X^- and the inactivated enzyme **9.26** is produced.

The initial steps in the inactivation of GABA-T by the naturally occurring inhibitor, gabaculin (**9.17**) (Scheme 9.2, upper part), are analogous with those described for Vigabatrin (**9.12**) (Scheme 9.1). Gabaculine (**9.17**) is recognized by GABA-T and is coupled to PLP to give the Schiff base **9.27**. Although **9.28**, formed by deprotonation of **9.27**, contains a dihydrobenzene ring showing some electrophilic character, **9.28** is not sufficiently reactive to alkylate GABA-T. As shown in Scheme 9.2, one of the highly activated protons at C2 in the dihydrobenzene ring of **9.28** is removed. Subsequent reprotonation of the complex by a protonated nucleophile on the enzyme (GABA-T) gives compound **9.29**, which inactivates GABA-T via tight, but non-covalent binding to the active site. A major driving

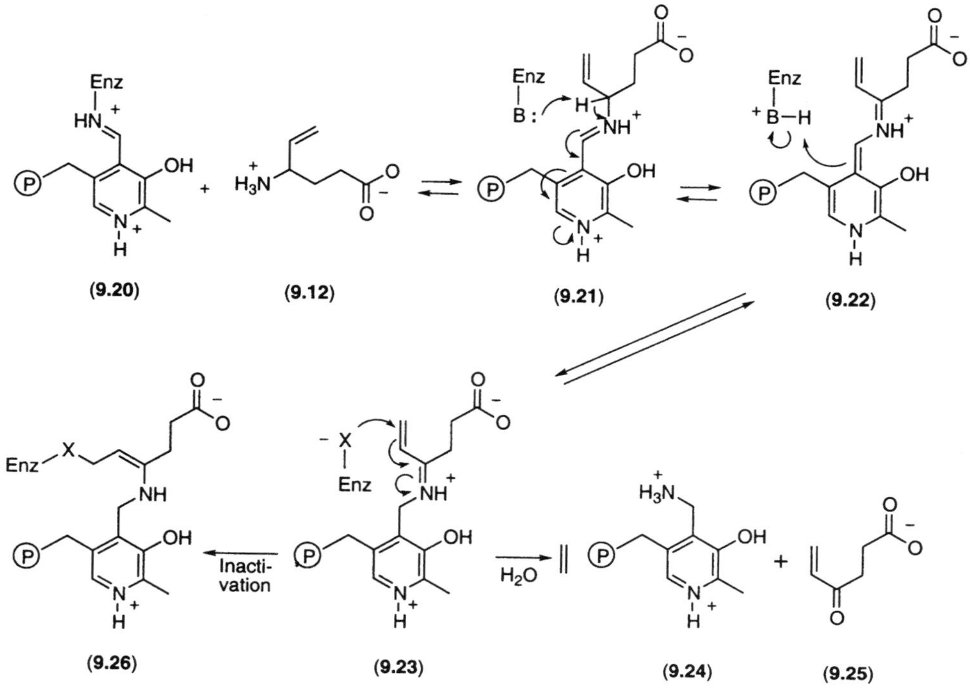

Scheme 9.1 Proposed inactivation mechanism of GABA-T by Vigabatrin (**9.12**).

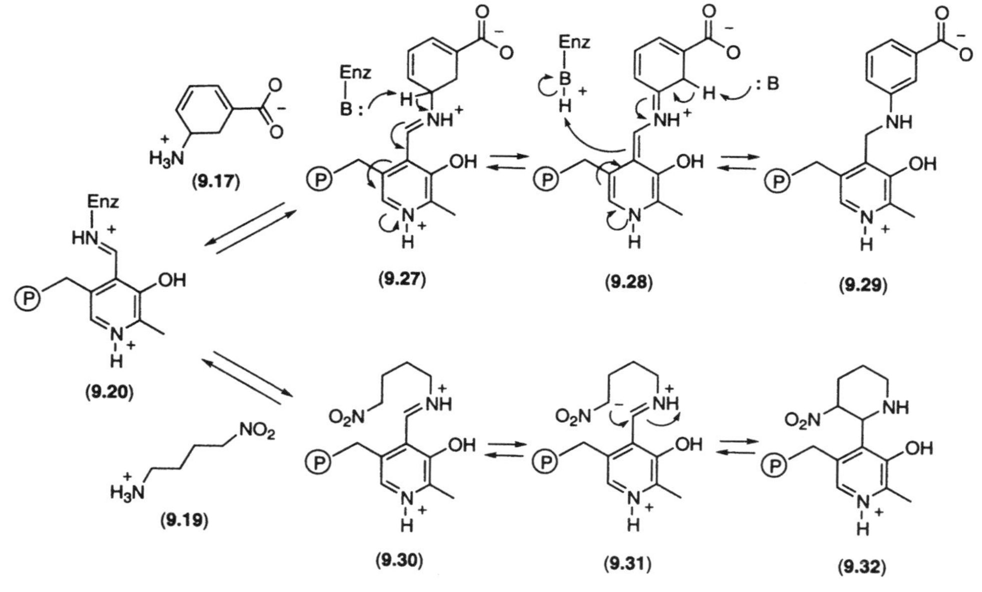

Scheme 9.2 Proposed inactivation mechanism of GABA-T by gabaculine (**9.17**) (upper part) and by 4-nitro-1-butanamine (**9.19**) (lower part).

force in the conversion of **9.28** into **9.29** is the aromatization of the dihydrobenzene ring of **9.28**.

The mechanism of action of the GABA-T inhibitor **9.19** is outlined in Scheme 9.2 (lower part). Like gabaculine (**9.17**), **9.19** reacts with PLP. This reaction produces **9.32**, which inhibits the action of GABA-T in a manner analogous with that described for compound **9.29**. The key step in the formation of **9.32** is the intramolecular nucleophilic reaction between the anionic nitromethylene and iminium group of **9.31**.

9.2.4 GABA uptake

The action of GABA at the synapses is terminated by reuptake into both pre-synaptic nerve terminals and surrounding glial cells (Figure 9.2). The GABA taken up into nerve terminals is available for reutilization, whereas GABA taken up in glial cells is metabolized to SSA by GABA-T and cannot be resynthesized to afford GABA again since glial cells lack GAD. The uptake process is catalyzed by sodium-coupled transport systems located in plasma membranes of nerve endings and glial cells and it has been demonstrated that both sodium and chloride ions are cotransported with GABA by the transporter. The GABA uptake data obtained from studies using cultured cells from mammalian CNS are consistent with heterogeneity of both neuronal and glial transport mechanisms. Molecular cloning studies have also shown that the GABA transporters are heterogenous and four different GABA transporter have, until now, been cloned. The four subtypes, which are homologs for the human and rat transporters, have been termed GAT-1, GAT-2, GAT-3 and BGT-1 (the betaine/GABA transporter). Studies of the neuronal vs. glial localization of GABA transporter mRNA have disclosed that whereas GAT-1, GAT-3 and BGT-1 mRNAs are present in both neurones and glial cells, GAT-2 is the only transporter being selectively expressed in non-neuronal cells.

9.2.4.1 Inhibitors of GABA uptake

A logical approach for increasing GABA neurotransmission would be blockade of the uptake systems in order to enhance the amount of GABA in the synaptic cleft. A selective blockade of glial uptake would be optimal, as this would ensure an elevation of the GABA concentration in the presynaptic nerve terminals. It has been established that neuronal and glial uptake mechanisms have dissimilar substrate specificities. The structural requirements for uptake inhibitors are also different from what is required for interaction with postsynaptic GABA receptors, as described in Section 9.2.2. Thus, selective interaction with the different GABA uptake sites is possible. Nipecotic acid (**9.7**) is an effective inhibitor of neuronal as well as glial GABA uptake, being twice as potent at the latter system. Furthermore, nipecotic acid has been shown to be a substrate for neuronal as well as glial GABA transport carriers making analyses of the pharmacology of this compound difficult. A number of cyclic amino acids structurally related to nipecotic acid, including guvacine (**9.8**) show a profile very similar to that of nipecotic acid. Whereas introduction of small substituents on the amino groups of nipecotic acid (**9.7**) or guvacine (**9.8**) results in compounds with reduced affinity for the GABA transport

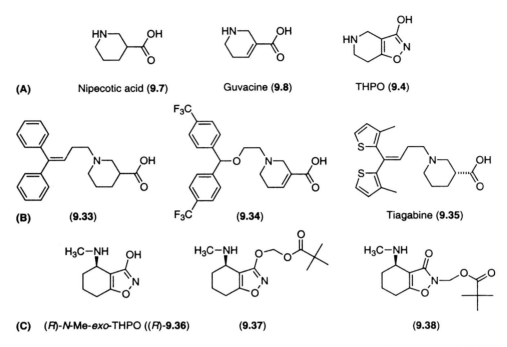

Figure 9.6 Structures of some GABA uptake inhibitors: (A) nipecotic acid, guvacine and THPO; (B) lipophilic analogs, (**9.33–9.35**); and (C) (R)-N-Me-exo-THPO ((R)-**9.36**) and two prodrugs of (R)-**9.36**.

carriers, N-(4,4-diphenyl-3-butenyl)nipecotic acid (**9.33**) and structurally related analogs, such as **9.34** (Figure 9.6B), are much more potent than the parent amino acids. In contrast to **9.7** and **9.8**, these lipophilic compounds are able to cross the blood–brain barrier and are potent anticonvulsants in animal models. Tiagabine (**9.35**) (Figure 9.6B), a structurally related compound, is now marketed as an add-on therapeutic agent for treatment of epilepsy.

The molecular mechanism underlying the interaction of the lipophilic analogs with GABA uptake systems is unknown. In contrast to the N-unsubstituted amino acids, these analogs do not seem to be substrates for the GABA transporters, although the competitive nature of action strongly suggest that they do interact directly with the carrier binding site. Molecular pharmacological studies of nipecotic acid (**9.7**) and guvacine (**9.8**) disclose high affinity for GAT-1 and GAT-2 and rather low affinity for GAT-3, whereas the lipophilic analogs, including tiagabine (**9.35**) interact selectively with GAT-1. A few compounds with moderate potency and selectivity for GAT-3 and BGT-1 have been identified. The GAT subtypes have different distribution in the brain and subtype selective compounds would be useful tools for studies of the physiological and pharmacological importance of the GAT subtypes, and may explain the different anticonvulsant profiles observed for different compounds.

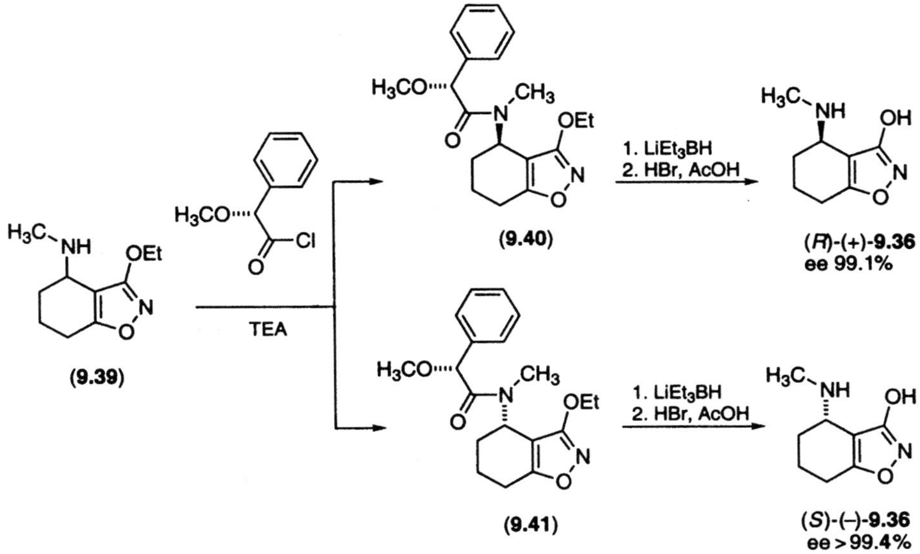

Scheme 9.3 Separation of the two enantiomers of N-Me-exo-THPO (9.36).

THPO has been used as a lead in the search for more glia-selective inhibitors. N-Me-*exo*-THPO (9.36) (Figure 9.6C) was developed as a GABA uptake inhibitor and the *R*-enantiomer of 9.36 has shown the highest degree of selectivity for the glial GABA transport system so far observed, with the *S*-form being inactive. Removal of the methyl group of (*R*)-N-Me-*exo*-THPO or replacement of this group by larger groups lead to pronounced loss of activity on the GABA transport. Since 9.36 is not active in mice after systemic administration, the prodrug approach was used to study the *in vivo* pharmacology of this compound. The *O*- and *N*-pivaloyl-oxymethyl derivatives, 9.37 and 9.38 (Figure 9.6C), respectively, were shown to be bioreversible derivatives of (*R*)-N-Me-*exo*-THPO ((*R*)-9.36) and showed potent anticonvulsant effect after subcutaneous administration in mice. These results underline the importance of the glial GABA uptake system as a potential thera-peutic target in convulsive disorders.

The enantiomers of N-Me-*exo*-THPO (9.36) were synthesized, as shown in Scheme 9.3, from 9.39 via the diastereomeric α-methoxyphenylacetamides, 9.40 and 9.41, which were separated using preparative HPLC. The absolute configuration of the *R*-enantiomer of 9.36 was established by an X-ray crystal-lographic analysis (Figure 9.7). In the low-energy conformation, as shown in Figure 9.7, (*R*)-nipecotic acid ((*R*)-9.7) adopts a chair conformation with the carboxylate group in equatorial orientation. The depicted conformation of THPO (9.4) is derived from the X-ray structure of its *O*-methyl derivative. THPO is much weaker than (*R*)-nipecotic acid as a GABA uptake inhibitor, but both compounds show a low degree of selectivity for glial vs. neuronal GABA uptake. The similarity of the conformations of THPO and of (*R*)-nipecotic acid may indicate that the two compounds interact with the GABA transport carriers in conformations similar to

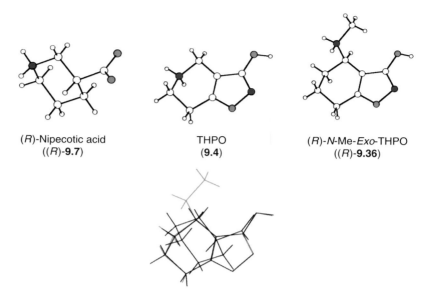

(R)-Nipecotic acid	THPO	(R)-N-Me-Exo-THPO
((R)-**9.7**)	(**9.4**)	((R)-**9.36**)

Figure 9.7 Comparison and superimposition of low-energy conformations of the GABA uptake inhibitors (R)-nipecotic acid ((R)-**9.7**) (blue), THPO (**9.4**) (green) and (R)-N-Me-exo-THPO ((R)-**9.36**) (red). The molecular structure of zwitterionic (R)-**9.7** was determined by an X-ray crystallographic analysis. The depicted molecular structure of cationic **9.4** is derived from the structure of O-Me-THPO hydrochloride, determined by an X-ray crystallographic analysis. The illustrated molecular structure of cationic ((R)-**9.36**) is based on an X-ray crystallographic analysis of the hydrobromide salt of ((R)-**9.36**).

those illustrated in Figure 9.7. The low-energy conformation of (R)-N-Me-exo-THPO ((R)-**9.36**) obviously is different from those of (R)-nipecotic acid and THPO. Since (R)-N-Me-exo-THPO shows a 13-fold higher selectivity as an inhibitor of glial vs. neuronal GABA uptake, this particular conformation of (R)-N-Me-exo-THPO may represent an important structural determinant for glia-selective GABA uptake inhibition.

9.2.5   GABA receptors

The GABA receptors have been divided into two main groups: (1) the ionotropic GABA$_A$ and GABA$_C$ receptors, which produce fast synaptic inhibition; and (2) the metabotropic (G-protein coupled) GABA$_B$ receptors, which produce slow and prolonged inhibitory signals. The classification of GABA receptors based on pharmacological characterization using selective ligands is outlined in Figure 9.8. Whereas BMC (**9.42**) and SR 95531 (**9.43**) are the classical antagonists at GABA$_A$ receptors, isoguvacine (**9.6**) and THIP (**9.3**) are specific GABA$_A$ receptor agonists. (R)-baclofen (**9.44**) is the classical GABA$_B$ receptor agonist and the corresponding phosphonic acid analog, (R)-phaclofen (**9.45**), was the first GABA$_B$ antagonist to be characterized. The GABA$_C$ receptors are insensitive to both BMC and baclofen, but

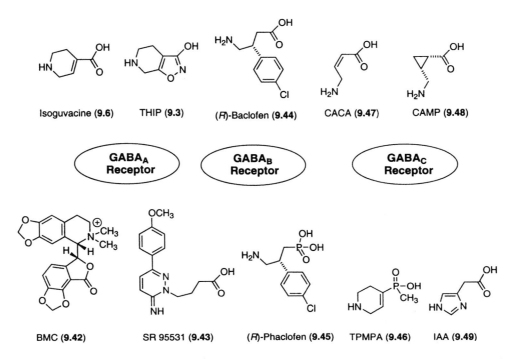

Figure 9.8 Schematic illustration of the different classes of GABA receptors and the structures of standard agonists (upper part) and antagonists (lower part) used for pharmacological characterization of these receptors.

are selectively antagonized by TPMPA (**9.46**), whereas CACA (**9.47**) and CAMP (**9.48**) are GABA$_C$ receptor agonists. Interestingly, the partial GABA$_A$ agonist, IAA (**9.49**) has been shown to be a potent antagonist at GABA$_C$ receptors.

The heterogeneity of GABA$_A$ receptors in the brain is large, because of the large number of different GABA$_A$ receptor subunits. At least 17 different subunits ($\alpha_{1-6}, \beta_{1-4}, \gamma_{1-4}, \delta, \varepsilon,$ and π) have been identified. The GABA$_A$ receptors are formed as a pentameric assembly of different subunits, making the existence of a very large number of such heteromeric GABA$_A$ receptors possible. The assembly, which in most receptors includes two α subunits, two β subunits and one γ or δ subunit, determines the pharmacology of the functional receptor. The GABA$_C$ receptors are the least characterized of the GABA receptors, but the membrane topology is assumed to be very similar to that of GABA$_A$ receptors. However, GABA$_C$ receptors are derived exclusively of ρ subunits (ρ_{1-3}) expressed primarily in the retina. The various isoforms of the ρ subunits can assemble into homomeric chloride channels showing a pharmacology different from the GABA$_A$ receptors.

The metabotropic GABA$_B$ receptors belong to the family of G-protein coupled receptors and more particularly to the subfamily C which comprises the metabotropic Glu receptors (see also Chapter 6). Two isoforms, GBR1 and GBR2, of the receptor protein have been isolated and more recent it has been shown that the two isoforms exist as a heterodimer and form a fully functional GABA$_B$ receptor.

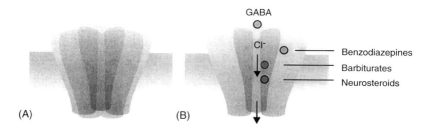

Figure 9.9 (A) Schematic model of the pentameric structure of the GABA$_A$ receptor complex; and (B) a schematic illustration of the GABA$_A$ receptor complex indicating the chloride ion channel and additional binding sites.

9.2.5.1 The GABA$_A$ receptor complex

The postsynaptic GABA$_A$ receptor is a receptor complex containing a number of modulatory binding sites for drugs such as benzodiazepines, barbiturates, and neurosteroids (Figure 9.9). The GABA$_A$ receptor regulates the influx of chloride ions in such a way that receptor activation causes hyperpolarization of the cell membrane and, thus, decreased sensitivity of the neurone to excitatory input. The complexity of the GABA$_A$ receptor function is comparable to that of the NMDA subtype of Glu receptor channels (see Section 9.3.1.3).

Site-directed mutagenesis studies have shown that the binding site for benzodiazepines is located at the interface between the α and γ subunit in the GABA$_A$ receptor complex, whereas the binding site for GABA and GABA$_A$ agonists is located at the interface between the α and β subunit. The potency and maximal response of ligands for the GABA binding site is highly subunit dependent. At some subunit combinations certain compounds may act as agonists and at other subunit combinations as antagonists or low efficacy partial agonists. Despite the fact that the GABA binding site is located at the interface between the α and β subunit, the pharmacological profile of the receptor seems to be determined by the interaction of all subunits present in the receptor. To study this in more detail more GABA$_A$ agonists, partial agonists and antagonists are needed with specific effects at the physiologically relevant GABA$_A$ receptors of different subunit compositions.

9.2.5.2 GABA$_A$ receptor ligands

The conformationally restricted analogs of GABA, muscimol (**9.2**), thiomuscimol (**9.50**) and DHM (**9.11**), are highly potent GABA$_A$ agonists (Figure 9.10). These compounds indicate that the 3-isoxazolol, the 3-isothiazolol and the 2-isoxazoline-3-ol heterocyclic systems are bioisosteres of the carboxyl group of GABA with respect to GABA$_A$ receptors. Whereas muscimol (**9.2**) interacts more effectively than GABA with GABA$_A$ receptors *in vivo* and *in vitro*, it binds less tightly than GABA to GABA$_B$ receptor sites and to GABA transport mechanisms. Thiomuscimol (**9.50**) does not affect GABA uptake *in vitro*, but as muscimol it is metabolized by GABA-T, and this metabolism reduces the value of these potent GABA$_A$ agonists for *in vivo* pharmacological studies.

A number of analogs of the structurally constrained GABA$_A$ agonist THIP (**9.3**) have been synthesized. As for the muscimol series, the 3-isoxazolol ring system has been replaced by other heterocyclic systems (Figure 9.10). With the exception of thio-THIP (**9.51**), which is a very weak GABA$_A$ agonist, none of these THIP analogs show significant GABA$_A$ receptor affinities, emphasizing the strict structural requirement for activation of GABA$_A$ receptors. THIP, which undergoes very limited metabolic decomposition *in vivo*, penetrates the brain–blood barrier. THIP shows non-opioid analgesic and anxiolytic effect and appears to improve the quality of sleep.

In general, the availability of antagonists with specific or highly selective effects on receptors is essential for elucidation of the physiological role of the receptors concerned. The fact that all GABA$_A$ antagonists, so far studied pharmacologically, are convulsants, makes it highly unlikely that such compounds are going to play an important role in future therapy. In certain diseases, where a reduction in the GABA$_A$ function is desired, low-efficacy partial GABA$_A$ agonists may have therapeutic interest (see Section 9.1.4).

4-PIOL (**9.53**) and the isothiazole analog (**9.54**) (Figure 9.11) have been shown to be low-efficacy partial agonists, with dominating antagonist profiles on brain tissue *in vitro*. In contrast to the desensitization observed after direct activation of GABA$_A$ receptors by full agonists, repeated administration of 4-PIOL (**9.53**) to cerebral cortical neurones did not cause significant desensitization of the GABA$_A$ receptors studied.

A number of analogs containing different substituent in the 4-position of the 3-isoxazolol ring of 4-PIOL (**9.53**) (Figure 9.11) has been synthesized in order to investigate the effect on the pharmacological profile. The results from these studies are listed in Figure 9.12 where the receptor pharmacology is represented by the K_i values from [^{3}H]muscimol binding studies and by IC$_{50}$ values from an electrophysiological model. Substituents in the 4-position of 4-PIOL analogs seem to be allowed in contrast to what has been found for the corresponding muscimol analogs. Introduction of a methyl or an ethyl group in the 4-position of muscimol to give **9.55** and **9.56** (Figure 9.11), respectively, leads to virtually inactive compounds. The methyl, ethyl and benzyl analogs of 4-PIOL (**9.57–9.59**)

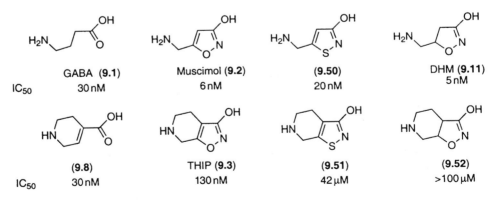

Figure 9.10 Structures of some GABA$_A$ receptor ligands with IC$_{50}$ values from [^{3}H]GABA binding.

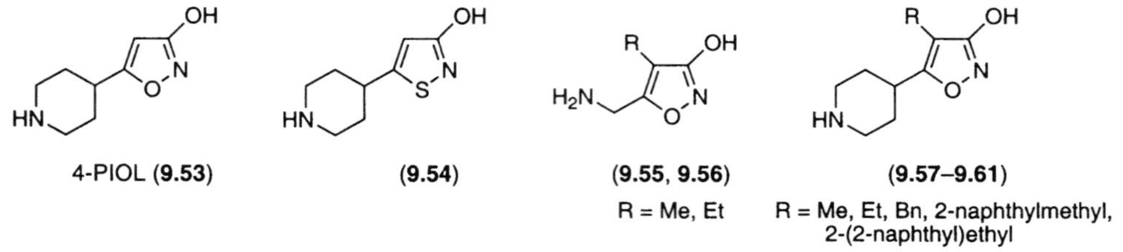

4-PIOL (**9.53**)   (**9.54**)   (**9.55, 9.56**)   (**9.57–9.61**)

                                                R = Me, Et   R = Me, Et, Bn, 2-naphthylmethyl,
                                                                  2-(2-naphthyl)ethyl

Figure 9.11 Structures of the partial GABA$_A$ receptor agonists 4-PIOL (**9.53**) and the thia analog (**9.54**), muscimol analogs (**9.55, 9.56**) and 4-PIOL analogues (**9.57–9.61**).

(Figure 9.12) show that larger substituents in the 4-position of the 3-isoxazolol ring of 4-PIOL affords compounds with higher affinity for the GABA$_A$ receptors. Extension of the aromatic system from a phenyl to a naphthyl group to give **9.60** markedly increases the affinity, with a corresponding increase in potency, whereas extension of the linker joining the 2-naphthyl group and the 3-isoxazolol ring to give compound **9.61** resulted in a 10-fold reduction in affinity relative to **9.60**.

Using whole-cell patch-clamp techniques on cultured cerebral cortical neurones in the electrophysiological testing, the functional properties of the 4-PIOL analogs (**9.57–9.61**) in the absence or in the presence of the specific GABA$_A$ receptor agonist isoguvacine (**9.6**) (Figure 9.8), were studied. The study showed that the structural modifications led to a change in the pharmacological profile of the compounds from low-efficacy partial GABA$_A$ receptor agonist activity to potent and selective antagonist effect. The 2-naphthylmethyl analog **9.60** showed an antagonist potency comparable with that of the standard GABA$_A$ antagonist SR 95531 (**9.43**) (Figure 9.12). These structure–activity studies seem to indicate that the binding modes of 4-PIOL (**9.53**) and muscimol (**9.2**) are different, as illustrated in Figure 9.13A. In this model illustrating the possible GABA$_A$ receptor interactions the 3-isoxazolol rings do not overlap (Figure 9.13B), implying that the 4-position in 4-PIOL does not correspond to the 4-position in muscimol. Thus, a large cavity at the 4-PIOL recognition site of the GABA$_A$ receptor seems to exist.

9.2.5.3   *Benzodiazepines and neurosteroids*

The GABAergic compounds acting at the benzodiazepine site or at the barbiturate site have been used as hypnotics for several decades. Agonists at these binding sites increase the chloride flux by modulation of the receptor response to GABA stimulation. Benzodiazepines increase the frequency of channel opening in response to GABA and barbiturates act by increasing mean channel open time. In the absence of GABA, the modulatory ligands do not produce any effect on the channel opening.

Not only drugs that have a benzodiazepine structure such as diazepam (**9.62**) and **9.63** can interact with the high-affinity benzodiazepine binding sites in the CNS, but also compounds such as β-carboline (**9.64**), imidazopyridine (**9.65**) and triazolopyridazine (**9.66**) as illustrated in Figure 9.14. The pharmacological profile of ligands binding to the benzodiazepine site spans the entire continuum from full and partial agonists, through antagonists, to partial and full inverse agonists.

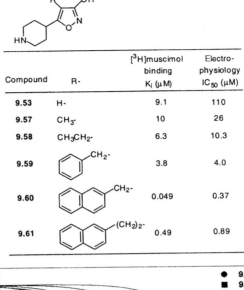

Compound	R-	[³H]muscimol binding K_i (μM)	Electro-physiology IC_{50} (μM)
9.53	H-	9.1	110
9.57	CH_3-	10	26
9.58	CH_3CH_2-	6.3	10.3
9.59	CH_2-	3.8	4.0
9.60	CH_2-	0.049	0.37
9.61	$(CH_2)_2$-	0.49	0.89

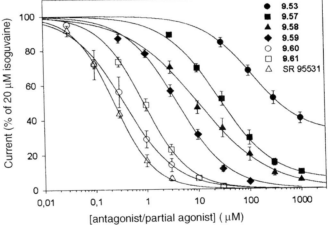

Figure 9.12 (Top) Receptor binding affinity (K_i values from [³H]muscimol binding on rat brain synaptic membranes) and *in vitro* electrophysiological activity (IC_{50} values from whole-cell patch clamp recording from cerebral cortical neurons) for a number of 4-PIOL analogs; (Bottom) effect of the partial agonists or antagonists on the response to 20 μM isoguvacine using whole-cell patch clamp recordings from cultured cerebral cortical neurons. 20 μM isoguvacine and varying concentrations of antagonist/partial agonist were applied simultaneously to the cells. The response to 20 μM isoguvacine alone has been set to 100%, and the other responses are expressed relative to this.

Antagonists do not influence GABA-induced chloride flux, but antagonize the action of benzodiazepine site agonists as well as of inverse agonist. The compounds with different efficacies produce a wide variety of behavioral pharmacological effects. The full benzodiazepine agonists show anxiolytic, anticonvulsant, sedative,

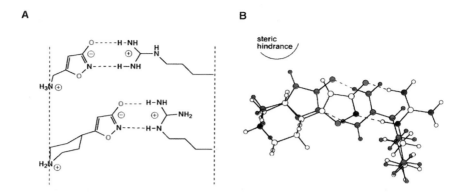

Figure 9.13 (A) Hypothetical model for the binding of muscimol and 4-PIOL to the GABA_A receptor; (B) a superimposition of the proposed bioactive conformations of muscimol (**9.2**) and 4-PIOL (**9.53**) binding to two different conformations of an arginine residue at the agonist binding site.

Diazepam (**9.62**)   Ro15-4513 (**9.63**)   DMCM (**9.64**)

Zolpidem (**9.65**)   CL218872 (**9.66**)

Figure 9.14 Structures of some ligands for the benzodiazepine site.

and muscle relaxant effects, whereas the inverse agonists produce anxiety and convulsions. Of particular therapeutic interest are the reports of compounds, which are partial agonists at the benzodiazepine site, displaying potent anxiolytic and anticonvulsive effects with markedly less sedation and muscle relaxation compared to conventional benzodiazepines.

The relationship between GABA_A receptor subunit composition and molecular pharmacology of benzodiazepines has been extensively studied and, as for GABA_A ligands, the benzodiazepines show highly subunit dependent pharmacological profiles. From such studies it may be possible to identify and localize distinct subtypes of $GABA_A$ receptors associated with different physiological and pathophysiological functions enabling development of novel compounds with more specific actions.

Neuroactive steroids are a novel class of positive allosteric modulators of the $GABA_A$ receptor that interact with a specific steroid recognition site on the receptor–ion channel complex. Neurosteroids are synthesized in the brain, whereas other neuroactive steroids with pharmacological effects in the CNS are not necessarily synthesized in the CNS tissue. Neurosteroids and neuroactive steroids are important endogenous agents for influencing brain function by modulation of the activation of $GABA_A$ receptors. They include pregnenolone (**9.67**) and reduced metabolites such as (**9.68**) and its 5β epimer (**9.69**) (Figure 9.15A). These steroids are rapidly biotransformed when administered exogenously due to metabolism of the 3-α-OH group at the 3-position. Thus, they exhibit rapid onset and short duration of action. Several synthetic analogs such as alphaxolone (**9.70**), ganaxolone (**9.71**) and **9.72** (Figure 9.15B) have been developed and show promising therapeutic effects. In general neuroactive steroids produce effects in animal models of CNS disorders similar to those of other positive allosteric modulators of the $GABA_A$ receptor without significant side-effects.

9.2.5.4 GABA_B receptor ligands

Of the two GABA receptor classes insensitive to BMC (**9.42**), the $GABA_B$ receptors have been most extensively studied. The $GABA_B$ receptors are coupled to G-proteins, which upon activation cause a decrease in calcium and an increase in potassium membrane conductance. The $GABA_B$ receptors seem to be pre-

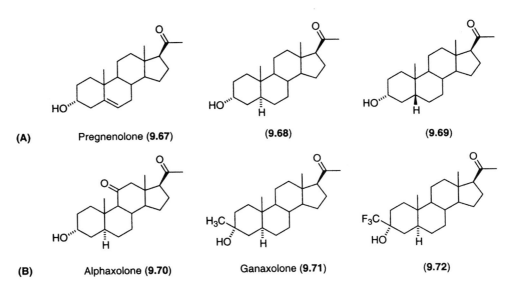

Figure 9.15 Structures of some (A) neurosteroids; and (B) neuroactive steroids.

dominantly located presynaptically and they modulate synaptic transmission by depressing neurotransmitter release, including Glu release. These receptors are activated by GABA and, in contrast to GABA$_A$ receptors, also by the GABA analog (R)-baclofen (**9.44**). Baclofen was developed as a lipophilic derivative of GABA, in an attempt to enhance the blood–brain barrier penetrability of the endogenous ligand. (R)-Baclofen is effective in certain types of spasticity and has been in clinical use as an antispastic agent before discovery of the GABA$_B$ receptor. The clinical effect is believed to be related to GABA$_B$ receptor mediated inhibition of the release of Glu from hyperactive Glu terminals.

Although, a number of phosphinic acid-based GABA$_B$ receptor agonists have been synthesized, the number of selective and potent agonists for the GABA$_B$ receptor is limited and (R)-baclofen remains one of the more potent and selective agonists for the GABA$_B$ receptor. Among the agonists synthesized, the phosphinic acid analog of GABA (**9.73**) and its methyl analog (**9.74**) (Figure 9.16A) are the most active, being 3- and 7-fold more potent than (R)-baclofen, respectively.

The phosphonate analog of (R)-baclofen, (R)-phaclofen (**9.45**) as well as saclofen (**9.75**) and 2-OH-saclofen (**9.76**) (Figure 9.16B) were introduced as the first GABA$_B$ antagonists with peripheral as well as central activity. In attempt to improve the pharmacology of the GABA$_B$ receptor agonist **9.73**, a new series of selective and potent GABA$_B$ antagonists, capable of penetrating the blood–brain

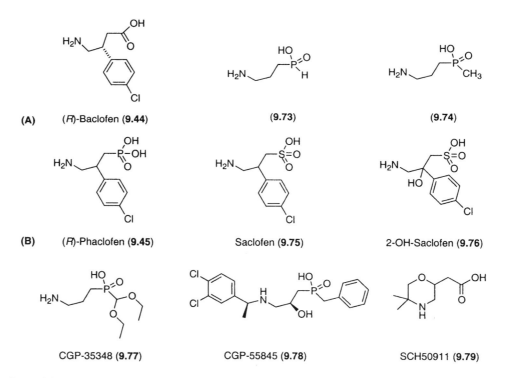

Figure 9.16 Structures of (A) GABA$_B$ receptor agonists and some examples of (B) GABA$_B$ receptor antagonists.

barrier after systemic administration, was discovered. One of the initial compounds in this series CGP-35348 (**9.77**) was succeeded by compound **9.78** (Figure 9.16B), showing very high affinities for the GABA$_B$ receptor. 2,5-Disubstituted-1,4-morpholines, exemplified by compound **9.79**, represent another structural class of GABA$_B$ receptor antagonists, which has been shown to be systemically active.

9.2.5.5   *GABA$_C$ receptor ligands*

The GABA$_C$ receptors do not respond to either BMC (**9.42**) or baclofen (**9.44**) (Figure 9.8). CACA (**9.47**) is a selective agonist for GABA$_C$ receptors but inactive at GABA$_A$ receptors, whereas the *trans*-isomer TACA (**9.80**) (Figure 9.17A) shows no preference. CAMP (**9.48**) is a selective GABA$_C$ agonist being inactive at GABA$_A$ receptors. All other known GABA$_A$ agonists seem to have some agonist/antagonist action at GABA$_C$ receptors, exemplified by THIP (**9.3**) and P4S (**9.81**) (Figure 9.17B), which are partial agonists at GABA$_A$ receptors and competitive antagonists at GABA$_C$ receptors. TPMPA (**9.46**) is a selective antagonist for GABA$_C$ receptors, at least 100 times more potent as an antagonist at GABA$_C$ receptors than at GABA$_A$ receptors. In contrast to the GABA$_A$ receptors the GABA$_C$ receptors are insensitive to barbiturates, benzodiazepines and neurosteroids.

9.3   GLUTAMIC ACID: EXCITATORY NEUROTRANSMITTER AND EXCITOTOXIN

Glu and a number of other endogenous acidic amino acids show excitatory effects when applied on central neurones. These excitatory amino acids also show neurotoxic properties when administered locally either at high concentrations for short periods or at lower concentrations for longer periods of time. This combination of neuroexcitatory activity and neurotoxic properties have been termed 'excitotoxicity' and seems to be a general phenomenon for excitatory amino acids.

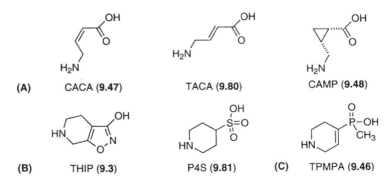

Figure 9.17 Structures of GABA$_C$ receptor (A) agonists; (B) partial agonists; and (C) an antagonist.

Glu is ubiquitously distributed in the CNS in high concentrations, and in addition to being the major excitatory neurotransmitter Glu participates in many metabolic processes and it is a precursor for the inhibitory neurotransmitter GABA. The high concentrations of Glu found in the CNS initially made it difficult to accept a transmitter role of Glu. Specific release and uptake mechanisms have, however, been identified and characterized, and these mechanisms can explain how the concentration-levels of Glu in the synaptic cleft is regulated. These highly efficient systems control the synaptic activity and prevent the above mentioned neurotoxicity of Glu in the normal mature brain. It is still unclear to what extent other acidic amino acids, such as (S)-aspartic acid or (S)-homocysteic acid, serve as endogenous neurotransmitters. Glu receptors are present in high numbers on most neurones in the CNS, reflecting the, atleast indirect, influence of Glu on virtually all physiological functions. Glu receptors play an important role in the synaptic plasticity associated with learning and memory functions, and these aspects open interesting therapeutic possibilities for Glu receptor agonists or other agents enhancing synaptic excitatory activity. Such agents may be used for improving cognition, learning and memory in certain pathological situations.

9.3.1   Classification of and ligands for Glu receptors

9.3.1.1   Receptor multiplicity

The Glu receptors are divided into two main classes (Figure 9.18, see also Figure 6.1) comprising a group of receptor-operated ion channels and a group of G-protein coupled receptors. Three types of ionotropic receptors have been identified, named N-methyl-D-aspartic acid (NMDA), 2-amino-3-(3-hydroxy-5-methyl-4-isoxazolyl)propionic acid (AMPA) and kainic acid (Kain) receptors. The group of metabotropic receptors (G-protein coupled receptors) is a very large and heterogeneous group of receptors subdivided into Group I, II and III. All receptor types are activated by Glu (**9.82**), and the three ionotropic receptors are named after selective agonists, whereas the metabotropic receptors have been classified according to pharmacology of ligands, second messenger coupling and sequence homology.

Figure 9.18 illustrates the number of subunits cloned within each class of receptors. At present, six NMDA receptor subunits (NR1, NR2A-NR2D, and NR3A), four AMPA-preferring subunits (GluR1-4) and five Kain preferring subunits (GluR5-7, KA1 and KA2) have been identified. The stoichiometry of subunits forming the functional ionotropic receptor complexes *in vivo* is still not clarified, but it is believed to be tetra- or pentameric structures of heteromeric nature. For the metabotropic receptors each circle in Figure 9.18 represents a single receptor protein (mGluR1-8). Each receptor protein is a functional unit, possibly with homo-dimers as the functional assembly *in vivo*.

In the following sections (9.3.1.2–9.3.1.7), some of the important ligands and characteristics of the individual receptor classes will be briefly covered. Examples covering more detailed medicinal chemistry studies are discussed in Section 9.3.2.

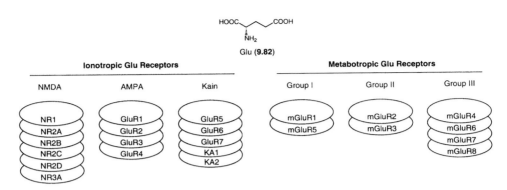

Figure 9.18 Schematic illustration of the multiplicity of excitatory amino acid receptors and the structure of Glu (**9.82**).

9.3.1.2   *Structure of ionotropic Glu receptors*

Cloning of the ionotropic Glu receptor subunits has disclosed the amino acid sequences of the receptor proteins, and the topology of these has been a matter of discussion. Studies defining the extra- and intracellular surfaces have now led to a model of the topology of the ionotropic Glu receptor comprising: a very large extracellular N-terminal domain, three transmembrane domains, one re-entry loop and an intracellular C-terminal (Figure 9.19). This model is based on a structure obtained from an X-ray crystallographic analysis of a soluble GluR2 binding domain consisting of the colored parts in Figure 9.19A (see also Figure 6.6). This soluble protein is formed by expression of a truncated form of the extracellular domain with the transmembrane domains, M1, M3 and the re-entry loop replaced by a hydrophilic linker (not shown). The protein exerts binding characteristics similar to the intact receptor protein. The binding site from this crystal structure is shown in Figure 9.19B, and the amino acid residues in the receptor protein binding to the Kain molecule (Figure 9.19C). The publication of this crystal structure with a ligand included has opened up new possibilities for structure-based design of ligands for these receptors.

In the following sections, important ligands for the different Glu receptors will be described. Most of these ligands have been developed prior to the appearance of the above mentioned crystal structure.

9.3.1.3   *NMDA receptor ligands*

The NMDA receptors have been characterized extensively and have been shown to be a receptor complex comprising a number of different binding sites (Figure 9.20), which can be manipulated pharmacologically. The NMDA receptor ion channel fluxes Na^+, K^+ and Ca^{2+} ions. Ca^{2+} ions have important intracellular functions as a second messenger, and Ca^{2+} also is implicated in the neurotoxicity observed after excessive receptor stimulation. NMDA (**9.83**), (*R*)-2-amino-2-(3-hydroxy-5-methyl-4-isoxazolyl)acetic acid [(*R*)-AMAA, **9.84**], (2*S*, 3*R*, 4*S*)-CCG (**9.85**) and (1*R*, 3*R*)-ACPD (**9.86**) (Figure 9.20A) are potent and selective agonists

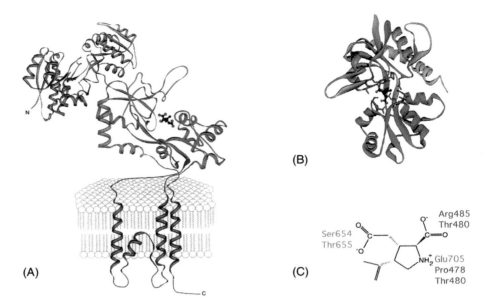

Figure 9.19 (A) Illustration of a single ionotropic Glu receptor subunit with a large extracellular amino-terminal domain, three transmembrane domains, a re-entry loop and an intracellular carboxy-terminal. The colored extracellular segments including Glu in the binding site is based on the crystal structure obtained of the soluble GluR2 binding core (see also Figure 6.6). (B) Model of the Glu binding core based on the crystal structure of the soluble binding core of GluR2 with the residues from the two extracellular segments involved in ligand binding indicated in blue and red. (C) Structure of Kain with numbers on interacting amino acid residues.

at the NMDA receptor. A great number of competitive NMDA receptor antagonists have been developed, most of which are analogs of (*R*)-2-amino-5-phosphono-valeric acid [(*R*)-AP5, **9.87**] or (*R*)-4-(3-phosphonopropyl)-2-piperazinecarboxylic acid [(*R*)-CPP, **9.88**] (Figure 9.20B). Most of these NMDA antagonists are phos-phono amino acids, in which the carboxy and phosphono groups are separated by four or six atoms, and for most of the compounds resolved, the activity resides in the *R*-form. (±)-*Cis*-LY233053 (**9.89**) represents an example of an NMDA antagon-ist with a tetrazole ring functioning as the distal acidic moiety.

Glycine (**9.90**) has been shown to be a co-agonist at the NMDA receptors. Thus, in order to get a response at the NMDA receptors, both the NMDA receptor site and the glycine site have to be activated simultaneously by agonists. Electrophysiological studies seem to indicate that a high extracellular glycine concentration, perhaps a saturating concentration, is normally found in the synapse. Thus, release and uptake of Glu seem to be the determining factor for triggering excitatory responses at NMDA receptors, whereas a more slow change in the glycine concentration may modulate the level of activity at these receptors. (*R*)-HA-966 (**9.91**) is a partial agonist at the glycine site, and the quinoxalinedione ACEA-1021 (**9.92**) represents a large group of competitive glycine site antagonists. It is important to note that this glycine site/receptor (sometimes referred to as the Glycine_B receptor) is excitatory in nature,

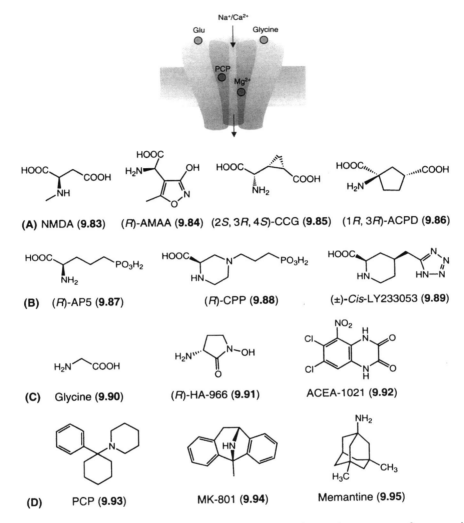

Figure 9.20 Schematic model of the NMDA receptor complex and structures of some selective (A) agonists; (B) competitive antagonists; (C) glycine site ligands; and (D) non-
competitive antagonists.

and not to be mistaken for the inhibitory, strychnine sensitive Glycine$_A$ receptor,
primarily found in the spinal cord.

Apart from a strict requirement for both Glu and glycine to activate the NMDA
receptors, another unusual factor is observed for this ligand gated ion channel. At
normal resting potentials, the NMDA receptors are blocked by Mg^{2+}, probably
binding to a site within the ion channel. When the neurone is partially depolarized,
e.g. by activation of other ionotropic Glu receptors on the same neurone, the Mg^{2+}
blockade is released, and the NMDA receptor ion channel can be activated to give
further depolarization. Thus, in some respects the NMDA receptors seem to function
as an amplification system working only at certain levels of activity of the neurones.

A site for non-competitive NMDA antagonists has been characterized, most often referred to as the phencyclidine (PCP, **9.93**) site. The action of PCP, MK-801 (**9.94**) (Figure 9.20D) and other non-competitive NMDA antagonists are use-dependent, meaning that repeated activation of the NMDA receptors by an agonist is needed to obtain effective antagonist activity of these antagonists. The interpretation of this phenomenon has been that these agents require access to the open ion channel in order to exert their use-dependent antagonism. The mechanism of use-dependency seems very interesting in relation to the treatment of neurodegenerative disorders. In principle, such non-competitive antagonists should elicit therapeutically useful antagonism at synapses with hyperactivity, as observed in neurodegenerative situations (Section 9.1), whereas less efficient antagonism are to be expected at synapses with normal synaptic activity. This would be expected to lead to reduced side effects of non-competitive NMDA antagonists as compared to competitive antagonists. Unfortunately, most non-competitive antagonists studied so far, have shown severe psychotomimetic side effects, which have prevented therapeutic applications. The amantadine analog Memantine (**9.95**), which show a low affinity to the PCP site compared to MK-801, is however very well tolerated in man. Memantine has been used for a number of years in the treatment of Parkinson's disease and is at present in the clinic for other indications, e.g. Alzheimer's disease.

Other binding sites, including at least two different binding sites for polyamines (blockade inside the ion channel and blockade or stimulation outside the ion channel), and a site for Zn^{2+} have also been identified at the NMDA receptor complex, but these sites are not further described here.

9.3.1.4   AMPA receptor ligands

Originally, the AMPA receptors were named Quis receptors after the naturally occurring compound quisqualic acid (Quis, **9.96**). Quite early it was however realized, that Quis is a non-selective Glu receptor agonist. Quis receptors were renamed to the AMPA receptors on the basis of the very potent and specific agonist activity of (*S*)-AMPA (**9.97**). Tritiated AMPA is used as the standard ligand for AMPA receptor binding studies. (*S*)-ACPA (**9.98**) is an analog of AMPA with even higher potency than AMPA. (*S*)-ACPA show very limited desensitization of AMPA receptors compared to AMPA itself. Willardiine is like Quis a naturally occurring compound with AMPA agonist activity and (*S*)-F-Willardiine (**9.99**) show potent and selective activity at AMPA receptors (Figure 9.21).

A very large and important group of competitive AMPA receptor antagonists is constituted by analogs of quinoxalinedione, with NBQX (**9.100**) being one of the early examples and still widely used as a pharmacological agent. Two more recent quinoxalinedione AMPA antagonists, Ro 48-8587 (**9.101**) and LY293558 (**9.102**), are systemically active. **9.101** has been radiolabeled as a tool for studies of the antagonist binding site. The isoxazole (*S*)-2-amino-3-[5-*tert*-butyl-3-(phosphono-methoxy)-4-isoxazolyl]propionic acid [(*S*)-ATPO, **9.103**], represents a group of selective AMPA antagonists derived from the structure of AMPA itself. More detailed structure activity studies on AMPA receptor agonists and antagonists are described in Sections 9.3.2.1 and 9.3.2.2, respectively.

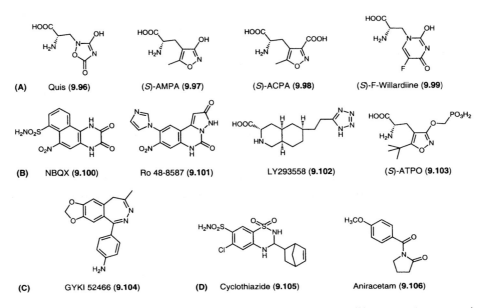

(A)   Quis (**9.96**)   (*S*)-AMPA (**9.97**)   (*S*)-ACPA (**9.98**)   (*S*)-F-Willardiine (**9.99**)

(B)   NBQX (**9.100**)   Ro 48-8587 (**9.101**)   LY293558 (**9.102**)   (*S*)-ATPO (**9.103**)

(C)   GYKI 52466 (**9.104**)   (D)   Cyclothiazide (**9.105**)   Aniracetam (**9.106**)

Figure 9.21 Structures of some selective AMPA receptor: (A) agonists; (B) competitive antagonists; (C) non-competitive antagonist; and (D) modulatory agents.

A number of compounds with non-competitive antagonist effects at AMPA receptors have been identified. GYKI 52466 (**9.104**) and other 2,3-benzodiazepines show potent and selective antagonist effects at AMPA receptors by interaction with an allosteric site. The rapid desensitization observed after application of agonists at AMPA receptors can be modulated by compounds such as the diuretic cyclothiazide (**9.105**) and the nootropic agent aniracetam (**9.106**). These compounds essentially block desensitization to agonists, thereby enhancing the excitatory activity, in some cases several-fold, depending on the initial level of desensitization observed for the individual agonist.

The AMPA receptors mediate fast excitatory activity, and AMPA antagonists have shown neuroprotective properties in numerous animal models. It is as yet unknown, whether such antagonists can be administered to man without severe side effects. In agreement with the previous discussions, AMPA receptors may have particular therapeutic interest (see also Section 9.3.2.4).

9.3.1.5 Kain receptor ligands

Studies using molecular cloning techniques have shown AMPA and Kain receptors to be closely related at the molecular level. Furthermore, these receptors show similar pharmacology, and only a limited number of selective Kain agonists are known. Kain (**9.107**) has been the standard agonist of choice for many years despite its non-selective action, and [^{3}H]Kain is the ligand generally used for binding studies of Kain receptors (Figure 9.22). Kain also shows relatively potent

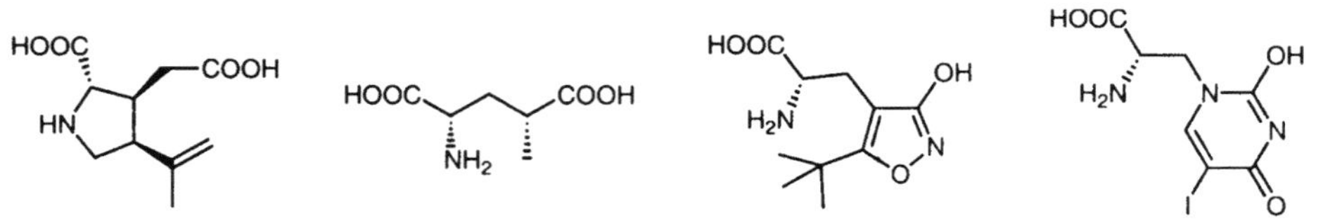

(A) Kain (**9.107**) (2*S*,4*R*)-4-Me-Glu (**9.108**) (*S*)-ATPA (**9.109**) (*S*)-I-Willardiine (**9.110**)

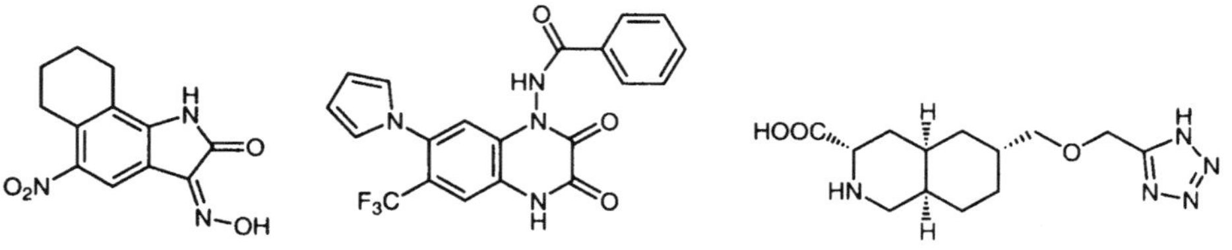

(B) NS-102 (**9.111**) LU97175 (**9.112**) LY294486 (**9.113**)

Figure 9.22 Structures of some Kain receptor (A) agonists and (B) antagonists.

interaction with AMPA receptors as well, and it is frequently used as agonist for studies of AMPA receptors, because Kain, in contrast to AMPA itself, does not desensitize AMPA receptors. (2*S*, 4*R*)-4-Me-Glu (**9.108**) shows selective affinity for the [^{3}H]Kain binding site and potent agonist activity at recombinant GluR5 and GluR6 receptors. More recently the AMPA derivative (*S*)-ATPA (**9.109**) has shown, apart from fairly weak AMPA agonist activity (Section 9.3.2.1), highly potent GluR5 agonist activity. Similarly does (*S*)-I-Willardiine (**9.110**), in contrast to (*S*)-F-Willardiine (**9.99**), show selective activity at GluR5. The agonist pairs AMPA/ATPA and F-/I-Willardiine indicate that in spite of close similarity in the structural requirements for activation of AMPA and Kain receptors, relatively small differences in at least the bulk tolerance can be used for the design of selective compounds.

Only a few antagonists at Kain receptors have been developed. NS-102 (**9.111**) has been reported to have affinity for [^{3}H]Kain binding site and antagonist activity at homomeric GluR6, but solubility problems limits its utility. LU97175 (**9.112**) and LY294486 (**9.113**) represent newer compounds with promising antagonist activities, at GluR5-7 and GluR5, respectively.

9.3.1.6 *Structure of metabotropic Glu receptors*

The metabotropic Glu receptors belong to family C of G-protein coupled receptors. The metabotropic Glu receptors have in analogy to the ionotropic Glu receptors a very large extracellular N-terminal domain, comprising the binding site for Glu and seven transmembrane spanning domains (see Section 6.2.1 and Figures 6.2 and 6.3). The binding of Glu in the extracellular domain lead to a closing of the two binding lopes, a concomitant conformational change of the receptor protein, and, by a yet unknown mechanism, to activation of the G-protein coupled to the receptor protein at the intracellular domains (see also Section 6.2.1 and Figures 6.3 and 6.12). An X-ray crystallographic structure of the extracellular ligand-binding region has been published for one of the subtypes of the metabotropic receptors (mGluR1). In analogy with the ionotropic Glu receptors (Section 9.3.1.2) this has furnished detailed new knowledge about the receptor binding site, which will be of importance for the development of new ligands.

Based on pharmacology, transduction pathways and amino acid sequences the metabotropic receptors has been divided into three groups: Group I consisting of mGluR1,5 stimulating phospholipase C and Group II (mGluR2,3) and Group III (mGluR4,6-8) both inhibiting the formation of cyclic AMP. This means that agonist stimulation of Group I receptors leads to cell excitation, whereas agonist stimulation of Group II and Group III receptors leads to cell inhibition. However, some of the metabotropic receptors are located presynaptically, and may function as autoreceptors. Thus, activation of such receptors inhibit the presynaptic release of Glu. The responses obtained through metabotropic receptors are generally slower than ionotropic receptor responses, and may be regarded as modulation of the fast excitatory tone set by the ionotropic Glu receptors.

9.3.1.7 *Metabotropic receptor ligands*

Characterization of metabotropic Glu receptors did not really proceed until after the cloning of the different subtypes in the early nineties. Thus, the research within this group of receptors has been going on for much shorter time than for the ionotropic Glu receptors. The focus on metabotropic receptors has however been enormous in recent years, among other things because of the little therapeutic success obtained after many years of research within the ionotropic area. Apart from Glu itself, (1*S*,3*R*)-ACPD (**9.114**), ibotenic acid (**9.115**) and Quis (**9.96**) were among the first potent metabotropic agonists (Figure 9.23A), though they are fairly non-selective.

Synthesis of the homologs of these and other Glu analogs (Figure 9.23B) did however afford compounds with more selective activity at metabotropic Glu receptors. Thus, (*S*)-2-aminoadipic acid [(*S*)-2-AA, **9.116**], was shown to be a

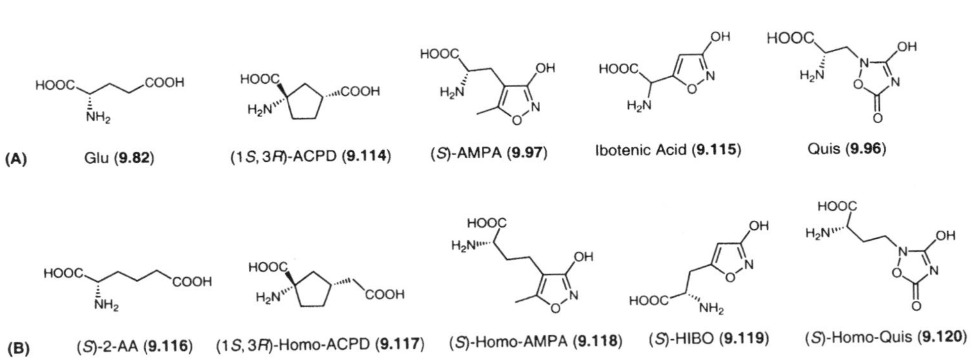

Figure 9.23 Structures of (A) Glu (**9.82**) and some Glu analogs and (B) corresponding homologs compounds showing activity at metabotropic Glu receptors.

mGluR2 and mGluR6 agonist, (1*S*, 3*R*)-Homo-ACPD (**9.117**) a Group I agonist, whereas (*S*)-Homo-AMPA (**9.118**) showed specific activity at mGluR6, and no activity at neither ionotropic Glu receptors or at other metabotropic Glu receptors. A number of homoibotenic acid (HIBO) analogs, including HIBO (**9.119**) itself show Group I antagonist activity and (*S*)-Homo-Quis (**9.120**) is a mixed Group I antagonist/Group II agonist. The activity of these and other Glu homologs indicate that Glu is interacting with the metabotropic receptors in an extended conformation. The effect of backbone extension of different Glu analogs is often unpredictable, but chain length are nevertheless a factor of utmost importance. A more detailed structure–activity study on HIBO analogs as Group I antagonists is described in Section 9.3.2.3.

Conformationally restricted analogs containing a Glu backbone or acidic phenylglycine analogs are two very important groups of compounds, which have afforded many analogs with selective activity at metabotropic receptors, including agonists as well as antagonists (Figure 9.24). The two Group I agonists ABHxD-I (**9.121**) (non-selective) and (*S*)-3,5-DHPG (**9.122**), are representatives of the two groups, and the two Group I antagonists (*S*)-4-CPG (**9.123**) and (*RS*)-AIDA (**9.124**) belong to the latter group.

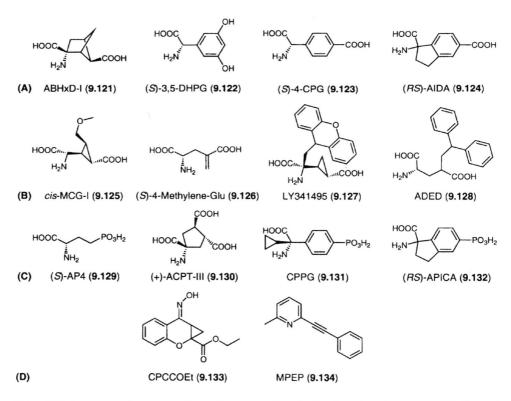

Figure 9.24 Structures of some metabotropic receptor ligands showing selectivity towards (A) Group I; (B) Group II or (C) Group III; and (D) noncompetitive antagonists.

The two Glu analogs *cis*-MCG-I (**9.125**) and (*S*)-4-Methylene-Glu (**9.126**) have shown fairly selective activity as Group II agonists, whereas the two related Glu analogs containing large lipophilic substituents LY341495 (**9.127**) and ADED (**9.128**) are converted into Group II antagonists.

At Group III metabotropic receptors the phosphonate Glu analog (*S*)-AP4 (**9.129**) and (+)-ACPT-III (**9.130**) are selective agonists, whereas CPPG (**9.131**) and (*RS*)-APICA (**9.132**) are selective antagonists.

The pharmacology of metabotropic ligands has evolved with the availability of the cloned receptors and thus, many subtype selective ligands have been discovered compared to ionotropic ligands. However, many of the above mentioned ligands have not been fully tested on all metabotropic (or ionotropic) subtypes, and the selectivity is therefore not fully investigated yet.

More recently a number of non-competitive antagonists at metabotropic Glu receptors has been discovered by high-throughput screening of compound libraries. These antagonists, represented by CPCCOEt (**9.133**) (see also Section 6.3.3 and Figure 6.12) and MPEP (**9.134**), are selective mGluR1 and mGluR5 antagonists, respectively, and show very high potency compared to the competitive antagonists.

The metabotropic receptors affect the activity of neurones and indirectly affect the activity of ion channels. Studies on animal models have shown both neuroprotective and neurotoxic properties of metabotropic agonists. This is related to the signal transduction mechanisms for the different subtypes, as mentioned in Section 9.3.1.6. Group I receptors being excitatory and Group II and III inhibitory, and also that some metabotropic receptors are presynaptically located, whereas other subtypes are postsynaptic in nature.

9.3.2   Ibotenic acid: a naturally occurring excitotoxin and lead structure

Many naturally occurring acidic amino acids have shown activity at excitatory amino acid receptors and have been used extensively as lead structures in the search for new and better ligands. The *Amanita muscaria* constituent ibotenic acid (**9.115**) shows potent activity at both NMDA receptors and certain metabotropic receptor subtypes, and it is a weak agonist at AMPA/Kain receptors. It is used as a pharmacological and neurotoxic agent, although chemical instability limits the utility in experimental pharmacology.

It is believed that Glu (**9.82**) interacts with the various Glu receptors in different conformations, suggesting that development of Glu analogs with restricted conformations may lead to compounds with selective action. Ibotenic acid is a conformationally restricted analog of Glu in which the 3-hydroxyisoxazole moiety functions as a bioisostere to the distal carboxyl group of Glu. Glu as well as ibotenic acid exist primarily on their fully ionized forms at physiological pH as illustrated in Figure 9.25. The similarity observed for the delocalization of charge on the distal carboxylate group of Glu and of the deprotonated 3-isoxazolol may explain the utility of this bioisosteric replacement.

Ibotenic acid has been used as the lead structure for the design of many compounds of importance in medicinal chemistry studies of different Glu receptors.

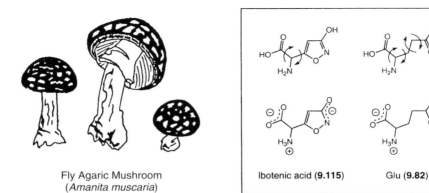

Fly Agaric Mushroom
(*Amanita muscaria*)

Ibotenic acid (**9.115**)   Glu (**9.82**)

Figure 9.25 Illustration of the structural flexibility of ibotenic acid (**9.115**) (isolated from the fly agaric mushroom) and of Glu (**9.82**), and delocalization of the three charges existing at physiological pH (pK$_a$ values: Ibotenic acid, 3.0, 5.0 and 8.2; Glu, 2.2, 4.3 and 10.0).

In the subsequent sections such structure–activity studies are illustrated for AMPA receptor agonists (Section 9.3.2.1), AMPA receptor antagonists (Section 9.3.2.2), Group I metabotropic antagonists (Section 9.3.2.3) and finally the principle of functional partial agonism (Section 9.3.2.4).

9.3.2.1   5-Substituted AMPA analogs

The tolerance for bulk in the 5-position of the isoxazole ring of AMPA analogs has been investigated by synthesis of a number of analogs with different substituents. Two series of compounds with 5-alkyl or 5-aryl substituents, respectively, are listed in Table 9.1. The influence on AMPA receptor pharmacology is represented by the IC$_{50}$ values from [^{3}H]AMPA binding studies and by the EC$_{50}$ values from an *in vitro* electrophysiological model. (*RS*)-AMPA (**9.136**) is obviously a very potent agonist, but the pharmacology of AMPA analogs is very dependent on the substituent in the 5-position of the isoxazole ring.

For the 5-alkyl substituted analogs a fairly simple structure–activity relationship seems to exist. Analogs with an increasing size of the substituent generally seem to lose activity. The compounds with small substituents are fairly potent (**9.136–9.138**), the butyl analog (**9.139**) is somewhat weaker, and the loss of activity is more dramatic for the analogs with branched substituents compared to the analogs with unbranched substituents. This is obvious from the isopentyl (**9.142**), neopentyl (**9.144**) and 4-heptyl (**9.145**) analogs, being very weak or inactive as AMPA agonists, indicating that there is a fairly strict limit for the size of the 5-substituent. On the basis of these compounds, the existence of a hydrophobic pocket at the receptor binding site capable of accommodating small substituents has been hypothesized. The demethylated analog (**9.135**) is an exception in terms of activity. It does show fairly high affinity for AMPA receptors, but is unexpectedly weak in the cortical slice preparation. However,

Table 9.1 Receptor affinity (IC$_{50}$ values from [^{3}H]AMPA binding) and *in vitro* electrophysiological activity (EC$_{50}$ values from the rat cortical slice preparation) for 5-alkyl and 5-aryl substituted AMPA analogs

		IC$_{50}$ (µM)	EC$_{50}$ (µM)			IC$_{50}$ (µM)	EC$_{50}$ (µM)
(9.135)	—H	0.27	900	(9.146)	phenyl	35	390
(9.136)	—CH$_3$	0.04	3.5	(9.147)	2-pyridyl	0.57	7.4
(9.137)	—CH$_2$-CH$_3$	0.03	2.3	(9.148)	pyridyl	>100	>1000
(9.138)	—CH$_2$-CH$_2$-CH$_3$	0.09	5.0	(9.149)	4-pyridyl	5.5	96
(9.139)	—CH$_2$-CH$_2$-CH$_2$-CH$_3$	1.0	32	(9.150)	pyrazinyl	1.2	11
(9.140)	—CH(CH$_3$)$_2$	0.19	9.0	(9.151)	tetrazolyl (NH)	72	>1000
(9.141)	—CH$_2$-CH(CH$_3$)$_2$	0.61	23	(9.152)	tetrazolyl (N-CH$_3$)	54	>1000
(9.142)	—CH$_2$-CH$_2$-CH(CH$_3$)$_2$	>100	>1000	(9.153)	tetrazolyl (N-CH$_3$)	0.03	0.92
(9.143)	—C(CH$_3$)$_3$ *(RS)-ATPA*	11	48	(9.154)	thienyl	0.28	5.8
(9.144)	—CH$_2$-C(CH$_3$)$_3$	55	420	(9.155)	thienyl	3.5	43
(9.145)	—CH(CH$_2$-CH$_2$-CH$_3$)$_2$	99	>1000	(9.156)	thiazolyl	0.09	2.3

electrophysiological experiments performed on dissociated neurones did show potent activity of **9.135**. This indicates that **9.135** may be a substrate for Glu uptake systems, which lead to low activity in intact test systems such as the cortical slice preparation. Glu itself is also found to be a very weak agonist in this electrophysiological model.

The picture concerning the structure–activity relationship is less clear for the 5-aryl substituted AMPA analogs. The 5-phenyl analog (APPA, **9.146**) is a fairly weak agonist, indicating that a phenyl group is too big a substituent in order to have potent AMPA agonist activity. However, APPA is pharmacologically interesting because it functions as a partial agonist, with an intrinsic activity of approximately 60% compared to other agonists. This aspect will be further discussed in Section 9.3.2.4. When the three pyridyl analogs 2-, 3-, and 4-pyridyl-AMPA (**9.147–9.149**) were examined, a very dramatic effect depending on the position of the pyridine nitrogen was observed. The 2-pyridyl analog **9.147** being a very potent agonist, **9.148** inactive and **9.149** fairly weak. The pyrazine analog **9.150** was also fairly potent, whereas the tetrazole analog (**9.151**) was quite weak. The tetrazole is obviously smaller in size, but it is however a quite acidic substituent, which may be unfavorable. The 2-methyl and 3-methyl-tetrazole analogs (**9.152** and **9.153**) were also very different in activity, **9.153** being the most potent AMPA agonist known so far. Also the 2-thienyl (**9.154**) and the 2-thiazole (**9.156**) analogs are very potent AMPA agonists, whereas the 3-thienyl (**9.155**) analog is fairly weak. These structures indicate that a heteroatom in the 2 position of the 5-substituent is of importance for the activity. The mechanism behind this dramatic effect of the heteroatom is not known. The heteroatoms may be involved in intra- and/or intermolecular hydrogen bonding to the receptor protein. These compounds also show that the size of the substituent is by no means the only factor of importance for potent receptor interaction.

9.3.2.2   *Isoxazole based AMPA receptor antagonists*

The AMPA receptor antagonists have been, and still are, of great interest as pharmacological tools and potential therapeutic agents, especially in relation to neurodegenerative disorders. In the search for compounds with AMPA antagonist activity many derivatives of AMPA itself have been prepared. Among the competitive NMDA receptor antagonists many acidic amino acids with a backbone longer than Glu have successfully been developed (Section 9.3.1.3). In analogy with this strategy the compound AMOA (**9.157**) was synthesized. This AMPA derivative is a selective AMPA receptor antagonist, though of fairly low potency. In order to improve the potency a number of analogs with different substituents and different distal acidic groups was synthesized. The *tert*-butyl analog ATOA (**9.158**) was found to be somewhat more potent than AMOA, and in analogy with the NMDA antagonists, the phosphonate analogs **9.159** and **9.160** proved to be significantly more potent than the carboxylate analogs. ATPO was shown to be the most potent analog, with a significant improvement of potency compared to AMOA and selective activity for AMPA receptors (Figure 9.26).

Due to the improved potency of ATPO, the compound was resolved by chiral HPLC to give the two enantiomers. The absolute configuration of the obtained enantiomers was established by an X-ray crystallographic analysis of the *R*-form (Figure 9.27A). The pharmacology of the two enantiomers was investigated on recombinant AMPA (GluR1, GluR1+2, GluR3 and GluR4) and Kain receptors (GluR5, GluR6 and GluR6+KA2) expressed in *Xenopus* oocytes. All activity was shown to reside in the *S*-form (**9.103**), with the *R*-form (**9.161**) being very weak or inactive on all receptor subtypes (Figure 9.27B–D). (*S*)-ATPO (**9.103**) was a fairly selective agonist at AMPA receptors, being approximately equipotent on GluR1-4, whereas it was somewhat weaker on the Kain preferring subtype GluR5. At GluR6 or GluR6+KA2 no activity was observed. GluR5 has previously shown pharmacology

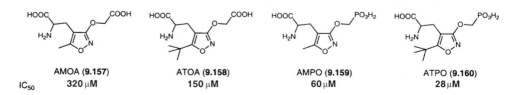

Figure 9.26 Structures of some competitive AMPA receptor antagonists with antagonist potencies from the rat cortical slice preparation (IC$_{50}$ values).

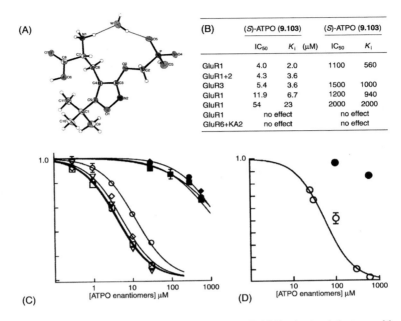

Figure 9.27 (A) Perspective drawing of (R)-ATPO·H₂O (**9.161**) obtained from an X-ray crystallographic analysis. Hydrogen bonds to the water molecule are indicated by thin lines. (B) Table with antagonist effects determined for the enantiomers of ATPO towards Kain induced activation of homo- and heteromeric Glu receptors expressed in *Xenopus* oocytes. (C) Concentration-dependent inhibition by (S)-ATPO (**9.103**) (open symbols) and (R)-ATPO (**9.161**) (closed symbols) of Kain induced responses in *Xenopus* oocytes expressing GluR1 (□), GluR1 + 2 (▽), GluR3 (◇), GluR4 (○) or (D) GluR5.

related to the AMPA receptor subtypes, in spite of its clear structural relationship to Kain receptor subtypes.

Development of subtype selective compounds is of importance in the understanding of the physiological and pathological importance of the receptor subtypes and may lead to valuable therapeutic compounds. The number of such compounds is still very limited and many of the older compounds have not been investigated on recombinant receptors at all. With the increasing knowledge on the structure of the receptor proteins and the availability of recombinant receptors for pharmacological testing, the issue of subtype pharmacology will be of great importance in the work to come.

9.3.2.3 Homoibotenic acid analogs as metabotropic antagonists

A number of 4-substituted analogs of (S)-HIBO (**9.119**) has been synthesized and was originally found to be selective and fairly potent AMPA receptor agonists. (S)-HIBO itself did, in analogy to the demethylated AMPA analog (**9.135**), show fairly high-affinity for AMPA receptors, but quite low activity in the functional test (Table 9.2). Other analogs with small substituents, (S)-methyl-(**9.162**) and

Table 9.2 Receptor binding affinity (IC_{50} values from [^{3}H]AMPA binding), *in vitro* electrophysiological activity (EC_{50} values from the rat cortical slice preparation) and activity at metabotropic Glu receptors (K_b values at cloned mGluRs expressed in chinese hamster ovary cells) of 4-alkyl-HIBO analogs

		[^{3}H]AMPA	Electrophys.	mGluR1	mGluR5	mGluR2	mGluR4
		IC_{50} (µM)	EC_{50} (µM)		K_b (µM)		
(S)-HIBO	(9.119)	0.80	330	250	490	>1000	>1000
(S)-Methyl-HIBO	(9.162)	0.32	18	190	180	>1000	>1000
(S)-Butyl-HIBO	(9.163)	0.48	17	110	97	>1000	>1000
Octyl-HIBO	(9.164)	>100	>500	>100	nd	>1000	>1000
Pentyl-HIBO	(9.165)	11	630	140	190	>1000	>1000
Hexyl-HIBO	(9.166)	>100	>1000	140	110	>1000	>1000
Heptyl-HIBO	(9.167)	>100	>500	160	990	>1000	>1000

(S)-butyl-HIBO (**9.163**) were fairly potent agonists, whereas the octyl-analog (**9.164**) was inactive (Table 9.2). These findings are in good agreement with the structure–activity relationships described for the 5-substituted AMPA analogs.

Testing on recombinant metabotropic receptors disclosed that these HIBO analogs also had antagonist activity at group I metabotropic receptors. The activity of (S)-Methyl-HIBO and (S)-Butyl-HIBO on mGluR1 and mGluR5 were approximately the same. This was interesting from a pharmacological point of view and also of potential therapeutic interest. The inactivity of Octyl-HIBO at AMPA receptors showed that there certainly is a size-limit for AMPA agonists, however the low solubility of Octyl-HIBO did not allow a full investigation in the metabotropic assays. In the search for compounds with selective activity on metabotropic receptors, Pentyl-, Hexyl- and Heptyl-HIBO (**9.165–9.167**) was synthesized. For Pentyl-HIBO a dramatic loss of activity on AMPA receptors was observed, and for Hexyl- and Heptyl-HIBO no AMPA agonist activity was left at all. However, all three compounds showed antagonist activity at metabotropic receptors, **9.165** and **9.166** with approximately the same activities at mGluR1 and mGluR5. Thus, Hexyl-HIBO can be characterized as a selective Group I receptor antagonist. Interestingly Heptyl-HIBO (**9.167**) show the same potency at mGluR1 as **9.165** and **9.166**, but a significantly lower activity at mGluR5. Thus, **9.167** is an antagonist selective for this mGluR1. *In vivo* studies in mice has shown Hexyl-HIBO to antagonize NMDA-induced convulsions. Unfortunately this antagonism was only observed when Hexyl-HIBO was given i.c.v., whereas peripheral administration (i.v.) did not lead to protection against the NMDA induced convulsions. This indicate that Hexyl-HIBO do not penetrate the blood–brain barrier, or alternative it may be metabolized systemically to an extent preventing blood–brain barrier penetration. The results does however, show that such metabotropic antagonists may have therapeutic potential.

9.3.2.4 Functional partial agonism

The partial agonism observed for racemic APPA (**9.146**) (Section 9.3.2.1) greatly stimulated the interest in this compound and a resolution procedure was developed to furnish the two enantiomers. Resolution was accomplished by diastereomeric salt formation using racemic APPA and (R)- or (S)-phenylethylamine (PEA). When (RS)-APPA was mixed with (S)-PEA and recrystallized from ethanol, the diastereomeric salt consisting of (R)-APPA and (S)-PEA precipitated and could be purified by repeated recrystallization, affording (R)-APPA after liberation from the salt. Analogously, (S)-APPA was obtained using (R)-PEA for the salt formation.

In contrast to the racemate, originally characterized as a partial agonist, (S)-APPA proved to be a full agonist at AMPA receptors, slightly more potent than the racemate (Figure 9.28A). (R)-APPA had no intrinsic activity at AMPA receptors when applied alone, but when co-applied with AMPA or (S)-APPA it antagonized the excitation evoked by these agonists. The dose–response curves of these two AMPA agonists could be shifted to the right in a parallel fashion, indicating that (R)-APPA was a competitive AMPA receptor antagonist (Figure 9.28A). These results reveal that the original partial agonism observed for (RS)-APPA was due to the interaction of a full agonist [(S)-APPA] and a competitive antagonist [(R)-APPA].

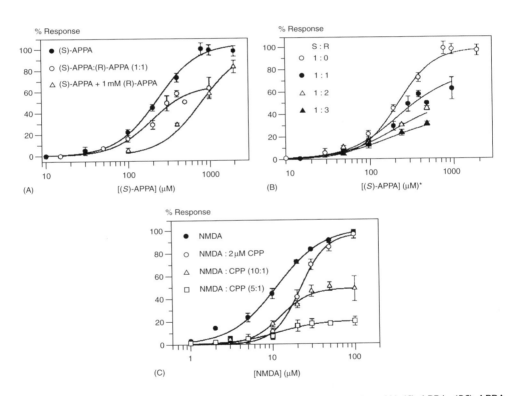

Figure 9.28 Dose–response curves from the rat cortical slice preparation. (A) (S)-APPA, (RS)-APPA (**9.146**) and parallel shift of the (S)-APPA curve with 1 mM (R)-APPA. (B) Curves obtained with fixed molar ratios of (S)- and (R)-APPA; 1:0, 1:1 (racemate), 1:2 and 1:3. *The X-axis represents the concentration of (S)-APPA, whereas the concentration of (R)-APPA is 0, 1, 2 or 3 times the concentration of (S)-APPA in the four different experiments. (C) Curves obtained with NMDA (**9.83**), fixed molar ratios of NMDA and CPP (**9.88**) (10:1 and 5:1) and rightward shift of the NMDA curve with 2 μM CPP.

Subsequently, dose–response curves were obtained using different ratios of (R)- and (S)-APPA. This is shown in Figure 9.28B for (S)-APPA alone and for different ratios of (S)-APPA/(R)-APPA [(1:1) (racemic APPA), (1:2) and (1:3)]. It is seen that with an increasing amount of the antagonist, the maximum response is depressed. The curves have not been extended further due to the rather low potency of the enantiomers. The figure illustrates the principle of functional partial agonism. This principle implicates that, in theory, any desired level of intrinsic activity can be obtained when mixing an agonist and a competitive antagonist in a fixed molar ratio. Functional partial agonism can be achieved using any pair of agonist and competitive antagonist. Furthermore, this principle can be applied not only to AMPA receptor ligands, but also to ligands of other ionotropic Glu receptors or other ionotropic neurotransmitter systems in general. The maximal activity attainable will depend on the relative potency of the two agents. It is important to notice the difference between these experiments using agonists and competitive antagonists, to achieve functional partial agonism, and the conventional pharmacological experiment designed to demonstrate competitive antagonism. In the latter case, a dose response curve for the agonist is determined in the presence of a fixed concentration of a competitive antagonist, which will shift the dose–response curve for the agonist to the right in a parallel fashion. In contrast to this, functional partial agonism is established using fixed molar ratios of the two components, i.e. the curves are obtained using increasing doses, at a fixed ratio, of both agonist and antagonist.

Another example of the principle of functional partial agonism is shown in Figure 9.28C using NMDA (**9.83**) and the competitive NMDA antagonist CPP (**9.88**). The high potency of these two compounds makes it possible to obtain full curves. Again, the figure shows the possibility of reaching any level of activity between 0 and 1, by choosing appropriate ratios of agonist and competitive antagonist.

Partial agonists may be therapeutically valuable in relation to Alzheimer's disease as described in Section 9.1.3 and may also prove to have therapeutic application in other disorders. For *in vivo* studies of functional partial agonism, a number of factors will have to be carefully considered. First of all, the level of efficacy desired for the disease in question is not known, and will have to be determined. If the two compounds, the agonist and the appropriate competitive antagonist, are administered systemically it is important to make sure that both compounds actually reach the site of action in the necessary concentrations. This means that absorption, metabolism, penetration and other factors will have to be taken into consideration for both compounds. At this point, the principle of functional partial agonism has been introduced – the future will show the applicability.

9.4   FUTURE DEVELOPMENTS

The cloning of the many GABA and Glu receptor subtypes and their pharmacological characterization has speeded up the development of selective ligands. More recently crystal structure determinations of binding cores has increased the structural knowledge about the receptor proteins and about the amino acid residues in the binding sites, and this has opened up the possibility of structure-based design. This may lead to a better understanding of the ligand–receptor interactions, receptor mechanisms and to the developments of more selective compounds. Many ligands have been developed as experimental tools and have been important for the understanding of many brain functions and pathophysiological aspects. However, the success as therapeutic agents, especially within the Glu area, is still very limited. The subtypes of receptors involved in the disorders described in Section 9.1 are still largely unknown, and thus, whether subtype-selective agents will be of therapeutic utility is also unknown. Determination of what subunits combinations are present *in vivo* and the physiological significance of these, combined with development of better subtype selective ligands may eventually lead to new therapeutic agents.

FURTHER READING

Armstrong, N. and Gouaux, E. (2000) Mechanisms for activation and antagonism of an AMPA-sensitive glutamate receptor: crystal structures of the GluR2 ligand binding core. *Neuron*, **28**, 165–181.

Bowery, N.G. and Enna, S.J. (2000) γ-Aminobutyric acid$_B$ receptors: first of the functional metabotropic heterodimers. *Perspectives Pharmacol.*, **292**, 2–7.

Bräuner-Osborne, H., Egebjerg, J., Nielsen, E.Ø., Madsen, U. and Krogsgaard-Larsen, P. (2000) Ligands for glutamate receptors: design and therapeutic prospects. *J. Med. Chem.*, **43**, 2609–2645.

Chebib, M., Johnston, G.A.R. (2000) GABA-activated ligand gated ion channels: Medicinal chemistry and molecular biology. *J. Med. Chem.*, **43**, 1427–1447.

Ebert, B., Madsen, U., Lund, T.M., Lenz, S.M. and Krogsgaard-Larsen, P. (1994) Molecular pharmacology of the AMPA agonist, (S)-2-amino-3-(3-hydroxy-5-phenyl-4-isoxazolyl)-propionic acid [(S)-APPA] and the AMPA antagonists, (R)-APPA. *Neurochem. Int.*, **24**, 507–515.

Enna, S.J. and Bowery, N.G. (eds.) (1997) *The GABA Receptors*. New Jersey: Humana Press Inc.

Frølund, B., Tagmose, L., Liljefors, T., Stensbøl, T.B., Engblom, C., Kristiansen, U. and Krogsgaard-Larsen, P. (2000) A novel class of potent 3-isoxazolol GABA$_A$ antagonists: design, synthesis, and pharmacology. *J. Med. Chem.*, **43**, 4930–4933.

Gasior, M., Carter, R.B. and Witkin, J.M. (1999) Neuroactive steroids: potential therapeutic use in neurological and psychiatric disorders. *Trends Pharmacol. Sci.*, **20**, 107–112.

Krogsgaard-Larsen, P., Frølund, B. and Frydenvang, K. (2000) GABA uptake inhibitors. Design, molecular pharmacology and therapeutic aspects. *Curr. Pharm. Design*, **6**, 1193–1209.

Kunishima, N., Shimada, Y., Tsuji, Y., Sato, T., Yamamoto, M., Kumasaka, T., Nakanishi, S., Jingami, H. and Morikawa, K. (2000) Structural basis of glutamate recognition by a dimeric metabotropic glutamate receptor. *Nature*, **407**, 971–977.

Madsen, U., Bräuner-Osborne, H., Frydenvang, K., Hvene, L., Johansen, T.N., Nielsen, B., Sánchez, C., Stensbøl, T.B., Bischoff, F., Krogsgaard-Larsen, P. (2001) New class of selective antagonists at Group I metabotropic glutamic acid receptors. *J. Med.Chem.*, **44**, 1051–1059.

Moroni, F., Nicoletti, F. and Pellegrini-Giampietro, D.E. (eds.) (1998) *Metabotropic glutamate receptors and brain functions*. London: Portland Press.

Nanavati, S.M. and Silverman, R.B. (1989) Design of potential anticonvulsant agents: mechanistic classification of GABA aminotransferase inactivators. *J. Med. Chem.*, **32**, 2413–2421.

Schoepp, D.D., Jane, D.E. and Monn, J.A. (1999) Pharmacological agents acting at subtypes of metabotropic glutamate receptors. *Neuropharmacology*, **38**, 1431–1476.

Zhang, D., Pan, Z.-H., Awobuluyi, M. and Lipton, S.A. (2001) Structure and function of GABA$_C$ receptors: a comparison of native versus recombinant receptors. *Trends Pharmacol. Sci.*, **22**, 121–132.

Chapter 10

Acetylcholine and histamine receptors and receptor ligands: medicinal chemistry and therapeutic aspects

Povl Krogsgaard-Larsen and Karla Frydenvang

10.1 ALZHEIMER'S DISEASE

Alzheimer's disease (AD) is a degenerative disorder of the human CNS that normally manifests in mid to late adult life with progressive cognitive, memory and intellectual impairment. The clinical features of the disease are accompanied by widespread loss of neocortical neurones (causing cerebral atrophy), by the presence of neurofibrillary tangles (composed, among other things, of paired helical filaments) in large pyramidal neurones, and by the presence of amyloid or senile plaques (extracellular fibrous protein deposits composed of a number of proteins including the amyloid β (Aβ) peptide).

The etiology of AD is complex. Epidemiological surveys have shown that genetic factors account for approximately 50% of the population variance for AD. These studies have also indicated that non-genetic factors including possibly head injury, reduced amounts of early childhood education, environmental exposure, etc. may be associated risk factors.

To date, no effective curative or preventive treatment for AD exists. However, since the central cholinergic neurones, which use acetylcholine (ACh) as neurotransmitter, for unknown reasons are particularly vulnerable in AD, and since these neurones play a key role in learning and memory processes in the brain, the synaptic processes associated with these neurones are potential therapeutic targets in AD (see subsequent sections). Partial and temporary symptomatic improvement of the cognitive deficits in AD actually can be achieved by the administration of inhibitors of the ACh-hydrolyzing enzyme acetylcholinesterase (AChE) (see Section 10.2.7).

In parallel with the attempts to develop cholinergic therapies for symptomatic treatment of Alzheimer patients, the biological mechanisms underlying AD are being extensively studied with the object of disclosing alternative targets for curative or preventive therapeutic interventions in the disease.

Recent insights from molecular genetic, molecular biological, and cell biological experiments have suggested that abnormalities in the processing of the membrane-bound β-amyloid precursor protein (β-APP) of unknown physiological function (Figure 10.1) are central to the pathogenesis of AD. This knowledge therefore provides a number of potential therapeutic targets for drug development.

There is a substantial body of evidence that the Aβ peptide formed by abnormal decomposition of β-APP is toxic to nerve cells, although it is an unresolved question,

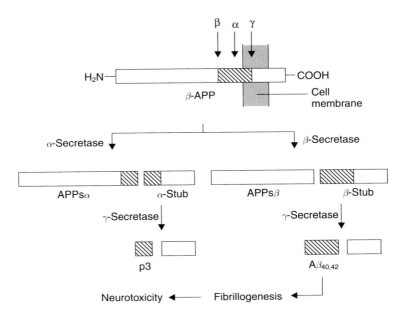

Figure 10.1 An outline of the enzymatic processes involved in the proteolytic cleavage of the membrane-bound β-APP leading to the formation of the toxic $A\beta_{40}$ and $A\beta_{42}$ peptides and other peptide fragments.

whether there are specific receptors for the $A\beta$ peptide. It has been shown that exposure to the $A\beta$ peptide activates apoptosis cell death pathways and potentiates the cytotoxic effects of excitatory amino acid neurotransmitters (see Chapter 9). However, one paradox that has not yet been resolved is that the neurotoxic effects of $A\beta$ peptide, when examined *in vitro*, are acute (within hours or days), whereas the progress of AD appears to be very slow, over many years.

In spite of this and a number of other unanswered questions, the enzymes involved in the proteolytic cleavage of β-APP have been, and continue to be, extensively studied as potential therapeutic targets in AD. In one pathway, β-APP is cleaved after amino acid residue 687 by a putative membrane-bound protease termed α-secretase at or near the cell membrane (Figure 10.1). This enzymatic pathway generates a soluble N-terminal fragment (APPsα) that may have a mild neurotrophic activity. The residual membrane-bound C-terminal fragment (α-stub) is then subsequently cleaved by a putative enzyme, γ-secretase, which is not yet fully characterized. This enzymatic cleavage, which takes place in the transmembrane domain of the α-stub, generates the 3-kDa fragment termed p3.

The alternate pathway involves an initial cleavage of β-APP by β-secretase at amino acid residue 671. This hydrolytic reaction generates a 99-amino acid C-terminal fragment (β-stub) and APPsβ, and the former peptide then undergoes a second cleavage in the transmembrane domain by γ-secretase at either residue 711 or 713 to liberate, respectively, $A\beta$ peptide of 40 amino acid residues ($A\beta_{40}$) or of 42 residues ($A\beta_{42}$) in length. Both of these peptides show neurotoxic effects.

release of ACh, full or partial GABA receptor blockade is expected to stimulate ACh release. In animal experiments, administration of $GABA_A$ receptor agonists or antagonists actually have been shown to impair or facilitate, respectively, learning and memory processes. The clinical implications of these observations are at present under investigation.

So far, the cholinergic synaptic receptors have been most extensively studied as therapeutic targets in AD, and the heterogeneity of muscarinic as well as nicotinic ACh receptors in the CNS may make it possible to identify subtypes of these receptors, which are of particular pharmacological relevance in AD (see sub-sequent section). On the basis of neurochemical evidence so far available, the post-synaptic M_1 receptors seem to be of primary therapeutic interest (Figure 10.2). Partial agonists at M_1 receptors probably have less predisposition to cause receptor desensitization than full agonists, making the former type of agonists more inter-esting from a therapeutic point of view. As a result of degeneration of ACh nerve terminals, such agents might be expected to act as agonists at the virtually 'empty' and, thus, presumably supersensitive postsynaptic M_1 receptors. In other brain regions, where the muscarinic synapses are normosensitive, partial M_1 agonists may have weak or, ideally, no effects.

Antagonists at presynaptic M_2 receptors, which function as autoreceptors mediating negative feed-back regulation of ACh release, might be useful drugs at the early stages of AD, and compounds with mixed M_1 agonist/M_2 antagonist profiles may prove to be of particular interest.

The presynaptically located nicotinic ACh receptors (Figure 10.2) are involved in a positive feed-back regulation of ACh release. Thus, activation of these receptors stimulates ACh release, and agonists, or preferentially partial agonists, at these receptors obviously have therapeutic interest in the early stages of AD, where ACh neurones are still functioning, though at reduced levels.

10.2.1   Muscarinic and nicotinic acetylcholine receptors and receptor ligands

As for other neurotransmitters, multiple receptors exist for ACh in the periphery as well as in the CNS (see Chapter 6). The ACh receptors are classified into two main groups: (1) the muscarinic; and (2) the nicotinic receptors (Figure 10.3). Whereas, the muscarinic acetylcholine receptors (mAChRs) belong to the group of G protein-coupled receptors, nicotinic acetylcholine receptors (nAChRs) are ligand-gated ion channels containing five subunits, which may be identical (homo-meric receptors) or different (heteromeric receptors).

Muscarine (**10.3**), which like muscimol and ibotenic acid (see Chapter 9) is a constituent of *Amanita muscaria*, to some extent reflects the structure of ACh (**10.2**) (Figure 10.3). The quaternary ammonium group is essential for the interaction of **10.3** with mAChRs, and the ether group appears to be strongly involved in the receptor binding of **10.3**. However, the relative importance of the other structural elements of **10.3** for receptor binding and activation has not yet been fully eluci-dated. The structure of nicotine (**10.4**), on the other hand, is very different from that of ACh (**10.2**), and the molecular basis of the very tight binding of **10.4** to nAChRs is still under investigation.

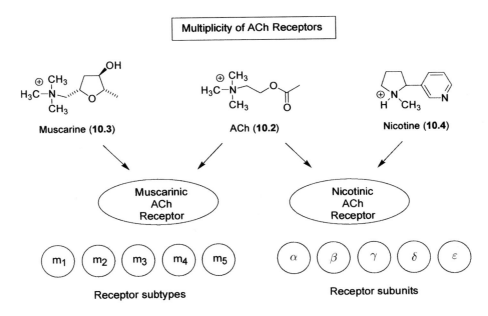

Figure 10.3 Structures of ACh (**10.2**) and the classical muscarinic and nicotinic ACh receptor agonists, muscarine (**10.3**) and nicotine (**10.4**), respectively, and an indication of the heterogeneity of ACh receptors.

Molecular cloning studies have revealed a high degree of heterogeneity of mAChRs (Figure 10.3). Five subtypes of such receptors (m_1-m_5) have been cloned and expressed in different model systems. So far, the correlation between these receptor subtypes, cloned from different tissues, and the mAChRs characterized using classical pharmacological methods (M_1-M_3) is not entirely clear, although m_1-m_3 are generally accepted to have pharmacological characteristics very similar to those of M_1-M_3, respectively (Figure 10.4).

Knockout animals, which typically are mice, are experimental animals, in which one, or perhaps two or three, genes have been deleted. In cases, where the deleted genes are coding for proteins of vital importance, the knockout mice only survive for short periods of time. However, in a number of cases, it has been possible to produce knockout mice lacking certain receptor or ion channel subtypes or enzymes as the results of deletion of the corresponding genes. Studies of the function and behavior of such animal models may provide important information about the physiological role of the particular biomechanisms.

In order to shed light on the functional roles of the mAChRs, knockout mice lacking one of the receptor subtypes m_1-m_5 have been produced. Mice lacking m_1 receptors had lost the ability to develop seizures after administration of muscarinic agonists and showed reduced hippocampal-based memory and learning as the most prominent behavioral alterations, as expected from pharmacological studies. In agreement with important roles of m_2 receptors in heart tissue and as cholinergic autoreceptors in the CNS (Figure 10.2), mice lacking m_2

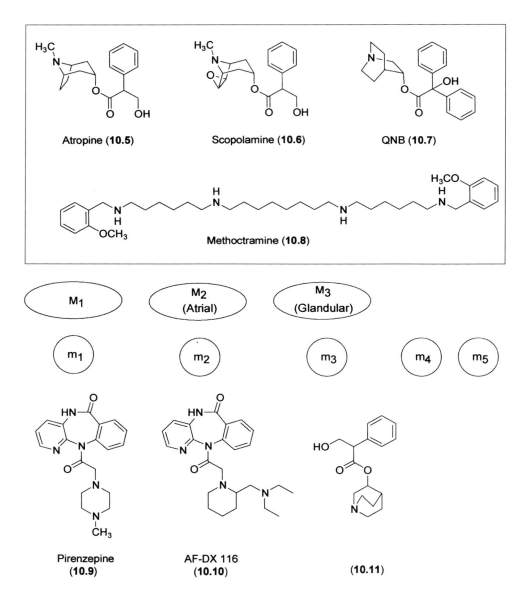

Figure 10.4 Multiplicity of muscarinic ACh receptors and structures of a number of non- or subtype-selective antagonists.

receptors did not show bradycardia or autoreceptor-mediated regulation of ACh release after administration of m_2-selective agonists (see Section 10.2.3). A prominent feature of m_3 receptor knockout mice was decreased mAChR-mediated salivation and smooth muscle contraction *in vitro*. Mice without m_4 receptors showed increased basal locomotor activity and reduced capacity to express mAChR-mediated analgesia, whereas m_5 receptor knockout animals, among other alterations, showed a pronounced decrease in mAChR-mediated dopamine release in the CNS.

These knockout animals are being intensively studied behaviorally and pharmacologically in order to validate these receptor subtypes as potential therapeutic targets.

Advances in molecular biology and selective probe design have resulted in the discovery of nine nAChR subunits expressed in the human CNS, and these receptor subunits are designated $\alpha_2-\alpha_7$ and $\beta_2-\beta_4$. Five additional nAChR subunits, which are expressed in the peripheral nervous system (PNS), are designated α_1, β_1, γ, δ, and ε (Figure 10.3). As mentioned previously, nAChR subunits oligomerize into both homopentameric and heteropentameric receptor subtypes. Each of these pentameric nAChRs possesses distinct ligand selectivity, pharmacological profile, and distribution in the CNS and the PNS. In the CNS and ganglia, α and β subunits assemble to form subtypes with the $(\alpha)_2(\beta)_3$ stoichiometry. Of major interest is the $\alpha_4\beta_2$ subtype, which exhibits very high affinity for the nAChR agonists nicotine (**10.4**), cytisine (**10.36**), and epibatidine (**10.37**) (see Section 10.2.5). Ganglionic nAChRs are known to consist of the following subtypes: $\alpha_3\beta_4$, $\alpha_3\alpha_5\beta_4$, and $\alpha_3\alpha_7\beta_x$. Finally, PNS nAChRs at the neuromuscular junction take the form of $\alpha_1\beta_1\delta\gamma$ or $\alpha_1\beta_1\delta\varepsilon$.

From the point of view of drug design, the region- or tissue-selective localizations of nAChRs are interesting, since nAChRs of different subunit composition will show more or less different affinities for structurally dissimilar nAChR agonists and antagonists, as exemplified for **10.4**, **10.36**, and **10.37**. These observations have greatly stimulated drug design programs in the nAChR field.

10.2.2   Muscarinic antagonists as pharmacological tools and therapeutic agents

The discovery that the alkaloids atropine (**10.5**) and scopolamine (**10.6**) (Figure 10.4) block the actions of ACh at muscarinic receptors and produce a number of therapeutically useful actions, including antispasmodic and antiparkinsonian effects, led to an extensive search for synthetic analogs of these natural products. Among various potent synthetic muscarinic receptor antagonists, quinuclidinyl benzilate (QNB, **10.7**) is used as a radioactive ligand for studies of muscarinic receptor sites. Like **10.5** and **10.6**, compound **10.7** does, however, bind tightly to all subtypes of muscarinic receptors, and this lack of selectivity makes these compounds inapplicable for studies of muscarinic receptor subtypes.

In contrast to these classical muscarinic receptor antagonists, pirenzepine (**10.9**) shows major affinity variations in different tissues. It binds weakly to muscarinic receptors in the heart but interacts strongly with such receptors in the cerebral cortex and sympathetic ganglia, whereas it shows intermediate affinity for receptors in salivary glands and in stomach fundic mucosa. Based on these pharmacological and binding studies, the muscarinic receptors were subdivided into two main classes: (1) M_1 receptors showing high affinity for **10.9**; and (2) a heterogeneous class of receptors (M_2) having much lower affinity for **10.9**.

The antagonist **10.9** did, however, not clearly distinguish between the muscarinic receptors previously classified together as M_2. An analog of **10.9**,

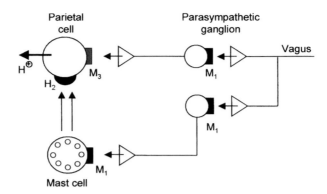

Figure 10.5 A schematic illustration of the muscarinic (M_1 and M_3) and histaminergic (H_2) receptors involved in acid secretion from parietal cells.

(11-[[2-[(diethylamino)methyl]-1-piperidinyl]acetyl]-5,11-dihydro-6*H*-pyrido[2,3-*b*]-benzodiazepin-6-one) (AF-DX 116, **10.10**) has, however, been shown to discriminate between M_2 receptor subtypes in peripheral tissues, showing high affinity for the M_2 receptors in the heart (M_2 atrial) and low affinity for the non-M_1 receptors in endocrine glands (M_3 glandular).

Whereas glandular M_3 receptors display low affinity for **10.9** as well for **10.10**, they are effectively blocked by compound **10.11** and related compounds, which show limited affinity for M_1 and for atrial M_2 receptors. These studies emphasize the different pharmacological characteristics of M_2 and M_3 receptors, and this difference has been supported by the observation that methoctramine (**10.8**) and related polyamines selectively block M_2 receptors (Figure 10.4).

Muscarinic antagonists were once the most widely used drugs for the management of peptic ulcer. Whereas the non-selective muscarinic antagonists atropine (**10.5**) or scopolamine (**10.6**) produce pronounced side effects, notably dry mouth, loss of visual accomodation and difficulty in urination, the M_1-selective antagonist pirenzepine (**10.9**) can be more safely used in the treatment of ulcer. Nevertheless, side effects do occur after administration of **10.9** to patients, and **10.9** has now largely been replaced by histamine H_2 antagonists (see Section 10.3.2) and, in particular, by proton pump inhibitors as antiulcer drugs.

According to our current knowledge, the antiulcer effects of **10.9** are based on different mechanisms of action. The main contribution results from the inhibition of acid secretion (Figure 10.5). Within the parasympathetic pathway, acid secretion is controlled by excitatory M_1 and M_3 receptors. M_1 receptors are located in the parasympathetic ganglion and at the histamine-containing mast cells. M_3 receptors, on the other hand, are located directly on the acid-producing parietal cells. A selective blockade of M_1 receptors therefore induces an inhibition of acid secretion via direct (ACh-mediated) and indirect (histamine-mediated) pathways. Selective M_3 antagonists obviously would be much less effective inhibitors of acid secretion, but compounds showing potent antagonist effects at M_1 as well as M_3 receptors would seem to be interesting as antiulcer agents. Such compounds actually have been developed but apparently have not been sufficiently effective

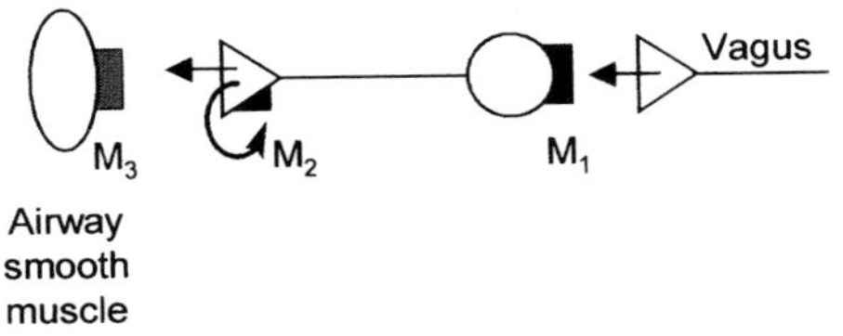

Figure 10.6 A schematic illustration of the muscarinic receptors (M_1, M_2 and M_3) involved in the regulation of the function of airway smooth muscles.

and safe to compete with histamine H_2 antagonists or proton pump inhibitors as drugs for the treatment of peptic ulcer.

There is a growing interest in mAChR antagonists for the treatment of broncho-pulmonary diseases. The airways receive a rich cholinergic innervation, and M_1 receptors are widely distributed in the respiratory tract. The cholinergic innervation of airway smooth muscle tissue contains M_1, M_2 and M_3 receptors (Figure 10.6). M_1 receptors located in the parasympathetic ganglia probably exert a facilitatory effect on neurotransmission, which is primarily under control of nAChRs (not illustrated). The release of ACh during vagal stimulation is controlled by a negative feed-back mechanism utilizing M_2 autoreceptors. Contraction of airway smooth muscle is primarily mediated by M_3 receptors.

Several clinical studies have disclosed that the M_1-selective antagonist piren-zepine (**10.9**) is not sufficiently effective for the treatment of chronic bronchitis or asthma because of its insufficient blockade of M_3 receptors located in the smooth muscle tissue. These aspects prompted the development of compounds showing high affinity for M_1 as well as M_3 receptors, but showing little, or preferentially no, antagonist effect at M_2.

Using pirenzepine (**10.9**) as lead structure, a series of analogs were synthe-sized and pharmacologically characterized. Within this group of compounds, BIBO 126 (**10.12**) showed the desired, though not the optimal, pharmacological profile being 40-fold more potent at the M_1 than at the M_2 receptor and showing

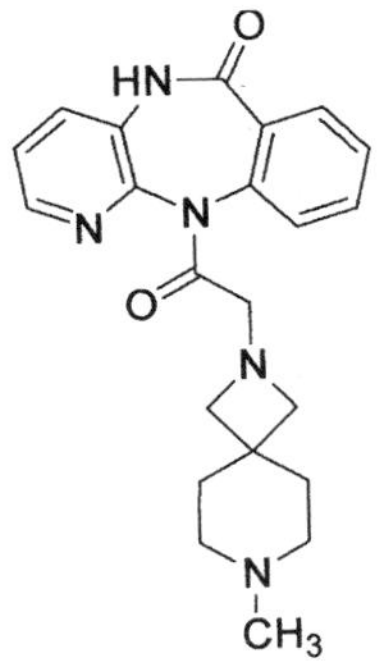

BIBO 126 (**10.12**)

similar affinity for M_1 and M_3 receptors. Compound **10.12** contains a spiro-diamino sidechain with protolytic properties similar to those of **10.9**, which has pK_a 2.1 and 8.2.

Compounds **10.12** and **10.9** have been subjected to comparative pharmacological studies in animals, and although these two compounds show significantly different receptor affinity profiles, their effects in functional assay system were similar. Nevertheless, the search for compounds showing the desired selectivities at M_1, M_2 and M_3 receptors continue in order to develop muscarinic antagonist drugs for the treatment of chronic bronchitis and nocturnal asthma.

10.2.3 Muscarinic agonists and partial agonists: bioisosteric design

The quaternary structure of ACh (Figure 10.7) and the rapid hydrolysis of its ester moiety in biological systems make ACh inapplicable for most types of pharmacological experiments and, of course, for clinical studies. Removal of one or more of the *N*-methyl groups of ACh with the object of obtaining cholinergic compounds capable of penetrating the blood–brain barrier (BBB) results in pronounced loss of activity.

Arecoline (**10.13**) which is a constituent of areca nuts, the seeds of *Areca catechu*, is a cyclic 'reverse ester' bioisostere of ACh, containing a tertiary amino group. In contrast to the findings for ACh, **10.13** is approximately equipotent with its quaternized analog, *N*-methylarecoline, as a muscarinic ACh receptor agonist.

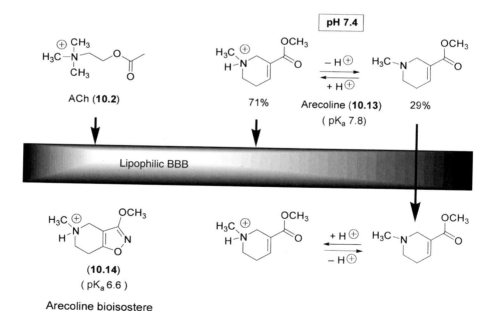

Figure 10.7 Structures of ACh (**10.2**) and the muscarinic agonists arecoline (**10.13**) and the isoxazole arecoline bioisostere **10.14**. The ability of **10.13** to penetrate the BBB is illustrated.

At pH 7.4, **10.13** is partially protonated, and using equation (10.1) the percentage ionization of **10.13** can be calculated to be 71 (Figure 10.7). Whilst **10.13** is assumed to bind to and activate muscarinic ACh receptors in its protonated form, the presence of a fraction of unionized molecules (29%) allows **10.13** to penetrate the BBB.

Analogously, the percentage of unionized acid in aqueous solution can be calculated using this equation. Thus, equation (10.1) can be used to calculate the percentage on acidic form of bases (ionized form) as well as acids (unionized form).

$$\% \text{Ionized} = \frac{100}{[1 + \text{antilog}(\text{pH} - \text{pK}_a)]} \qquad (10.1)$$

Compound **10.13**, which actually is a partial agonist at both M_1 and M_2 receptors, has been shown to improve cognitive functions significantly when infused (i.v.) in Alzheimer patients, and **10.13** facilitates learning in normal young humans. These effects of **10.13** are, however, shortlived reflecting rapid *in vivo* hydrolysis of the ester group of this compound. Furthermore, the pronounced side effects of **10.13** probably reflect the ability of this muscarinic agonist to activate peripheral and central M_2 receptors in addition to the desired partial agonist effect on central M_1 receptors.

Bioisosteric replacements of the carboxyl group of GABA analogs by the 3-isoxazolol group or structurally related heterocyclic units with protolytic properties similar to that of the carboxyl group have led to a number of specific and very potent $GABA_A$ agonists. Similar bioisosteric replacements in the molecule of glutamic acid have led to heterocyclic amino acids with specific actions at subtypes of central glutamic acid receptors (see Chapter 9). These findings prompted the development of the arecoline bioisostere 3-methoxy-5-methyl-4,5,6,7-tetrahydro-isoxazolo[4,5-c]pyridine (**10.14**) containing the hydrolysis-resistant ester isostere 3-methoxyisoxazole (Figure 10.7).

Like **10.13**, the isoxazole bioisostere **10.14** interacts potently with central M_1 as well as M_2 receptors, but the latter compound is a more selective ligand for M_1 receptor sites than is **10.13**, and the partial agonist character of **10.14** is more pronounced than that of the lead compound, **10.13**. Compared with **10.13**, the bicyclic bioisostere **10.14** has a lower pK_a value (6.6) and a higher $\log P$ value, and these physico-chemical properties can explain why **10.14** very easily penetrates the BBB.

Compound **10.14** has been used as a 'second lead' for the design and development of a number of effective muscarinic agonists showing different degrees of M_1 selectivity and pharmacological profiles ranging from antagonists through low-efficacy agonists to full agonists. Like **10.14**, 3-methoxy-5,6,7,8-tetrahydro-4H-isoxazolo[4,5-c]azepine (**10.21**) is a partial muscarinic agonist, **10.21** being markedly more potent than **10.14**. The 'pharmacological importance' of the O-alkyl groups of these compounds is reflected by the observation that the O-ethyl analog (**10.22**) is a competitive muscarinic antagonist, whereas the O-isopropyl analog (**10.23**) shows the characteristics of a non-competitive antagonist.

Oxotremorine (**10.15**) is a very potent partial muscarinic agonist, which shows some selectivity for autoreceptors of the M_2 type. Extensive structural modifications of **10.15** have led to compounds with a broad spectrum of pharmacological

(10.15)   (10.16)   (10.17)   (10.18)

(10.19)   (10.20)   (10.14)   (10.21)

(10.22)   (10.23)   (R)-(10.24)   (S)-(10.24)

(S)-(10.25)   (10.26)

effects ranging from full agonists to antagonists at central and/or peripheral muscarinic receptors.

The potent peripheral actions of **10.15**, including the effects on cardiovascular mechanisms, probably reflect its preferential activation of M_2 receptors. Attempts have been made to design analogs of **10.15** with pharmacological profiles relevant to AD. One of these analogs (BM5, **10.16**) has been characterized as an M_1 agonist/M_2 antagonist (see Section 10.2). An evaluation of the potential of **10.16** as a therapeutic agent in AD must await further behavioral pharmacological studies.

The naturally occurring heterocyclic cholinergic agonist pilocarpine (**10.17**) is widely used as a topical miotic for the control of elevated intraocular pressure associated with glaucoma. The bioavailability of pilocarpine is, however, low, and based on studies in animal models it has been suggested that this compound does not easily penetrate the BBB. Compound **10.17** is a partial muscarinic agonist showing an *in vitro* pharmacological profile very similar to that of arecoline (**10.13**).

Impairments of position discrimination learning in animals could be overcome by systemically administered **10.13** as well as **10.17** at doses lower than those producing marked autonomic effects. These observations are interesting in relation to AD and have focused behavioral pharmacological interest on prodrugs of **10.17** showing improved bioavailability (see Chapter 14).

The compounds **10.18–10.20** show very high affinity for mAChRs. The 3-amino-1,2,4-oxadiazole **10.18**, which interacts non-selectively with mAChR subtypes, probably is the most potent muscarinic agonist known. The arecoline (**10.13**) bioisosteres, the 2-ethyltetrazole (**10.20**) and the 3-hexyloxy-1,2,5-thiadiazole (**10.19**) analogs have been reported to preferentially activate M_1 receptors vs. M_2 receptors. Compound **10.19** has been evaluated clinically as a potential drug for the treatment of AD.

Compound **10.19** did improve the symptoms of Alzheimer patients but only after administration of doses, which also provoked cholinergic side effects. During the clinical studies of **10.19** it was, quite surprisingly, observed that the compound was capable of reducing the psychotic symptoms of AD patients, which in addition suffered from schizophrenia. These observations disclosed an involvement of the central mAChRs in schizophrenia, possibly reflecting an interaction between cholinergic and dopaminergic neurones.

Thus, whereas treatment of AD patients with muscarinic agonists or partial agonists has been shown not to be straightforward due to apparently unavoidable peripheral cholinergic side effects, such compounds are potential therapeutic agents in schizophrenia.

More recently, the (R)- and (S)-forms of 5,7-dimethyl-3-propargyloxy-4,5,6,7-tetrahydroisothiazolo[4,5-c]pyridine (**10.24**) were synthesized (see Scheme 10.1) and characterized as mAChR ligands *in vitro*. Both of these enantiomers of **10.24** bind tightly to muscarinic receptor sites, and they were both shown to be approximately an order of magnitude more potent at M_1 than at M_2 receptors. (R)-**10.24** typically showed a 3–5 fold higher affinity for muscarinic receptor sites than (S)-**10.24**. This surprisingly low degree of stereoselectivity may reflect that the part of these molecules carrying the chiral center does not bind tightly to the receptor proteins during the interactions with the mAChRs.

Although the propargyloxy side chain present in **10.24** and **10.25** appears to be optimal for binding of this group of compounds to mAChRs, the triple bond can be reduced to a double bond (**10.33** and **10.35** in Scheme 10.1) without significant loss of receptor affinity. Furthermore, compound **10.26**, in which the triple bond of **10.25** has been replaced by a nitrile group, binds tightly to muscarinic receptors, though weaker than **10.25**.

10.2.4 Muscarinic agonists and partial agonists: synthetic and structural aspects

The syntheses of a number of partial muscarinic agonists containing the bicyclic 4,5,6,7-tetrahydroisothiazolo[4,5-c]pyridine heterocyclic system are outlined in Scheme 10.1. The synthetic strategy has been to first build up the six-membered rings containing the nitrogen atoms, which become the basic groups of the target compounds **10.24–10.26**, **10.33**, and **10.35**, and containing functional groups

Scheme 10.1 (i) CH$_2$=CH-CN, C$_2$H$_5$OH; (ii) KOC(CH$_3$)$_3$, toluene, ClCOOC$_2$H$_5$; (iii) H$_2$SO$_4$ (85%), 60–70 °C; (iv) C$_6$H$_5$CH$_2$NH$_2$, xylene, reflux; (v) H$_2$S, DMF, Br$_2$; (vi) CH$_2$=CH-CH$_2$Br, (C$_4$H$_9$)$_4$N·HSO$_4$, K$_2$CO$_3$, KOH/CH$_3$OH; (vii) HCOOH, CH$_2$O, reflux; (viii) HBr/ AcOH (33%); (ix) (Boc)$_2$O, K$_2$CO$_3$; (x) CN-CH$_2$-Cl, (C$_4$H$_9$)$_4$N·HSO$_4$, K$_2$CO$_3$; (xi) HCl, ether, NaOH; (xii) CH≡C-CH$_2$Br, (C$_4$H$_9$)$_4$N·HSO$_4$, K$_2$CO$_3$; (xiii) HCOOH, CH$_2$O, reflux.

suitable for the construction of the 3-isothiazolol unit annulated with the six-membered ring.

Nucleophilic addition of the amino group of the starting material **10.27** to acrylonitrile gives the dinitrile **10.28**. In the presence of the strong base potassium *tert*-butoxide, a carbanion in the α-position of the unsubstituted chain is formed, and this anion attacks the nitrile group of the methylated chain to form a cyclic product containing an imino group. This imino group is hydrolyzed under mild conditions to give the keto group of **10.29**, and partial hydrolysis of the nitrile group of **10.29** under more drastic conditions gives compound **10.30**. Treatment of **10.30** with benzylamine converts the keto group into an enamino group with the double bond conjugated with the amide group, and this intermediate, **10.31**, can now be transformed into the bicyclic compound, **10.32**. Thus, by treatment of **10.31** with hydrogen sulfide, the benzylamino group is replaced by a mercapto group, and this group and the amide group undergo an oxidative cyclization reaction in the presence of bromine to give **10.32**. The hydroxy groups of **10.32** or the corresponding Boc-protected derivative, **10.34**, are alkylated using the appropriate alkylation reagents, and acid hydrolyses of the alkylation products remove the *N*-protecting groups to give the final compounds **10.24–10.26**, **10.33**, and **10.35**.

(*R*)-**10.25** and (*S*)-**10.25** were prepared by optical resolution of **10.25** using (2*R*,3*R*)-*O*,*O*′-dibenzoyltartaric acid and (2*S*,3*S*)-*O*,*O*′-dibenzoyltartaric acid, respectively, for diastereomeric salt formation. The absolute stereochemistry of

(S)-**10.25** was established by an X-ray crystallographic analysis of its (2S, 3S)-O,O'-dibenzoyltartaric acid salt (Figure 10.8). Since (R)-**10.24** and (S)-**10.24** were synthesized from (R)-**10.25** and (S)-**10.25**, respectively, by N-methylation, these chemical transformations unequivocally established the absolute configuration of the enantiomers of **10.24**. In the crystals of the (2S, 3S)-O,O'-dibenzoyltartaric acid salt of (S)-**10.25**, two conformationally different forms of the cation of (S)-**10.25** were observed (Figure 10.8), probably reflecting a low-energy barrier for rotating the propargyloxy side chain of the molecule.

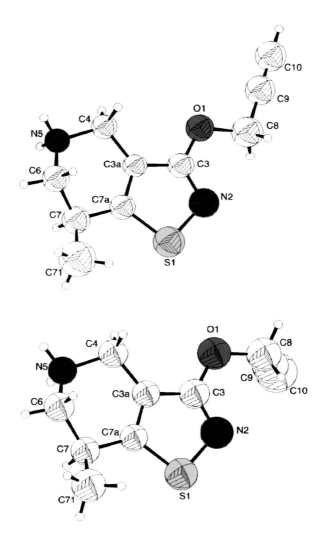

Figure 10.8 Perspective drawings of the two conformationally different cations of compound (S)-**10.25** crystallized as a salt with (2S,3S)-O,O'-dibenzoyltartaric acid. Spheres representing the isotropic or equivalent isotropic displacement parameters of the non-hydrogen atoms are shown at the 50% probability level. Hydrogen atoms in calculated positions are represented by spheres of arbitrary size.

10.2.5   Nicotinic agonists and partial agonists: bioisosteric design

A large number of naturally occurring alkaloids interact potently with nAChRs in the CNS and the PNS, and many of these compounds are generally described as very toxic compounds. The toxicological, or rather pharmacological, effects of these toxins are mediated by nAChRs with different subunit composition (see Section 10.2.1). The classical nAChR agonists, nicotine (**10.4**) and cytisine (**10.36**) show particularly high affinity for the $\alpha_4\beta_2$ subtype of nAChRs, which comprise the majority of nicotinic cholinergic receptors in the brain. Thus radiolabeled **10.4** and **10.36** (^{3}H-nicotine and ^{3}H-cytisine) are useful tools for studies of this class of nAChRs.

Epibatidine (**10.37**) was isolated from the skin of the poisonous frog, *Epipedobates tricolor*, and represents a new class of amphibian alkaloids, which probably serves the role in nature to protect the frog from potential predators. Compound **10.37** is a non-opioid analgesic, which is several hundred times more potent than morphine. **10.37** binds strongly to central nAChRs of the $\alpha_4\beta_2$ subtype, which mediate its analgesic effects, and **10.37** therefore is a very potent inhibitor of the receptor binding of ^{3}H-nicotine and ^{3}H-cytisine. The concentration of **10.37** in the frog skin is low, and less than 0.5 mg of this compound was isolated from the skin of 750 frogs, emphasizing the need for the development of effective methods for the synthesis of this compound (see Section 10.2.6).

Anatoxin-a (**10.38**) was first isolated from the freshwater blue-green algae, *Anabaena flosaquae*. This toxin, which possesses a 9-azabicyclo[4.2.1]nonane skeleton, is a highly potent nAChR agonist and an effective inhibitor of the receptor binding of ^{3}H-nicotine. The high potency of this nAChR ligand and its unique structural characteristics make **10.38** a useful tool for studies of nAChRs.

Bioisosteric replacements of the pyridine ring of nicotine (**10.4**) have been reported, and the 3-methylisoxazole bioisostere ABT-418 (**10.39**) has been shown to be a potent nAChR agonist. This compound has been extensively characterized in different *in vitro* assay systems and animal models, and it shows beneficial effects in

Nicotine
(**10.4**)

Cytisine
(**10.36**)

Epibatidine
(**10.37**)

Anatoxin-a
(**10.38**)

ABT-418
(**10.39**)

Altinicline
(**10.40**)

(**10.41**)

(**10.42**)

Alzheimer patients. Like nicotine (**10.4**), the analog, (S)-5-ethynyl-3-(1-methyl-2-pyr-rolidinyl)pyridine (altinicline, **10.40**), is a potent agonist at the $\alpha_4\beta_2$ nAChR subtype, but shows less effects than **10.4** at the peripheral and ganglionic $\alpha_3\beta_4$ nAChR subtype. This subtype-selectivity of **10.40** may explain its limited peripheral side effects, and **10.40** is undergoing clinical trials for the treatment of Parkinson's disease.

A large number of analogs of the naturally occurring potent nAChR ligands have been synthesized and pharmacologically characterized, as exemplified by **10.41** and **10.42**. Compound **10.41**, which is a ring homolog of **10.37** binds effectively to nAChRs, though somewhat weaker than **10.37**. Compound **10.42**, which is a conformationally restrained analog of **10.4** is essentially inactive, indicating that the conformations attainable by the nicotine structural element of **10.42** apparently do not reflect the receptor-active conformation(s) of nicotine (**10.4**). In structure–activity studies along these lines, it must, however, be kept in mind that the additional structure element incorporated into the nicotine analog **10.42** may interfere with its binding to the active site of the receptor.

10.2.6   Nicotinic agonists: synthetic aspects

The pronounced pharmacological interest in epibatidine (**10.37**) has prompted the development of several synthetic methods for the preparation of this unique compound. The synthetic sequence outlined in Scheme 10.2 is an effective route to **10.37**, which has been optimized for the production of the target compound on large scale.

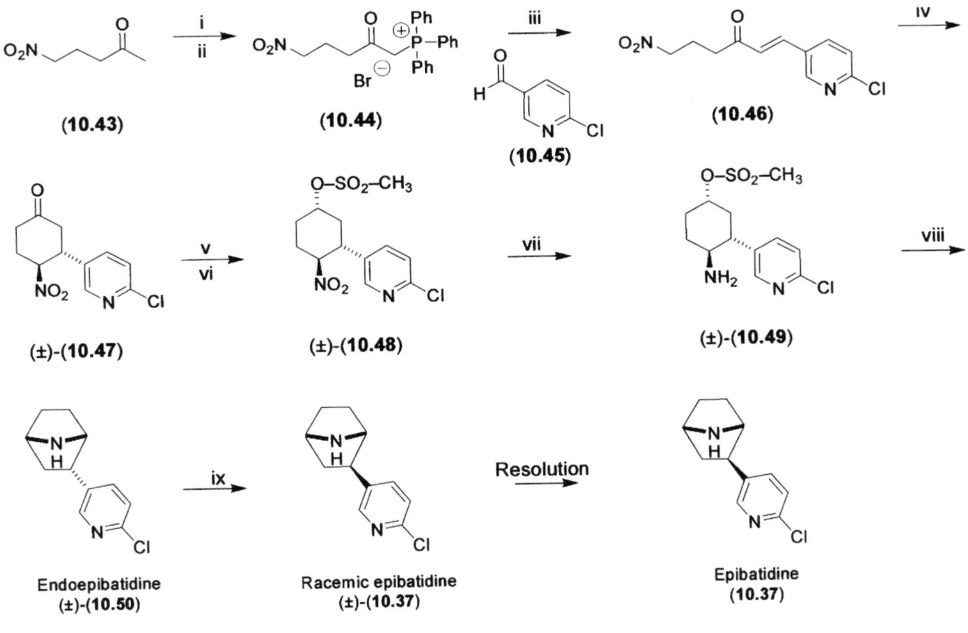

Scheme 10.2 (i) Br$_2$, CH$_3$OH; (ii) (Ph)$_3$P, benzene; (iii) CH$_2$Cl$_2$, NaOH; (iv) KF/Al$_2$O$_3$, THF, 25 °C; (v) NaBH$_4$, C$_2$H$_5$OH; (vi) CH$_3$SO$_2$Cl, CH$_2$Cl$_2$, pyridine; (vii) SnCl$_2$·2H$_2$O, C$_2$H$_5$OH; (viii) toluene; (ix) KOC(CH$_3$)$_3$, HOC(CH$_3$)$_3$.

The methyl group of the starting material **10.43** was selectively brominated, and treatment of the bromomethyl ketone intermediate with triphenylphosphine gave the quaternized salt **10.44**. A Wittig reaction of the phosphorane, generated from **10.44**, with the chloropyridine aldehyde **10.45** provided the α, β-unsaturated ketone **10.46**. Under weakly basic conditions, the anion, formed at the carbon α to the nitro group, underwent a nucleophilic addition to the double bond, producing the cyclized compound **10.47** with the indicated relative stereochemistry. Reduction of the keto group of **10.47** to give a secondary alcohol group proceeded in a stereoselective manner, and after treatment of the alcohol intermediate with methanesulfonyl chloride, compound **10.48** was obtained. Reduction of the nitro group of **10.48** provided amine **10.49**, still as a racemate but with the relative stereochemistry shown. Compound **10.49** easily underwent an intramolecular nucleophilic substitution reaction, with methanesulfonate as the leaving group, to give the *endo* isomer of epibatidine, endoepibatidine (**10.50**). Treatment of **10.50** with strong base induced epimerization to give the corresponding *exo* isomer, which is epibatidine (**10.37**), obtained in the racemic form but with the correct relative stereochemistry. Using different optically active carboxylic acids, racemic **10.37** was resolved to give epibatidine (**10.37**), which was shown to be identical with **10.37** isolated from frog skin (see Section 10.2.5).

10.2.7   Acetylcholinesterase inhibitors

Inhibitors of AChE allow a build up of ACh at the nerve endings resulting in a prolonged activation of cholinergic receptors. Treatment with such inhibitors has been useful in myasthenia gravis, a disease associated with the rapid fatigue of

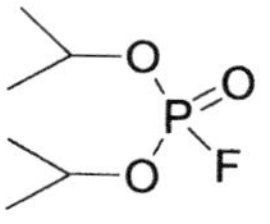

(10.51)

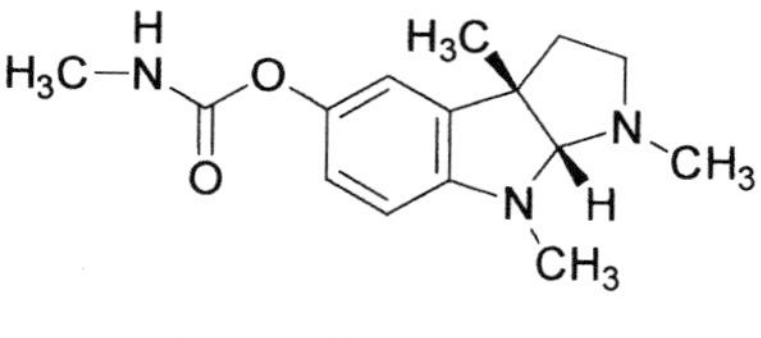

Physostigmine **(10.52)**
(pK_a 1.8; 7.9)

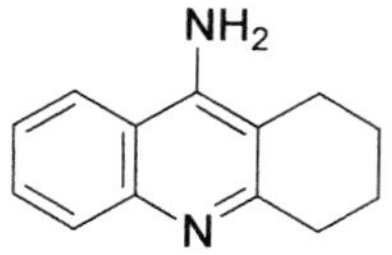

Tacrine **(10.53)**
(pK_a 10.0)

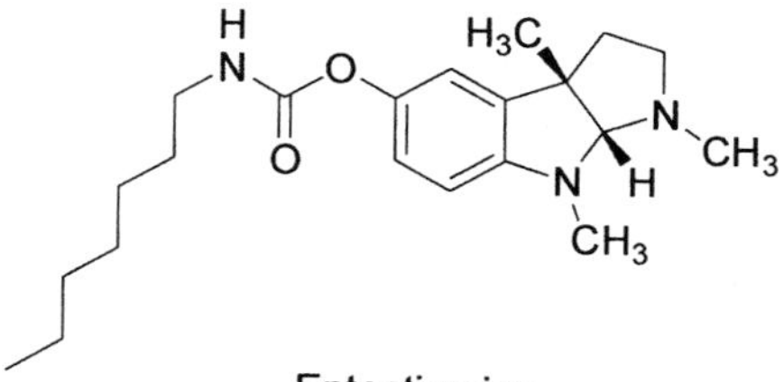

Eptastigmine
(10.54)

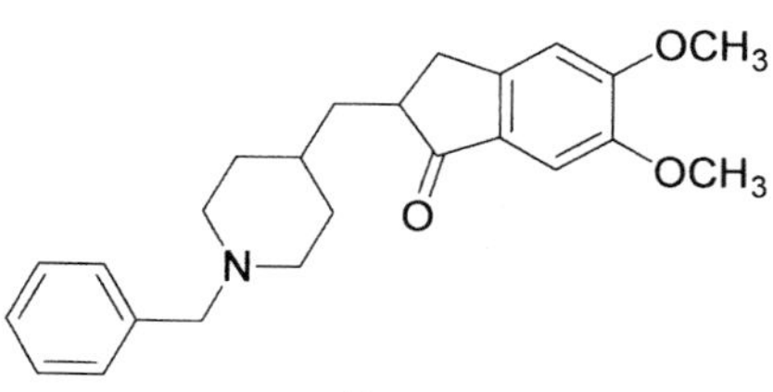

Donepezil
(10.55)

muscles and also in the treatment of glaucoma, where stimulation of the ciliary body improves drainage from the eye and, thus, decreases intraocular pressure.

Two main classes of AChE inhibitors have been developed: (1) irreversible organophosphorus inhibitors, such as dyflos (**10.51**); and (2) carbamoylating, but reversible, inhibitors, such as physostigmine (eserine, **10.52**). The former class of compounds has a long duration of action in the body, and after a single dose of drug the activity of AChE only returns after resynthesis of the enzyme. Due to dangers of overdosage they are only used therapeutically for the treatment of a limited number of glaucoma patients. A variety of volatile organophosphorus AChE inhibitors have been produced on large scales for use as nerve gasses in war, whereas other less volatile compounds of this category have been used as insecticides.

Inhibitors of the latter class including **10.52** are protonated at physiological pH and are bound at the anionic site of AChE. The relative positions of the ammonium and carbamate groups allow a transfer of the carbamoyl group onto the serine hydroxyl group at the esteratic site of the enzyme. The carbamoylated enzyme is hydrolyzed to regenerate the enzyme with a half-life of less than one hour. Kinetic studies originally gave the impression that **10.52** and related carbamates were acting as simple reversible competitive inhibitors of AChE.

Inhibitors of AChE, notably **10.52**, have been studied clinically in AD. Treatment of Alzheimer patients with **10.52** have marginally improved learning and memory, but these positive effects have been accompanied by unacceptable side effects. Although amines like **10.52** are capable of penetrating the BBB (see Figure 10.7), they are likely to enhance the activity at virtually all cholinergic synapses in the periphery and the CNS. Thus, stimulation of all nicotinic and muscarinic ACh receptors may explain the complex therapeutic effect/side effect profiles observed after administration of **10.52** to AD patients.

9-Amino-1,2,3,4-tetrahydroacridine (tacrine, THA, **10.53**) is a non-selective but reversible inhibitor of AChE. In spite of its strongly basic character (pK$_a$ 10.0) and, thus, high degree of protonation at physiological pH, **10.53** is capable of penetrating the BBB to some extent, probably as a result of the lipophilic character of its phenyl and cycloalkyl ring structures.

Clinical studies of **10.53** in Alzheimer patients have shown improvements in learning and memory, at least in certain groups of patients. These promising effects have been proposed to reflect selective effects of **10.53** on brain AChE. Since **10.53** also has pharmacological effects unrelated to the inhibition of AChE, the mechanism(s) underlying its clinical effects in AD are not fully understood.

Eptastigmine (**10.54**) is more lipophilic than **10.52**, and **10.54** actually showed very promising effects in AD patients. However, the development of this derivative of **10.52** as a therapeutic agent was stopped after two patients developed aplastic anemia during the phase III clinical trials. Donepezil (**10.55**) is structurally unrelated to **10.52** and is described as a 'second-generation' AChE inhibitor. In clinical trials, **10.55** has been shown to be devoid of the problems associated with the administration of tacrine (**10.53**) to AD patients, and **10.55** offered modest improvement in cognitive processes for at least a few months in almost 50% of the patients studied. These data illustrate the limited therapeutic effects in AD of AChE inhibitors.

10.3 HISTAMINE RECEPTORS

Histamine (2-(imidazole-4-yl)ethylamine) (**10.64**), which is biosynthesized by decarboxylation of the basic amino acid histidine, is involved as a chemical messenger in a variety of complex biological actions. In mammals, it is mainly stored in an inactive bound form in many body tissues, from which it is released by different stimuli and mechanisms. Histamine exerts its biological functions via activation of specific receptors, and during the past 2–3 decades three pharmacologically distinct histamine receptors designated H_1, H_2 and H_3 have been characterized (Figure 10.9). Like the H_1 and H_2 receptors, the H_3 receptor, and also the very recently cloned H_4 receptor, have been shown to belong to the group of G protein-coupled receptor (see Chapter 6).

Activation of H_1 receptors stimulates the contraction of smooth muscles in many organs such as the gut, the uterus, and the bronchi. Contraction of the bronchi leads to restriction of the passage of air into and out of the lungs as in asthma. Stimulation of H_1 receptors on smooth muscles in for example fine blood vessels does, however, cause muscle relaxation, and the resulting vasodilation may result in severe fall in blood pressure. Furthermore, histamine increases the permeability of the capillary walls so that more of the plasma constituents can escape into the tissue space, leading to the formation of oedema. This series of events is manifest in the well-known redness and wheal associated with histamine release, the so-called 'triple response'. Histamine is also involved in the removal of the products of cell

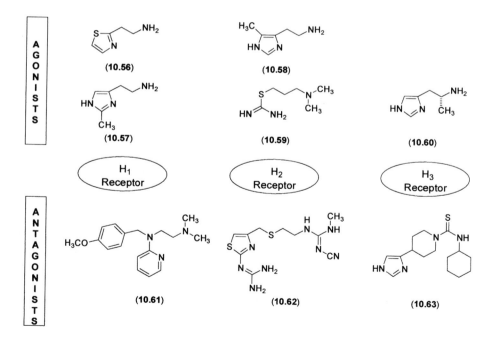

Figure 10.9 A schematic illustration of the multiplicity of histamine receptors and the structures of a number of subtype-selective agonists and antagonists.

damage during inflammation. Under these circumstances, the liberation of histamine is accompanying the production of antibodies and their interaction with foreign proteins. Under extreme circumstances, however, the effects of histamine can become pathological, leading to exaggerated responses with distressing results, as may occur in some allergic conditions.

A number of selective and very potent antagonists at H_1 receptors are now available. Such compounds, including mepyramine (**10.61**), are structurally very different from histamine. These 'antihistamines' are typically developed via lead optimization of accidentally discovered compounds capable of blocking the effects of histamine on the perfused lung or the isolated ileum or trachea from guinea pigs or on human bronchi. A number of these competitive H_1 antagonists are used clinically.

Compounds showing selective agonist activity at subtypes of histamine receptors are essential as tools for pharmacological studies of histamine receptors. In order to develop such agonists, the molecule of histamine has been subjected to extensive structural modifications. Most of these histamine analogs, in which the imidazole ring and/or the 2-aminoethyl side chain have been alkylated or otherwise structurally modified, show very weak histamine agonist activity. These systematic structural variations of histamine have, however, led to receptor subtype-selective agonists. Thus, 2-methylhistamine (**10.57**) and, in particular, 2-(thiazol-2-yl)ethylamine (**10.56**) are selective agonists at H_1 receptors, though weaker than histamine itself. On the other hand, 5-methylhistamine (**10.58**) selectively activates H_2 receptors. Similarly, S-[3-(N,N-dimethylamino)propyl]isothiourea (dimaprit, **10.59**), in which the imidazole ring of histamine has been bioisosterically replaced by an S-alkylisothiourea group showing similar protolytic properties, is a highly selective H_2 receptor agonist. These two H_2 agonists have been useful tools in connection with the elegant design and development of selective H_2 receptor antagonists such as **10.62** (see Section 10.3.2).

Studies in recent years have established that histamine is acting as a neurotransmitter in the CNS. Whilst H_1 and H_2 receptors seem to be predominantly localized on postsynaptic membranes of central neurones, H_3 receptors appear to function predominantly as presynaptic receptors, possibly as histamine autoreceptors. Although H_3 receptors have also been detected in some peripheral organs, this class of histamine receptors exists primarily in the CNS. Very recently, a fourth G protein-coupled histamine receptor, H_4, has been identified and pharmacologically characterized. This H_4 receptor exhibits a very restricted localization and is found primarily in intestinal tissue, spleen and immune active cells, such as T cells, suggesting a therapeutic potential for H_4 receptor ligands in allergic and inflammatory diseases. The H_4 receptor shows signal transduction mechanisms and pharmacological characteristics similar to those of H_3 receptors.

The physiological role of the central histamine neurotransmitter system is far from being elucidated, but it has been suggested that it plays a role in cerebral circulation, energy metabolism, and states of wakefulness. These aspects have focused pharmacological interest on agonists as well as antagonists at H_3 receptors. Interestingly, stereoselectivity of agonists is much more pronounced at H_3 receptors than either H_1 or H_2 receptors, and (R)-α-methylhistamine (**10.60**) has been shown to be a selective and very potent H_3 receptor agonist (Figure 10.9). Whilst a number of H_2 antagonists interact potently with H_3 receptors, highly selective H_3 antagonists, notably thioperamide (**10.63**), have recently been described. The availability of such compounds is likely to stimulate studies of the precise role of histamine in the CNS.

10.3.1 Protolytic properties of histamine and histamine analogs

Studies of the protolytic properties of histamine have played an important part in the design of selective H_2 antagonists (see subsequent section) and in the interpretation of structure–activity relationships for subtype-selective histamine receptor agonists. At physiological pH (7.4) the primary amino group (pK_a 9.8) of histamine is almost fully ionized, whereas the monobasic imidazole ring (pK_a 6.0) is only about 4% protonated (see equation (10.1), Section 10.2.3). Thus, in aqueous solution at physiological pH only ca. 4% of histamine exists as the resonance-stabilized dication **10.65**. The ionized side chain of **10.65** exerts a negative inductive ($-I$) effect on the protonated imidazole ring. This electron-withdrawing effect reduces the electron density at the nearest ring nitrogen atom (N3) and, thus, facilitates the dissociation of a proton from this atom to form the monocation **10.66**, named the N^τ–H tautomer. The methyl group of the H_2 receptor-selective agonist **10.58** exerts a positive inductive ($+I$) effect on the heterocyclic ring. This electron-repelling effect of the methyl group, which increases the electron density at N1, further stabilizes the N1–H bond in **10.67** and, consequently, the N^τ–H tautomer **10.68** after dissociation of a proton from the dication **10.67**.

Based on extensive structure–activity studies of histamine analogs, it is assumed that the monocationic N^τ–H tautomer **10.66** is the active form of histamine at H_1 as well as H_2 receptors. The protonated primary amino group and the lone pair of electrons at N3 in **10.66** are essential for the binding of histamine to H_1 receptors, whereas the protonated primary amino group and the N1–H group are essential molecular components for the binding of **10.66** to H_2 receptors.

10.3.2 H_2 and H_3 receptor antagonists: design and therapeutic aspects

Histamine (**10.64**) has a physiological function in regulating the secretion of acid in the stomach where, acting on the H_2 receptor, it stimulates the parietal cells to produce hydrochloric acid (see Figure 10.5). This probably is a protective mechanism, since the acid controls the local bacterial population. Under different conditions, the regulation of acid secretion by histamine or other chemical messengers may run out of control, and under such circumstances excessive acid secretion can lead to the formation of gastric and/or duodenal ulcers.

These aspects prompted the design and development of selective antagonists at H_2 receptors, and this field of drug research has been one of the most active and successful areas in medicinal chemistry. Systematic structural modifications of histamine led to the discovery of burimamide (**10.69**) as a selective but relatively weak H_2 receptor antagonist. The low activity of **10.69** was explained in terms of non-optimal protolytic properties of its imidazole ring, which is substantially more basic (pK_a 7.2) than is the ring of histamine. Consequently, the degree of protonation of the imidazole ring of **10.69** is more than an order of magnitude higher than that of histamine at physiological pH. This increased basic character of the ring of **10.69** reflects a $+I$ effect of the alkyl side chain, and, furthermore, this electron-repelling effect favors the dissociation of the proton from N1 in **10.70** by increasing the electron density at N3. Thus, the N^π–H tautomer **10.71** will be the dominating neutral form of burimamide. Since burimamide appears to bind to the H_2 receptor in a neutral form, and since the imidazole ring of burimamide is assumed to bind to the site of the H_2 receptor, which binds the imidazole ring of histamine, the N^π–H tautomer **10.71** of burimamide was considered nonoptimal for effective receptor binding.

This reasoning prompted modifications of the structure of burimamide in order to obtain compounds, which more closely resembled histamine. Introduction of a sulphur atom into the side chain and a methyl group into position 5 of the ring of burimamide gave metiamide (**10.72**), which showed greater potency and selectivity as an H_2 receptor antagonist than did burimamide. Introduction of the sulphur atom converted the $+I$ effect of the side chain of burimamide into a $-I$ effect, whereas the C5 methyl group exerts a $+I$ effect. As a consequence of these structural modifications, the electron densities at C5-N1 and at C4-N3 in metiamide were, respectively, increased and decreased as compared with burimamide. Thus, the facilitated dissociation of the N3-H proton from protonated metiamide (**10.73**) gives the desired N^τ–H tautomer (**10.72** or **10.74**) as the dominating neutral form of metiamide.

(10.69)　　　　　　(10.70)　　　　　　(10.71)

(10.72)　　　　　　(10.73)　　　　　　(10.74)

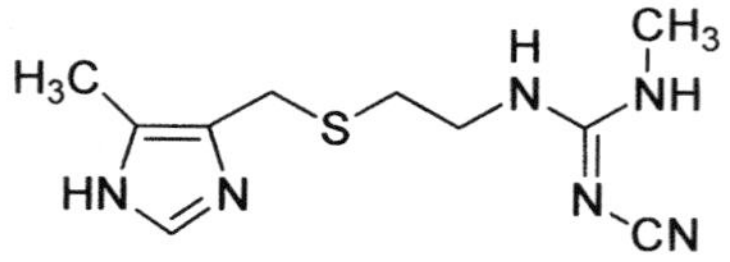

Cimetidine (**10.75**)

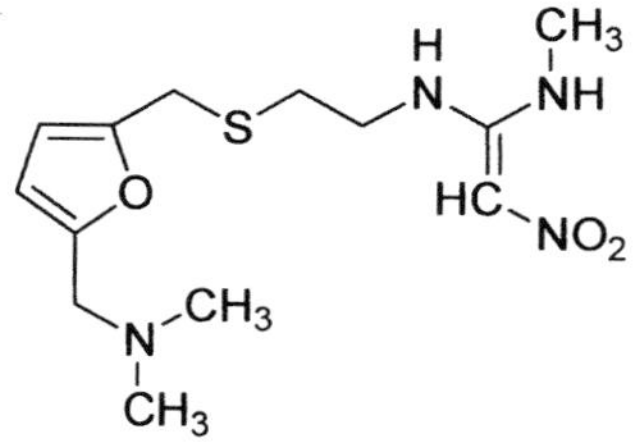

Ranitidine (**10.76**)

Side effects, such as agranulocytosis, of metiamide (**10.72**) led to the replacement of its thiourea unit by the structurally related cyanoguanidine group to give cimetidine (**10.75**), which is more active than **10.72** as an H_2 antagonist and less toxic. Cimetidine turned out to be a successful drug, and, since its introduction some two decades ago, several million patients suffering from diseases caused by unnaturally high gastric secretion of hydrochloric acid have derived benefit from its therapeutic use. In recent years, a wide variety of other H_2 antagonists, notably ranitidine (**10.76**), have been introduced in the human clinic. The structural basis of the proposed interaction of the 2-guanidinothiazole and the 2-dimethylamino-methylfuran groups of **10.62** and **10.76**, respectively, with the imidazole-binding part of the H_2 receptor is not fully understood.

The cloning of the H_3 receptor, and its proposed involvement in a number of diseases and pathological conditions such as asthma, migraine, hypertension, septic shock, and in learning and memory degenerative disorders like AD have prompted an intense search for H_3 receptor ligands, primarily H_3 antagonists.

Since the discovery of thioperamide (**10.63**) as a potent and selective H_3 antagonist, a number of 4(5)-substituted imidazole derivatives have been designed,

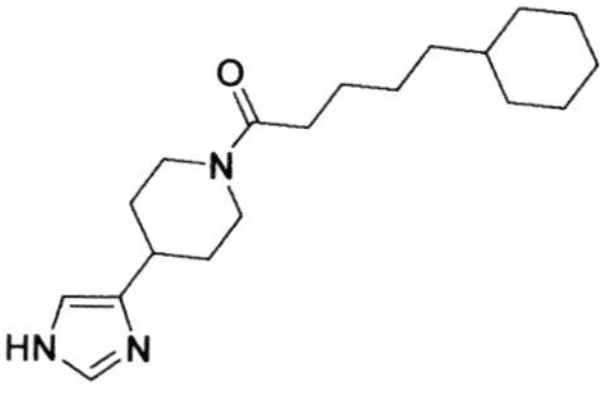

GT-2016 (**10.77**)

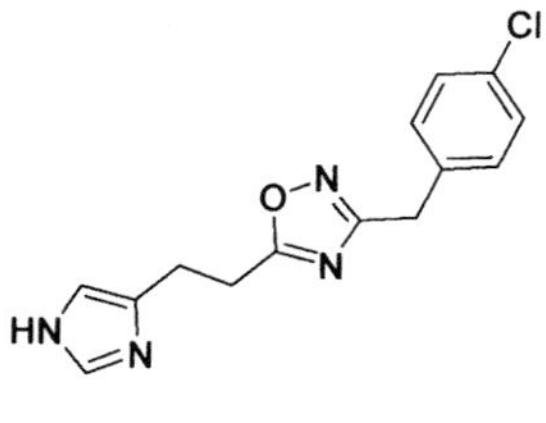

GR 175737 (**10.78**)

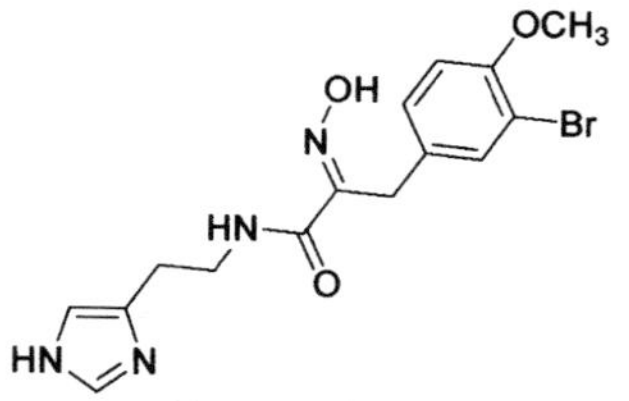

Verongamine (**10.79**)

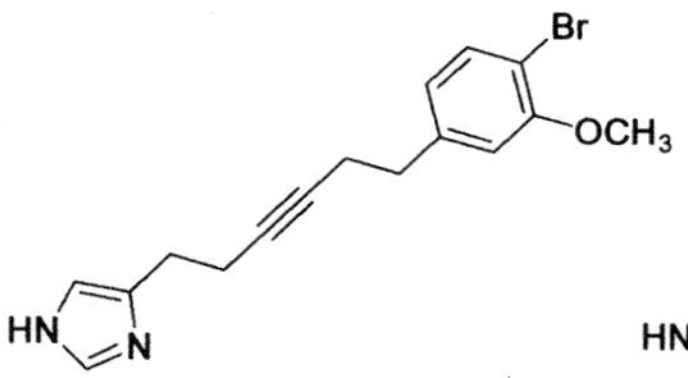

(**10.80**)

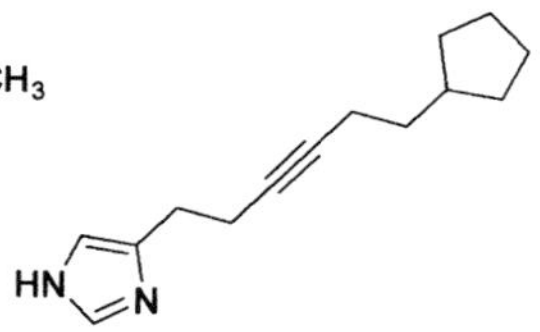

(**10.81**)

synthesized and pharmacologically evaluated. Some of the more prominent new H$_3$ receptor antagonists are GT-2016 (**10.77**) and GR 175737 (**10.78**) which show receptor affinities in the low nanomolar range.

Verongamine (**10.79**) is, so far, the only natural product that has been reported to possess H$_3$ antagonist effect. **10.79** only binds to H$_3$ receptors with moderately high affinity (IC$_{50}$ = 500 nM), and due to the presence of polar groups in the molecule, **10.79** does not easily penetrate the BBB. Based on molecular modeling studies, the compounds **10.79** and **10.80** were shown to adopt very similar energy-minimized conformations, and based on these studies, a series of lipophilic and highly potent H$_3$ antagonists were designed. Within this group of acetylenic imidazole derivatives, compound **10.81** turned out to be almost three orders of magnitude more potent than the lead compound, **10.79**. These compounds are undergoing further pharmacological evaluation as potential therapeutic agents.

FURTHER READING

Ali, S.M., Tedford, C.E., Gregory, R.,Yates, S.L. and Phillips, J.G. (1998) New acetylene based histamine H$_3$ receptor antagonists derived from the marine natural product verongamine. *Bioorg. Med. Chem. Lett.*, **8**, 1133–1138.

Arneric, S.P. and Brioni, J.D. (1999) *Neuronal Nicotinic Receptors: Pharmacology and Therapeutic Opportunities*. New York: Wiley-Liss.

Birdsall, N.J.M., Nathanson, N.M. and Schwarz, R.D. (2001) Muscarinic receptors: it's a knockout. *Trends Pharmacol. Sci.*, **22**, 215–219.

Brown, J.H. (ed.) (1989) *The Muscarinic Receptors*. Clifton, New Jersey: The Humana Press.

Cooper, D.G., Young, R.C., Durant, G.J. and Ganellin, C.R. (1990) Histamine receptors. In *Comprehensive Medicinal Chemistry*, Vol. 3, edited by C. Hansch, P.G. Sammes, J.B. Taylor and J.C. Emmett, pp. 323–421. Oxford: Pergamon Press.

Eberlein, W.G., Engel, W., Hasselbach, K.M., Mayer, N., Mihm, G., Rudolf, K. and Doods, H. (1992) Tricyclic compounds as selective muscarinic antagonists: structure activity relationships and therapeutic implications. In *Trends in Receptor Research*, edited by P. Angeli, U. Gulini and W. Quaglia, pp. 231–249. Amsterdam: Elsevier.

Fisher, A. (ed.) (1996) *Muscarinic Agonists and the Treatment of Alzheimer's Disease*. Heidelberg: Springer-Verlag.

Kovalainen, J.T., Christiaans, J.A.M., Kotisaari, S., Laitinen, J.T., Männistö, P.T., Tuomisto, L. and Gynther, J. (1999) Synthesis and *in vitro* pharmacology of a series of new chiral histamine H$_3$-receptor ligands: 2-(R and S)-amino-3-(1H-imidazol-4(5)-yl)propyl ether derivatives. *J. Med. Chem.*, **42**, 1193–1202.

Leurs, R., Watanabe, T. and Timmerman, H. (2001) Histamine receptors are finally 'coming out'. *Trends Pharmacol. Sci.*, **22**, 337–339.

Pedersen, H., Bräuner-Osborne, H., Ball, R.G., Frydenvang, K., Meier, E., Bøgesø, K.P. and Krogsgaard-Larsen, P. (1999) Synthesis and muscarinic receptor pharmacology of a series of 4,5,6,7-tetrahydroisothiazolo[4,5-c]pyridine bioisosteres of arecoline. *Bioorg. Med. Chem.*, **7**, 795–809.

Schmitt, J.D. and Bencherif, M. (2000) Targeting nicotinic acetylcholine receptors: advances in molecular design and therapies. *Annu. Rep. Med. Chem.*, **35**, 41–51.

St George-Hyslop, P.H., McLaurin, J. and Fraser, P.E. (2000) Neuropathological, biochemical and genetic alterations in AD. *Drug News Perspect.*, **13**, 281–288.

Szántay, C., Kardos-Balogh, Z., Moldvai, I., Szántay, C. Jr., Temesvári-Major, E. and Blaskó, G. (1996) A practical enantioselective synthesis of epibatidine. *Tetrahedron*, **52**, 11053–11062.

Timmerman, H. (1990) Histamine H$_3$ ligands: just pharmacological tools or potential therapeutic agents? *J. Med. Chem.*, **33**, 4–11.

Wess, J., Buhl, T., Lambrecht, G. and Mutschler, E. (1990) Cholinergic receptors. In *Comprehensive Medicinal Chemistry*, Vol. 3, edited by C. Hansch, P.G. Sammes, J.B. Taylor and J.C. Emmett, pp. 423–491. Oxford: Pergamon Press.

Chapter 11

Dopamine and serotonin receptor and transporter ligands

Klaus P. Bøgesø and Benny Bang-Andersen

11.1 RECEPTORS AND TRANSPORTERS FOR DOPAMINE AND SEROTONIN

Dopamine (DA) and serotonin (5-hydroxytryptamine, 5-HT) are both important neurotransmitters in the human brain. A schematic drawing of a neurotransmitter synapse representative for both DA and serotonin is shown in Figure 11.1. Neurotransmitters are released from vesicles into the synaptic cleft where they subsequently can activate a number of postsynaptic receptors (PR). The neurotransmitters may also activate a number of autoreceptors (AR) which regulate the synthesis and release of the transmitters, and generally, activation of autoreceptors leads to inhibition of neurotransmitter synthesis and release. The autoreceptors can be localized both presynaptically or somatodendritically (on the cell bodies). The concentration of neurotransmitter in the synapse may also be regulated by active reuptake into the presynaptic terminal by transporters (T).

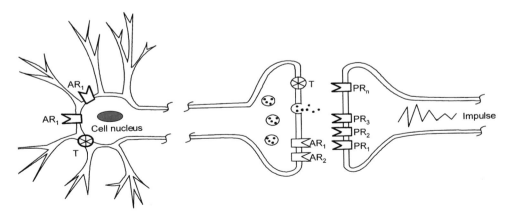

Figure 11.1 Neurotransmitter synapse. PR: Postsynaptic receptor; AR: Autoreceptor; T: Transporter.

11.2 DOPAMINE AND SEROTONIN RECEPTOR LIGANDS

11.2.1 Molecular biology and structure of receptors for dopamine and serotonin

Subtypes of DA receptors were not known until Kebabian and Calne in 1979 suggested that the DA receptor, which stimulated adenylyl cyclase, and the receptor that did not stimulate adenylyl cyclase were distinct categories of receptors and should be designated D-1 and D-2, respectively. The same year, Peroutka and Snyder suggested the existence of two different serotonin receptor subtypes based on differential drug potencies for serotonin receptor sites labeled with [3H]5-HT and [3H]spiroperidol, respectively. In both of these cases, the subtypes were identified by the use of classical pharmacological techniques, but since the late 1980s, the application of molecular biological techniques has had a major impact on the identification of additional subtypes of these receptors.

The DA and serotonin receptor subtypes known today are shown in Figures 11.2 and 11.3, respectively. All of these receptors are putative 7-TM G-protein-coupled receptors (see Chapter 6) except for the 5-HT$_3$ receptor, which is a ligand-gated ion channel regulating the permeability of Na$^+$ and K$^+$ ions. Selective ligands have been developed for the majority of these receptors of which the 7-TM receptors in particular have proven to be drug targets for a number of psychiatric disorders.

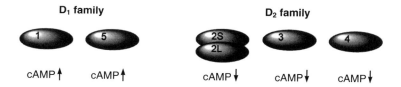

Figure 11.2 Dopamine (DA) receptor classification. cAMP↑: Activation of receptor stimulates adenylyl cyclase which results in an increase in the intracellular concentration of cyclic adenosine monophosphate (cAMP); cAMP↓: Activation of receptor inhibits adenylyl cyclase which results in a decrease in the intracellular concentration of cAMP.

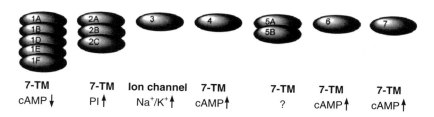

Figure 11.3 Serotonin (5-hydroxytryptamine, 5-HT) receptor classification. 7-TM and ion channel: Classification of receptor type; cAMP↑ and cAMP↓: see legend to Figure 11.2; PI↑: Activation of receptor stimulates phospholipase C which results in an increase in the intracellular turnover of phosphatidylinositol (PI) biphosphate; Na$^+$/K$^+$: Activation of receptor increases the permeability of sodium and potassium ions into the cell.

The 7-TM receptors are 350–550 amino acid peptides that have seven regions consisting of 20–25 hydrophobic amino acids, which form helices through the nerve cell membrane. Between the helices there are loops of varying length (three extracellular and three intracellular). The third intracellular loop is longer and is believed to interact with the G-protein. The N-terminal end is extracellular, while the carboxy terminal end is intracellular (for further discussions on 7-TM receptors, see Chapter 6).

11.2.1.1   Dopamine receptor subtypes

The DA receptor subtypes are divided into two families based on structural and pharmacological similarities (Figure 11.2): The D_1 family (D_1 and D_5 receptors) and the D_2 family (D_2, D_3 and D_4 receptors). Activation of D_1 and D_5 receptors leads generally to stimulation of adenylyl cyclase while inhibition is observed after D_2, D_3 and D_4 receptor activation. In addition, there are two isoforms of the D_2 receptor named D_{2S} (short) or D_{2L} (long).

Dopamine D_1 and D_2 receptors are expressed in regions associated with motor, limbic and neuroendocrine function, and D_2 antagonists and agonists are used in the treatment of schizophrenia and Parkinson's disease, respectively. The more recently identified receptor subtypes D_3, D_4, and D_5 have more restricted distributions. D_3 and D_4 receptors are primarily localized in limbic regions of the brain associated with emotion, whereas little to no expression is seen in striatal regions associated with motor function. The D_5 receptor has very limited distribution in the human brain. The involvement of the different DA receptor subtypes in the treatment of schizophrenia will be discussed in more detail in the following.

11.2.1.2   Serotonin receptor subtypes

A total of 14 serotonin receptor subtypes grouped in seven families are known (Figure 11.3). The receptors of the $5\text{-}HT_1$ family are all negatively coupled to adenylyl cyclase, while the $5\text{-}HT_4$, $5\text{-}HT_6$ and $5\text{-}HT_7$ receptors are all positively linked to adenylyl cyclase. All members of the $5\text{-}HT_2$ family are linked to phosphatidylinositol (PI) turnover (i.e. stimulation leads to an increased production of inositol phosphates and increased concentration of intracellular Ca^{2+}). Signal transduction pathways for $5\text{-}HT_5$ receptors remain to be defined unequivocally.

All of the serotonin receptor subtypes are expressed in the human brain but several of the subtypes are also found in the periphery. The $5\text{-}HT_{1A}$ receptor is involved in modulation of emotion and mood, and partial $5\text{-}HT_{1A}$ agonists such as buspirone have anxiolytic and antidepressant activity. The $5\text{-}HT_{1B}$ and $5\text{-}HT_{1D}$ (formerly called $5\text{-}HT_{1D\beta}$ and $5\text{-}HT_{1D\alpha}$ in humans) receptors are autoreceptors that regulate neurotransmitter release, and they may prove to be interesting targets for antidepressant or anxiolytic drugs. The $5\text{-}HT_{2A}$ receptor is found both in the CNS and the periphery. In the periphery, it is widely distributed and mediates contractile responses in bronchial, gastrointestinal, urinary, uterine and vascular smooth muscle. Platelet aggregation and increased capillary permeability are also $5\text{-}HT_{2A}$ mediated actions. Therefore, $5\text{-}HT_{2A}$ antagonists such as ketanserin have shown potential as antihypertensive and antiplatelet aggregating drugs. In the brain, the 5-HT$_{2A}$ receptor is found in cortical areas, in parts of the limbic system and in the basal ganglia. Therefore, 5-HT$_{2A}$ receptors are important targets for development of antipsychotic drugs. The 5-HT$_{2C}$ (formerly called 5-HT$_{1C}$) receptor is predominantly localized in the brain, and their dysregulation may contribute to particular symptoms of anxiety and depression. In addition, antagonism of 5-HT$_{2C}$ receptors may be important for the effect of antipsychotic drugs and may also be responsible for their potential to increase weight gain. The 5-HT$_3$ receptor is widely distributed in the periphery (cardiovascular and gastrointestinal systems) but it is also found in the brain. The nausea and gastrointestinal discomfort often seen in the first weeks of treatment of depressed patients with Selective Serotonin Reuptake Inhibitors (SSRIs, see also Section 11.3.2.2) is probably caused by activation of 5-HT$_3$ receptors. Along similar lines antagonists for the 5-HT$_3$ receptor are used to control vomiting in e.g. cancer patients. Interestingly, 5-HT$_3$ antagonists are effective in certain animal models of schizophrenia and anxiety. The 5-HT$_6$ and 5-HT$_7$ receptors are mainly expressed in the brain. Several antidepressant and antipsychotic drugs bind with high affinity to these receptors but no clear picture has been found between the affinity of these compounds for these receptors and their clinical profile.

As already mentioned, selective ligands have been described for many of the dopamine and serotonin receptor subtypes but it is not within the scope of this chapter to review all of these ligands. In the following, we have chosen to concentrate on ligands which have shown a potential as antipsychotic or antidepressant drugs or which have been important in the discovery of these drugs.

11.2.2 Antipsychotic drugs

11.2.2.1 Classical antipsychotic drugs

Antipsychotic drugs are primarily used to treat schizophrenia and a number of other psychotic disorders, such as e.g. schizoaffective disorder. These disorders are distinguished from each other on the basis of characteristic clusters of symptoms and, in the case of schizophrenia, the characteristic symptoms can be arranged into two broad categories – positive and negative. The positive symptoms appear to reflect an excess or distortion of normal function (i.e. delusion, hallucinations, disorganized thinking, disorganized behavior and catatonia), whereas the negative symptoms appear to reflect a diminution or loss of normal functions (i.e. affective flattening, poverty of speech and an inability to initiate and persist in goal-directed activities). However, in recent years, more and more interest has been devoted to the importance of cognitive deficits as the core of schizophrenia, and in future the diagnostic schema for schizophrenia may very well also include cognitive symptoms (i.e. impairment of memory, executive function and attention).

Reserpine (**11.1**, Figure 11.4), which is the principal active indole alkaloid of the roots of *Rauwolfia serpentina*, was first described as an antihypotentive and tranquillizing agent, whereas chlorpromazine (**11.2**, Figure 11.5) was described as an antihistaminergic agent. It was subsequently discovered in the 1950s that both reserpine and chlorpromazine were effective in the treatment of mainly the

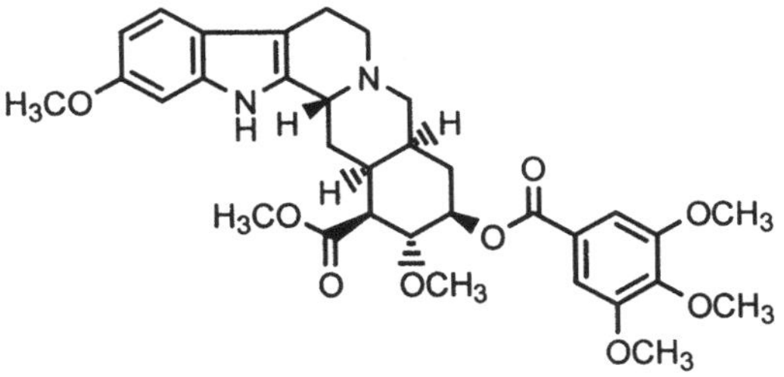

Reserpine (11.1)

Figure 11.4 Reserpine.

positive symptoms of schizophrenia. However, the use of both compounds was associated with severe side effects such as parkinsonian symptoms (i.e. tremor, muscle rigidity and akinesia), dystonia, akathisia and tardive dyskinesia, which subsequently were known as extrapyramidal symptoms (EPS). It was later shown that the two compounds had very different mechanisms of action despite their similar clinical effects. Reserpine blocks unselectively the accumulation of the monoamines norepinephrine (NE), DA and 5-HT by synaptic vesicles (vesicular pool). The monoamines will subsequently leak out of the vesicles and into the presynaptic neurone, where the enzymes monoamine oxidase-A and -B (MAO-A and MAO-B) will deaminate them. As a result, the synaptic cleft will be depleted for any of these monoaminergic neurotransmitters. On the contrary, chlorpromazine is a postsynaptic dopamine receptor antagonist. However, the net effect of both reserpine and chlorpromazine is the same – no or reduced neurotransmission in dopaminergic synapses.

Observations along these lines resulted in the 1960s in the formulation of the 'dopamine hypothesis of schizophrenia', which has provided a theoretical framework for understanding the biological mechanisms underlying this disorder. In its simplest form, the DA hypothesis states that schizophrenia is associated with a hyperdopaminergic state. The hypothesis is still valid today although a number of other hypotheses have been formulated during the years, which focus on other neurotransmitter systems or which in addition to the dopamine system includes other neurotransmitter systems (see Sections 11.2.2.2 and 11.2.2.3). It is believed that reserpine and chlorpromazine exert their effect on positive symptoms by reducing the dopamine hyperactivity in limbic areas of the brain, whereas the EPS results from the reduction of dopaminergic neurotransmission in striatal areas. The striatum is known as the motor system of the brain and is, e.g. closely related to parkinsonism. The neurochemical origin of this disease is also linked to reduced neurotransmission in dopaminergic synapses although due to degeneration of the cells.

Today, the term classical antipsychotic drugs is linked to compounds that show effect in the treatment of the positive symptoms of schizophrenia at similar doses that induce EPS. In addition, the classical antipsychotic drugs are without effect on negative and cognitive symptoms, and today it is generally agreed that these compounds may even worsen these symptoms. It has been argued that the

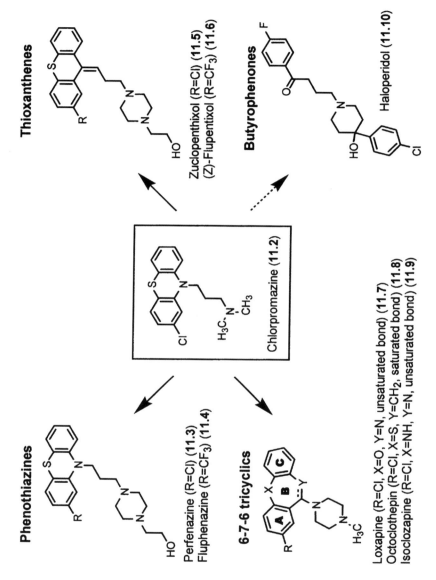

Thioxanthenes

Zuclopenthixol (R=Cl) (**11.5**)
(Z)-Flupentixol (R=CF₃) (**11.6**)

Butyrophenones

Haloperidol (**11.10**)

Chlorpromazine (**11.2**)

Phenothiazines

Perfenazine (R=Cl) (**11.3**)
Fluphenazine (R=CF₃) (**11.4**)

6-7-6 tricyclics

Loxapine (R=Cl, X=O, Y=N, unsaturated bond) (**11.7**)
Octoclothepin (R=Cl, X=S, Y=CH₂, saturated bond) (**11.8**)
Isoclozapine (R=Cl, X=NH, Y=N, unsaturated bond) (**11.9**)

Figure 11.5 Classical antipsychotic drugs.

worsening of negative and cognitive symptoms may be a consequence of EPS, and the separation of the dose–response curves for antipsychotic action and EPS is the foremost important property of the newer antipsychotic drugs (see Section 11.2.2.2).

The use of reserpine as an antipsychotic drug was, in addition to EPS, limited by its hypotensive action. Furthermore, the complicated structure of reserpine made it a rather poor target for structural manipulation in order to make an antipsychotic drug without EPS and hypotensive action, and today, reserpine is mainly used as an experimental tool.

However, the structure of chlorpromazine with its phenothiazine backbone was an excellent lead for medicinal chemists (Figure 11.5). After the discovery of chlorpromazine in the beginning of the 1950s, medicinal chemists modified the structure of chlorpromazine without changing the phenothiazine backbone, and these modifications led to a number of drugs such as perphenazine (**11.3**) and fluphenazine (**11.4**) (Figure 11.5). Medicinal chemists around the world also replaced the phenothiazine backbone with other tricyclic structures, and these modifications led to other classes of classical antipsychotic drugs such as the thioxanthenes and the 6-7-6 tricyclics. The thioxanthene backbone was in particular investigated by H. Lundbeck A/S, and this work has resulted in drugs such as zuclopenthixol (**11.5**) and (Z)-flupentixol (**11.6**) (Figure 11.5). The 6-7-6 tricyclic backbone has also led to a number of classical antipsychotic drugs such as loxapine (**11.7**), octoclothepin (**11.8**) and isoclozapine (**11.9**) (Figure 11.5). The R group, which is found in all of these compounds, is called the 'neuroleptic substituent'. For further discussions on the 'neuroleptic substituent' see Chapter 4, Section 4.9.2.

In the late 1950s, researchers at Janssen discovered an entirely new class of classical antipsychotic drugs without a tricyclic structure, namely the butyrophenones. Haloperidol (**11.10**, Figure 11.5) is the most prominent representative of this class of compounds, and today haloperidol is considered the archetypical classical antipsychotic drug for both preclinical experiments and clinical trials.

The classical antipsychotic drugs were all discovered by the use of *in vivo* (animal) models, because today's knowledge about receptor multiplicity and receptor-binding techniques as screening models were not available at that time. However, many of the *in vivo* models, which were used at that time, would today be considered to be predictive of various side effects. For example, antagonism of methyl phenidate-induced stereotypies was used as a model predictive of antipsychotic action whereas catalepsy, which is the syndrome in rats that corresponds to EPS in humans, was used to predict EPS. However, today it is known that both stereotypies and catalepsy are mediated via antagonism of striatal D_2 receptors, and both models are therefore essentially EPS models. With only these models available at that time, it was difficult to find new antipsychotic drugs without the potential to induce EPS.

Examination of the classical antipsychotic drugs by today's range of receptor-binding techniques and other more advanced biochemical methods has revealed that these drugs are postsynaptic D_2 receptor antagonists, and this accounts for both their antipsychotic action and their potential to induce EPS. However, these drugs also display affinity for a large number of other sites and receptors, which may contribute to their antipsychotic action and to some extent to their adverse effects.

11.2.2.2   Newer antipsychotic drugs

Isoclozapine (**11.9**, Figure 11.5), which has the 'neuroleptic chloro substituent' in benzene ring **A**, is a classical antipsychotic drug. On the contrary, clozapine (**11.11**, Figure 11.6), which has the chloro substituent in benzene ring **C** (Figure 11.5), has revolutionized the pharmacotherapy of schizophrenia. In the middle of the 1960s, it was shown that clozapine was effective in the treatment of the positive symptoms

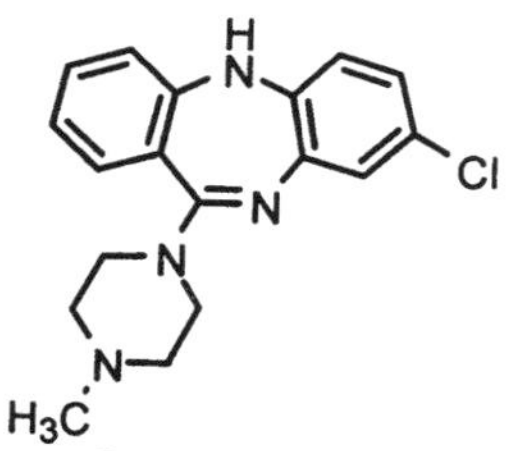

Clozapine (**11.11**)

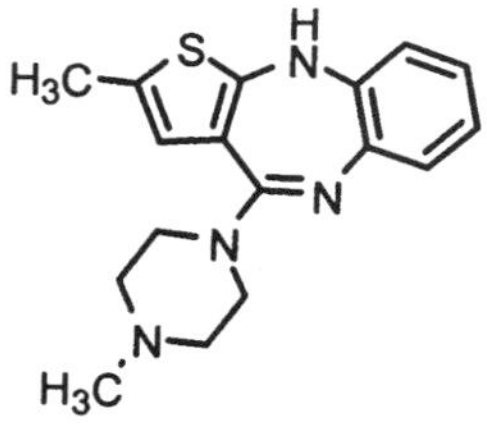

Olanzapine (**11.12**)

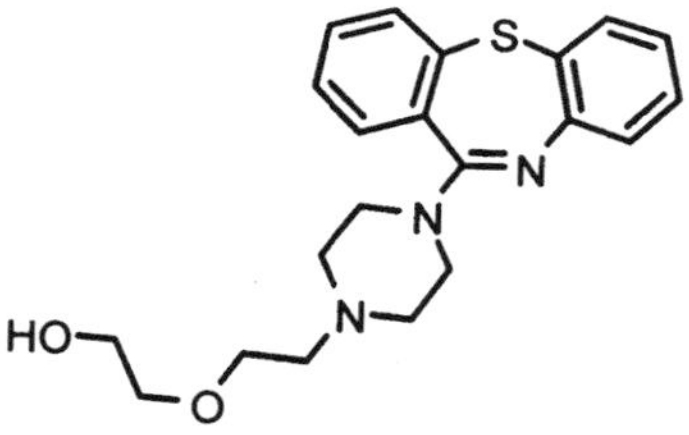

Quetiapine (**11.13**)

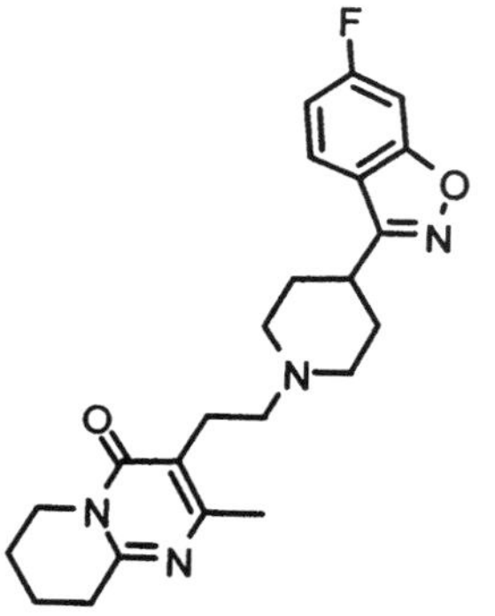

Risperidone (**11.14**)

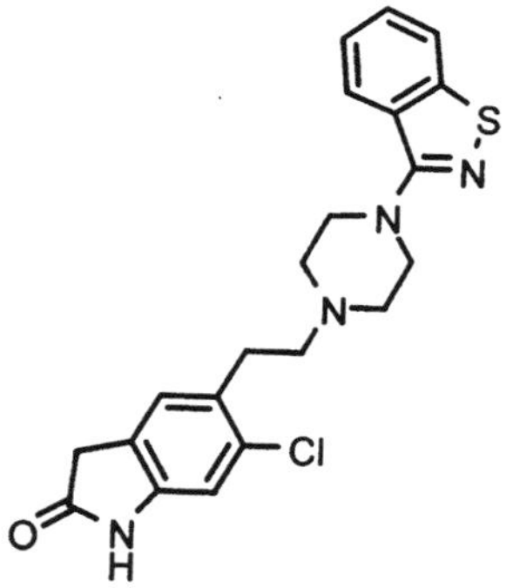

Ziprasidone (**11.15**)

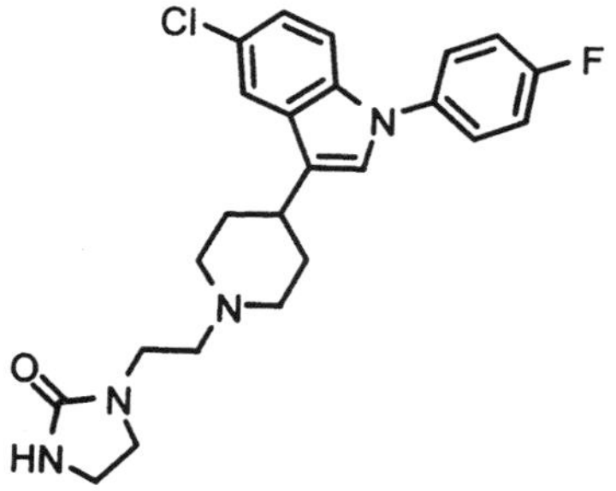

Sertindole (**11.16**)

Figure 11.6 Newer antipsychotic drugs.

of schizophrenia and free of inducing EPS in humans. However, the judgement at that time among pharmacologists and clinicians was that a compound without EPS could not be an effective antipsychotic drug. It was not until its 'second' discovery in the 1980s by clinicians in the United States of America that clozapine was judged to be the drug of the future, and this view was further substantiated in the years to come. Very importantly, it was shown that clozapine to some extent was effective in the treatment of negative and cognitive symptoms, and also in the treatment of refractory schizophrenia (individuals who do not respond adequately to classical antipsychotic drugs which is estimated to be as high as one-third of the treated). Unfortunately, clozapine can cause potentially fatal agranulocytosis in a small percentage of individuals (1–2%), which necessitates periodic monitoring of the blood picture of individuals undergoing treatment with the drug. Therefore, much effort has been directed toward the identification of new antipsychotic drugs with a clozapine-like clinical profile but without the potential to cause agranulocytosis.

This search has resulted in a number of new antipsychotic drugs such as olanzapine (**11.12**), quetiapine (**11.13**), risperidone (**11.14**), ziprasidone (**11.15**) and sertindole (**11.16**) (Figure 11.6). A closer look at the structure of these compounds reveals that olanzapine and quetiapine were obtained by structural modification of clozapine, whereas risperidone and ziprasidone were obtained from the butyrophenones. However, sertindole is quite different in chemical structure, and the discovery of sertindole are discussed in Section 11.2.2.2.1.

Binding profiles and catalepsy data for the newer antipsychotic drugs as well as for the classical antipsychotic drug haloperidol are shown in Table 11.1. All compounds have 'mixed' receptor profiles except for quetiapine, which in our hands is a relative selective α_1 ligand (others find it to be a more balanced 5-HT_2/α_1 ligand). With this exception, the general tendency is that these drugs like all classical antipsychotics display relatively high affinity for D_2 receptors (classical and newer antipsychotics are antagonists at D_2 receptors). However, when compared to

Table 11.1 Receptor profile and EPS potential of antipsychotic drugs

Compound	Receptor binding K_i(nM)							In vivo ED_{50} (μmol/kg)
								Catalepsy max., sc
	D_1	D_2	D_3	D_4	5-HT_{2A}	5-HT_{2C}	α_1	
Classical antipsychotic drug								
Haloperidol (**11.10**)	15	0.82	1.1	2.8	28	1500	7.3	0.37
Newer antipsychotic drugs								
Risperidone (**11.14**)	21	0.44	14	7.1	0.39	6.4	0.69	20
Olanzapine (**11.12**)	10	2.1	71	32	1.9	2.8	7.3	37
Quetiapine (**11.13**)	390	69	1100	2400	82	1500	4.5	>80
Ziprasidone (**11.15**)	9.5	2.8	n.t.	73	0.25	0.55	1.9	>97
Sertindole (**11.16**)	12	0.45	2.0	17	0.20	0.51	1.4	>91
Clozapine (**11.11**)	53	36	310	30	4.0	5.0	3.7	460

Sources: Data from Arnt, J. and Skarsfeldt, T. (1998) Do Novel Antipsychotics Have Similar Pharmacological Characteristics? A Review of the Evidence. *Neuropsychopharmacology*, **18**, 63–101 and Lundbeck Screening Database; n.t. not tested.

haloperidol, these newer antipsychotics display an increased affinity for 5-HT_2 ($5\text{-HT}_{2A/2C}$) receptors and α_1-adrenoceptors relative to their D_2 affinity, and this difference in affinity for D_2 and 5-HT_2 receptors has been used to rationalize their different propensity to induce EPS at therapeutic doses. Another argument, which has proven to distinguish classical and newer antipsychotic, is that all of these compounds to some extent have a preference for limbic as compared to striatal regions of the brain (see also below). In line with this evidence, the newer antipsychotics are either inactive or much weaker than haloperidol in the catalepsy model, and it has subsequently been shown that this tendency correlate quite well with their different propensity to induce EPS in humans.

Clozapine and the other new antipsychotic drugs are often called 'atypical antipsychotics' but the term 'newer antipsychotics' is preferred, as they cannot be seen as a homogeneous class. Although a number of common limitations have become apparent for these drugs, they have their own advantages and limitations. For example, all the drugs except clozapine display limited effect in the treatment of refractory schizophrenia. Several of the drugs have also a strong tendency to increase weight gain. But whereas clozapine and olanzapine are known to increase weight gain rather dramatically, ziprasidone is more or less without this effect. Some of the drugs but in particular ziprasidone and sertindole exert some prolonging effect on the QT interval in the surface electrocardiogram. A prolonged QT-interval is a reflection of abnormally prolonged repolarization of cardiac tissue and has been associated with a risk for development of ventricular arrhythmias. Thus, there is still room for improved antipsychotic drugs for the treatment of schizophrenia as none of these newer antipsychotics are perfect.

11.2.2.2.1   Sertindole discovery

In the 1970s, H. Lundbeck A/S had successfully marketed a number of what is today known as classical antipsychotic drugs, and the medicinal chemistry program at H. Lundbeck A/S was still aimed at finding new antipsychotic drugs by manipulation of the phenothiazine or thioxanthene structures. However, in 1975 the first compounds were synthesized in a project aimed at finding new NSAIDs (nonsteroidal anti-inflammatory drugs), and fortunately the compounds were also examined in a few *in vivo* models predictive of antipsychotic and antidepressant action. It was found that the two racemic *trans*-1-piperazino-3-phenylindanes **11.17** and **11.18** (Figure 11.7) were relative potent in the methyl phenidate model, which as already mentioned was seen as a model predictive of antipsychotic action but today mostly is seen as a model for EPS and *in vivo* D_2 antagonism. However, when at the same time it was found that these compounds were about a factor of ten weaker in the catalepsy model (predictive of EPS), these compounds were seen as prototypes of a new class of antipsychotic drugs with a promising side effect profile, notably with respect to EPS.

In 1980, the *trans*-racemate tefludazine (**11.19**, Figure 11.7) was selected from this series as a development candidate with potential antipsychotic action. Tefludazine displayed a similar ratio as the two lead compounds in the methyl phenidate vs. the catalepsy model but tefludazine was at least a factor of 100 more potent in these *in vivo* models. After the discovery of the multiplicity of dopamine

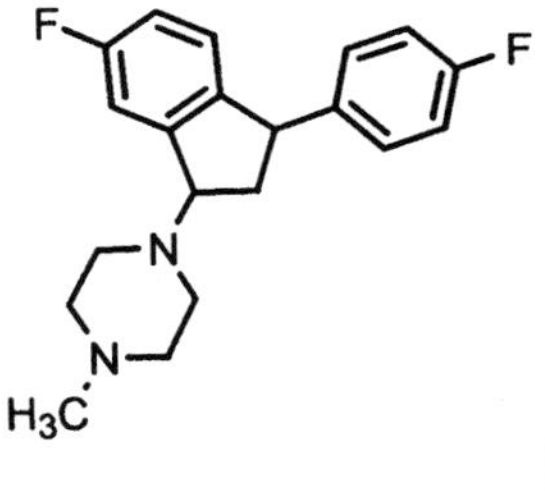

11.17 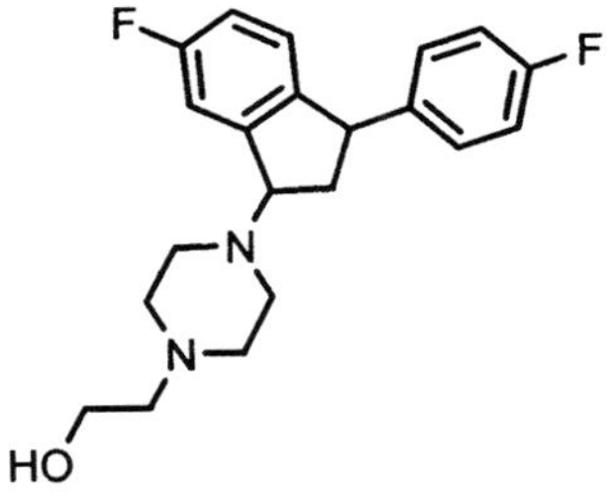   **11.18**

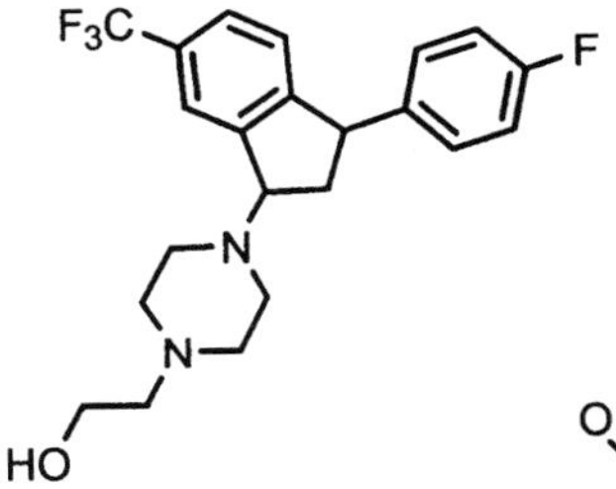

Tefludazine (**11.19**) 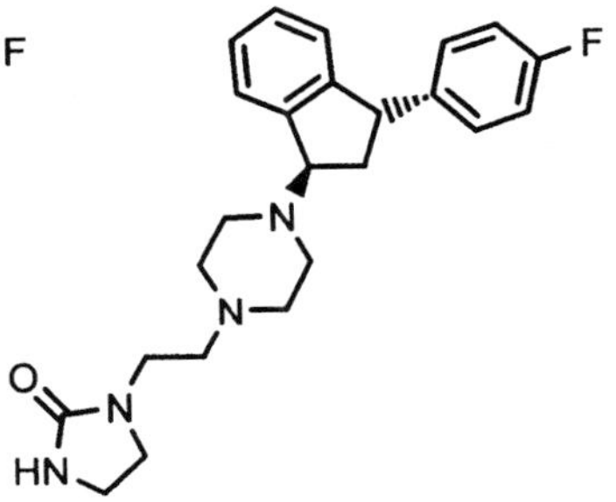   Irindalone (**11.20**)

Figure 11.7 Selected *trans*-1-piperazino-3-phenylindanes.

and serotonin receptors in 1979, many pharmaceutical companies around the world, including H. Lundbeck A/S, implemented receptor-binding assays for D_1, D_2, 5-HT$_1$, 5-HT$_2$ receptors. Thus, it was subsequently shown that the most prominent feature of tefludazine was its high affinity for D_2 and 5-HT$_2$ receptors. It was also shown that tefludazine was a potent *in vivo* D_2 antagonist (methyl phenidate model) and an extremely potent and long-acting *in vivo* 5-HT$_2$ antagonist (quipazine model).

During the 1980s, an electrophysiological *in vivo* model for evaluation of limbic vs. striatal selectivity was introduced at H. Lundbeck A/S. This was a chronic model where rats were treated with a drug for three weeks before the number of active dopamine neurones were measured in the ventral tegmental area (VTA) and in substantia nigra pars compacta (SNC) from where neurones project to limbic and striatal areas, respectively. After treatment with classical antipsychotic drugs such as chlorpromazine and haloperidol, neurones in both areas were completely inhibited (by equal doses), whereas clozapine selectively inactivated the dopamine neurones in the VTA. At H. Lundbeck A/S, it was demonstrated that this model had the potential to predict the therapeutic window between antipsychotic action and EPS of putative new antipsychotic drugs. It was subsequently shown that tefludazine displayed some selectivity in this model. The dose–response curves for inhibiting the neurones in the VTA as compared to the SNC were separated by a factor of three, which substantiated the preclinical evidence for tefludazine as a development candidate. Unfortunately, due to toxicological findings in dogs, the development of this compound was discontinued in Phase I.

It was subsequently discovered that removal of the 'neuroleptic substituent' in the indan benzene ring (i.e. the trifluoromethyl group in **11.19**), reduced the D_2 antagonism, whereas the 5-HT$_2$ antagonism was retained. Concurrent replacement of the hydroxyethyl side chain with the more bulky 1-ethyl-2-imidazolidinone side chain, resulted in irindalone (**11.20**, Figure 11.7), which was a very potent and selective 5-HT$_2$ antagonist. Irindalone was developed as a potential antihypertensive drug, but in 1989 the development was discontinued in Phase II for strategic reasons. Irindalone was, in contrast to tefludazine, developed as the pure ($1R, 3S$)-enantiomer. This configuration of the 1-piperazino-3-phenylindanes is generally associated with receptor antagonistic properties, while other stereoisomers are uptake inhibitors (see Section 11.3.3 and Figure 11.17).

A general disadvantage of the piperazinoindanes is their stereoisomerism, which complicates all stages of drug discovery and development process. Therefore, the corresponding piperazino-, tetrahydropyridino- and piperidino-indoles were designed, but their synthesis was not straightforward. These compounds could eventually be synthesized, and it was discovered that the piperidinoindole moiety bioisosterically substituted for the *trans*-piperazinoindan moiety with respect to D_2 and 5-HT$_2$ antagonism. One of the compounds synthesized in this series was sertindole (**11.16**, Figure 11.6), which incorporates structural elements from both tefludazine (neuroleptic substituent) and irindalone (imidazolidinone side chain). Despite high affinity for both D_2 and 5-HT$_2$ receptors, sertindole displayed the *in vivo* profile of a selective 5-HT$_2$ antagonist. Therefore, it was very surprising that sertindole in the VTA/SNC model displayed very selective inhibition of dopamine neurones in the VTA as compared to the SNC. It was found that the dose–response curves were separated by a factor of 100, and sertindole was subsequently pushed through development and marketed in 1996 for the treatment of schizophrenia. Sertindole was temporarily withdrawn in 1998 because of uncertainties regarding the connection between QT prolongation and the ability to induce potentially fatal cardiac arrhythmias in humans. The suspension was lifted early 2002.

11.2.2.3 *Future perspectives*

Clozapine (**11.11**) still remains the golden standard of the industry with respect to clinical effect, and much effort has been put into trying to understand the mechanisms behind the superiority of clozapine. It has been shown that clozapine displays affinity for a large number of receptor subtypes in the human brain such as a substantial number of the DA and the serotonin receptor subtypes. Thus, besides the newer antipsychotics already discussed, which are 'mixed' D_2/5-HT$_2$ antagonists displaying affinity for quite a few other receptor subtypes as well, one of the important strategies of the industry has been to develop more selective ligands. One of the goals has been to retain antipsychotic action but diminish adverse effects, and this approach has resulted in a number of development candidates (most prominent representative in parentheses) with the following profiles (Figure 11.8): Selective D_1 antagonists (SCH-23390, **11.21**), D_2/D_3

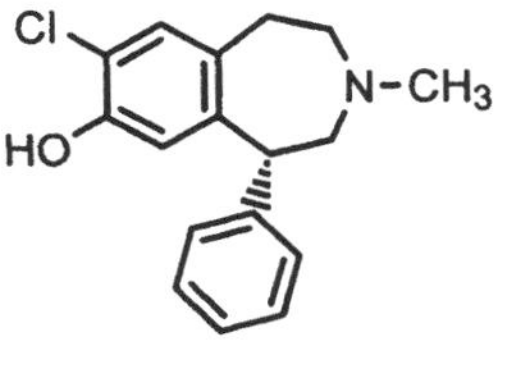

SCH-23390 (**11.21**) 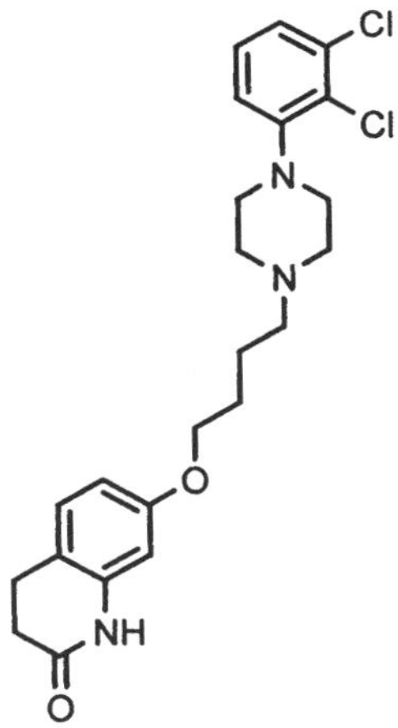   Aripiprazole (**11.22**) 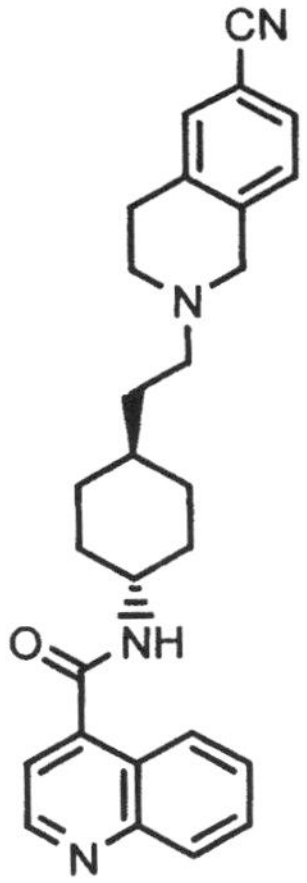   SB-277011-A (**11.23**)

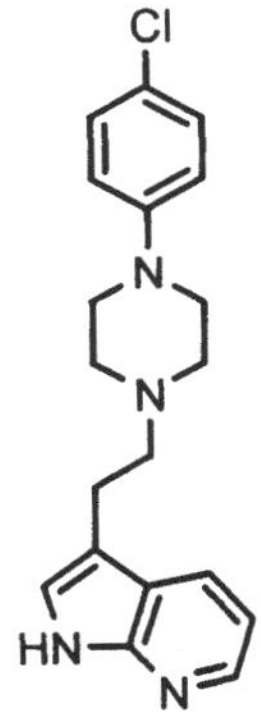

L-745,870 (**11.24**) 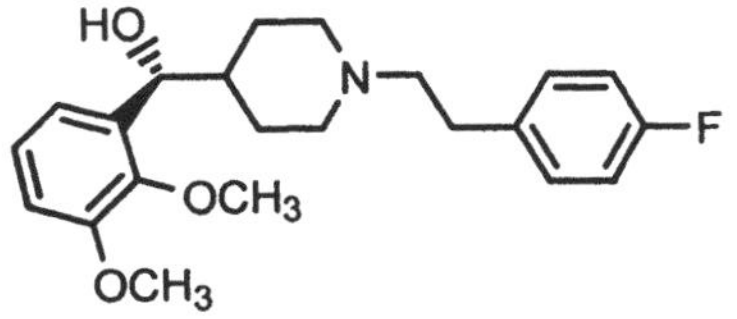   M-100,907 (**11.25**) 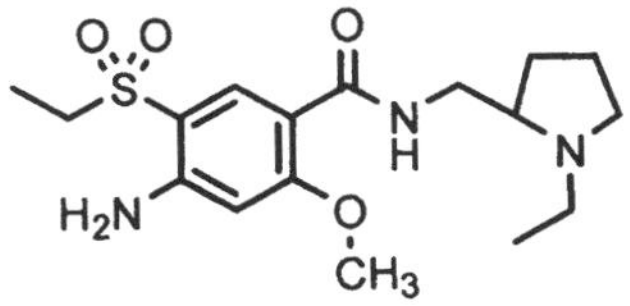   Amisulpride (**11.26**)

Figure 11.8 Selective dopamine and serotonin ligands developed as potential antipsychotics.

(partial) agonists (aripiprazole, **11.22**), selective D_3 antagonists (SB-277011-A, **11.23**), selective D_4 antagonists (L-745,870, **11.24**) and selective 5-HT$_{2A}$ antagonists (M-100,907, **11.25**). Years ago, the industry also aimed at selective D_2 antagonists but today there are no signs of such compounds in the pipeline of pharmaceutical companies. The benzamide class of antipsychotics was developed as selective D_2 antagonists, and today amisulpride (**11.26**) is probably the most interesting compound from this class as it has been shown to be effective against both positive and negative symptoms of schizophrenia. Other compounds from this class include raclopride and remoxipride, of which the latter has been marketed but withdrawn because of fatal aplastic anemia. It has later been shown that the benzamides often have affinity for D_3 and D_4 receptors, too, but that they are rather selective for DA vs. serotonin receptors.

The next generation of marketed antipsychotics may very well be a presynaptic D_2/D_3 (partial) agonist or a subtype selective DA antagonist possibly combined with some $5-HT_{2A}$ antagonism. Aripiprazole and M-100,907 are currently undergoing Phase III clinical trials for the treatment of schizophrenia, and whereas positive results have been published for aripiprazole, it has recently been shown that M-100,907 was without effect in the treatment of acute schizophrenia, although it may still be effective as an add-on in chronic treatment. Aripiprazole is actually a partial D_2/D_3 agonist, which in functional *in vivo* models manifests itself as presynaptic D_2 agonism and postsynaptic D_2 antagonism but the hypothesis behind this is not discussed here. Furthermore, a number of D_1 antagonists have undergone clinical trials during the years but there are still no drugs on the market from this class of compounds, whereas selective D_3 antagonists still undergo clinical trials, and no results have yet been published. The D_4 antagonists will receive a little more attention, as the D_4 receptor probably has been the most investigated target for schizophrenia during the 1990s.

The 'dopamine D_4 hypothesis of schizophrenia' is based on two principal observations, namely the localization of D_4 receptors in limbic areas of the brain (the site of antipsychotic action) and the 'selective' affinity of clozapine for D_4 receptors over D_2 receptors. In our hands, clozapine is not found to be selective for D_4 receptors (Table 11.1), and also other groups have questioned the selectivity. However, manipulation of D_4 receptors could be beneficial in the treatment of schizophrenia and would not be expected to cause EPS.

It has recently been shown that clozapine is a silent antagonist at D_4 receptors whereas a number of D_4 ligands, which initially were postulated to be selective D_4 antagonists, notably L-745,870 (**11.24**), indeed are partial D_4 agonists in some *in vitro* efficacy assays. Thus, L-745,870 may not have been the most appropriate compound for the clinical evaluation of D_4 antagonism in the treatment of schizophrenia. In the future, more will be learned about the efficacy (intrinsic activity) at DA and serotonin receptors of the different compounds which have undergone clinical trials during the years, and this may foster new medicinal chemistry programs in order to make new and better antipsychotic drugs. Also non-dopaminergic and/or non-serotonergic targets have attracted attention over the years, and certainly the glutamatergic system will be in focus in the future. However, these new targets still have to prove that they may give drugs with antipsychotic action in the clinic.

11.3 DOPAMINE AND SEROTONIN TRANSPORTER LIGANDS

11.3.1 Molecular biology and structure of transporters for biogenic amines

Termination of the neurotransmission in the dopaminergic and serotonergic synapses is effected by the rapid reuptake of the neurotransmitters into the presynaptic terminal (Figure 11.1). The knowledge regarding the structure and function of the transporter molecules has increased dramatically in recent years

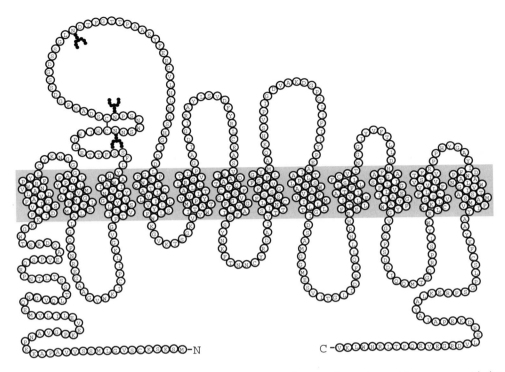

Figure 11.9 Illustration of the human DA transporter showing the amino acid sequence and the putative 12 transmembrane α-helices. N- and C-terminal ends are intracellular. By courtesy of Lene Nørregaard, University of Copenhagen.

following the cloning of the 5-HT and DA transporters (5-HTT and DAT) from several species. These transporters, as well as the norepinephrine transporter (NET), are important drug targets notably for antidepressant drugs. But they are also the target for the psychostimulant drug cocaine, and it is possible that both environmental and endogenous toxins are transported into the neurone by the transporters.

The transporter molecules for the biogenic amines are peptides consisting of 600–700 amino acids. They all contain 12 stretches of 20–24 hydrophobic residues, and it is therefore suggested that they have 12 membrane-spanning helices.

Both the N- and C-terminal ends are believed to be located intracellularly. All the loops are relatively short except the second extracellular loop, which is long. While the secondary structure of these proteins is known, their tertiary structure is still unknown due to lack of X-ray crystallographic data.

The highest homology among the cloned human transporters is found between DAT (Figure 11.9) and NET. This is not surprising considering the close structural resemblance of the transmitters DA and NE, and this has clear implications for the design of selective DA uptake inhibitors (see below).

The localization of the transporters generally parallels the localization of the DA, NE and serotonin neurones, respectively. Subtypes of the three transporters are not known. However, polymorphic variants are known of both the DAT and the 5-HTT genes.

Inhibition of reuptake of the biogenic amines is either studied by measuring the inhibition of the uptake of the tritiated amines in brain slices, in synaptosomes or in suitable cell lines expressing cloned transporters, alternatively, by displacement of tritiated selective inhibitors of the transporters.

11.3.2   Antidepressant drugs

11.3.2.1   First generation drugs

The pharmacotherapy of depression started in the late 1950s with the introduction of the two drugs iproniazid (11.27) and imipramine (11.29, Figure 11.10). Iproniazid was originally an antituberculosis drug, but it was noticed that the drug had an antidepressant effect. Structural modifications of the tricyclic antipsychotic drugs (with chlorpromazine (11.2, Figure 11.5) as a prototype) led to the 6-7-6 tricyclic compound imipramine. It was subsequently discovered that iproniazid was an unselective, irreversible inhibitor of the enzymes MAO-A and MAO-B which

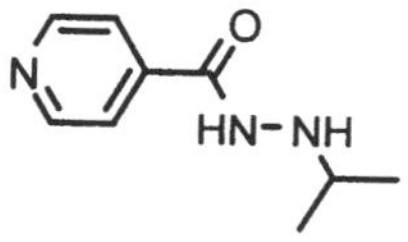

Iproniazid (11.27)

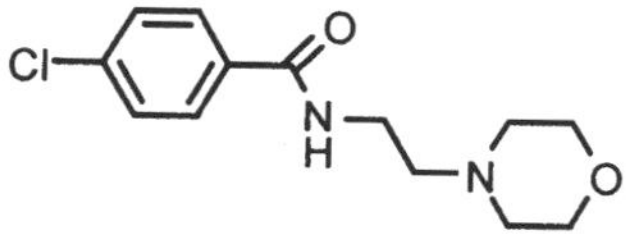

Moclobemide (11.28)

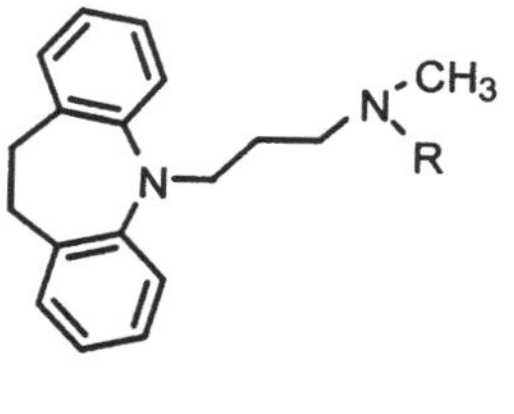

Imipramine (R=CH3) (11.29)
Desipramine (R=H) (11.30)

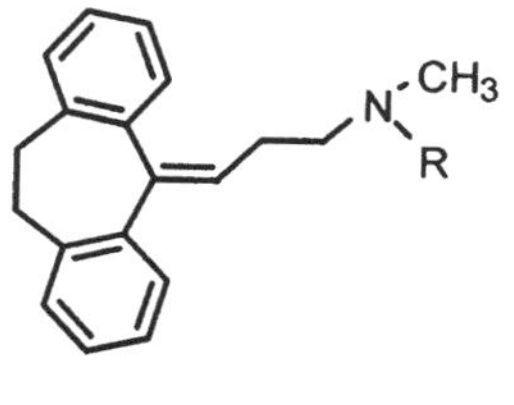

Amitriptyline (R=CH3) (11.31)
Nortriptyline (R=H) (11.32)

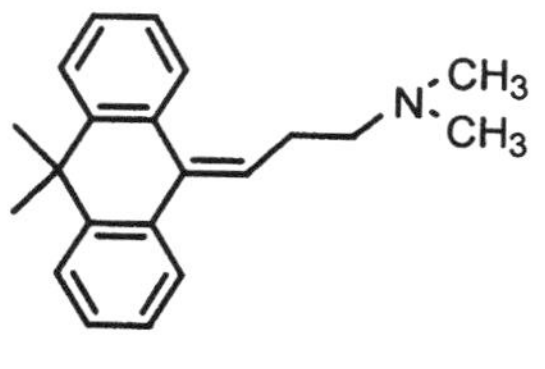

Melitracen (11.33)

Figure 11.10 Antidepressant drugs from MAO-inhibitor and tricyclic classes.

deaminate the monoamines NE, DA and 5-HT. Imipramine was found to block the transporters for NE and 5-HT. Both mechanisms led to an increase of the concentrations of NE and 5-HT in the synapse. These observations led to the so-called 'amine hypothesis of depression', saying that, for unknown reasons, there is a decreased availability of these neurotransmitters in depression.

Although the discovery of these two different classes of drugs was of major therapeutic importance, it quickly turned out that both types had serious side effects. Treatment with MAO inhibitors could induce a hypertensive crisis because of a fatal interaction with foodstuffs such as cheese, containing tyramine. It was therefore necessary to introduce dietary restrictions during treatment with MAO inhibitors. Reversible MAO-A (responsible for the breakdown of NE and 5-HT) inhibitors have been developed later (such as moclobemide (**11.28**)), but such drugs are still not totally devoid of the 'cheese-effect' because the tyramine potentiation is inherent to blockade of MAO-A in the periphery. The MAO inhibitors are therefore only used to a small extent in the antidepressant therapy of today.

A major problem with the tricyclic antidepressants such as imipramine (**11.29**), desipramine (**11.30**), amitriptyline (**11.31**), nortriptyline (**11.32**) and melitracen (**11.33**) is that, due to their fundamental tricyclic structures, in addition to their blockade of 5-HTT and/or NET, they also block a number of postsynaptic receptors notably for NE, acetylcholine and histamine (Figure 11.11). Therefore, they may induce a number of anticholinergic and cardiovascular side effects, such as dryness of the mouth, constipation, confusion, dizziness, orthostatic hypotension, tachycardia or arrhytmia, and sedation. Moreover, they are toxic in overdose.

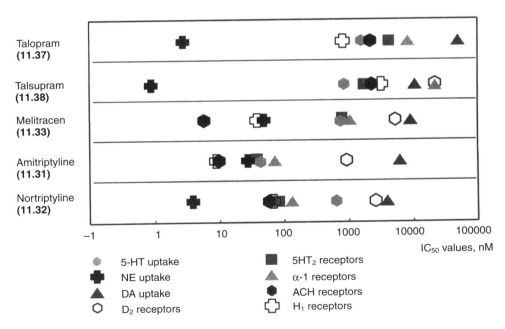

Figure 11.11 Receptor profiles of talopram and talsupram vs. tricyclics.

So, even if these drugs represented a major therapeutic break-through, it quickly became clear that there was a need for better and more safe drugs.

11.3.2.2   The selective serotonin reuptake inhibitors (SSRIs)

As can be seen from Figure 11.11, nortriptyline (**11.32**) is a relative selective NE uptake inhibitor, while the corresponding dimethyl derivative, amitriptyline (**11.31**), is a mixed 5-HT/NE uptake inhibitor with concomitant high affinity for the postsynaptic receptors mentioned above. The same is true for the corresponding pair imipramine/desipramine. Paul Kielholz coupled these observations to the clinical profiles of these drugs, and Arvid Carlsson noticed that the tertiary amine drugs, which were mixed 5-HT and NE uptake inhibitors, were 'mood elevating', while the secondary amines, being primarily NE uptake inhibitors, increased more 'drive' in the depressed patients. Because the foremost quality of an antidepressant drug should be mood elevation (elevation of drive before mood could induce a suicidal event), Carlsson advocated for the development of selective serotonin reuptake inhibitors. Consequently, a number of companies started discovery programmes aimed on designing such drugs in the early 1970s.

11.3.2.2.1   Citalopram discovery

In the middle of the 1960s, chemists at H. Lundbeck A/S were looking for more potent derivatives of the tricyclic compounds amitriptyline, nortriptyline and melitracen which the company had developed and marketed in the years before. The trifluoromethyl group had in other in-house projects proved to increase potency in thioxanthene derivatives with antipsychotic activity (see Figure 11.5), and it was therefore decided to attempt to synthesize the 2-CF$_3$ derivative (**11.35**) of melitracen (Figure 11.12). The precursor molecule **11.34** was readily synthesized, but attempts to ring-close it in a manner corresponding to the existing melitracen method, using concentrated sulfuric acid, failed. However, another product was formed which through meticulous structural elucidation proved to be the bicyclic phthalane (or dihydroisobenzofuran) derivative **11.36**. Fortunately, this compound was examined in test models for antidepressant activity, and was very surprisingly found to be a selective NET inhibitor. Some derivatives were synthesized, among them two compounds that later got the INN (International Nonproprietary Name), names talopram (**11.37**) and talsupram (**11.38**). These compounds are still among the most selective NE uptake inhibitors (SNRIs) ever synthesized (Figure 11.11 and Table 11.3).

Both talopram and talsupram were investigated for antidepressant effect in clinical trials but were stopped in Phase II for various reasons, among which were an activating profile in accordance with their potent NE uptake inhibition and the suggestion from Carlsson of rather looking for selective serotonin uptake inhibitors. A project was therefore started in early 1971 with the aim of developing an SSRI from the talopram structure.

It may look strange to use an SNRI as template structure for an SSRI. However, in the first series synthesized, two compounds (**11.40** and **11.41**, Table 11.2) without dimethylation of the phthalane ring showed a tendency for increased 5-HT uptake, and in accordance with the structure–activity relationships mentioned above

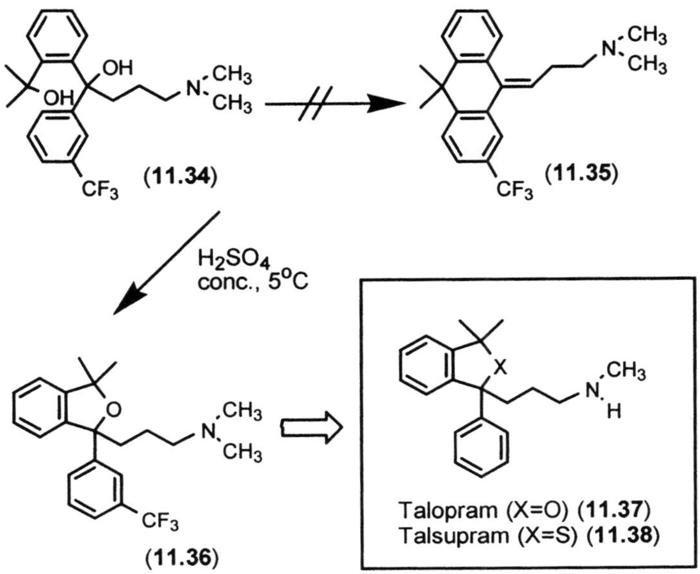

Figure 11.12 Discovery of phenylphthalane antidepressants.

Table 11.2 5-HT and NE uptake inhibition of selected talopram derivatives

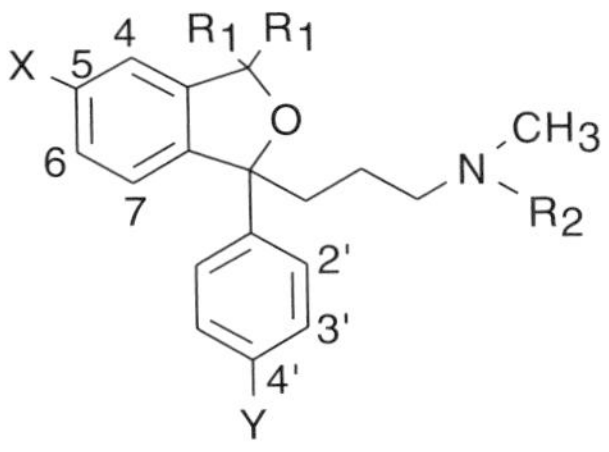

Compound	R_1	R_2	X	Y	5-HT uptake (in vitro) Rabbit blood pl. IC_{50} (nM)	NE uptake (in vivo) Mouse heart ED_{50} (μmol/kg)
Talopram (11.37)	CH_3	H	H	H	3400	2.2
(11.39)	CH_3	CH_3	H	H	53000	5
(11.40)	H	H	H	H	1300	43
(11.41)	H	CH_3	H	H	600	66
(11.42)	H	CH_3	H	Cl	110	170
(11.43)	H	CH_3	Cl	H	220	>200
(11.44)	H	CH_3	Cl	Cl	24	>80
(11.45)	H	CH_3	H	Br	310	NT
(11.46)	H	CH_3	H	CN	54	23
(11.47)	H	CH_3	CN	Cl	10	>80
Citalopram (11.48)	H	CH_3	CN	F	38	>40

Source: Data from Lundbeck Screening Database.

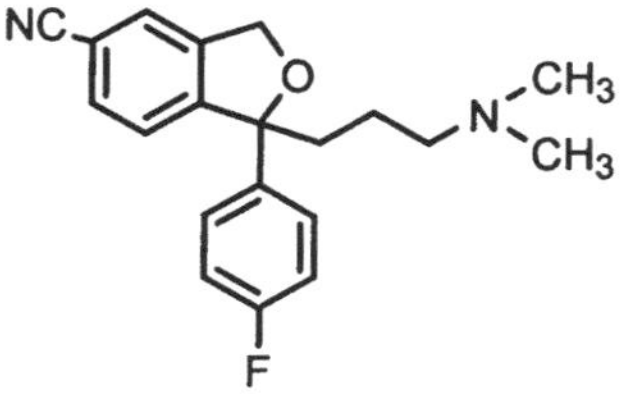

Citalopram (**11.48**)
14.1.1976

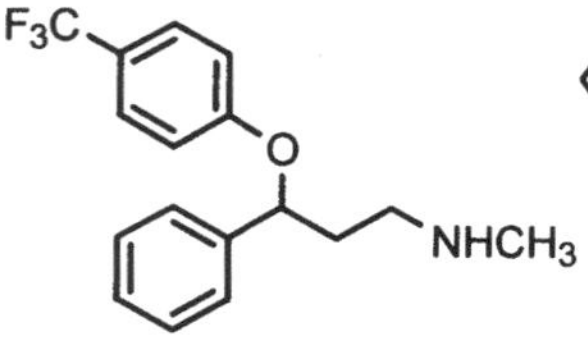

Fluoxetine (**11.49**)
10.1.1974

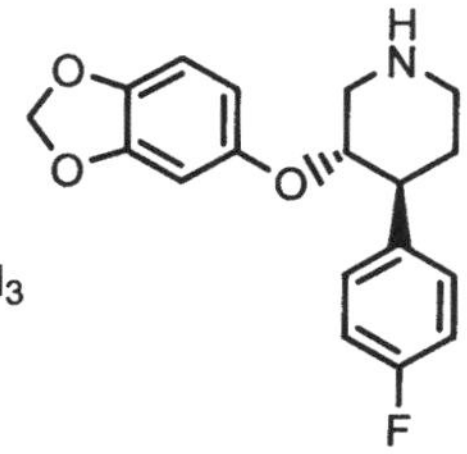

Paroxetine (**11.50**)
30.1.1973

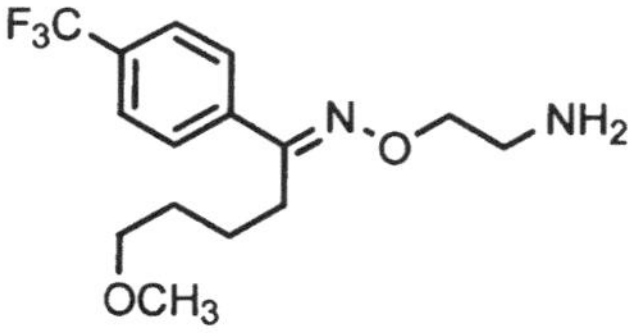

Fluvoxamine (**11.51**)
20.3.1975

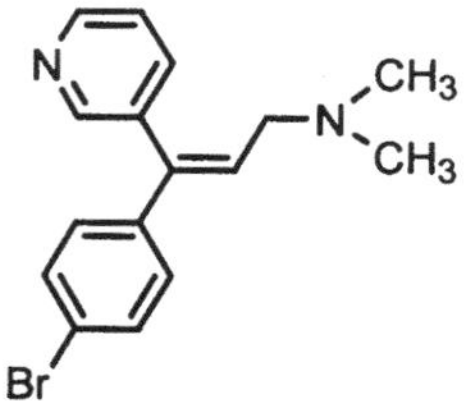

Zimelidine (**11.52**)
28.04.1971

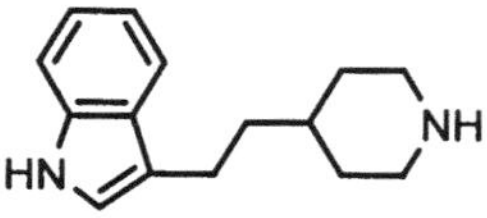

Indalpine (**11.53**)
12.12.1975

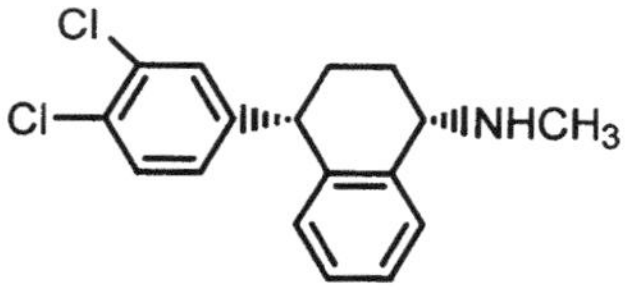

Sertraline (**11.54**)
1.11.1979

Figure 11.13 Selective serotonin reuptake inhibitors (SSRIs).

for tricyclics, the *N,N*-dimethyl derivative **11.41** was the more potent. Therefore, compound **11.41** became a template structure for further structural elucidation.

In this phase of the project, test models for measuring neuronal uptake were not available, so 5-HT uptake inhibition was measured as inhibition of tritiated 5-HT into rabbit blood platelets, while inhibition of NE uptake was measured *ex vivo* as inhibition of tritiated NE into the mouse heart (Table 11.2). Although these models were not directly comparable, they were acceptable as long as the goal was development of selective compounds.

Chlorination of the template structure **11.41**, further increased 5-HT uptake and decreased NE uptake inhibition (**11.42** and **11.43**), again in accordance with observations by Carlsson that halogenation both in zimelidine (**11.52**, Figure 11.13) (see below) derivatives and in the 2-chloro derivative of imipramine (clomipramine) increased 5-HT uptake. And indeed, the dichlorinated **11.44** derivative proved to be a selective 5-HT uptake inhibitor! So the goal of obtaining an

SSRI from an SNRI was actually achieved very fast (in 1971), when less than 50 compounds had been synthesized.

Structure–activity relationships were further explored, and it was established that high activity generally was found in 5, 4'-disubstituted compounds where both substituents were halogen or other electron-withdrawing groups. Cyano-substituted compounds were obtained by reaction of the bromo precursors (e.g. **11.45**) with CuCN. One of the cyano-substituted compounds was (**11.48**), later known as citalopram. The compound was synthesized for the first time in August 1972. It was feared that the cyano group might be metabolically labile, but this was subsequently shown not to be the case neither in animals nor in humans. Citalopram displayed the best overall preclinical profile and was consequently selected for development. The 5-cyano substituent in citalopram also proved to be surprisingly chemically stable, e.g. it was not attacked by Grignard reagents, which led to a new and patentable process for its production.

Citalopram was launched in Denmark in 1989, and it has since been registered in 73 countries worldwide. Citalopram is a racemate, having an asymmetric carbon at the 1-position. When it was synthesized in 1972, classical resolution via diastereomeric salts was the only realistic alternative for separation of the enantiomers. However, it is generally difficult to make salts of citalopram, and the few salts which were successfully prepared from chiral acids showed no resolution after recrystallizations. Finally, an intermediate was resolved in this way, and the resolved intermediate could then be transformed into the pure S- and R-enantiomers. Subsequent testing showed that all the 5-HT uptake inhibition resided in the S-enantiomer. The high stereospecificity was later rationalized in the 5-HTT pharmacophore model discussed in Section 11.3.2.2.3. The pure S-enantiomer has subsequently been developed (INN name escitalopram) and is successfully produced by Simulated Moving Bed (SMB) separation of enantiomers.

11.3.2.2.2   Other SSRIs

In Figure 11.13 are shown the seven SSRIs that have reached the market. The dates are the priority dates of the first patent applications. However, the two first compounds on the market were both withdrawn due to serious, although rare, side effects. Zimelidine (**11.52**) was found to induce an influenza-like symptom in 1–2% of the patients, which in rare cases (1/10 000) resulted in the so-called Guillain-Barré syndrome. The drug was withdrawn in 1983 after $1\frac{1}{2}$ years on the market. Indalpine (**11.53**) induced agranulocytosis in 1/20 000 patients and was withdrawn in 1984.

As it appears from Figure 11.13, all the marketed SSRIs (except sertraline) was discovered in the first half of the 1970s, meaning that the companies had no detailed information regarding the structural classes their competitors were developing. Accordingly, rather diverse (at least at first sight) structures were developed. However, they were all selective serotonin inhibitors (Table 11.3), although their selectivity ratios vary significantly, citalopram/escitalopram being the most selective compounds. The SSRIs generally have low affinity for receptors for DA, NE and 5-HT and other neurotransmitters, although exceptions exist. With regard to interaction with P450 enzymes there are important differences, e.g. paroxetine and fluoxetine having significant affinity for CYP2D6.

Table 11.3 The effect of SSRIs, talopram and talsupram on the inhibition of uptake of 5-HT, NE and DA

Compound	Uptake inhibition IC$_{50}$ (nM)			Ratio	
	5-HT	NE	DA	NE/5-HT	DA/5-HT
Citalopram (**11.48**)	3.9	6100	40000	1560	10300
Escitalopram (S)-(**11.48**)	2.1	2500	65000	1200	31000
R-citalopram (R)-(**11.48**)	275	6900	54000	25	200
Indalpine (**11.53**)	2.1	2100	1200	1000	570
Sertraline (**11.54**)	0.19	160	48	840	250
Paroxetine (**11.50**)	0.29	81	5100	280	17600
Fluvoxamine (**11.51**)	3.8	620	42000	160	11000
Zimeldine (**11.52**)	56	3100	26000	55	460
Fluoxetine (**11.49**)	6.8	370	5000	54	740
Talopram (**11.37**)	1400	2.5	44000	0.0017	0.00006[a]
Talsupram (**11.38**)	770	0.79	9300	0.0010	0.00008[a]

Note

a NE/DA; Data from Hyttel, J. (1994) Pharmacological Characterization of Selective Serotonin Reuptake Inhibitors (SSRIs). *Int. Clin. Psychopharmacology*, **9** Suppl. 1, 19–26 and Lundbeck Screening Database.

11.3.2.2.3   *The 5-HTT pharmacophore model*

Despite very different molecular structures, the SSRIs all bind to the serotonin transporter. As information about the 3D-structure of the transporter was lacking, development of a pharmacophore model was of major interest. Generally, published pharmacophoric models for 5-HT-uptake inhibitors only include one aromatic moiety and the basic nitrogen atom in the construction of the pharmacophore. The distance between these pharmacophoric elements is comparable to the distance found in serotonin itself. The second phenyl ring found in many 5-HT-uptake inhibitors shows no spatial correlation in these models.

Recently, we have developed a pharmacophore model of the 5-HT uptake site based on extensive conformational studies and superimpositions of SSRIs and other uptake inhibitors (Figure 11.14). In contrast to previous models, this model operates with two aromatic ring binding sites, and a site point 2.8 Å away from the nitrogen atom in the direction of the lone pair as fitting points. This site point mimics a hypothetical hydrogen-binding site on the 5-HT transporter. The basic nitrogen atom of the SSRIs is not always superimposable. However, when the site points are used instead, very good superimpositions are obtained. Many SSRIs have aromatic substituents (cyano, trifluoromethyl, chloro, methylendioxo etc.), and these substituents all occupy the volume marked with yellow on Figure 11.14.

The model has been validated with a number of 5-HT-uptake inhibitors in addition to the compounds in Figure 11.13. However, importantly the model explains the more than 100-fold stereoselectivity of citalopram enantiomers. It is possible to find a conformation of R-citalopram that is superimposable on the active conformation of S-citalopram, however, the energy penalty is 2.8 kcal/mol. This corresponds closely to a 100-fold affinity difference. The enantiomers of fluoxetine show no stereoselectivity and this is explained in a similar way.

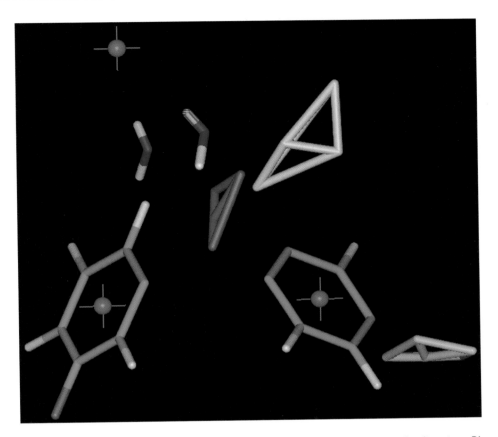

Figure 11.14 Pharmacophore model of the 5-HT uptake site. Green: Phenyl ring binding sites. Blue: Nitrogen atoms. Pink: Transporter interaction site-point. Yellow: Allowed volume for SSRI substituents. White: Forbidden volume at 5-HTT, allowed at NET. Red: Possible hydrogen bond acceptor site. For further discussions on pharmacophore models see Chapter 4.

As mentioned above, the SNRI talopram was transformed into the SSRI, citalopram, by making relatively small changes in the molecule. A similar observation was made by researchers at Eli Lilly in their fluoxetine series, because the SSRI profile of this compound could be changed into an SNRI profile by replacing the *p*-trifluoromethyl group of fluoxetine with an *O*-methyl (tomoxetine) or an *O*-methoxy (nisoxetine (**11.55**)) substituent (Figure 11.15). Later other SNRIs such as reboxetine (**11.56**) and viloxazine (**11.57**) were developed. Talopram, nisoxetine and tomoxetine can be acccomodated without problems in the SSRI model in low-energy conformations, leading to the conclusion that the change in profile must be due to unfavorable steric interactions of the SNRIs substituents at the 5-HTT site. Superimposition studies confirmed that the 3,3-dimethyl substituents of talopram, the methyl and methoxy groups of tomoxetine and nisoxetine, and the ethoxy groups of reboxetine and viloxazine all occupy the same volume (marked as the

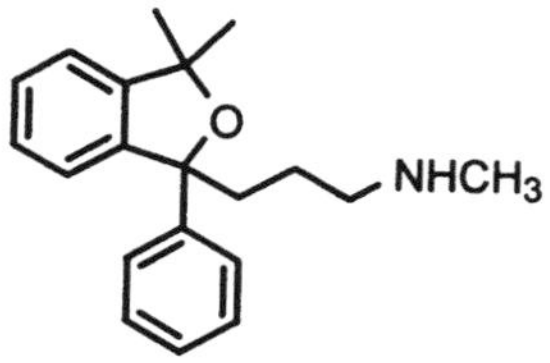

Talopram (**11.37**)
SNRI
0.0018

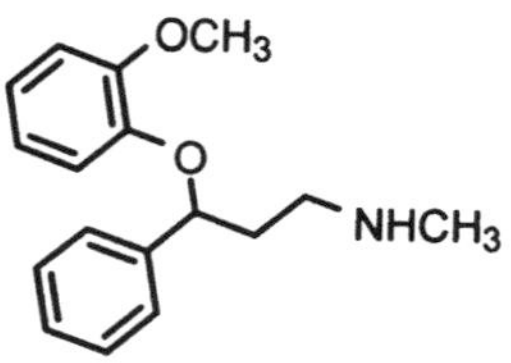

Nisoxetine (**11.55**)
SNRI
0.0054

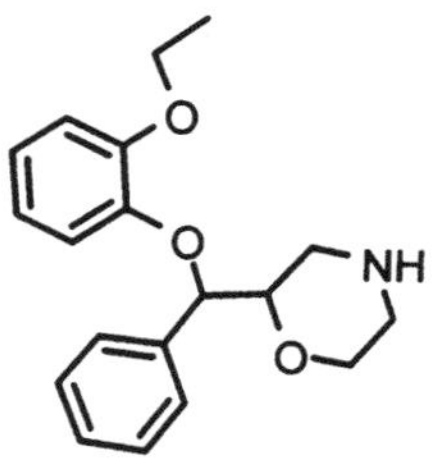

Reboxetine (**11.56**)
SNRI
0.0039

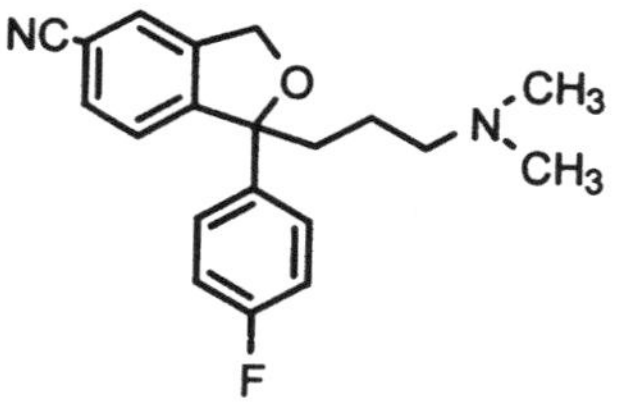

Citalopram (**11.48**)
SSRI
1560

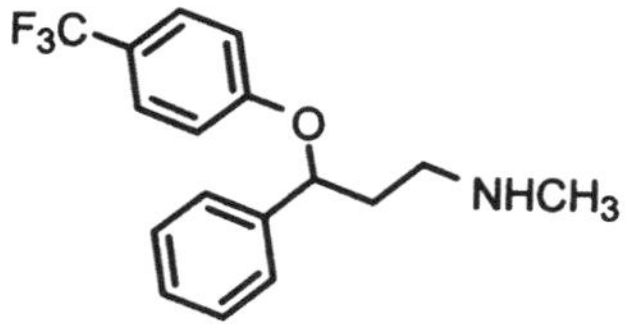

Fluoxetine (**11.49**)
SSRI
54

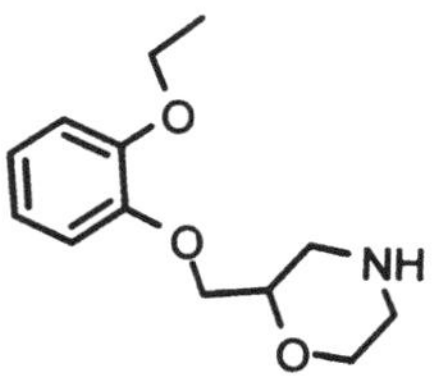

Viloxazine (**11.57**)
SNRI
0.022

Figure 11.15 Structurally related SNRIs and SSRIs. NET/5-HTT IC_{50} ratio shown.

white pyramidal structure on Figure 11.14) in space. This volume is therefore 'forbidden' at the 5-HTT site.

Certain aspects, such as the original observation of a change from mixed inhibitors in tricyclics with dimethylamino group to NE uptake inhibitors in corresponding monomethyl derivatives still remain to be explained. The amine group in SSRIs varies from primary to secondary and tertiary amines, including heterocyclic amines.

11.3.2.3 *Unmet needs and new treatment strategies*

Due to their high safety in use, the SSRIs have been extremely successful, and a number of new indications (e.g. panic disorder, obsessive compulsive disorder, social phobia) have been registered for many of the drugs in addition to major depression. However, there are still two major problems in the treatment of depression: Slow onset-of-action (4–6 weeks) in the patients and treatment resistance in up to 30% of the patients.

While the reasons for treatment resistance remain unclear, hypotheses regarding the slow onset of SSRIs have been formulated. The SSRIs exert their antidepressant effect through the stimulation of various postsynaptic receptors by the serotonin that is accumulating as a consequence of the uptake inhibition. However, extracellular 5-HT will not only increase in projection areas but also in the cell body region (the raphé region). The resulting stimulation of somatodendritic 5-HT_{1A} receptors here (see Figure 11.1, T = 5-HTT and $AR_1 = 5\text{-HT}_{1A}$ receptors) will inhibit synaptic 5-HT release, thereby counteracting the acute effect of SSRIs. These receptors desensitize over a time period congruent with the delay in antidepressant effect of SSRIs. 5-HT uptake inhibition with concomitant 5-HT_{1A} blockade may therefore result in a faster onset of action of SSRIs. Animal experiments with combinations of SSRIs and 5-HT_{1A} antagonists, and preliminary clinical trials with combinations of SSRIs and pindolol (a β-blocker with additional 5-HT_{1A} antagonistic effect) seem to confirm this hypothesis.

11.3.3   Dopamine uptake inhibitors

In relation to drug development, there has been less focus on dopamine uptake inhibitors than on 5-HT and NE uptake inhibitors. This is due to their inherent stimulatory effect that may complicate development and may lead to a risk of drug addiction and abuse. However, compounds with a different pharmacokinetic profile than cocaine (which is a mixed DA, NE and 5-HT uptake inhibitor) may on the other hand be useful for treatment of the same conditions in cocaine abusers. Moreover, in certain conditions (e.g. Parkinson's disease) and as an additional element in antidepressants DA uptake inhibition may be useful. In fact, two antidepressants, nomifensine (**11.58**) and bupropion (**11.65**) (Figure 11.16) has significant DA uptake inhibition, although nomifensine is an even more potent NE uptake inhibitor, and bupropion is a relatively weak DA/NE uptake inhibitor. Nomifensine did have a stimulant antidepressant profile, but was withdrawn in 1986 due to induction of acute haemolytic anemia. Bupropion is both used as antidepressant and for the treatment of smoking cessation. Another mixed uptake inhibitor is mazindol (**11.61**) that is used in the treatment of obesity.

11.3.3.1   *Structural considerations*

Besides nomifensine, bupropion and mazindol, a number of pharmaceutical companies developed mixed inhibitors of DA, NE and 5-HT uptake in the 1980s (Figure 11.16). However, these efforts did not lead to new drugs in any of the cases, probably due to the problems with development of stimulating drugs mentioned above.

All of these compounds are potent inhibitors of DA and NE uptake, and with the exception of nomifensine, bupropion and **11.64** they are also 5-HT-uptake inhibitors. Optimum activity is invariably found in compounds with 3',4'-dichloro-substitution. Furthermore, it was reported that the 3',4'-dichlorophenyl ring had a similar spatial orientation in the more potent enantiomer (S-configuration in all cases). Based on these facts, we proposed a 'qualitative' pharmacophore model for DA-uptake inhibitors consisting of a phenyl ring (ring A, with an optimal 3',4'-dichloro-substitution) and a nitrogen atom held by a molecular framework in a position to each other that mimics the fully extended (antiperiplanar) conformation of DA. A further common structural element is the second phenyl ring 'B', held in an optimal position to ring 'A' and the nitrogen atom by the molecular framework.

The 3-phenyl-1-indanamines is a rare example of how a single scaffold by extensive substitution and stereo SAR studies can be used for drug development

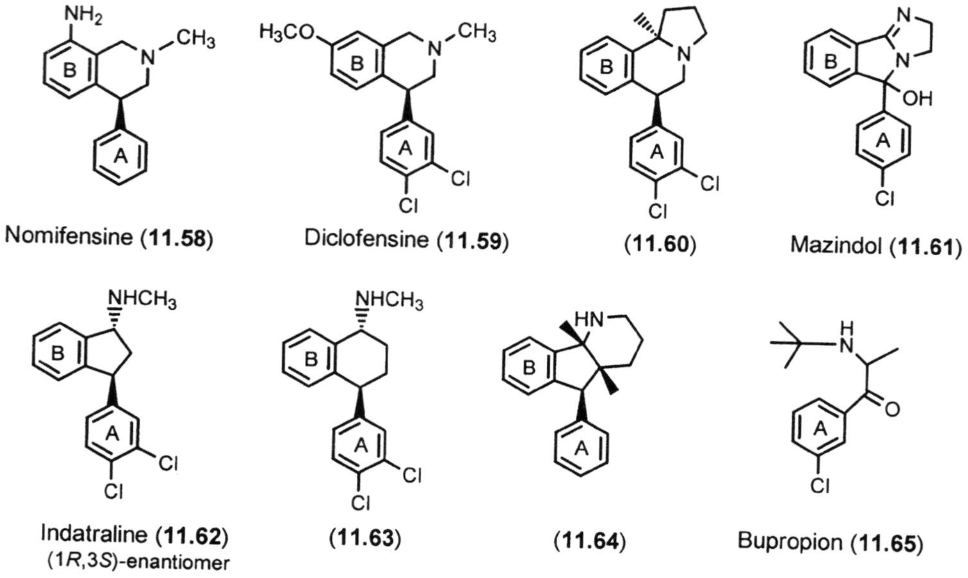

Nomifensine (**11.58**)   Diclofensine (**11.59**)   (**11.60**)   Mazindol (**11.61**)

Indatraline (**11.62**)   (**11.63**)   (**11.64**)   Bupropion (**11.65**)
(1*R*,3*S*)-enantiomer

Figure 11.16 Dopamine uptake inhibitors.

on both transporters and receptors for the same neurotransmitters. The 3-D SAR of this class of compounds is shown in Figure 11.17, and has been described in detail elsewhere (Bøgesø, further reading). Briefly, small amine derivatives (notably dimethyl or monomethyl) are inhibitors of 5-HT, NE and DA uptake with *cis*-isomers being predominantly 5-HT (and NE) uptake inhibitors, while *trans*-isomers such as indatraline (**11.62**) are potent inhibitors of all three transporters (note that a corresponding SAR is observed in the tetralines where sertraline is an SSRI, while the *trans*-isomer, **11.63**, Figure 11.16, is a mixed inhibitor of all three transporters). (1*R*, 3*S*)-3-Phenyl-1-piperazinoindans are potent antagonists of DA, 5-HT$_2$ and α_1 receptors with the highest activity confined to 6, 4′-disubstituted compounds (see also Section 11.2.2.2.1 and Chapter 4). The (1*S*, 3*R*)- and (1*R*, 3*R*)-enantiomers are potent DA and NE uptake inhibitors (maximal activity in 3,4-dichloro substituted derivatives), while the (1*S*, 3*S*)-enantiomers are inactive.

As mentioned, cocaine (**11.66**, Figure 11.18) is an equally potent inhibitor of the uptake of DA, NE and 5-HT. Although its euphorigenic effects are mainly believed to be associated with its DA potentiating effects, it is possible that the increased levels of NE and 5-HT also contribute both to the positive (euphoric) and to the negative (anxiogenic effect) of cocaine in humans. Another element, which has been suggested to be important for cocaine euphoria, is the rapid (and short-lasting) rate of DAT occupancy and the resulting DA increase that follows cocaine intake. The DA-uptake inhibitors have, therefore, been in focus in the treatment of cocaine abuse. An ideal drug would bind to the cocaine binding site without affecting the transport of DA itself. A way to search for such a compound could

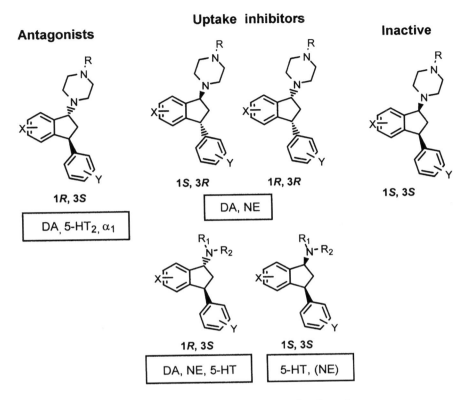

Figure 11.17 Stereo SAR of 3-phenyl-1-indanamines.

be to look for compounds with a high affinity for the binding site of a cocaine ligand and a low potency for inhibiting uptake of tritiated DA.

The cocaine scaffold has therefore, especially in recent years, also been subject to extensive SAR studies, including syntheses of an abundance of derivatives. Many groups have found that the ester bond between the phenyl ring and the tropane amine can be deleted, thus increasing stability and also potency. One of these compounds is WIN 35,428 (**11.67**) which is also used as a binding ligand for DAT in a tritiated form. Further increase in potency and stability is obtained in brasofensine (**11.68**) which has the optimal 3,4-dichloro-substitution and where the methylester is replaced by an methyl oxime ether. This compound is in development for the treatment of Parkinson's disease. Very interesting studies have shown that the basic nitrogen of the tropane ring, which was considered to be an essential pharmacophoric element, can be replaced with both oxygen (O-914, **11.69**) and carbon (O-1414, **11.70**) without consequence for DAT uptake inhibition. Whether a similar replacement is possible in other DAT inhibitors still remains to be shown.

Finally, straight chain analogs of the piperazinoindans are also potent and selective DA uptake inhibitors. One of these compounds (vanoxerine, GBR 12,909, **11.71**) has been investigated in depression, but with negative results, implicating

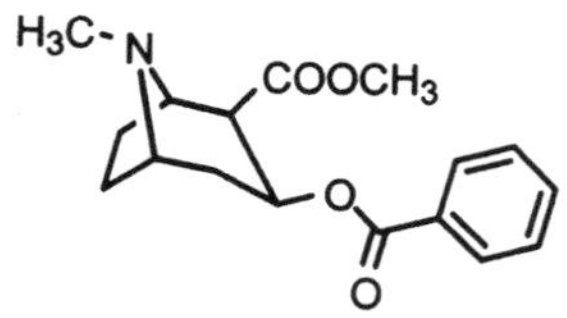

Cocaine (**11.66**)

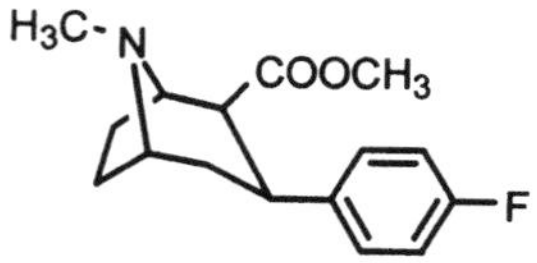

WIN 35,428 (**11.67**)

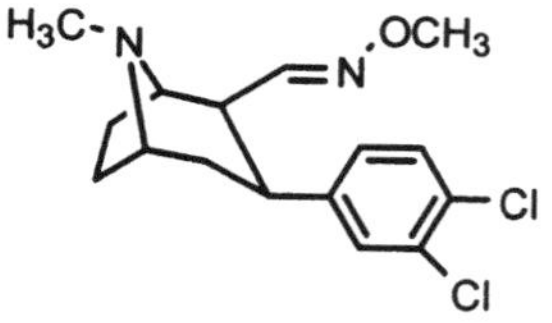

Brasofensine (**11.68**)

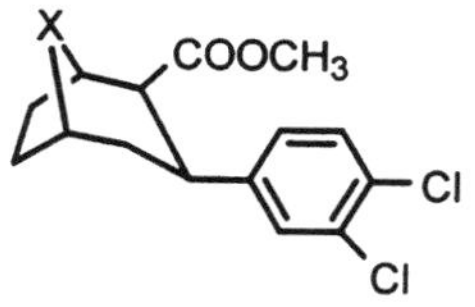

O-914 (X=O) (**11.69**)
O-1414 ($X=CH_2$) (**11.70**)

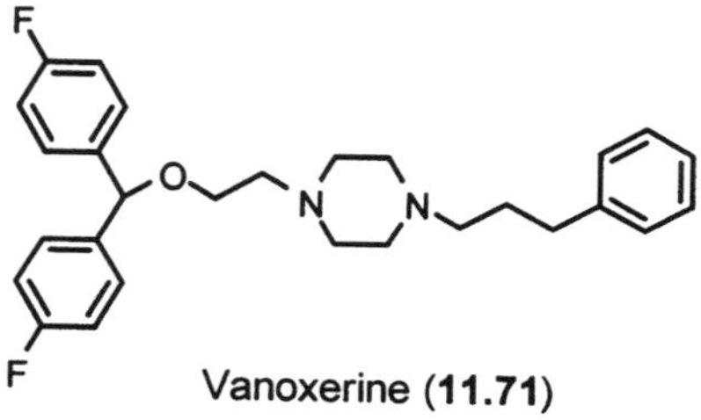

Vanoxerine (**11.71**)

Figure 11.18 Dopamine uptake inhibitors derived from cocaine and vanoxerine.

that concomitant 5-HT and/or NE uptake inhibition probably is a prerequisite for antidepressant action.

FURTHER READING

Arnt, J. and Skarsfeldt, T. (1998) Do novel antipsychotics have similar pharmacological characteristics? A review of the evidence. *Neuropsychopharmacology*, **18**, 63–101.

Barnes, N.M. and Sharp, T. (1999) A review of central 5-HT receptors and their function. *Neuropharmacology*, **38**, 1083–1152.

Bøgesø, K.P. (1998) *Drug Hunting: The Medicinal Chemistry of 1-Piperazino-3-Phenylindanes and Related Compounds*. Copenhagen, Denmark. Copy may be obtained from author.

Emilien, G., Maloteaux, J.-M., Geurts, M., Hoogenberg, K. and Cragg, S. (1999) Dopamine receptor-physiological understanding to therapeutic intervention potential. *Pharmacology & Therapeutics*, **84**, 133–156.

Hrib, N.J. (2000) The dopamine D_4 receptor: a controversial therapeutic target. *Drug of the Future*, **25**, 587–611.

Kinon, B.J. and Lieberman, J.A. (1996) Mechanisms of action of atypical antipsychotic drugs: a critical analysis. *Psychopharmacology*, **124**, 2–34.

Meador-Woodruff, J.H., Damask, S.P., Wang, J., Haroutunian, V., Davis, K.L. and Watson, S.J. (1996) Dopamine receptor mRNA expression in human striatum and neucortex. *Neuropsychopharmacology*, **15**, 17–29.

Pinder, R.M. and Wieriga, J.H. (1993) Third-generation antidepressants. *Medicinal Research Reviews*, **13**, 259–325.

Rowley, M., Bristow, L.J. and Hutson, P.H. (2001) Current and novel approaches to the drug treatment of schizophrenia. *J. Med. Chem.*, **44**, 477–501.

Snyder, S.H. (1996) *Drugs and the Brain*. New York: Scientific American Library; 18, W.H. Freeman and Company.

Chapter 12

Enzymes and enzyme inhibitors

Robert A. Copeland and Paul S. Anderson

12.1 INTRODUCTION

Every aspect of cell biology, from intermediate metabolism to protein synthesis to catabolism, requires the chemistry of bond forming and bond breaking reactions at various steps. The majority of these common chemical reactions, however, proceed at spontaneous rates that are too slow to support life. Hence, all living organisms rely on the catalytic power of enzymes to accelerate reaction rates, and thus sustain life.

While the importance of enzymatic catalysis in normal physiology cannot be overstated, aberrant catalysis can also play an important role in a variety of human diseases. A significant number of genetic disorders, for example, result in the overexpression or mutation-based gain of function for key enzymes of metabolic pathways. Other diseases, such as cancers and inflammatory diseases, involve aberrant hyperproliferation of specific cell types. The metabolic pathways that fuel cell proliferation all involve enzyme catalysis, making the enzymes of these pathways attractive targets for chemotherapeutic intervention. Enzymatic catalysis is required not only for human life, but also for life in micro-organisms (e.g. viral, bacterial and protozoan life) and larger parasites that infect human beings. Hence, essential enzyme functions within these organisms are also attractive targets for infectious disease therapies.

It is not surprising, then, that the abolition of aberrant enzyme activity, through the administration of small molecule enzyme inhibitors, is a common strategy for pharmaceutical intervention in human diseases. In fact, a recent survey demonstrates that nearly 30% of all drugs in current clinical use elicit their pharmacological effects by inhibition of specific enzyme targets. As new targets are identified through the recent advances in genomic and proteomic sciences, the proportion of drugs that act through enzyme inhibition is likely to increase further. Hence, a significant effort is put forth by the pharmaceutical community to target key enzymes for inhibition by small molecular weight, orally bioavailable drugs. Table 12.1 gives some sense of the breadth of enzyme targets that are currently being pursued for this purpose.

A critical step towards the identification and optimization of small molecule inhibitors of specific enzymes is a thorough understanding of the reaction mechanism of the target enzyme, and of the chemical and structural basis for ligand interactions with the enzyme. In this chapter, we present an introduction to some of the key features of enzymatic catalysis and enzyme–inhibitor interactions that

Table 12.1 Some examples of enzymes that are targets for current drugs and experimental therapeutic agents

Compound	Target enzyme	Clinical use
Acetazolamide	Carbonic anhydrase	Glaucoma
Acyclovir	Viral DNA polymerase	Herpes
AG7088	Rhinovirus 3C protease	Common Colds
Allopurinol	Xanthine oxidase	Gout
Argatroban	Thrombin	Heart disease
Aspirin	Cyclooxygenases	Inflammation
Amoxicillin	Penicillin binding proteins	Bacterial infections
Captopril, Enalapril	Angiotensin converting enzyme	Hypertension
Carbidopa	Dopa decarboxylase	Parkinson's disease
CELEBREX, VIOXX	Cyclooxygenase-2	Inflammation
Clavulinate	β-lactamase	Bacterial resistance
Digoxin	Sodium, potassium ATPase	Heart disease
Efavirenz, Nevirapine	HIV-1 reverse transcriptase	AIDS
Episteride, Finasteride	Steroid 5α-reductase	Benign prostate hyperplasia, Male pattern baldness
Fluorouracil	Thymidylate synthase	Cancer
Leflunomide	Dihydroorotate dehydrogenase	Inflammation
Lovastatin	HMG-CoA reductase	Cholesterol lowering
Methotrexate	Dihydrofolate reductase	Cancer, Inflammation
Nitecapone	Catechol-O-methyltransferase	Parkinson's disease
Norfloxacin	DNA gyrase	Urinary tract inflections
Omeprazole	H$^+$, K$^+$-ATPase	Peptic ulcers
PALA	Aspartate transcarbamoylase	Cancer
Sorbinol	Aldose reductase	Diabetic retinopathy
Trimethoprim	Bacterial Dihydrofolate reductase	Bacterial Infections
VIAGRA	Phosphodiesterase	Erectile Dysfunction

Source: Adapted and expanded from Copeland, R.A. (2000) *Enzymes: A Practicle Introduction to Structure, Mechanism and Data Analysis*, 2nd edition. New York: Wiley-VCH.

form the basis of enzymology-based drug discovery. We shall see that enzymes function to accelerate specific chemical reactions through common thermodynamic mechanisms. These mechanisms involve a sequential series of enzyme–ligand binding interactions that facilitate the chemical transformations of the substrate molecule to the reaction product. Small molecules that mimic these specific binding interactions prove to be high-affinity ligands for the enzyme, and thus provide a basis for inhibitor design. We shall see further that to facilitate the chemical transformations of the substrate, enzymes often undergo dynamic structural changes during catalysis. These conformational transitions, within the ligand binding site and elsewhere on the enzyme molecule, create novel structural features that can be targeted by small molecule inhibitors.

12.2 CHEMICAL MECHANISMS OF ENZYME CATALYSIS

Speed and reaction fidelity are two requirements of biochemical reactions for the sustainment of life. Hence, enzymes have evolved to facilitate these reactions by greatly accelerating the reaction rates and by acting on specific reactant molecules (referred to as substrates). In this section, we shall explore the structural and chemical mechanisms by which enzymes achieve reaction rate acceleration and substrate specificity. In all of the discussion that follows, it is important for the reader to recognize that enzymes, like all other catalysts, cannot alter the thermo-dynamics of chemical reactions; rather they can only accelerate the rates at which these reactions occur. Recall that the Gibb's free energy of a reaction is a path-independent function, depending only on the initial and final states of the reaction system. Since the reactants (substrates) and products of the uncatalyzed and enzyme–catalyzed reactions are identical, it must be true that ΔG of both reactions is the same:

$$\Delta G_{\text{uncatalyzed}} = \Delta G_{\text{enzyme-catalyzed}} \qquad (12.1)$$

Thus, as stated above, the catalytic power of enzymes results from their ability to recognize specific substrates and to accelerate the rate at which these molecules are converted to reaction products. These common features of enzyme catalysis can be understood in terms of the reaction pathway through which enzyme reactions proceed, and particularly in terms of the attainment of the transition state of the reaction.

12.2.1   Transition-state theory in enzyme catalysis

All chemical reactions proceed through a high energy, short-lived virtual state commonly referred to as the *transition state* of the reaction. This concept is well illustrated by the reaction of an alkyl halide with a hydroxide ion to form an alcohol (Figure 12.1A). As the reaction proceeds the carbon–halide bond is ruptured and a new carbon–oxygen bond is formed. One can imagine that at some moment during the reaction, the reactive carbon exists in a pseudo-pentacoordinate state in which partial bonds exist simultaneously with both the halide and the oxygen atoms; this species is the transition state. Clearly, such a state would be extremely unstable, occurring at a very high free energy and for a very short time (typical transition state half-lives are ca. 10^{-13} s). Nevertheless, the reaction must attain this transition state to proceed to products. As illustrated in the free energy diagram in Figure 12.1B, attainment of the transition state represents the most energetically costly step in the reaction pathway, and thus limits the rate at which the system proceeds from the reactant state to the product state.

All enzymes accelerate the rates of chemical reactions by a common mechanism: by lowering the energy barrier to attaining the reaction transition state. Let us consider a simple enzymatic reaction in which a single substrate molecule is converted into a single product. The enzyme catalyzed reaction proceeds through a number of intermediate states. First, the free enzyme and substrate molecules must encounter one another,

$$E + S \underset{K_{\text{S}}}{\rightleftharpoons} ES$$

A

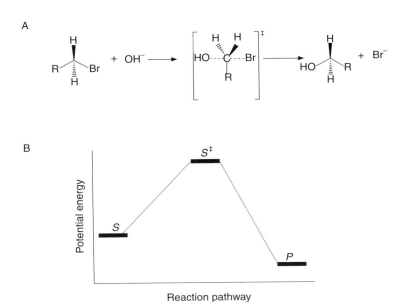

B

Figure 12.1 (A) Reaction of an alkyl halide with hydroxide ion, illustrating the reaction transition state; and (B) free energy diagram for the reaction profile of a simple chemical reaction.

through diffusion-controlled collision, and bind each other to form an initial

y complex is referred to as the *ES* or Michaelis
onditions the formation of the *ES* complex is
of the free enzyme and substrate in solution and
he binary complex, K_S.

(12.2)

boratory conditions, the equilibrium favors the *ES*
stabilization of the system. This gain in binding
the energetic cost of attaining the transition state.
elis complex, structural rearrangements of the
ng pocket where substrate binds) induce changes
ning the substrate molecule into its transition state
state is greatly stabilized within the context of the
the free form, by a combination of effects to be
overall effect, however, is to diminish the energy
tion energy, $\Delta G^{\ddagger}$). From the bound transition state,
, or through intervening intermediate states, to the
bound product state, *EP*, and finally to release of the product molecule and
recovery of the free enzyme. Each step subsequent to *ES* formation represents

a microequilibrium characterized by a forward and reverse rate constant. These individual steps are often difficult to measure experimentally. Hence, a single forward rate constant, referred to as k_{cat}, is used to collectively represent the rate of forward progress from the ES state to the final free product and free enzyme state. Thus, a minimum reaction scheme for a simple, single substrate enzymatic reaction is as follows:

$$E + S \underset{K_S}{\rightleftharpoons} ES \xrightarrow{k_{cat}} E + P$$

The term K_S represents the dissociation constant for the binary enzyme–substrate complex and can be related to the free energy of binding, ΔG_{ES} as follows:

$$\Delta G_{ES} = -RT \ln\left(\frac{1}{K_S}\right) \tag{12.3}$$

where R is the ideal gas constant and T represents temperature in degrees Kelvin. The term k_{cat} reflects the rate of transition from the bound substrate ground state to the transition state, and can be related to a free energy difference between these two states as:

$$\Delta G_{k_{cat}} = RT\left(\ln\left(\frac{k_B T}{h}\right) - \ln(k_{cat})\right) \tag{12.4}$$

where k_B is the Boltzman constant and h is Planck's constant. The overall activation energy is the energy difference between the free enzyme and substrate state and the transition state, which is given by combining equations (12.3) and (12.4):

$$\Delta G^{\ddagger} = -RT \ln\left(\frac{k_{cat}}{K_S}\right) + RT \ln\left(\frac{k_B T}{h}\right) \tag{12.5}$$

From equation (12.5) we see that the ratio k_{cat}/K_S, which has units of a second order rate constant, is a good measure of the overall rate of the enzyme–catalyzed reaction. The catalytic efficiency of an enzyme is thus measured by the ratio of this second-order rate constant to the second-order rate constant for the uncatalyzed reaction ($[k_{cat}/K_S]/[k_{uncatalyzed}]$). By this measure, some enzymes achieve a rate enhancement of some 10^{17} over the uncatalyzed reaction! We also see from equation (12.5) that the binding energy associated with formation of the ES complex is used to offset partially the energetic cost of attainment of the transition state. One strategy that enzymes use to lower the activation barrier of reaction is to partition the energy among several binding complexes, including the ES complex, the EP complex and various intermediate species (Figure 12.2). As we shall see in the next section, however, enzymes also use specific chemical strategies to stabilize the transition state itself. The overall effect, from a combination of factors, is to substantially lower the reaction activation energy, as schematically illustrated in Figure 12.2.

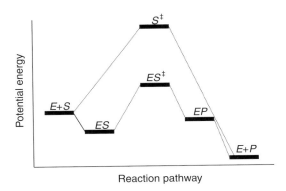

Figure 12.2 Free energy diagram for a simple enzyme–catalyzed reaction, illustrating the reduction in activation energy required to reach the transition state.

In the laboratory, it is most often the case that enzyme reactions are studied under conditions of low concentrations of enzyme and high concentrations of substrate ($[S] \gg [E]$). Under these conditions, product formation is linear with time early in the reaction, until about 10–20% of the substrate has been consumed. During this initial linear phase, the reaction rate or velocity is measured as the slope of the linear product vs. time progress curve. The reaction velocity depends on the concentration of ES complex in the system. In the early phase of the reaction, the velocity is constant (i.e. the progress curve is linear) because the system is at a steady state with respect to the concentration of ES complex, rather than at equilibrium (i.e. the rate of formation of the ES complex is the same as its rate of disappearance so that the concentration remains constant for the duration of the measurement period). Because the system is not in equilibrium under these conditions, the thermodynamic dissociation constant in the above equations must be replaced with a steady-state kinetic term, K_M (also known as the Michaelis constant). If one were to measure the steady-state velocity as a function of substrate concentration for a simple enzyme reaction under these laboratory conditions, the results would appear as illustrated in Figure 12.3A. At low substrate concentrations the velocity increases quasi-linearly with increasing substrate concentration. However, the system saturates at higher substrate concentrations, eventually reaching a maximum velocity, V_{max}, at infinite substrate concentration. This saturable, hyperbolic behavior was first described by Michaelis and Menten and later adapted for a steady-state treatment by Briggs and Haldane. The following equation describes the dependence of steady-state enzyme velocity on substrate concentration, and is known as the Michaelis–Menten equation in honor of the scientists who first defined it.

$$v = \frac{V_{max}[S]}{K_M + [S]} \qquad (12.6)$$

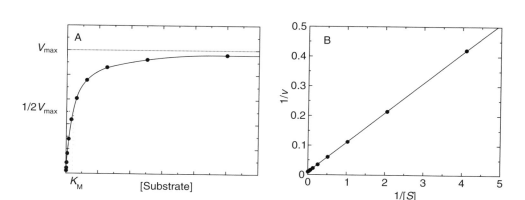

Figure 12.3 (A) Reaction velocity as a function of substrate concentration for a simple enzyme catalyzed reaction; and (B) the same data as in (A) plotted in double reciprocal form.

The term K_M, like K_S, has units of molarity as does the substrate concentration. If we were to fix the substrate concentration at the same numerical value as K_M, and rearrange equation (12.6), we would obtain:

$$v = \frac{V_{max}[S]}{2[S]} = \frac{1}{2} V_{max} \qquad (12.7)$$

Equation (12.7) provides a working definition of K_M: K_M is that substrate concentration that yields a velocity equal to half of the maximum velocity under steady-state conditions. Hence, this kinetic term relates to the concentration of substrate required to half saturate the system under steady-state conditions, even though it cannot be equated with a true equilibrium dissociation constant.

The term V_{max} in the above equations can be related to k_{cat} as follows:

$$k_{cat} = \frac{V_{max}}{[E]} \qquad (12.8)$$

Thus, enzyme reactions can be quantified in terms of the kinetic parameters k_{cat}, K_M and k_{cat}/K_M. These kinetic constants are obtained by experimentally measuring the reaction velocity as a function of substrate concentration at a fixed, known concentration of enzyme. The resulting data are fit directly to the Michaelis–Menten equation by non-linear regression analysis to obtain estimates of K_M and V_{max}. Alternatively, the data are plotted in double reciprocal form with $1/v$ plotted on the y-axis and $1/[S]$ on the x-axis, producing a linear function. The slope of the linear fit in such plots provides an estimate of the ratio K_M/V_{max} while the y-intercept provides an estimate of $1/V_{max}$ (Figure 12.3B). These double reciprocal plots (also known as Lineweaver–Burk plots) were commonly used in the days prior to the widespread use of personal computers with non-linear curve fitting capacity, and they remain popular today.

As described above, the kinetic constant K_M provides a measure of ground state substrate affinity for the enzyme, while the second order rate constant k_{cat}/K_M provides a measure of the efficiency of transition state lowering by the enzyme, hence a measure of overall catalytic efficiency.

12.2.2   Active site structure stabilizes the transition state

Almost all enzymes in biology are proteins and are thus composed of polypeptide chains of the 20 natural amino acids. The specific details of the 3D-structure into which the polypeptide chain folds defines the tertiary structure of the protein and, in the case of enzymes, also defines the structural details of the binding pocket into which the substrate molecule binds and is chemically transformed into product. This chemically reactive ligand binding pocket is referred to as the enzyme active site. The detailed structure of this active site determines the range of ligand structures that can be bound and the types of chemical transformations that can take place. Generally, the active sites of enzymes are small, mainly hydrophobic pockets that are well shielded from bulk solvent. Initial substrate binding to the active site is generally reversible and is mediated by common reversible chemical interactions with amino acid side chains and main chain atoms within the active site; these interactions include hydrogen bonding, hydrophobic interactions, van der Waals forces, etc. The topology and nature of the amino acid side chains contained within the active site also dictate the chemical reactivity of the enzyme. In many cases, the repertoire of chemical reactivities provided by the natural amino acids is augmented by incorporation of a non-protein co-factor (e.g. hemes, flavins, metal ions, pyridoxal phosphate, etc.) within the enzyme active site. These co-factors provide additional electrophilic, nucleophilic and redox chemistry components for catalysis.

One of the hallmarks of enzymes·is that they catalyze very specific chemical reaction of particular substrate molecules. This high degree of substrate specificity was recognized early in the development of enzymology, and led to the suggestion that there is a complementary structural relationship between the substrate molecule and the enzyme active site. The earliest version of this hypothesis was articulated by Emil Fisher and is referred to as the 'lock and key' model of enzyme catalysis. In this model, the enzyme active site is viewed as a static structure that has evolved to exactly complement the structure of the substrate – in terms of molecular volume, 3D shape and electrostatic distribution – in much the same way that the disposition of tumblers in a lock exactly complement the structure of the correct key. The original version of this model views the enzyme active site as complementary to the ground-state structure of the substrate, as the model was formulated prior to the development of transition state theory. Today, however, it is clear that the active site structure of enzymes, while demonstrating binding affinity for ground-state substrate, have evolved to best complement the structure of the reaction transition state. Indeed, this is well illustrated by studies of substrate specificity for a variety of enzymes. For example, Table 12.2 summarizes the results of steady-state measurements of peptide hydrolysis by the protease pepsin for a series of synthetic peptides of varying amino acid sequence. What is clear from these data is that the K_M varies very little throughout the range of peptide

Table 12.2 Substrate specificity of pepsin for synthetic peptides demonstrating selectivity based on transition state, rather than ground-state structure

Peptide[a]	K_M (mM)	k_{cat} (s^{-1})	k_{cat}/K_M (mM^{-1}s^{-1})
Cbz-G-H-F-F-OEt	0.8	2.4300	3.04000
Cbz-H-F-W-OEt	0.2	0.5100	2.55000
Cbz-H-F-F-OEt	0.2	0.3100	1.55000
Cbz-H-F-Y-OEt	0.2	0.1600	0.80000
Cbz-H-Y-F-OEt	0.7	0.0130	0.01860
Cbz-H-Y-Y-OEt	0.2	0.0094	0.04700
Cbz-H-F-L-OMe	0.6	0.0025	0.00417

Source: Data from Bender M.L., Bergeron, R.J. and Komiyama, M. (1984) *The Bioorganic Chemistry of Enzymatic Catalysis.* New York: Wiley.
Note
a   One letter code for amino acid residues is used here. Cbz is carbobenzyloxy, OEt is an ethyl ester of the carboxyl terminus of the peptide and OMe is a methyl ester of the carboxyl terminus of the peptide.

structures studied; yet there is almost a 1000-fold variation in the efficiency of catalysis among these peptidic substrates. Hence, the enzyme is discriminating among these potential substrates not on the basis of their ground state structures, but rather on the basis of best fit between the enzyme active site and the transition-state structure of the substrate.

Thus, the enzyme active site is structurally adapted to facilitate the bond distortions of the substrate that lead to strong interactions between the enzyme and the reaction transition-state. To achieve this transition-state complementarity, hence transition-state stabilization, enzymes use a number of structural and chemical strategies. A few of the more common of these strategies are described briefly in the following sections.

12.2.3   Strategies for transition-state stabilization

There is a variety of strategies used by enzymes to stabilize the transition state-structure and thus accelerate the reaction rate. Four common strategies that are discussed are approximation, covalent catalysis, acid/base catalysis and conformational distortions.

12.2.3.1   *Approximation*

The term approximation refers to the bringing together of the substrate molecules and reactive groups of the enzyme active site into the required proximity and orientation for facile catalysis. Consider a reaction involving bond formation between two substrate molecules, A and B to form a single product, A-B. For this reaction to occur in solution the two substrate molecules must encounter one another through diffusion-controlled collisions. Not only must the two substrates encounter one another, they must do so in an orientation that allows the appropriate bond distortions to occur so that the reaction transition state can be attained. In solution, both substrate molecules will be solvated, and at least some, energetically costly, desolvation will need to occur before bond formation can ensue.

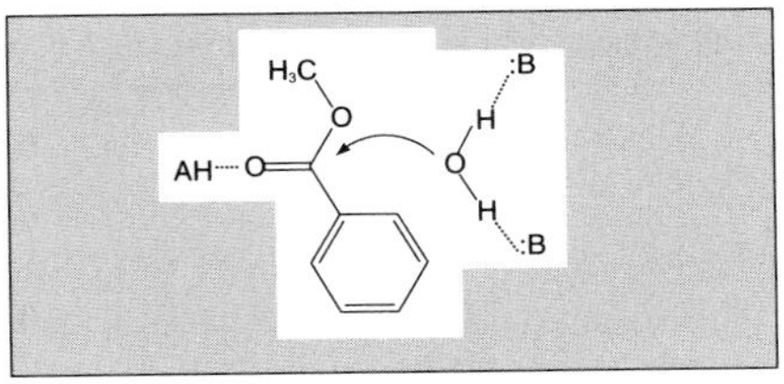

Figure 12.4 Schematic representation of an enzyme active site for a two substrate $(A + B)$ reaction illustrating the orbital alignments that take place within the active site. In this illustration, a water molecule is positioned properly for nucleophilic attack of an ester substrate. Two basic groups (:B) from the enzyme anchor the water molecule in the proper orientation for reaction.

Binding to the enzyme active site ameliorates all of these effects. The mere act of binding brings the two substrate molecules into close proximity with one another within the enzyme active site. The specific set of interactions between the enzyme and substrate molecule that stabilize the *ES* complex also ensure a specific orientation of the bound substrate that best favors the molecular orbital distortions that lead to the transition-state structure. For a bisubstrate reaction as we are considering here, binding of A and B within the enzyme active site not only brings the two molecules into proximity with one another, but also aligns them in a specific orientation to facilitate catalysis (Figure 12.4). The cost of desolvation is offset in the enzyme–catalyzed reaction by the favorable binding energy associated with *ES* complex formation. Thus, a number of energetic advantages are realized by bringing the substrate molecules together within the solvent-shielded environment of the enzyme active site. These advantages are collectively referred to as approximation effects, and provide some means of overcoming the energy barrier to transition-state formation.

12.2.3.2 *Covalent catalysis*

Another mechanism for promoting bond distortions that lead to the transition-state structure is to form a covalent bond between an atom of the substrate and a reactive group within the enzyme active site. The resulting covalent intermediate resembles the transition-state structure of the substrate, thus helping to overcome a significant portion of the activation barrier to catalysis. The covalent species formed during catalytic turnover must be transient, so that both a bond forming and bond breaking step must occur along the reaction pathway. Often one finds that the overall reaction rates of enzymes that utilize covalent catalysis are rate limited by one of these two reaction steps; i.e. either covalent intermediate formation or breakdown is the slowest step in catalysis. Hence, the covalent intermediates formed by these enzymes are relatively long-lived and can often be trapped and studied by crystallographic and other biophysical methods. Covalent catalysis in enzymes is generally mediated by nucleophilic and electrophilic catalysis, and more rarely by redox chemistry.

Nucleophilic catalysis refers to the situation where electrons are donated from an active site nucleophile to a substrate atom, resulting in bond formation. Amino acid side chains that can act as reactive nucleophiles include: serine, cysteine, aspartate, lysine, histidine and tyrosine; examples of enzymes forming covalent intermediates between substrates and each of these active site residues are known. A good example of nucleophilic catalysis comes from the reaction mechanism of the family of hydrolytic enzymes known as the serine proteases. These enzymes hydrolyze amide bonds within peptides and proteins through a mechanism involving acylation and deacylation of the active site serine. Serine is not a particularly good nucleophile by itself, but the serine proteases have evolved a specific mechanism for enhancing the nucleophilicity of this amino acid side chain. Within the active sites of all serine proteases is a triad of amino acids made up of aspartic acid, histidine and serine, as illustrated for α-chymotrypsin in Figure 12.5A. The hydroxyl group of the serine forms a hydrogen bond with one of the ring nitrogens of the histidine residue. The other ring nitrogen of this histidine forms a hydrogen bond with the

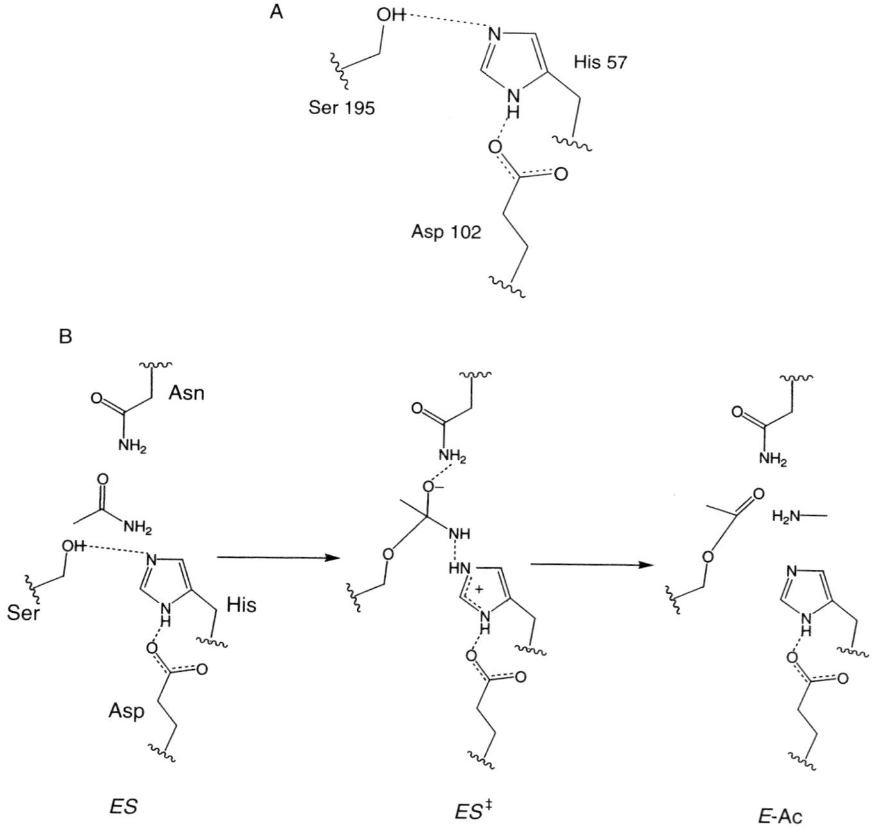

Figure 12.5 (A) The catalytic triad of Ser, His, Asp as aligned in the active site of the serine protease α-chymotrypsin; and (B) schematic representation of the reaction pathway for the serine proteases.

aspartic acid residue. In this way, the side chain oxygen atom of the serine is made much more nucleophilic and is able to attack the amide bond of the substrate peptide. This is a good example of the concept, described above, of active site topography dictating chemical reactivity for enzymes. The mechanism of acyl transfer for the serine proteases is illustrated in Figure 12.5B. The peptide substrate binds within the enzyme active site to form the initial Michaelis complex. This is followed by nucleophilic attack of the scissile peptide bond by the active site serine, resulting in formation of a tetrahedral transition state containing a charged oxygen species (an oxyanion). The oxyanionic nature of the transition state requires specific charge neutralizing interactions with other amino acid residues within the enzyme active site (another example of active site structure designed to stabilize the transition state). The transition state next decays with proton donation from the active site histidine residue to the newly formed amine of the C-terminal peptide fragment of the substrate. This C-terminal product is released from the enzyme, but the N-terminal fragment remains covalently bound to the active site serine. The departure of the C-terminal peptide product creates a cavity through which a water molecule can enter and attack the remaining acyl-serine group within the active site. This leads to deacylation of the enzyme, release of the N-terminal peptide product, and recovery of the free enzyme species.

Electrophilic catalysis involves covalent intermediate formation between cationic electrophiles in the enzyme active site and electron-rich atoms in the substrate or co-factor molecule. None of the natural amino acids are good electrophiles, so enzymatic electrophilic catalysis is generally mediated by enzyme co-factors, especially metal ions. Other co-factors that are common in electrophilic catalysis include pyridoxal phosphate and *in situ* formation of lysine-substrate Schiff bases. As with nucleophilic catalysis, the main advantage to covalent adduct formation is that the resulting intermediate resembles the structure of the reaction transition state, and thus helps to overcome the activation barrier to transition-state formation. In some cases, the enzymatic electrophile does not directly attack the substrate molecule, but rather serves to enhance the nucleophilicity of an attacking co-factor. This is a common strategy for many zinc metalloenzymes where a metal-coordinated water molecule serves as the attacking species. In the matrix metalloproteases, for example, the active site zinc ion serves two roles in catalysis of peptide bond hydrolysis. First, it serves to enhance the nucleophilicity of a co-ordinated water molecule that attacks the peptidic substrate. Second, the zinc ion helps to neutralize the oxyanion formed during bond rupture by forming a partial co-ordinate bond, as illustrated in Figure 12.6.

12.2.3.3   Acid/base chemistry

Enzyme reactions generally require some proton transfer step(s) during turnover, and these are facilitated by acidic and basic groups within the enzyme active site. Most often these acid/base functionalities are derived from the amino acid side chains of aspartic acid, glutamic acid, histidine, cysteine, tyrosine and lysine, and from the free amino and carboxyl termini of the protein. Acid/base groups can participate directly in critical proton donation or abstraction from substrate molecules, as we have already seen for the active site histidine of the serine proteases (Figure 12.5B).

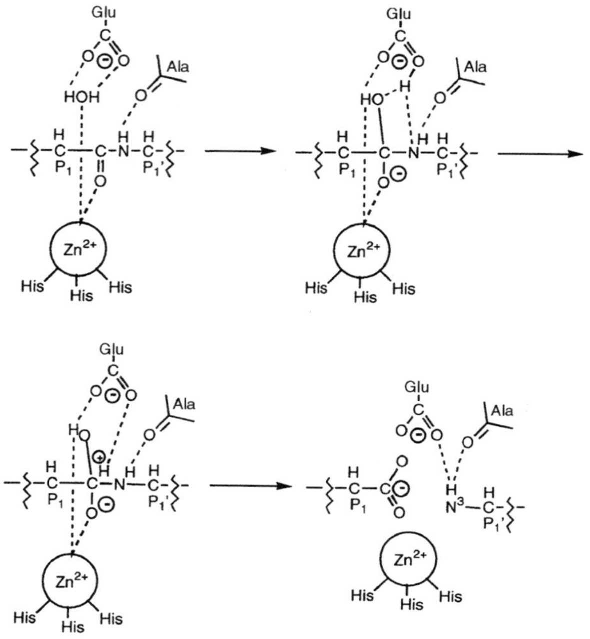

Figure 12.6 Role of the active site zinc in the reaction mechanism of the matrix metalloproteases. Redrawn and modified from Whittaker, M., Floyd, C.D., Brown, P., and Gearing, A.J.H. (1999) Chem. Rev., 99, 2735–2776. Figure kindly provided by Dr Carl P. Decicco.

These groups can also play more subtle roles in stabilizing transition-state structures by helping to polarize specific chemical bonds, as seen, for example, for the active site glutamic acid of the matrix metalloproteases (Figure 12.6).

12.2.3.4 Conformational distortions

As already discussed, the bond distortions required to bring the ground-state substrate molecule to the transition-state structure represent the highest energetic barrier to reaction progress. Once bound in the enzyme active site, the ground-state substrate molecule must be forced to adopt the transition-state structure. One way that enzymes accomplish this is by introducing strain into the system through conformational distortions of the enzyme active site. There is clear experimental evidence for enzyme conformational adjustments subsequent to substrate binding. How can these conformational changes be used to stabilize the bound transition-state? One hypothesis for this is known as the induced strain model. In this model, the most stable form of the enzyme is one in which the active site topography is most complementary to the transition-state structure of the reaction (i.e. in its lowest energy conformation, the active site is preorganized to best complement the reaction transition-state structure). Substrate binds to the enzyme active site in its ground-state configuration. To accommodate this ligand, the enzyme adjusts its conformation to maximize favorable contacts with the bound substrate. However, this altered conformation of the enzyme is thermodynamically unfavorable, occurring at a higher potential energy than the resting state of the enzyme. Hence, the system relaxes back to the lowest energy state of the enzyme and in so doing forces bond distortions of the bound substrate that lead to the transition state. Product formation and release then follow and the enzyme is returned to its un-ligated lowest energy conformation. These concepts are schematically illustrated in Figure 12.7.

The conformational distortions associated with transition-state stabilization typically involve a number of steric and electronic changes in the active site structure. Thus, changes not only in protein packing but also in hydrogen bonding patterns, van der Waals interactions, and charge distribution can participate in the induction of strain to the ground-state substrate and/or in the stabilization of the transition-state structure. The serine proteases again offer a good example of this latter concept. Acylation of the active site serine and formation of the bound transition state produces an oxyanion from an uncharged peptidic substrate. Conformational adjustments of the active sites of serine proteases involve movements of key residues to produce new hydrogen bonding interactions that help to stabilize this developing charge on the oxygen atom. Thus, hydrogen bonding patterns, hydrophobic interactions, charge distribution, etc. within the enzyme active site may appear unfavorable for substrate interactions, but are in fact situated for optimal interactions with the transition state.

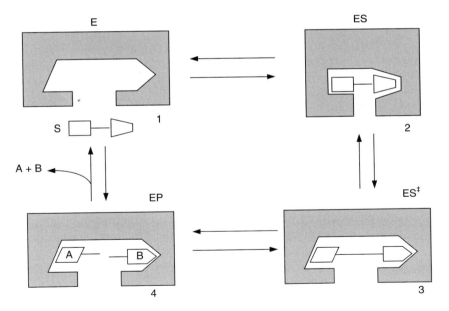

Figure 12.7 Schematic representation of the induced strain model of enzyme catalysis. Figure reprinted from Copeland, R.A. (2000) Enzymes: A Practical Introduction to Structure, Mechanism and Data Analysis, 2nd edition. New York: Wiley-VCH. With permission of the publisher.

The strategies discussed here for transition state stabilization are commonly used in concert with one another to optimize enzyme–transition state interactions. As we shall see in the following sections, some of these same strategies can be exploited in ligand design to enhance the binding affinity of small molecule inhibitors.

12.3   REVERSIBLE ENZYME INHIBITORS

The majority of enzyme inhibitors that are used as drugs in human medicine are simple reversible inhibitors of their target enzyme. The term reversible inhibitor implies that there is a reversible equilibrium established between the enzyme and inhibitor that can be characterized by a rate constant for binary enzyme–inhibitor complex formation, a rate constant for binary complex dissociation, and an equilibrium dissociation constant for the enzyme–inhibitor complex. The dissociation constant for an enzyme–inhibitor complex is often represented by the special symbol K_i to indicate that we are dealing with an inhibitory ligand. If we consider a simple, one substrate enzyme reaction we find that there are a number of potential ways that an inhibitor could interact with an enzyme species. The various equilibria associated with these potential interactions are summarized in Figure 12.8.

In Figure 12.8, the free enzyme (E) can combine with substrate to form the ES complex with a corresponding dissociation constant, K_S. The ES complex can then go on to form product through a series of chemical steps collectively described by k_{cat}. Alternatively, the free enzyme can combine with the inhibitor molecule (I) to form the binary EI complex with dissociation constant K_i. The EI complex can potentially bind substrate to form the ternary ESI complex. The dissociation constant for substrate release from the ESI complex is, however, not necessarily the same as for release from the ES complex. Hence, in our illustration the substrate dissociation constant for the ESI complex is modified by the term α. The ESI ternary complex could also be formed by inhibitor binding to the binary ES complex. In this case, the inhibitor dissociation constant would be modified by the same α term as just described. In principle, the ESI complex could go on to form product at a reduced rate relative to the uninhibited enzyme, a situation referred to as partial inhibition. However, most of the enzyme inhibitors that are used as drugs are not of this type, and for the remainder of our discussion we shall assume that saturation of the appropriate enzyme species with inhibitor leads to a complete loss of catalytic activity.

Thus K_i represents the inhibitor dissociation constant for the EI complex while αK_i represents the inhibitor dissociation constant for the ESI complex. The various equilibria illustrated in Figure 12.8 lead to three potential kinetic modes of enzyme inhibition: competitive inhibition; non-competitive inhibition; and uncompetitive inhibition (Figure 12.9). The nature and characteristics of these three inhibitor modalities are discussed next.

12.3.1   Competitive inhibition

An inhibitor that binds exclusively to the free enzyme, displaying no affinity for the binary ES complex, is referred to as a competitive inhibitor. The terminology comes

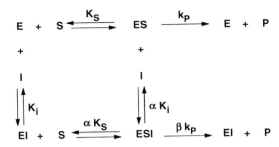

Figure 12.8 Equilibrium scheme for enzyme turnover in the presence and absence of reversible inhibitors. Figure reprinted from Copeland, R.A. (2000) *Enzymes: A Practical Introduction to Structure, Mechanism and Data Analysis*, 2nd edition. New York: Wiley-VCH. With permission of the publisher.

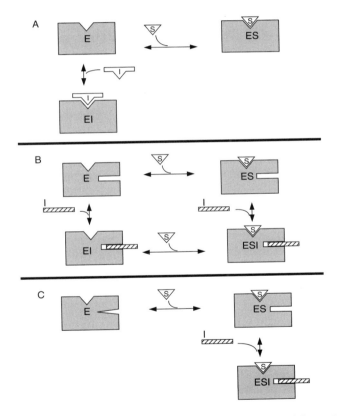

Figure 12.9 Cartoon representations of the three major modes of inhibitor interactions with enzymes: (A) competitive inhibition; (B) non-competitive inhibition; (C) uncompetitive inhibition. Figure reprinted from Copeland, R.A. (2000) *Enzymes: A Practical Introduction to Structure, Mechanism and Data Analysis*, 2nd edition. New York: Wiley-VCH. With permission of the publisher.

from the fact that the free enzyme can combine with either inhibitor or substrate molecules, but not both simultaneously. Hence, the inhibitor and substrate compete for the same form of the enzyme, and bind in a mutually exclusive fashion.

The competitive relationship between inhibitor and substrate binding in this case suggests to many researchers that the two molecules share a common binding site on the enzyme; i.e. that competitive inhibitors bind within the enzyme active site, sterically blocking substrate binding, as illustrated schematically in Figure 12.9A. Structural analysis of enzyme–inhibitor complexes often confirms this inference for competitive inhibitors. However, it is important to realize that it is also possible for a competitive inhibitor to bind to the enzyme in a binding pocket distal to the active site and to affect substrate binding through induction of a conformational change that is propagated to the active site (an allosteric mechanism). Hence, although often the case, kinetic determination of competitive inhibition alone cannot be viewed as *prima facie* evidence for a commonality of binding sites for the inhibitor and substrate molecules.

In the presence of a competitive inhibitor, the velocity equation (i.e. the Michaelis–Menten equation) is modified as follows:

$$v = \frac{V_{\max}[S]}{[S] + K_M\left(1 + \dfrac{[I]}{K_i}\right)} \tag{12.9}$$

We see from equation (12.9) that as the concentration of a competitive inhibitor is increased, the apparent value of K_M is increased by the term $(1 + [I]/K_i)$ with no concomitant effect on $V_{\max}$. Thus, if one were to generate a double reciprocal plot of velocity as a function of substrate concentration at several concentrations of a competitive inhibitor, one would expect that the slopes $(K_M/V_{\max})$ of the lines would be influenced by the presence of inhibitor but not the y-intercepts $(1/V_{\max})$. The resulting plot would therefore be characterized by a series of lines that intersect at the y-axis, as illustrated in Figure 12.10A; this is the classical signature of a competitive inhibitor. The value of the dissociation constant K_i is determined by fitting the untransformed velocity data (as in Figure 12.3A) to equation (12.9). Alternatively, K_i can also be determined from the x-intercept obtained by linear fitting of a replot of the apparent K_M value (determined by fitting the velocity data to equation (12.6)) as a function of $[I]$.

A general way to assess the effects of any inhibitor on enzyme activity is to plot the fractional activity (v/v_0) as a function of inhibitor concentration (under conditions of fixed enzyme and substrate concentrations) on a semi–log scale, in what is commonly referred to as a dose-response plot. The diminution of activity with increasing inhibitor concentration can be fit to a Langmuir isotherm as follows:

$$\frac{v}{v_0} = \frac{1}{1 + \dfrac{[I]}{IC_{50}}} \tag{12.10}$$

where v is the velocity observed at inhibitor concentration $[I]$, v_0 is the velocity observed in the absence of inhibitor, and IC_{50} is the concentration of inhibitor

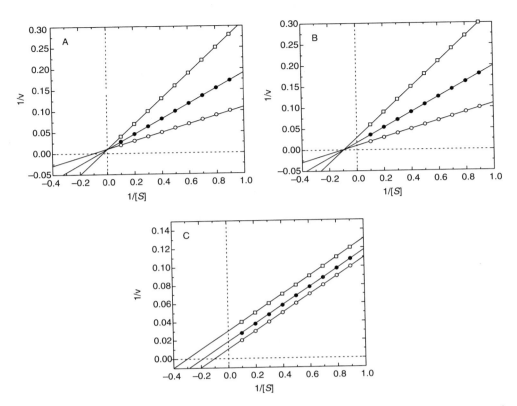

Figure 12.10 Double reciprocal plots for the three major modes of inhibitor interactions with enzymes: (A) competitive inhibition; (B) non-competitive inhibition (with $\alpha = 1$); and (C) uncompetitive inhibition.

required to reduce the observed velocity to half of that seen in the absence of inhibitor (i.e. $0.5v_0$). The IC_{50} value is related to the inhibitor K_i in different ways, depending on the inhibitor modality. For competitive inhibitors the relationship is:

$$IC_{50} = K_i\left(1 + \frac{[S]}{K_M}\right) \tag{12.11}$$

Thus, from equation (12.11) we see that the IC_{50} of a competitive inhibitor increases with increasing concentration of substrate. This is another classic signature of competitive inhibition that can be used to diagnose this form of inhibition. Figure 12.11 illustrates this concept, demonstrating the shift in IC_{50} for a competitive inhibitor studied at substrate concentrations of $0.1\,K_M$ and $10\,K_M$.

Because they bind in the enzyme active site, structural analogs of substrates, products, reaction intermediates and transition-state species generally behave as competitive inhibitors. These molecules provide good starting points for drug design, and numerous examples of active site-directed competitive inhibitors can be found among the drugs in clinical use.

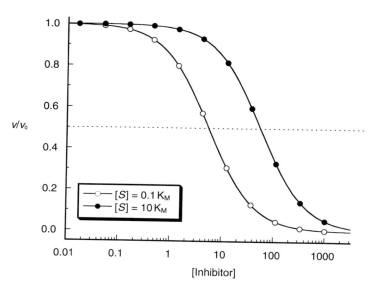

Figure 12.11 Concentration–response plots for competitive inhibition of an enzyme-catalyzed reaction studied at two fixed concentrations of substrate: $[S] = 0.1\,K_M$ (open circles) and $[S] = 10\,K_M$ (closed circles). The dashed line at $v/v_0 = 0.5$ indicates the level at which 50% inhibition of enzymatic activity is achieved.

The antiproliferative drugs methotrexate and trimethoprim are good examples of active-site directed, competitive enzyme inhibitors. Both compounds inhibit the enzyme dihydrofolate reductase (DHFR), which catalyzes a critical step in the biosynthesis of deoxythymidine. Inhibition of DHFR blocks deoxythymidine biosynthesis, which in turn blocks cellular proliferation. Hence, inhibitors of DHFR are useful as inhibitors of cellular proliferation for cancer, inflammatory diseases, and as antibiotics.

The chemical structure of the substrate of DHFR, dihydrofolate, is illustrated in Figure 12.12A. Hoping to engage similar sets of active site interactions, initial attempts to identify inhibitors of this enzyme focused on compounds that were structural analogs of this substrate. From these efforts, the antiproliferative drug methotrexate (Figure 12.12B) was discovered. Kinetic analysis revealed methotrexate to be a competitive inhibitor of DHFR with a K_i of $<1\,nM$ ($<1 \times 10^{-9}\,M$). Indeed, when the crystal structures of DHFR with dihydrofolate and methotrexate were solved, they revealed a very similar binding mode for the two ligands, with a remarkable number of common interactions within the enzyme active site (Figure 12.13). For example, hydrogen bonds are formed between the side chain carboxylate of Asp 27 and two amine groups of the ligands. A network of hydrogen bonds connects Trp 22 with heteroatom interactions within the ligand through an intervening active site water molecule. Another active site water interacts with a ligand amine and with active site residues Thr 113, Trp 30, and Tyr 111.

The crystal structure of the DHFR-methotrexate complex reveals that the majority of enzyme–inhibitor interactions are localized to the first ring (i.e. the

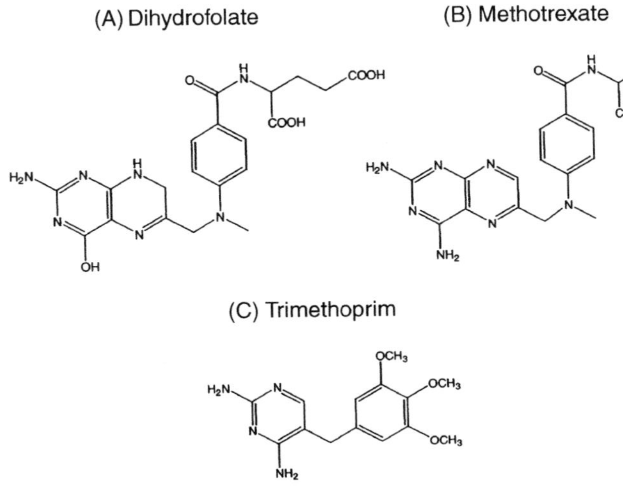

(A) Dihydrofolate   (B) Methotrexate

(C) Trimethoprim

Figure 12.12 Chemical structures of ligands of the enzyme dihydrofolate reductase: (A) the substrate dihydrofolate; (B) the inhibitor methotrexate; and (C) the inhibitor trimethoprim.

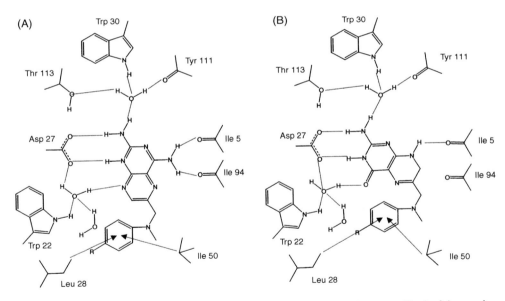

Figure 12.13 Schematic representations of the active site interactions between dihydrofolate reductase and the ligands (A) methotrexate; and (B) dihydrofolate. Figure adapted and redrawn from data in Klebe, G. (1994) J. Mol. Biol., **237**, 212–235.

2,4-diaminopyrimidine) of the pteridine ring system. This conclusion was also drawn prior to the crystal structure on the basis of structure–activity relationship (SAR) studies, in which the structure of the lead inhibitor is systematically varied to define the minimum structural unit required for inhibition (this minimal structure is referred to as the *pharmacophore*). Once the 2,4-diaminopyrimidine system was identified as the pharmacophore for DHFR inhibition, systematic substitutions off this ring system were investigated, leading to the discovery of trimethoprim (Figure 12.12C). Trimethoprim is a very potent inhibitor of the DHFR from *E. coli* ($K_i = 1.35\,$nM; $1.35 \times 10^{-9}\,$M). Testing of this compound with mammalian forms of DHFR revealed that trimethoprim was a selective inhibitor of the bacterial enzyme (e.g. the K_i for the human enzyme is $170\,000\,$nM). Today both methotrexate and trimethoprim are prescribed as antiproliferative agents. Methotrexate is used in cancer and inflammatory disease therapies, while trimethoprim is used for treatment of infectious diseases.

Another example of a clinically relevant competitive enzyme inhibitor is lovastatin, a drug that is used to control cholesterol levels in the blood. Cholesterol is a major constituent of the atherosclerotic plaques that can build up on the inner walls of arteries, leading to coronary heart disease. Controlling circulating cholesterol levels is a valuable method for preventing plaque buildup. About half of the cholesterol in the body comes from dietary intake, and the other half results from *de novo* biosynthesis in the liver. The biosynthesis of cholesterol, starting from acetyl-coenzyme A, requires 20 enzymatic steps. The rate-limiting step in the overall synthetic pathway is the conversion of 3-hydroxy-3-methylglutaryl coenzyme A (HMG-CoA) to mevalonic acid by the enzyme 3-hydroxy-3-methylglutaryl coenzyme A reductase (HMG-CoA reductase). Inhibition of HMG-CoA reductase blocks *de novo* cholesterol biosynthesis, thus leading to a significant reduction in total body cholesterol.

The reaction mechanism of HMG-CoA reductase is illustrated in Figure 12.14A. The enzyme binds HMG-CoA (**12.1**: $K_M = 10\,\mu$M; $1 \times 10^{-5}\,$M) and reduces the

Figure 12.14 (A) Reaction mechanism of the enzyme HMG-CoA reductase; (B) ring opening reaction of lovastatin leading to the active enzyme inhibitor. Note the structural similarity between the active inhibitor and intermediate **2** of the HMG-CoA reductase mechanism.

thiolester to intermediate **12.2**, using NADPH as a redox co-factor. This is followed by base-catalyzed elimination of the coenzyme A thiol, leaving behind the aldehyde, **12.3**. The aldehyde is then reduced to the alcohol by another equivalent of NADPH, leading to the product, mevalonic acid (**12.4**).

Lovastatin (also known as mevinolin) is a natural product that was isolated from a number of fungi by different laboratories. The Merck group, for example, isolated lovastatin from *Aspergillus terreus* and demonstrated that this molecule was a potent inhibitor of cholesterol biosynthesis *in vitro*. Lovastatin turns out to be a prodrug (i.e. an inactive species that is metabolically converted to an active compound) that undergoes a ring-opening reaction to form the active species illustrated in Figure 12.14B. This active form of lovastatin bears a striking resemblance to the intermediate species **12.2** of the reaction pathway of HMG-CoA reductase (Figure 12.14A). The compound was indeed found to be a very potent competitive inhibitor of HMG-CoA reductase with a K_i value of 0.64 nM (6.4×10^{-10} M).

Structural mimics of reaction pathway intermediates and transition states, such as lovastatin, are generally found to be extremely potent (i.e. tight binding) enzyme inhibitors. This is not surprising since, as discussed above, the enzyme active site is evolved to best compliment the structure of the reaction transition state. A number of enzyme inhibitors have been developed on the basis of this concept. Additional examples of clinically relevant reaction intermediate-based inhibitors are the drugs captopril and enalapril, two inhibitors of angiotensin-converting enzyme (ACE) which are used in the treatment of hypertension.

The octapeptide angiotensin II is a powerful modulator of hypertension, acting to increase blood pressure in two distinct ways: (1) the peptide is itself a vasoconstrictor; and (2) it stimulates the release of the hormone aldosterone which facilitates the excretion of potassium ions and the retention of sodium and water in cells. Both the electrolyte changes and vasoconstriction caused by angiotensin II contribute to raising blood pressure. Angiotensin II is generated *in vivo* by proteolytic cleavage of the C-terminal dipeptide His-Lys from the decapeptide precursor angiotensin I. The conversion of angiotensin I to angiotensin II is catalyzed by the zinc metalloenzyme ACE. The ACE proteolytic activity additionally contributes to hypertension by hydrolyzing, thus inactivating, the vasodilating nonapeptide, bradykinin. Hence, inhibition of ACE would reduce blood pressure by blocking the pressure raising effects of angiotensin II and by sparing the pressure lowering peptide bradykinin from proteolytic inactivation.

Angiotensin-converting enzyme, like other zinc carboxypeptidases, catalyzes peptide bond cleavage by forming a co-ordinate bond between the zinc ion and the oxygen atom of the carbonyl group of the amide bond to be hydrolyzed (an example of electrophilic catalysis). This co-ordination to zinc polarizes the carbonyl bond, making it more susceptible to nucleophilic attack by an active site water molecule, whose nucleophilicity is itself enhanced by a near-by active site base. The zinc co-ordinated intermediate then leads to a transition state in which the carbonyl carbon is tetrahedral, making bonds to both the zinc co-ordinated oxygen and the oxygen of the attacking water molecule (Figure 12.15A). Both captopril and enalapril inhibit ACE by mimicking the zinc-co-ordinated transition-state structure. The sulphydryl group of captopril (Figure 12.15B) co-ordinates to the active site zinc. Additional active site interactions are made with the methyl,

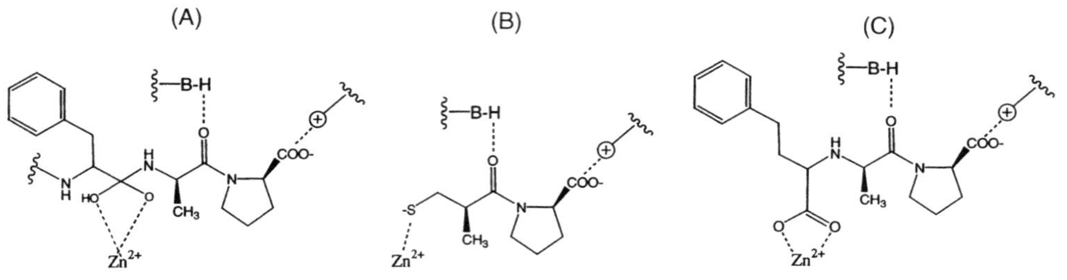

Figure 12.15 Schematic representation of the ACE active site interactions with (A) the substrate tetrahedral intermediate; (B) captopril; and (C) enalaprilate.

carbonyl and carboxylate groups as illustrated in Figure 12.15B. These combined interactions mimic the structure of the reaction intermediate leading to a tight binding enzyme–inhibitor complex with a K_i of 1.7 nM (1.7×10^{-9} M). Captopril was the first selective ACE inhibitor to be used as an antihypertension drug. However, uncomfortable side effects, such as rashes and loss of taste, were found with captopril, owing to the sulphydryl group within this molecule. This sulphydryl group was replaced by a carboxyl group, and other groups were added to make additional interactions with the enzyme active site in the molecule known as enalaprilate (Figure 12.15C). Enalaprilate is a very potent inhibitor of ACE, displaying a K_i of 0.18 nM (1.8×10^{-10} M). The free carboxylate of enalaprilate, however, limits membrane transport of the molecule into cells. To overcome this limitation, the drug is administered as the ethyl ester form, known as enalapril, which is converted to enalaprilate *in vivo* by the enzymatic action of various esterases (this is another example of a prodrug). Today both captopril and enalapril are prescribed for the treatment of hypertension.

12.3.2 Non-competitive inhibition

Non-competitive inhibition refers to the situation where the inhibitory molecule has binding affinity for both the free enzyme and the enzyme–substrate binary complex. Hence, it is possible to form a ternary *ESI* complex with a non-competitive inhibitor. Here the affinity of the inhibitor for the free enzyme is quantified in terms of the dissociation constant K_i and the affinity for the *ES* complex is quantified in terms of αK_i (see Figure 12.8). If the inhibitor has equal affinity for both *E* and *ES*, the value of α is 1. If the inhibitor binds preferentially to *E* or to *ES* then the value of α is greater than or less than 1, respectively (these latter two cases are sometimes referred to as *mixed inhibition* in some of the biochemical literature). The general velocity equation for non-competitive inhibition is given by:

$$v = \frac{V_{\max}[S]}{[S]\left(1 + \dfrac{[I]}{\alpha K_i}\right) + K_M\left(1 + \dfrac{[I]}{K_i}\right)}$$

(12.12)

The apparent values of both V_{max} and K_M are affected by the presence of a non-competitive inhibitor. Hence, double reciprocal plots at varying non-competitive inhibitor concentration results in a nest of lines that converge beyond the y-axis above, on, or below the x-axis, depending on whether α is >1, equal to 1, or <1, respectively (Figure 12.10B). Since non-competitive inhibitors can bind to the ES complex, the IC_{50} for these inhibitors is not significantly influenced by substrate concentration. Non-competitive inhibitors that display similar affinity for the free enzyme and ES complex can offer a pharmacological advantage over competitive inhibitors in situations where the cellular concentrations of substrates are high relative to K_M. In such cases, the cellular effect of the inhibitor is not diminished by a need to compete with high concentrations of substrate for the free enzyme. Also, some enzymes bind macromolecular substrates and catalyze multiple turnover events without substrate dissociation (this is referred to as precessive catalysis). An example of a precessive enzyme reaction is the sequential addition of nucleotides to a growing nucleic acid strand by DNA and RNA polymerases. For enzymes like these, the ES complex, rather than the free enzyme, may be the predominant species in cells. Hence, non-competitive inhibitors might show an advantage over competitive inhibitors in these situations.

Examples of clinically useful non-competitive enzyme inhibitors come from the class of AIDS (Acquired Immune Deficiency Syndrome) drugs known as non-nucleoside reverse transcriptase inhibitors (NNRTI's). The HIV virus has been clearly established as the causative agent in AIDS. The HIV belongs to a family of viruses referred to as *Retroviridae*, which contain an RNA-based genetic system. To replicate the virus must reverse-transcribe its RNA into DNA by the action of an enzyme known as reverse transcriptase (RT), and then incorporate this DNA into the genome of the infected host cell. Hence, the viral life cycle is critically dependent on the enzymatic activity of the RT, and inhibition of this enzyme should block replication.

The HIV RT is a member of the DNA polymerase family of enzymes. It consists of a heterodimer of two protein subunits, p51 and p66. Each of these subunits folds into a classic polymerase structure consisting of three subdomains that are arranged in a way that resembles a human hand; the three subdomains are referred to as the fingers, palm and thumb subdomains (Figure 12.16). Under *in vitro* conditions HIV RT utilizes an RNA or DNA template to direct complementary base incorporation into a small DNA primer strand. Deoxynucleotide triphosphates (dNTP; ATP, TTP, GTP, CTP) are utilized as the source of bases for DNA primer extension; which dNTP is used for a particular turnover cycle depends on the next base to be incorporated into the growing DNA strand, dictated by the next base of the complementary template. Thus, the enzyme utilizes two substrates *in vitro*: a template–primer complex (TP) and the four dNTP's. Results of kinetic studies suggest that these substrates bind to the enzyme in a preferred order, leading to the following reaction sequence:

$$E + TP \underset{K_{TP}}{\rightleftharpoons} E-TP \underset{K_{dNTP}}{\rightleftharpoons} E-TP-dNTP \xrightarrow{k_{cat}} E-TP_{(n+1)}$$

The enzyme is highly precessive so that $TP_{(n+1)}$ release does not readily occur. Thus, multiple rounds of dNTP incorporation occur on the enzyme-bound primer

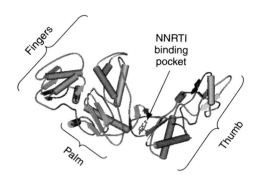

Figure 12.16 Crystal structure of HIV-1 reverse transcriptase with the inhibitor efavirenz bound to the NNRTI binding pocket. The structure of the p66 subunit only is shown. Note the three subdomains referred to as the fingers, palm and thumb subdomains. Structural data from Ren, J. Milton, J., Weaver, K.L., Short, S.A., Stuart, D.I. and Stammers, D.K. (2000) *Structure (London)*, **8**, 1089–1094.

until the full length of the template has been complimented. The rate limitation on k_{cat} can be either the chemistry of phosphodiester bond formation itself, or a rate-limiting conformational change of the enzyme that is required for dNTP incorporation. Competitive inhibitors can block binding of *TP* or of dNTP. Non-competitive inhibitors can act subsequent to substrate binding by: (1) disrupting the chemistry of phosphodiester bond formation; (2) blocking a catalytically required conformational transition of the enzyme; or (3) altering the reaction pathway so as to change the rate-limiting step in catalysis.

Early attempts to inhibit HIV RT relied on competitive inhibitors that were nucleoside analogs. Some of these compounds were clinically useful, but these inhibitors generally lack specificity for the viral polymerase over mammalian nucleoside-utilizing enzymes. Hence, side effects associated with the use of these inhibitors limited their clinical utility. Random screening of compound libraries identified several non-nucleoside-based inhibitors of RT that were non-competitive with respect to both TP and dNTP's; two of these compounds, nevirapine (Viramune) and efavirenz (Sustiva) have been studied in detail and are currently used in the treatment of AIDS patients (see Figure 12.17 for the chemical structures of these molecules).

Nevirapine is a selective inhibitor of HIV RT, showing no ability to inhibit the polymerases from mammalian cells. The K_i for nevirapine inhibition of RT has been reported to range from 19 to 400 nM, depending on assay conditions and *TP* composition. All of the kinetic studies reported in the literature agree, however, that nevirapine is a non-competitive inhibitor of RT, displaying equal affinity for the free enzyme (*E*), the enzyme–TP binary complex (*E–TP*) and the *E–TP–dNTP* ternary complex (*E–TP–dNTP*). The crystal structure of HIV RT complexed to nevirapine has been solved. The structure reveals that the inhibitor binds in a deep hydrophobic pocket close to, but not overlapping, the active site of polymerization. The binding site contains two tyrosine residues, Tyr 181 and Tyr 188, that make hydrophobic contact with the inhibitor. These hydrophobic interactions contribute

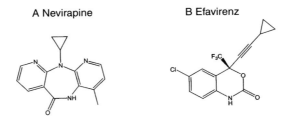

Figure 12.17 Chemical structures of the HIV-1 reverse transcriptase inhibitors (A) nevirapine; and (B) efavirenz.

to the binding energy for the inhibitor; as expected mutation of Tyr 181 to Ile disrupts this hydrophobic interaction resulting in a large reduction in inhibitor affinity. The binding pocket for nevirapine exists on the p66 subunit of the enzyme only. This observation is consistent with equilibrium binding data that suggest a single inhibitor binding site per heterodimer. The binding pocket is situated near the interface between the 'palm' and 'thumb' subdomains of the p66 subunit and may therefore play a role in conformational changes that affect the disposition of these subdomains during catalysis. This observation led to the speculation that the NNRTI's inhibit RT by blocking a catalytically required conformational transition of the enzyme. Subsequent presteady-state kinetic studies suggest that it is more likely that these inhibitors slow down, but do not block entirely the chemical steps in primer extension. The main effect of the NNRTI's may be to alter the nature of the rate-limiting step in catalysis subsequent to substrate binding.

Efavirenz is also an NNRTI that acts as a non-competitive inhibitor of HIV RT. Kinetic and equilibrium binding studies suggest that efavirenz binds to the same pocket on the enzyme as nevirapine. This suggestion has recently been verified by crystallographic determination of the structure of the RT-efavirenz complex. The structure reveals interactions between efavirenz and Tyr 181 and Tyr 188, as with nevirapine. Additional hydrophobic interactions with efavirenz are made with Trp 229, Phe 227, Leu 100 and Val 106. The inhibitor also makes ring-edge contacts with Tyr 318 and Val 179 and hydrogen bonding interactions with the mainchain carbonyl of Lys 101. All of these interactions contribute to the binding energy for this inhibitor. Unlike nevirapine, efavirenz shows a preference for binding to the ternary E–TP–dNTP complex over the free enzyme. The K_d values for efavirenz complexes of the various enzyme forms are as follows: $K_E = 170 \pm 5$ nM; $K_{E–TP} = 30 \pm 2$ nM; $K_{E–TP–dNTP} = 4 \pm 0.5$ nM. Therefore, efavirenz is best described as a mixed-type non-competitive inhibitor.

Today both nevirapine and efavirenz are used in combination with other AIDS drugs to control viral levels in AIDS patients. Both inhibitors are well tolerated by patients and are very effective in blocking viral replication. The rapidity of viral replication and the infidelity of the HIV replication system result in a high rate of mutation in all HIV proteins including the RT. Mutations that confer resistance to inhibition are a significant problem for all AIDS drugs, including the NNRTI's. In this regard efavirenz appears to have some advantage over other NNRTI's. In clinical trials and in patient treatment with NNRTI's the most common mutation found to develop in RT is a change of Lys 103 to Asn. This residue is within the NNRTI binding pocket and makes van der Waals contacts with some inhibitors. The K103N mutation results in a 40-fold reduction in nevirapine affinity for the enzyme. In contrast, the affinity of efavirenz for the K103N mutant enzyme is reduced by only six-fold. The crystal structure of the RT-efavirenz complex may provide a structural rationale for the reduced resistance against this inhibitor. The topography of the inhibitor binding pocket is altered by the mutation. The binding configuration of efavirenz appears to be more adaptable to these structural changes than that of nevirapine and other NNRTI's. Thus tight binding interactions are maintained by efavirenz with this pocket in the mutant form of RT where similar interactions are lost by the other NNRTI's. Nevertheless, continued research will be required to provide additional drugs, hopefully ones that are more refractory to target mutations, for the treatment of this devastating disease.

12.3.3 Uncompetitive inhibition

An uncompetitive inhibitor is one that binds exclusively to the *ES* complex, displaying no affinity for the free enzyme. The inhibitor binding pocket is only revealed in the presence of enzyme-bound substrate. This can occur due to conformational changes in enzyme structure that accompany substrate binding, opening up a previously occluded binding pocket (Figure 12.9C). Alternatively, the inhibitor binding pocket could be composed of structural elements from both the enzyme and the substrate molecules, so that the binding pocket, *per se*, does not exist except in the context of the *ES* complex.

The velocity equation for uncompetitive inhibition is as follows:

$$v = \frac{V_{max}[S]}{[S]\left(1 + \frac{[I]}{\alpha K_i}\right) + K_M} \tag{12.13}$$

Algebraic rearrangement of equation (12.13) demonstrates that both V_{max} and K_M are influenced by the same factor $(1 + [I]/\alpha K_i)$. In double reciprocal plots, the y-intercept $(1/V_{max}(1 + [I]/\alpha K_i))$ varies with uncompetitive inhibitor concentration, but the slope $(K_M(1 + [I]/\alpha K_i)/V_{max}(1 + [I]/\alpha K_i))$ is unaffected, since the inhibitor concentration term cancels. Thus, the classic signature of an uncompetitive inhibitor is a double reciprocal plot composed of parallel lines (Figure 12.10C).

Because uncompetitive inhibitors bind exclusively to the *ES* complex, the IC_{50} of these inhibitors decreases with increasing substrate concentration as follows:

$$IC_{50} = \alpha K_i \left(1 + \frac{K_M}{[S]}\right) \tag{12.14}$$

Thus, in the exact opposite direction as for competitive inhibitors, the IC_{50} of uncompetitive inhibitors shifts to lower values with increasing substrate concentrations.

As with non-competitive inhibitors, uncompetitive inhibitors can have pharma-cological advantages for target enzymes that catalyzed precessive reactions or for which cellular substrate concentrations are high relative to K_M.

The steroid 5α-reductase inhibitor epristeride provides a clinically interesting example of uncompetitive enzyme inhibition. The androgen dihydrotestosterone (DHT) mediates a number of male sexual characteristics. The DHT is produced by the reduction of testosterone by the enzyme steroid 5α-reductase. A genetic deficiency in this enzyme was identified in association with a population of pseudo-hermaphrodites in the Dominican Republic. These individuals do not display normal male genitalia until the onset of puberty; hence they are raised as females until then. Other phenotypical characteristics of these individuals include no male pattern baldness, mild or no acne, and underdeveloped prostates. These observa-tions led to the suggestion that inhibitors of steroid 5α-reductase might be clinically useful in the treatment of benign prostate hyperplasia, a non-cancerous enlargement of the prostate that affects a significant proportion of men over 50 years old.

The reaction mechanism of steroid 5α-reductase is illustrated in Figure 12.18. The enzyme binds the redox co-factor NADPH first and then binds testosterone to form a ternary enzyme-NADPH-testosterone complex. Hydride transfer to the β-carbon of the testosterone double bond then occurs; the enolate intermediate thus formed is stabilized by an acid group within the enzyme active site. The α-carbon of the enolate is then protonated by an active site base, leading to

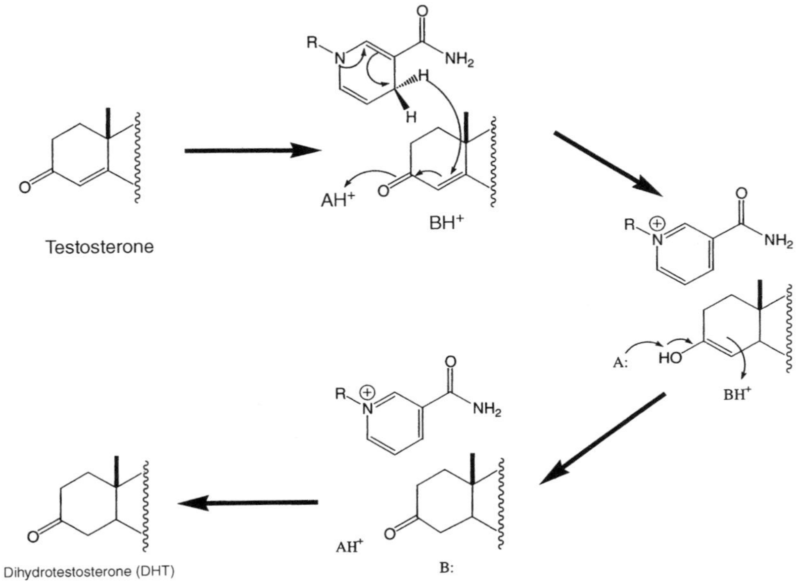

Figure 12.18 Reaction mechanism of the enzyme steroid 5α-reductase. Redrawn and modified from Harris, G.S. and Kozarich, J.W. (1997) *Current Opinion Chem. Biol.*, 1, 254–259.

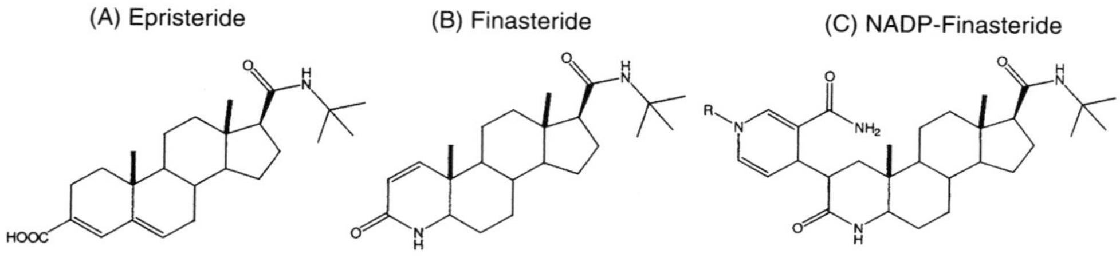

(A) Epristeride   (B) Finasteride   (C) NADP-Finasteride

Figure 12.19 Chemical structures of inhibitors of steroid 5α-reductase: (A) epristeride; (B) finasteride; and (C) the covalent NADP-finasteride complex.

the product, DHT. The DHT and then the $NADP^+$ co-factor are released to regenerate the free enzyme.

Epristeride (Figure 12.19A) was designed to mimic the testosterone enolate intermediate of the steroid 5α-reductase reaction pathway. The carboxylate functionality of the inhibitor electronically resembles the enolate. The pK_a of the carboxylate is 4.8, so that it is the anion form that is responsible for inhibition under physiological conditions. Kinetic and equilibrium binding studies demonstrated that epristeride is an uncompetitive inhibitor with respect to the NADPH co-factor, binding to the enzyme only after formation of the NADPH–enzyme binary complex, with a K_d of ca. 25 nM (2.5×10^{-8} M). This is expected from the reaction mechanism if the inhibitor is indeed functioning as a reaction intermediate mimic. Surprisingly, the inhibitor was also found to be uncompetitive with respect to testosterone. The interpretation of this observation is that the inhibitor binds to the enzyme form that results from release of the DHT product, prior to $NADP^+$ release.

Epristeride demonstrated the expected lowering of DHT levels upon oral dosing. In healthy volunteers this compound reduced circulating levels of DHT by 25–54%. The drug was not pursued in further clinical trials, however, most likely because more potent inhibitors of steroid 5α-reductase, such as finasteride (see below), were contemporaneously identified.

12.4   OTHER TYPES OF INHIBITORS

While many drugs behave as simple reversible enzyme inhibitors, compounds that inhibit enzyme by other mechanisms can also demonstrate clinical utility. Space does not permit an exhaustive review of all forms of enzyme inhibition. However, three other inhibitor modes that have led to a number of clinically useful drugs are slow, tight-binding inhibitors, covalent enzyme modifiers, and mechanism-based enzyme inhibitors. Examples of these inhibition modes will be described here.

12.4.1   Slow, tight-binding inhibitors

Simple, reversible inhibitors bind to enzymes rapidly, typically at diffusion-limited rates, and likewise dissociate from the enzyme on a relatively fast time scale. Some inhibitors, however, bind slowly to enzymes either because their rate of binding is limited by a chemical event or because binding is associated with a rate-limiting conformational change of the enzyme. There are a number of examples of inhibitors that bind to the enzyme initially with modest affinity but then induce a conformational change in the enzyme leading to much tighter binding affinity (the inhibitor equivalent of the induced fit model discussed above for substrate interactions). In this case, the onset of inhibition is slow relative to the rate of enzyme turnover so that the product progress curve for the enzyme goes from a linear function in the absence of inhibitor, to a curvilinear form in the presence of the inhibitor. The non-linear character of the progress curve results from an initial rate of turnover characteristic of the weak, initial enzyme interaction with the inhibitor, and a second rate of turnover that results from the final inhibitor binding species (Figure 12.20). Hence, the accumulation of product with time is a function of three parameters: the initial velocity of reaction, the final velocity of reaction, and a rate constant associated with the transition between these enzyme–inhibitor complexes. The true affinity of the inhibitor for the enzyme can thus only be assessed after this final equilibrium has been established.

The selective inhibitors of cyclooxygenase-2 (COX2) are excellent contemporary examples of drugs in clinical use that function by slow, tight-binding enzyme inhibition. The COX2 is one of two isozymes of cyclooxygenase that catalyze the conversion of arachidonic acid to prostaglandin H_2. Prostaglandin H_2 and its metabolites serve a protective function in the GI and kidneys but also stimulate the pain, swelling, and fever associated with inflammation. The activity of the COX1 isozyme is mainly responsible for the protective functions of prostaglandin production while COX2 activity is associated with inflammatory response. Traditional anti-inflammatory drugs, such as aspirin and ibuprofen, inhibit both COX1

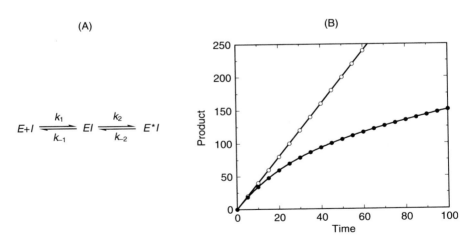

Figure 12.20 (A) A two-step reaction mechanism involving initial inhibitor binding to an enzyme followed by a conformational transition of the enzyme that results in much tighter inhibitor binding. The symbols E and E^* represent the two distinct conformational states of the enzyme. (B) Product appearance time courses for an enzyme in the absence (open circles) and presence (closed circles) of an inhibitor conforming to the mechanism illustrated in (A).

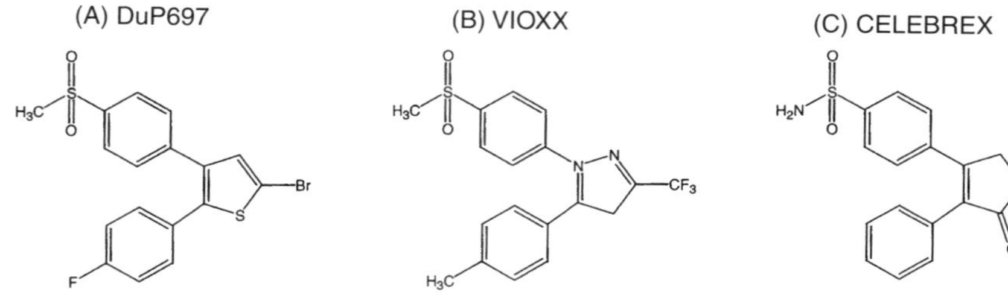

Figure 12.21 Chemical structures of COX-2 selective inhibitors that function by a slow, tight-binding mechanism: (A) DuP697; (B) VIOXX; and (C) CELEBREX.

and COX2. Prolonged use of these drugs is associated with GI and renal ulceration as a result of COX1 inhibition. Hence, selective inhibitors of COX2 provide a clear mechanism for anti-inflammatory therapy without untoward side effects.

The first selective COX2 inhibitor to be described was the experimental compound DuP697 (Figure 12.21A). This compound proved to be an excellent anti-inflammatory agent in animal models without associated ulcerogenicity. Detailed kinetic analysis of DuP697 inhibition of COX1 and COX2 demonstrated an unexpected mechanism for isozyme selectivity. The compound binds to both COX1 and COX2 with equal, modest affinity ($K_i \sim 5\,\mu M$). Inhibitor binding induces a slow conformational change in COX2, but not COX1, that increases inhibitor affinity by >10-fold. Thus, the isozyme-selective induction of a conformational change in the enzyme leads to potent inhibition of COX2 that is not seen for COX1. This observation led several groups to investigate structural analogs of DuP697, resulting in improved potency and selectivity based on this same isozyme-selective conformational transition. Ultimately, two COX2 selective inhibitors, based on this inhibition mechanism, have been brought to the clinic for the treatment of inflammatory diseases: VIOXX and CELEBREX (Figure 12.21B and C). Both compounds are structurally related to DuP697 and both demonstrate the same slow, tight-binding inhibition of COX2 but not COX1. These compounds have quickly become the standard of care for anti-inflammatory therapies and provide a great benefit to patients due to the amelioration of GI and renal side effects with these new medicines.

12.4.2   Covalent enzyme modifiers

Many chemically reactive compounds can interact with specific amino acid side chains within proteins to covalently modify them, in a process referred to as affinity labeling. When the amino acid side chain is critical to the catalytic mechanism of the enzyme, covalent modification leads to irreversible inactivation. Generally, compounds that covalently modify enzymes in this way do so too indiscriminately to be useful as drugs. In some cases, however, covalent modifiers (also referred to as affinity labels) have been discovered that are highly selective for a specific enzyme active site. A classical example of this is the anti-inflammatory drug aspirin.

Aspirin (acetylsalicylic acid) and its analogs have been used, in one form or another, to treat pain, fever and general inflammation since the time of Hippocrates. The anti-inflammatory activity of aspirin results from its ability to block prostaglandin biosynthesis by inhibiting the cyclooxygenase isozymes COX1 and COX2 (see above). Aspirin irreversibly inactivates these enzymes by acetylation of an active site serine residue within the arachidonic acid binding pocket. The additional bulk added to the serine by acetylation sterically blocks arachidonic acid entry into this binding pocket, thus acting as an irreversible competitive inhibitor.

A more recent example of a enzyme-selective covalent modifier is the compound AG7088, an experimental drug that inhibits the 3C protease of human rhinovirus, the causal agents of common colds in humans.

Rhinovirus are members of the *picornavirus* family of RNA viruses that rely on proteolytic processing of a viral polyprotein for replication. One viral protease that is critical for replication is the 3C protease. This enzyme is a cysteine protease, using an active site cysteine as the attacking nucleophile for peptide bond hydrolysis. Inhibition of this enzyme will therefore block viral replication, potentially leading to a rapid resolution of the infection.

The Agouron group solved the crystal structure of the rhinovirus 3C protease and used this structural information for inhibitor design. The first inhibitor to be designed was based on a short peptide representing the canonical substrate sequence on the N-terminal side of the 3C protease cleavage site. The last residue in this peptide (i.e. the group immediately preceding the scissile bond of the substrate) was replaced by an aldehyde group that binds to the active site cysteine to create a tetrahedral carbon structure resembling the transition state of the reaction. This proved to be a potent inhibitor of the enzyme, with a K_i of 6 nM. Reduction of the aldehyde to the corresponding alcohol resulted in a complete loss of binding affinity. This suggested that small molecule, non-covalent inhibitors were unlikely to be effective against this enzyme. Based on these results the Agouron group focused their efforts on finding better, irreversible modifiers of the active site cysteine. Replacement of the aldehyde group with an α,β-unsaturated ethyl ester provided the peptide with a Michael acceptor that could readily undergo nucleophilic attack by the active site cysteine. Optimization of the rest of the peptide led to compound AG7088 (Figure 12.22A). The kinetics of AG7088 inhibition of the protease indicated that the compound first binds reversibly and then more slowly inactivates the enzyme by forming a covalent species. Thus, the compound acts as a slow binding, irreversible inhibitor, conforming to the mechanism:

$$E + I \underset{k_{\text{off}}}{\overset{k_{\text{on}}}{\rightleftharpoons}} EI \xrightarrow{k_{\text{inact.}}} E - I$$

The affinity of such compounds cannot be measured by an equilibrium dissociation constant, as there is no back reaction. Instead, affinity is quantified in terms of the second order rate constant obtained from the ratio $k_{\text{obs}}/[I]$, where k_{obs} is the observed pseudo-first order rate constant for inactivation (measured as described above for slow, tight-binding inhibitors); the second order rate constant for AG7088

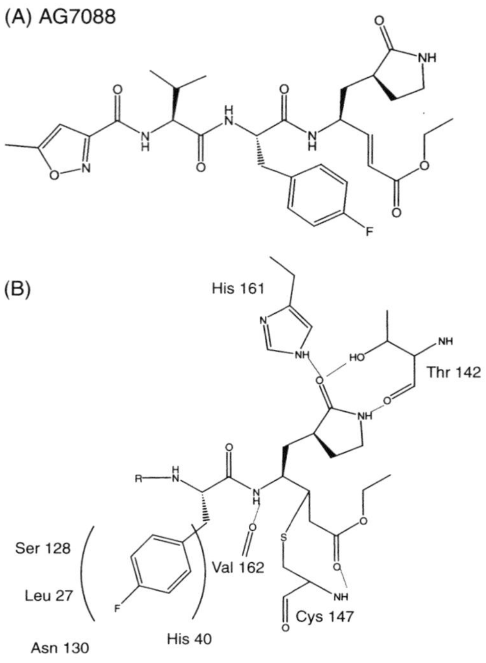

Figure 12.22 (A) Chemical structure of the rhinovirus 3C protease inhibitor AG7088; and (B) schematic representation of the covalent species formed between AG7088 and the active site cysteine of the rhinovirus 3C protease.

inactivation of the 3C protease is $1\,470\,000\,\text{s}^{-1}\,\text{M}^{-1}$. The crystal structure of AG7088 bound to the 3C protease confirmed the expected mechanism of covalent inhibition. The side chain sulfur of the active site cysteine forms a covalent bond to the β-carbon of the formerly unsaturated ethyl ester group (see Figure 12.22). The affinity of the inhibitor is further augmented by hydrophobic interactions with leucine and asparagine residues and by hydrogen bonding interactions with histidine, threonine and serine side chains, as well as with mainchain heteroatoms of a valine and the active site cysteine in the binding pocket. AG7088 not only shows activity as an enzyme inactivator *in vitro*, it also demonstrates good inhibition of viral replication in cellular assays. In HeLa and MRC-5 cells the mean EC_{50} for inhibition of viral replication was 23 nM, while the compound showed no toxicity for these cells at concentrations as high as 100 μM. This compound has now entered human clinical trials to determine its safety and effectiveness at treating common colds.

12.4.3   Mechanism-based enzyme inhibitors

Mechanism-based inhibitors are molecules that themselves are inactive as enzyme inhibitors, but resemble the substrate or product of the enzyme reaction enough to be recognized and acted upon by the enzyme. The chemical transformation of the molecule within the enzyme active site results either in covalent modification of the enzyme or of a cofactor, leading to inactivation, or *in situ* formation of an extremely tight-binding non-covalent inhibitor. This form of inhibition is distinct from affinity labeling in that mechanism-based inhibition relies on the normal chemistry of enzymatic catalysis to transform the compound into an active inhibitor. Affinity labels, on the other hand, rely on the inherent chemical reactivity of the labeling molecule itself. Mechanism-based inhibitors, therefore, are usually very specific for a particular target enzyme, making this form of inhibition attractive for drug applications (see Chapter 9).

A recent example of a clinically useful mechanism-based enzyme inhibitor is the drug finasteride, an inhibitor of steroid 5α-reductase. Inhibitors of this enzyme, as described earlier, have potential application in the treatment of benign prostate hyperplasia, male pattern baldness, and severe acne. Finasteride (Figure 12.19B) is a structural analog of testosterone and binds to the enzyme within the testosterone binding pocket. The compound was initially described as a reversible slow, tight-binding inhibitor of steroid 5α-reductase. More detailed kinetic and chemical studies, however, revealed that the molecule actually functions through an unusual form of mechanism-based inhibition. Like testosterone, finasteride binds to the enzyme–NADPH binary complex to form a ternary complex. The NADPH reduction of and hydride transfer to finasteride then occurs within the active site of the enzyme with formation of a lactam enolate of finasteride, analogous to the testosterone enolate reaction intermediate. This species then attacks the electrophilic pyrimidine of the $NADP^+$ cofactor, leading to a covalent NADP-finasteride adduct (Figure 12.19C). This adduct occupies both the NADPH and testosterone binding pockets simultaneously as a bisubstrate inhibitor. The favorable binding interactions with both substrate binding pockets leads to very high affinity inhibition; the estimated K_d for the NADP-finasteride adduct is 0.3 pM (3×10^{-13} M) with an estimated half-life for dissociation of >30 days! Hence, in practice finasteride acts essentially as an irreversible inactivator of steroid $5\ \alpha$-reductase.

Finasteride demonstrates good efficacy for the treatment of benign prostate hyperplasia. Patients treated with this drug for 36 months had a median reduction in prostate volume of 27% (relative to pretreatment volume) with correlated improvements in urinary flow rates and other symptoms. The drug is currently prescribed for this indication and is also undergoing clinical trials for the treatment of prostate cancer. Finasteride has also demonstrated clinical efficacy in the treatment of male pattern baldness, promoting hair growth in a significant portion of treated men. The drug is currently prescribed for this indication as well.

12.5   SUMMARY

In this chapter, we have briefly introduced the chemical mechanisms by which enzymes catalyze the critical biochemical reactions of life. Strategies for substrate recognition and transformation to the reaction transition state were discussed in the context of achieving reactant specificity and reaction rate acceleration. Blocking the pathogenic activity of enzymes with small molecular weight inhibitors forms the mechanistic basis for a large proportion of currently prescribed drugs. We saw that the same structural determinants of substrate binding and chemical transformation can be exploited to design potent enzyme inhibitors that compete with the natural substrate for the free enzyme. Other modes of reversible enzyme inhibition were also introduced and clinically relevant examples of each inhibitor modality were discussed. Examples of other types of enzyme inhibitors, such as slow, tight-binding inhibitors, covalent modifiers and mechanism-based inhibitors were also presented. These examples give some sense of the diversity of strategies available for the chemotherapeutic use of enzyme inhibition. As we enter the twenty-first century, new technologies are enhancing our ability to identify pathogenic targets associated with human diseases. A significant portion of these to-be-discovered targets is likely to be enzymes. Hence, continued study of the catalytic mechanisms and methods for inhibition of these proteins will remain a mainstay of pharmaceutical science for the foreseeable future.

FURTHER READING

Chan, C.-C., Boyce, S., Brideau, C., Charleson, S., Cromlish, W., Ethier, D., Evans, J., Ford-Hutchinson, A.W., Forrest, M.J., Gauthier, J.Y., Gordon, R., Gresser, M., Guay, J., Kargman, S., Kennedy, B., Leblanc, Y., Leger, S., Mancini, J., O'Neill, G.P., Ouellet, M., Patrick, D., Percival, M.D., Perrier, H., Prasit, P., Rodger, I., Tagari, P., Therien, M., Vickers, P., Visco, D., Wang, Z., Webb, J., Wong, E., Xu, L.-J., Young, R.N., Zamboni, R. and Riendeau, D. (1999) Rofecoxib [Vioxx, MK-0966; 4-(4′-methylsulfonylphenyl)-3-phenyl-2-(5H)-furanone]: A potent and orally active cyclooxygenase-2 inhibitor. Pharmacological and biochemical profiles. *J. Pharmacol. Exp. Ther.*, **290**, 551–560.

Copeland, R.A. (2000) *Enzymes: A Practical Introduction to Structure, Mechanism and Data Analysis*, 2nd edition. New York: Wiley-VCH.

Copeland, R.A., Williams, J.M., Giannaras, J., Nurnberg, S., Covington, M., Pinto, D., Pick, S. and Trzaskos, J.M. (1994) Mechanism of selective inhibition of the inducible isoform of prostaglandin G/H synthase. *Proc. Natl. Acad. Sci. USA*, **91**, 11202–11206.

Drews, J. (2000) Drug discovery: A historical perspective. *Science*, **287**, 1960–1964.

Fersht, A. (1999) *Structure and Mechanism in Protein Science*. New York: Freeman.

Harris, G.S. and Kozarich, J.W. (1997) Steroid 5α-reductase inhibitors in androgen-dependent disorders. *Current Opinion Chem. Biol.*, **1**, 254–259.

Levy, M.A., Brandt, M., Heys, R., Holt, D.A. and Metcalf, B.W. (1990) Inhibition of rat liver steroid 5α-reductase by 3-androstene-3-carboxylic acids: mechanism of enzyme–inhibitor interactions. *Biochemistry*, **29**, 2815–2824.

Mathews, D.A., Dragovich, P.S., Webber, S.E., Fuhrman, S.A., Patick, A.K., Zalman, L.S., Hendrickson, T.F., Love, R.A., Prins, T.J., Marakovits, J.T., Zhou, R., Tikhe, J., Ford, C.E., Meador, J.W., Ferre, R.A., Brown, E.L., Binford, S.L., Brothers, M.A., DeLisle, D.M. and Worland, S.T. (1999) Structure-assisted design of mechanism-based irreversible inhibitors of human rhinovirus 3C protease with potent antiviral activity against multiple rhinovirus serotypes. *Proc. Natl. Acad. Sci. USA*, **96**, 11000–11007.

Purich, D.L. (ed.) (1996) *Contemporary Enzyme Kinetics and Mechanism*, 2nd edition. San Diego: Academic Press.

Ren, J., Milton, J., Weaver, K.L., Short, S.A., Stuart, D.I. and Stammers, D. K. (2000) Structural basis for the resilience of efavirenz (DMP-266) to drug resistance mutations in HIV-1 reverse transcriptase. *Structure (London)*, **8**, 1089–1094.

Segel, I.H. (1975) *Enzyme Kinetics*, 2nd edition. New York: Wiley.

Silverman, R.B. (1992) *The Organic Chemistry of Drug Design and Drug Action*. San Diego: Academic Press.

Spence, R.A., Kati, W.M., Anderson, K.S. and Johnson, K.A. (1995) Mechanism of inhibition of HIV-1 reverse transcriptase by nonnucleoside inhibitors. *Science*, **267**, 988–993.

Chapter 13

Metals in medicine: inorganic medicinal chemistry

Ole Farver

13.1 INTRODUCTION

Bioinorganic chemistry lies in the interface between inorganic chemistry and biology, and although biology is generally associated with organic chemistry, in fact most of the chemical elements from hydrogen to bismuth bear potential in drug design (Figure 13.1). Thus, inorganic chemistry is beginning to have a larger impact on modern medicine. Given the enormous variety and range in reactivity of inorganic compounds, the application of inorganic chemistry in improving human health opens for a whole new research field. While still in its infancy, bioinorganic chemistry is destined to play an increasingly important role in modern medicinal chemistry since essential as well as non-essential and toxic elements can be utilized in drug design.

Pharmaceuticals may control metabolism of essential elements in two ways:

1 Supply of specific drugs with target properties may enable delivery or removal of elements to/from specific sites.
2 The natural physiological pathways may be blocked by the drug.

A general problem associated with the use of inorganic compounds as pharmaceuticals is the poor characterization of the compounds with respect to toxicity *in vivo*. The issues of understanding the reaction mechanisms and identification

IA	IIA	IIIB	IVB	VB	VIB	VIIB	VIIIB	VIIIB	VIIIB	IB	IIB	IIIA	IVA	VA	VIA	VIIA	VIIIA
H																	He
Li	Be											B	C	N	O	F	Ne
Na	Mg											Al	Si	P	S	Cl	Ar
K	Ca	Sc	Ti	V	Cr	Mn	Fe	Co	Ni	Cu	Zn	Ga	Ge	As	Se	Br	Kr
Rb	Sr	Y	Zr	Nb	Mo	Tc	Ru	Rh	Pd	Ag	Cd	In	Sn	Sb	Te	I	Xe
Cs	Ba	*La*	Hf	Ta	W	Re	Os	Ir	Pt	Au	Hg	Tl	Pb	Bi	Po	At	Rn
Fr	Ra	*Ac*	Th	Pa	U												

Figure 13.1 The periodic table of the elements. Selected elements which are important in bioinorganic chemistry are highlighted: **bulk biological elements**; *essential elements*; possibly **essential trace elements**. Other elements may be used in drugs or as probes.

of target centers are together with the toxicity problem central aspects that have to be addressed before potential new drugs can be applied. This underlines the major point: *Specific biological activity of inorganic compounds can be achieved by proper design.*

Metals are commonly found as natural constituents in proteins where they perform a wide spectrum of specific functions associated with biological processes. Metalloproteins with catalytic properties are called metalloenzymes. They implement chemical transformations of certain molecules called substrates, and it is interesting to note that almost half of all enzymes in the human organism are depending on the presence of one or more metal ions. Obviously, these metal ions are key pharmaceutical targets for drugs. Inorganic chemistry thus has a huge potential in modern pharmacology as it introduces a new realm of compounds. It is noteworthy that metal ions control some of the fundamental biochemical processes such as RNA and DNA replication. From an 'inorganic' point of view co-ordination chemistry in biological systems (metalloproteins and -enzymes) is particularly interesting, and this applies to both the thermodynamic (structure and binding) and the kinetic (reactivity) aspects.

13.1.1   Essential and non-essential elements

Elements are called essential if their absence causes irreversible damage to the organism or if the optimal function of the organism is impaired. Otherwise they are labeled non-essential. The chemistry behind the way the human body utilizes the elements is fascinating, but even the mechanisms of how essential elements are supplied from the diet are poorly understood.

Which elements are essential or beneficial and which are non-essential or even toxic for a certain organism? These questions are continuously being discussed. The elements as such are not good or evil and we recognize a general concentration dependence of the action of all elements. As the diagram in Figure 13.2 indicates, there is a dose/effect response curve different for each element. Many substances may even have an ambivalent effect which illustrates the saying of Paracelsus: *The dose makes the poison.*

Homeostasis which means maintenance of an optimal concentration of beneficial elements, as well as detoxification, i.e. transport of non-beneficial elements out of the system, require a delicate balance between processes of uptake, utilization, and excretion. As far as the essential elements are concerned, too low concentrations will result in deficiency diseases. Excess of an otherwise beneficial element as well as addition of a toxic compound will cause poisoning of the organism (Figure 13.2). This could either be due to unwanted redox reactions where damaging byproducts such as the hydroxyl radical is formed or by non-specific binding to certain centers which may lead to inhibition of the normal physiological processes.

As far as the non-essential (or toxic) elements are concerned, the concentration region in the left-hand side of Figure 13.2 (a) can be applied since these elements show no toxic effect in a certain limited concentration range. This provides us with an opportunity to apply the compounds pharmacologically, e.g. killing certain cell

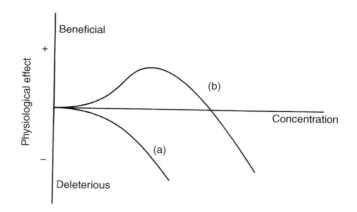

Figure 13.2 Dose/effect diagram. An organism's response to (a) non-essential or toxic and (b) essential elements. Note that at sufficiently small concentrations, toxic compounds are tolerated. Essential elements become toxic at elevated concentrations.

types or micro-organisms that are more sensitive to a particular element. Examples are drugs based on Pt(II) and Au(I) complexes. These metal ions are otherwise highly toxic and should be administered with the utmost care. The toxicity may also depend on a certain oxidation state. Arsenic, for example is generally considered being a highly toxic substance, but As(III) compounds are much more toxic than As(V) compounds.

13.1.2   History

Inorganic compounds have been applied in medicine for thousands of years. The ancient Egyptians and Hebrews are supposed to have utilized copper for sterilization of water (3000 years B.C.E.). About the same time the Chinese used gold for medical purposes – including the noble purpose of obtaining a state of immortality (youth elixir). Calomel (Hg_2Cl_2) has been a well-known diureticum since the renaissance and was used until the 1950s. P. Ehrlich's arsenic compounds were the first successful pharmaceuticals for treating syphilis. Another drug worth mentioning is AuCN which was used as a relatively efficient drug against tuberculosis. Gold therapies are applied even today in treatment of rheumatoid arthritis, both as injections of gold thiolates and orally as aurarofin (Section 13.8.6). It is, however, noteworthy that serendipity has played a major role in the discovery of all these treatments. Introduction of Pt(II) complexes that have revolutionized treatment of several malignant tumor species is an excellent example. Platinum compounds and their mechanism of action (as far as they are known today) will be discussed in Section 13.8.5.

For modern rational drug design and development, it is of utmost importance to understand the reaction mechanism of the inorganic compounds, including identification of the target centers. And indeed, a huge world of inorganic drugs, which have not yet been explored is now slowly opening.

13.2 CLASSIFICATION OF INORGANIC PHARMACEUTICALS

Inorganic drugs may be divided into three different categories (Figure 13.3):

1   *Active complexes*: In this case, it is the entire complex, metal ion and ligands, which determines the action. Many inert positively charged co-ordination compounds act as neurotoxins by blocking acetylcholine receptors. *Cis*-platinum and other uncharged Pt(II) and Ru(II) complexes are active as antitumor drugs (Section 13.8.5). Bi(III) complexes with sulphur containing ligands are used in the treatment of gastrointestinal diseases. These compounds will be dealt with later in more detail (Section 13.8.8). Insoluble salts of certain heavy metals can be applied as X-ray contrast compounds, such as $BaSO_4$. The rare earth gadolinium (Gd) is used in NMR diagnostics. The $[Xe]4f^7$ electron configuration of Gd^{3+} with its 7 unpaired electrons makes the ion highly paramagnetic. However, due to pronounced toxicity gadolinium compounds are administered as chelate compounds protecting the organism, e.g. as the $GdEDTA^-$ complex. Tin co-ordinated to protoporphyrin inhibits heme oxygenase degradation of a certain iron-heme product to bilirubin. The latter compound is the most frequent cause of neonatal jaundice.

Active complexes
- Cr, Co, Rh (neuromuscular blockers)
- Pt, Ru (anticancer drugs)
- Gd (NMR probes)
- Co (vitamin B_{12})
- Al, Zr (antiperspirant)
- Ba (x-ray contrast)
- Sn (jaundice)
- Bi (antiulcer and -bacterial agents)

Active elements
- Li (manic-depressive psychosis)
- F (tooth paste)
- Ag, Hg (antimicrobial compounds)
- ^{99m}Tc, ^{111}In (radiodiagnostica)
- Au (rheumatoid arthritis)

Active ligands
- *Delivered by a metal ion*
  - Ca, Mg, Al (antacid compounds)
  - Fe (antihypertensiva)
  - Ti, Au (anticancer)
- *Delivered to a metal ion*
  - Bleomycin (Fe)
  - Penicillamine (Cu)
  - Desferrioxamine (Fe, Al)
  - Bisphosphonates (Ca)

Figure 13.3 Classification of inorganic drugs. Adapted from P.J. Sadler (1991).

2   *Active elements*: In this case, the metal ion is decisive for the action of the drug while the anion or ligand only serves to keep the metal ion in solution or simply as a counter ion. The effect of lithium in the manic-depressive psychosis is well known even if not fully understood. Interestingly, the lithium ion is counteracting both phases of the cyclic course of this disease (Section 13.8.1). The cariostatic effect of fluoride is well established although the mechanism is still unclear. Formation of a particularly resistant crystalline layer of tooth enamel (fluoroapatite) is one possibility. Inhibition of caries-promoting enzymes by fluoride ions is another widely accepted idea. Silver(I) and mercury(II) are potential antibacterial agents, and silver sulfadiazene is still used clinically (Section 13.8.6). Technetium (the ^{99m}Tc isotope) is applied in radiodiagnostics. The γ-active isotope has a half-life of 6 h. Tc is mainly administered as a $Tc^{VII}(CNR)_6^+$ complex. The significance of gold in treating rheumatoid arthritis is discussed further in Section 13.8.6.

3   *Active ligands*: Many ligands can be delivered to or from a metal ion in the organism. The classic iron(III) co-ordination compound, nitroprusside $[Fe^{III}(CN)_5NO]^{2-}$, with its $[Ar]d^5$ electron configuration, relatively easily releases NO which functions as an hypotensive agent causing smooth muscle relaxation. The half life of the very reactive NO radical is only 6 sec. Some selected chelates are presented in Section 13.6.

13.3   THE HUMAN BODY AND BIOINORGANIC CHEMISTRY

The living organism may be considered being an open system in a steady state where energy input and output maintain a dynamic flow equilibrium (a dissipative system). Besides energy flux, life requires a constant exchange of material, which in principle could comprise all elements of the periodic table (Figure 13.1). The occurrence of a given element in an organism depends on several factors. First of all, how available the element is in nature, i.e. abundance and accessibility. But elements which are rarer or more difficult to obtain may be accumulated actively by the organism, nonetheless. In the latter case, energy consuming processes are required. The composition of elements in the human body is given in Table 13.1.

Table 13.1 requires some comments: The large quantities of hydrogen and oxygen simply reflect the amount of 'inorganic' water. 'Organic' carbon comes in second. Calcium is the first metallic element to be encountered, and its primary function is stabilization of the skeleton. The table also demonstrates rather large quantities of the metals potassium, sodium, and magnesium, and furthermore the non-metallic elements nitrogen, sulfur, phosphorous, and chlorine are abundant.

Now follows iron and zinc as the first representatives of the transition metals, though in much smaller quantities. They constitute together with the non-metallic elements fluorine and silicon, which are important for our bone structure, the transition to the genuine trace elements. Here we set the boundary, quite arbitrarily, to less than 1 g per 70 kg body weight. Many trace elements are essential, which as stated above, means that the organism will be irreversibly damaged by eliminating them from the food. Elements in Table 13.1 which are marked by an asterix, some of

Table 13.1 Constitution of the human organism (adult 70 kg)

Element	Mass (g)	Recommended daily dose (mg)
oxygen	45500	
carbon	12600	
hydrogen	7000	
nitrogen	2100	
calcium	1050	800–1200
phosphorous	700	800–1200
sulfur	175	10
potassium	140	2000–5500
chlorine	105	3200
sodium	105	1100–3300
magnesium	35	300–400
iron	4.2	10–20
zinc	2.3	15
silicon	1.4	
rubidium*	1.1	
fluorine	0.8	1.5–4.0
bromine*	0.2	
strontium*	0.14	
copper	0.11	1.5–3
aluminium*	0.1	
lead*	0.08	
antimony	0.07	
cadmium*	0.03	
tin*	0.03	
iodine	0.03	0.15
manganese	0.03	2–5
vanadium*	0.02	
selenium	0.02	0.05–0.07
barium*	0.02	
arsenic*	0.01	
boron*	0.01	
nickel*	0.01	
chromium	0.005	0.05–0.2
cobalt	0.003	0.2
molybdenum	<0.005	ca. 0.1

Source: Recommended Dietary Allowance, RDA.
Note
* The elements marked by * are either non-essential or their function is unknown.

which occurring in rather large concentrations, probably are not essential like rubidium, strontium, bromium, and aluminium. The reason why these elements occur is their close chemical resemblance with essential ones: $Rb^+ \sim K^+$, $Br^- \sim Cl^-$, $Al^{3+} \sim Fe^{3+}$. Certain elements which are known to be toxic, even in very small quantities, like arsenic, lead, and cadmium require special attention. It has been discussed whether these elements in minimal amounts (Figure 13.2 (a)) could be, if not essential to the organism, then at least beneficial. It is not inconceivable at all that during evolutionary pressure all elements have obtained some physiological function.

It is also noteworthy that elements like silicon and titanium which are found in abundance in many minerals forming the earth's crust play such a marginal role in biological systems. The reason is, of course, that these elements are practically non-available in aqueous solution at pH 7. On the other hand, a rather exotic metal like molybdenum is relatively soluble at neutral pH as $Mo^{VI}O_4^{2-}$, and molybdenum has found an important function as an essential metal in certain enzymes (Section 13.8.3).

Now, which elements are essential, which are beneficial without being indispensable, and which are exclusively toxic? From the previous section this seems to be a difficult question. And it is! Maybe the best answer is given by Paracelsus, referred to above, that it is the amount which determines the effect.

The diagram in Figure 13.2 demonstrates that too low concentration of essential elements will cause deficiency effects. The same element in too large quantity, however, will lead to poisoning whether this is caused by excessive uptake or excretion failure. Toxication of this nature can be treated by 'inorganic' chemistry using e.g. chelate therapy. Synergistic processes where one chelate binds the unwanted element while another transports it out of the organism has proven particularly effective. Menkes' and Wilson's diseases are caused by impaired copper uptake and defect copper excretion, respectively. In both cases, chelate therapy is used in treatment of the patients.

Since the human body functions by uptake, accumulation, transport, and storage of chemical compounds the arbitrary differentiation between 'organic' and 'inorganic' matter is irrelevant and just a historical relic. The double helix structure of DNA, for instance, could not be stabilized without the presence of mono- and divalent cations that compensate for the electrostatic repulsion between the negatively charged phosphate groups. Electric nerve impulses as well as more complex trigger mechanisms are initiated by rapid bursts of ions across membranes. Particularly Na^+, K^+, and Ca^{2+} ions are used to trigger cellular responses. Degradation of organic molecules requires acid and base catalysis which at physiological pH could not take place without the presence of either Lewis acids like the zinc(II) ion or Lewis bases that could be inorganic anions. Electron transfer is essential for all energy conversion processes in organisms, and here redox active transition metals like iron and copper become indispensable. The metal ions may be bound in small proteins and undergo redox transformations without catalyzing chemical changes in substrates. Instead the current carriers pass electrons to or from redox active iron and copper containing enzymes which are involved in specific biological functions. The reduction potentials of the metal ions co-ordinated to biological ligands embedded in a protein will usually differ markedly from potentials of the particular metal ion complexes in aqueous solution.

From the previous, it is evident that all fundamental biological processes proceed in reactions that often involve inorganic substances in central roles. It is thus obvious that inorganic chemistry holds a huge potential for developing new pharmaceuticals which may influence physiological processes. All this requires a detailed knowledge of interactions between metal ions and organic molecules; a field also known as co-ordination chemistry. Stability and kinetics of metal ion complexes will therefore be a central subject in this chapter describing inorganic drugs.

13.4   CO-ORDINATION CHEMISTRY

According to Lewis' definition, all metal ions as such are Lewis acids since they can co-ordinate to free electron pairs (i.e. Lewis bases). The outcome of this reaction is called a co-ordination compound or a complex between the central metal ion (Lewis acid) and the electron donor (Lewis base). A complex is thus composed of ions or molecules which may exist individually in solution, but in combination they produce the co-ordination compound. The ions or molecules co-ordinated to the central metal ion are called ligands and make up the co-ordination sphere. The number of points at which ligands are attached to the metal ion is called the co-ordination number. The different categories of ligands are shown in Table 13.2.

13.4.1   Chelate effect

Ligands (Lewis bases) with several binding sites are called polydentate ligands (chelates) and form particularly stabile complexes: metal-chelates. The most advantageous situation occurs when 5- or 6-membered rings can be formed. One of the important factors controlling the stability of a complex is the chelate effect: The stability of a co-ordination compound increases with the number of binding centers of the ligands. Amino acids, peptides and proteins contain many metal binding groups which make them excellent chelates. Besides peptide NH and C=O groups, many side chains may serve as complexing agents for metal ions. These include thiolate in cysteine, the imidazole ring of histidine, carboxylates of glutamic acid and aspartic acid, and the amino side chain of lysine.

The rationale behind the chelate effect is quite straightforward. As soon as a metal ion co-ordinates to one of the binding centers in a multidentate ligand, the chance for co-ordination of other potential donor groups enhances since these cannot get very far away and only need to swing into position. If two independent molecules having access to much larger volume of the solution should bind, the second ligand must find its way to the metal ion by diffusion in a bimolecular

Table 13.2 Ligand types

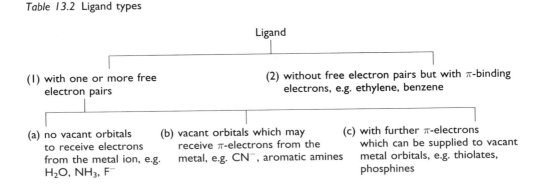

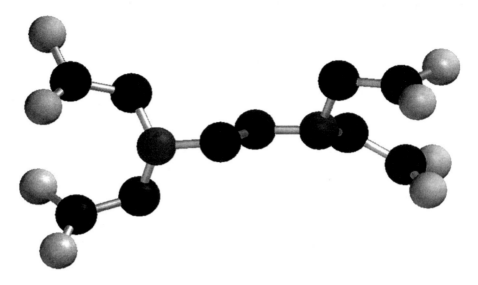

Figure 13.4 Structure of the free EDTA molecule. Carbon atoms are black, oxygen light gray, and nitrogen dark gray. Hydrogen atoms are not shown.

process. The difference in rates between the two processes, uni- vs. bimolecular, would typically be of an order of 10^4. A favorable entropic factor further adds to the stability since chelation is accompanied by release of non-chelating ligands like water from the co-ordination sphere. An example of a good chelate is shown in Figure 13.4, where the six possible donor groups in EDTA are all more or less in the correct position for metal ion co-ordination.

A closely related effect is termed the macrocyclic effect. It simply relates to the notion that a complex with a cyclic polydentate ligand has greater thermodynamic stability when compared with a similar non-cyclic ligand. Important examples are afforded by the porphyrin and corrin rings. As a consequence, macrocyclic complexes provide bioinorganic groups of widespread occurrence and utility in nature, being found in e.g. crown ethers, cryptands (alkali metals), cytochromes (iron), chlorophyll (magnesium), and coenzyme-B_{12} (cobalt).

Based on a large number of experimental data on the stability of divalent metal ion complexes with a given ligand, a certain trend has been demonstrated which is relatively insensitive to the choice of ligands. This variation is also known as the Irving–Williams series:

$$Ca^{2+} < Mg^{2+} < Mn^{2+} < Fe^{2+} < Co^{2+} < Ni^{2+} < Cu^{2+} > Zn^{2+}$$

The order is partly related to the decrease in ionic radii across the series which leads to stronger electrostatic effects and in addition to changes in crystal field stabilization energies. The latter is discussed in Section 13.4.3.

13.4.2   Hard and soft acids and bases (HSAB principle)

Metal ions may be divided into two categories:

1   Those which bind strongly to bases binding strongly to the proton; i.e. bases in the ordinary sense of the word (Class a metals).
2   Those binding preferentially to large polarizable or unsaturated bases that usually show insignificant basicity towards the proton (Class b metals).

This division is obviously not absolute and intermediate examples exist. Nevertheless, the division is reasonably distinct and has proven to be quite useful. We may now divide the bases into two categories: (1) Those which are polarizable or 'soft' bases; and (2) those which are not, the 'hard' bases. There are cases where a base is soft and at the same time binds to the proton with high affinity, e.g. the sulfide ion. However, generally it is true that hardness of a base is correlated with good proton binding. Among the bases with the central atom from main groups V, VI, and VII of the periodic table (which constitute the majority of all bases), those with nitrogen, oxygen, and fluorine are the hardest in their respective groups and at the same time the most basic towards the proton (F^-, OH^-, NH_3).

For Class a metal ions the order of complex stability is the following:

$$F^- > Cl^- > Br^- > I^-$$
$$O \gg S > Se > Te$$
$$N \gg P > As > Sb > Bi$$

while for Class b metal ions the order is virtually the opposite:

$$F^- < Cl^- < Br^- < I^-$$
$$O \ll S \sim Se \sim Te$$
$$N \ll P > As > Sb > Bi$$

It is now obvious that Class a metal ions co-ordinate best to the least polarizable (hardest) atoms of the group while Class b metal ions prefer the more polarizable (softer) atoms within the same family. It is also noteworthy that the softest (most polarizable) atom from a group does not necessarily form the most stable complexes with Class b metal ions. The reason is that many bases in general are poor ligands for all metal ions. Still, complexes between soft bases with Class b metal ions will in all cases be far more stable than their complexes with class a metals.

In Table 13.3, all metal ions which exhibit some importance in the bioinorganic chemistry are classified. The division of these Lewis acids was performed using the above mentioned criterion by comparing the stability of complexes with bases containing nitrogen vs. phosphorus, oxygen vs. sulfur, and fluorine vs. iodine.

It is quite straightforward to catagorize the two types of Lewis acids as in Table 13.3. The general feature of a Class a metal ion is a small ionic radius, high positive charge, and/or valence electrons that cannot be distorted easily. Class b metal ions are in contrast associated with low oxidation state, large ionic radius,

Table 13.3 Classification of Lewis acids

Hard	Soft
H^+, Li^+, Na^+, K^+	Cu^+, Ag^+, Au^+, Tl^+, Hg_2^{2+}
Mg^{2+}, Ca^{2+}, Sr^{2+}, Mn^{2+}	Pd^{2+}, Cd^{2+}, Pt^{2+}, Hg^{2+}
Al^{3+}, La^{3+}, Gd^{3+}, Cr^{3+}, Co^{3+}, Fe^{3+}, As^{3+}	Tl^{3+}, Au^{3+}
Si^{4+}, Ti^{4+}, Os^{4+}	
Borderline	
Fe^{2+}, Co^{2+}, Ni^{2+}, Cu^{2+}, Zn^{2+}, Sn^{2+}, Pb^{2+}, Sb^{3+}, Bi^{3+}, Ru^{2+}, Os^{2+}	

and/or relatively easily distorted outer electrons. Since features of Class a metals thus may be characterized by small polarizability they are called hard (Lewis) acids while Class b type metal ions having higher polarizability are called soft (Lewis) acids. This leads to a useful corollary which is as simple as it is useful:

Hard acids prefer to coordinate to hard bases, while soft acids prefer soft bases

This rule has proven to be extremely useful for estimating the stability of co-ordination compounds including complex formation between metal ions and biomolecules. Obviously other properties like the net charge of the ligand, steric factors, and resonance effects will influence the stability of the complex. Nonetheless, the stability order for soft acid complexes with Lewis bases is as follows:

$$S \sim C > I > Br > Cl > N > O > F$$

For hard acids, the division is even sharper since generally only complexes with oxygen or fluorine donor atoms will exist in aqueous solution. It should also be noted that the order of the above Lewis bases is exactly the same as the one for increasing electronegativity.

In the classification, polarizability was used as the decisive property, but other effects that are correlated with polarizability could well be responsible. For example, high ionization potentials are usually identified with small polarizability while a low ionization potential gives rise to larger polarization, and further the ionization potential is directly related to electronegativity. Also unsaturated bases which may accept π-electrons from the Lewis acid or easily reducible bases which could promote electron transfer to the metal ion are associated with a high degree of polarizability. The Hard and Soft Acid and Base (HSAB) principle will be widely applied in the following.

13.4.3   Kinetics: inert and labile complexes

Any complex formation takes place in a substitution reaction by replacement of one ligand by another. Following the terminology for organic reactions, we use the terms nucleophilic and electrophilic substitution. A nucleophilic reagent is one which donates electrons while an electrophilic reagent receives electrons.

These terms are synonymous with Lewis' base and acid definition, respectively. In a kinetic process, a good nucleophile is one which reacts rapidly with electrophilic reagents like a metal ion, and vice versa. Thus, any substitution reaction is fundamentally an acid–base reaction.

What primarily determines the rate of a substitution reaction, is the ratio between charge and size (charge density) of the metal ion, but when transition metals are involved also the d-electron structure should be taken into account. The term labile will be used for very reactive complexes while less reactive ones are called inert. Obviously, there is no sharp division between inert and labile co-ordination compounds. A useful definition of a labile system is one where the reaction is complete within the time of mixing (i.e. $<1\,\mathrm{min}$). The term inert is used for complexes that react sufficiently slow to be monitored by traditional spectroscopic methods, or which react too slowly to be studied at all. Care should be taken not to confuse the term labile (kinetic) with the thermodynamic designation, stable. It is often true that thermodynamically stable compounds react slowly whereas unstable compounds react rapidly. However, this is not an absolute requirement. Hg(II) as well as Fe(II) form very stable complexes with cyanide, $Hg(CN)_4^{2-}$ and $Fe(CN)_6^{4-}$ but the mercury complex exchanges its ligands extremely rapidly and must be categorized as labile. The iron complex, on the other hand, is inert. Other pertinent examples are many cobalt(III) complexes which are rather unstable but will nevertheless persist in solution for weeks and must thus be categorized as inert.

Knowledge of the kinetic properties of complexes will obviously be decisive in the design of drugs. If a pharmaceutical in form of an organic molecule is transferred to a target site by means of a metal ion, it is not advantageous to choose a metal ion that forms highly inert complexes. On the other hand, it is an absolute necessity that a complex formation between Pt(II) and DNA bases must lead to products sufficiently inert in order to have the adequate time to affect the division of tumor cells.

From information about the electronic structure of metal ion complexes, some general rules for the reactivity of these compounds can be stated. What characterizes transition metals is the partial occupancy of the d-orbitals. Following the crystal field theory the five d-orbitals split in the presence of the electrostatic field provided by the ligands (crystal field). Those orbitals lying in the direction of the ligands are raised in energy compared to the orbitals pointing away from the ligands. In an octahedral field the d-orbitals split as follows from Figure 13.5.

The doubly degenerate energy levels are denominated e while the triply degenerate levels are called t_2. The energy difference, Δ_O, is called the ligand field splitting. The two high energy d-orbitals of an octahedral complex are thus type e-orbitals while the three lower lying orbitals are of the t_2 type. The first three d electrons will go into each of the three t_2-orbitals (Hund's rule). The next electrons will enter either into the e-orbitals or pair up with electrons of the t_2-orbitals. The choice depends on the magnitude of the energy separating the two levels, Δ_O, and the energy required for pairing electrons in the same orbital. If the ligand field splitting is small, the electrons will preferentially occupy different orbitals with parallel spin and form a high-spin complex. If the splitting is large, the electrons will enter the t_2-orbitals forming a low-spin complex. For an octahedral iron(II) co-ordination compound, i.e. a d^6 system, there are thus two possibilities: $t_2^4 e^2$ (high spin) and t_2^6 (low spin) depending upon the magnitude of Δ_O. For aqua complexes

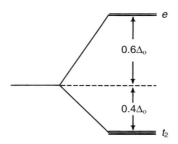

Figure 13.5 Crystal splitting of the *d*-orbitals. The diagram shows the splitting of a set of *d*-orbitals in a metal ion complex having an octahedral symmetry. The energy difference between the *e* and t_2 orbitals is designated Δ_O.

of divalent metal ions from the first transition series, the value of Δ_O is about 100 kJ/mol while the energy difference becomes twice as large for the trivalent aqua ions from the same series. When other ligands replace water, Δ_O changes as well, i.e. Δ_O is also a function of the ligands. The order of increasing splitting is called the spectrochemical series and is empirically found to be:

$$I^- < Br^- < Cl^- < F^- < OH^- < H_2O < NH_3 < NO_2^- < CO < CN^-$$

Those ligands associated with high splitting are called strong-field ligands, and those that give rise to low splitting energies are called weak-field ligands. For octahedral complexes with divalent metal ions of the first transition series the borderline between high-spin and low-spin complexes may be found after ammonia. Weak-field ligands from iodide to ammonia thus give rise to high-spin complexes while the remaining co-ordination compounds will be of the low-spin type. For trivalent metal ions of the same series, the border between strong-field and weak-field ligands lies between water and ammonia. From ammonia to cyanide the octahedral complexes will be of the low-spin type. For the transition metals of the second and third transition series the situation is much simpler. Due to the much larger ligand field splitting no high-spin octahedral complexes have ever been encountered with these elements. Tetrahedral complexes of the first transition series are always of the high spin type, as the result of a much smaller crystal field splitting, $\Delta_T (= 4/9 \times \Delta_O)$.

By preferentially filling up the lower lying t_2-orbitals the d electrons will stabilize the system relative to an average arrangement of the electrons among all available orbitals. The gain in binding energy obtained by distributing the charges in a non-symmetrical way is called crystal field stabilization energy (CFSE). The reason becomes quite obvious when looking at Figure 13.5. The e-orbitals clearly have higher energy than the t_2-orbitals. Taking an arbitrary zero when each orbital is randomly occupied, i.e. a spherically symmetric distribution, we may assign an energy of $-2/5 \times \Delta_O$ to the three t_2-orbitals and $+3/5 \times \Delta_O$ to the e-orbitals. We can now calculate the stabilization energies for complexes with any number of d electrons by assigning the appropriate energy to each electron. For example a d^5 high-spin octahedral complex will acquire a CFSE of $(-3 \times 2/5 + 2 \times 3/5) \times \Delta_O$

equal to 0. On the other hand, the corresponding low-spin d^5 complex will be stabilized by $-5 \times 2/5 \times \Delta_O$ or $-2 \times \Delta_O$. Thus, the latter will be considerably less reactive than the former.

The reactivity of octahedral complexes may now be predicted quite simply: The main group metal ions (alkali and alkaline earth metals) with d^0 electron structure together with the d^{10}-systems have no CFSE and in general thus exchange ligands extremely rapidly. Also d^1, d^2 and d^9 complexes having only a slight excess of electrons in the t_2-orbitals are expected to react fast. The same applies to high-spin d^4, d^5, d^6, and d^7 complexes. The d^3 system and low-spin complexes with d^4, d^5, and d^6 configuration are predicted to be substitution inert with d^6 being the least reactive. Finally, the d^8 configuration deserves a special comment since this system leads to very stable and inert square planar compounds. Platinum(II) complexes belong to this group and are discussed in detail in Section 13.4.5.

It was mentioned earlier that the thermodynamically stable $Hg(CN)_4^{2-}$ complex is substitution labile. It follows nicely the above notion, since Hg(II) has d^{10} electron configuration (CFSE = 0). In the corresponding inert $Fe(CN)_6^{4-}$ low-spin complex the Fe(II) iron has d^6 configuration (CFSE = $-12/5 \times \Delta_O$), and the reactivity is once more in accordance with the prediction based on CFSE. Cu(II) (d^9) and Zn(II) (d^{10}) co-ordination compounds are found frequently in enzyme systems where their large reactivity is fully exploited.

13.4.4   Redox reactions

The classical definition of oxidation is a process in which oxygen has been gained, while a reduction reaction is one where oxygen has been lost. This definition has now been replaced with the concepts electron loss (oxidation) and electron uptake (reduction). A reduction–oxidation (redox) reaction is thus a process in which changes in oxidation states or oxidation numbers take place, and the alleged electron transfer is a sort of book-keeping for balancing the equations. Mechanistically, it is often difficult to discern between atom or group transfer and plain electron transfer processes.

Many transition metals exist in several stable oxidation states which render them particularly interesting also in biological redox chemistry. Redox reactions play a central role in biochemistry; pertinent examples are photosynthesis and respiration where cascades of electron transfer reactions are coupled to synthesis of high-energy molecules like adenosine triphosphate (ATP) and similar compounds. The photosynthetic turnover of CO_2 is quite impressive with production of about 200 billion tons of carbohydrate annually. This production of reduced carbon compounds is accompanied by evolution of oxygen (O_2) following oxidation of two water molecules. However, one of the expenses for living under oxygen rich conditions is the danger of unwanted radical formations. Oxygen easily gets reduced to hydrogen peroxide, and in the presence of reducing metal ions like Fe^{2+} or Cu^+ further reactions may take place like the Fenton reaction, generating hydroxyl radicals:

$$Fe^{2+} + HO_2^- \rightarrow FeO^+ + \cdot OH$$

In the presence of other reductants, this hydroxyl radical production can even become a catalytic reaction, promoting DNA strand scission through attack on the sugar–phosphate backbone. Free metal ions with redox properties should be avoided, and supplement of e.g. iron(II) as nutritional additive is therefore not unproblematic. Fortunately, the organism possesses numbers of effective chelates, proteins like albumin, transferrin, etc. that to a certain limit will sequester redox-active iron- and copper ions. Other major biochemical targets of oxygen seem to be lipids and proteins. Thus, elevated levels of oxygen are clearly toxic for mammals leading first to coughing and soreness of the throat and eventually to pulmonary edema and irreversible lung and other tissue damage.

13.4.5   The *trans*-effect

As mentioned in Section 13.4.3, Pt(II) (low-spin d^8 electron configuration) preferentially forms square planar complexes which are both stable and inert. Many other low-spin d^8 systems also form square planar complexes, e.g. Ni(II), Pd(II), Au(III), and Ir(I). The kinetics of this type of co-ordination compounds have been investigated thoroughly, and it was shown that all of these complexes generally undergo nucleophilic substitution.

That these four-co-ordinated complexes are square planar rather than tetrahedral, which is otherwise the preferred geometry, was observed early in the twentieth century. The fact that a compound like $Pt(NH_3)_2Cl_2$ could be produced in two forms demonstrated that the geometry could not be tetrahedral. One form was produced by reacting $PtCl_4^{2-}$ with ammonia while the other form could be obtained by heating solid $[Pt(NH_3)_4]Cl_2$. Since the complexes were monomeric, it was concluded that they were *cis/trans* isomers. Further studies demonstrated that the first reaction led to a *cis* configuration and the latter to the *trans* isomer. The rationale behind this behavior which also applies to the function of '*cis*-platinum' as an antitumor agent is called the *trans*-effect, and the concept correlates many of the reactions of square planar Pt(II) complexes.

The utility of this *empirical* rule can be illustrated by the synthesis of *cis*- and *trans*-$Pt(NH_3)_2Cl_2$ which is in keeping with the concept of the *trans*-effect (Figure 13.6). In the upper row, we begin with $PtCl_4^{2-}$; in the second row the starting material is $Pt(NH_3)_4^{2+}$. The negatively charged chloride ion has a greater labilizing effect on a group sitting opposite to it (*trans* position) than on a group in *cis* position. Also, this labilizing effect is usually larger for a negative ligand than it is for a neutral σ-bonding molecule like ammonia. In the upper reaction scheme of Figure 13.6, the second ammonia molecule will enter in a *cis* position since the chloride ion has a larger *trans* directing effect than that of ammonia. In the lower reaction series, the ammonia molecule opposite the chloride ion will be the most labile one and the result will be that Cl^- ion number two enters into the *trans* position. The empirical rule is thus quite useful, and in the section on *cis*-platinum (13.8.5) we shall see why the *trans* form is inactive as a cytostatic drug.

Briefly the *trans*-effect can be outlined as follows: The rate of substitution of a ligand is determined by the nature of the substituent at the opposite end of the diagonal (in *trans* position). Thus, while the chemical bond between the metal ion and any substituent is little affected by the character of neighboring

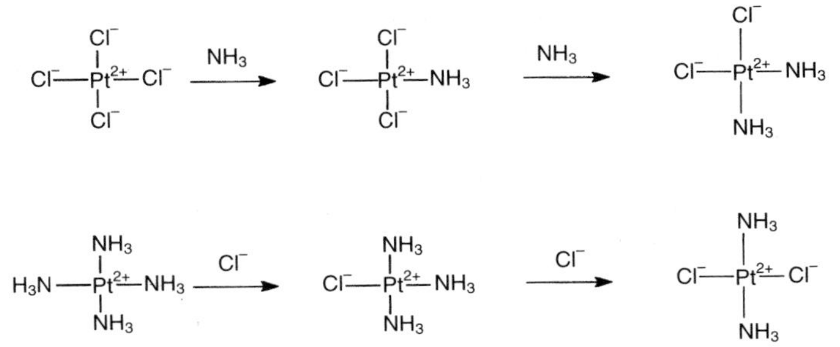

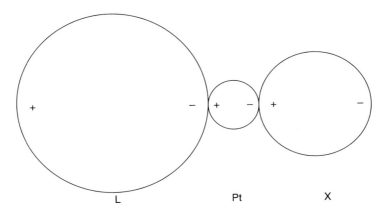

Figure 13.6 Illustration of the *trans*-effect. Synthesis of *cis*- and *trans*-[PtCl$_2$(NH$_3$)$_2$]. In the upper reaction, the second ammonia molecule enters a *cis*-position because the *trans*-directing influence of the chloride ion is larger than that of ammonia. In the lower process, a chloride ion replaces the most labile ammine ligand which is opposite, the chloro group.

molecules (*cis* position), it is greatly influenced by those farther away in the *trans* position. The approximate order of increasing *trans*-effect for typical ligands is

$$H_2O < OH^- < NH_3 < Cl^- < Br^- < I^- < NO_2^- < NO < CO < CN^-$$

It is worth emphasizing that the *trans*-effect is an empirical rule and based on kinetic effects and thus does not reflect the thermodynamic stability of a complex. The effect can nevertheless be dramatic. A complex containing a ligand with a large *trans*-directing effect may undergo substitution at rates a factor of 10^6 or higher compared with a ligand lower in the *trans*-effect series.

The *trans*-effect is relatively easily explained in terms of ligand polarizability (Figure 13.7). It is therefore not surprising that the above series of *trans*-directing

Figure 13.7 Trans-effect. Distribution of charge-induced dipoles in L-Pt-X of *trans*-[PtA$_2$LX]. The two A ligands are not depicted.

ligands correlate with the classification of Lewis bases presented in Section 13.4.2. We consider the *trans*-effect of L on the ligand X in *trans*-PtA$_2$LX (the A ligands are not shown). The primary positive charge on the platinum(II) ion induces a dipole in L, which in turn induces a dipole in the metal ion. However, this dipole is oriented in such a way to repel donor electrons on the Lewis base, X. Thus, the Pt-X bond will be weakened (and lengthened). The theory explains immediately the correlation between *trans*-influence of L and its polarizability, e.g. $Cl^- < I^- < CN^-$. Further, it predicts that the effect will be larger if the metal ion is itself polarizable. This agrees with the observation that Pt(II) is stronger influenced than e.g. Ni(II) or Pt(IV).

13.4.6   Plasma mobilization index

It will often be of interest to predict how a given pharmaceutical influences the metal ion balance in an organism. This may, however, be quite complicated as several potential chelates usually are present, as for example amino acids, proteins, and inorganic anions in the blood plasma. In principle, the effect can be calculated by simulation of the multiple equilibria present in the biological fluid from known stability constants for the metal ion with the different ligands together with the ligands' acid–base properties. The useful concept of a plasma mobilization index (PMI) was introduced by May and Williams in 1977, but we shall define the concept in a slightly different manner. The metal ions in a biological system are assumed to be distributed among states involving metal–protein and metal–small molecule complexes, all in equilibrium. We now let $[M_{TOT}]$ indicate the concentration of all forms in which a given metal ion exists in the biological fluid containing some chelating drug, while $[M_P]$ denotes the total concentration of the metal ion in normal fluid. The PMI is now defined as

$$PMI = \frac{[M_{TOT}]}{[M_P]} \tag{13.1}$$

An example, using computer simulation based on known stability constants, is shown in Figure 13.8 where PMI curves are calculated for copper(II) and Zn(II) in plasma in the presence of the strongly chelating agent, *d*-penicillamine (D-PEN (see Section 13.6.2)). Here it is obvious that administrating even very small amounts of D-PEN (concentration $\sim 1\,\mu M$) the PMI for copper(II) is increased by a factor of 10 ($\log_{10} PMI = 1$) and there will be a ten-fold increase in mobilizing copper(II) ions with a possibility of either passing it on to some tissue or excreting it. Zinc(II) ions, in contrast, are influenced to a much smaller degree by D-PEN as can be seen from Figure 13.8. More complicated schemes involving several protein and small molecule complexes can of course be calculated in a similar way.

It is, however, often possible to perform a good estimate by the following simple approximate considerations. Let us as an example take Fe(III) in blood plasma (pH 7.4). Here the iron(III) is primarily bound to transferrin (Tr) which is present in a concentration of $10^{-8}\,M$. The stability constant for the Fe(III) transferrin complex is $10^{20}\,M^{-1}$. Suppose now that some iron(III) chelating drug (L) is

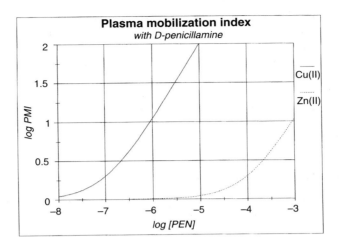

Figure 13.8 Plasma mobilization index curves. Simulated PMI curves calculated for d-penicillamine (D-PEN) using stability constants from the literature. Full line: Cu(II); broken line: Zn(II).

introduced which is essentially fully deprotonated at physiological pH ($pK_a < 6$) with a binding constant, K_L. We now have the following competing processes:

$$Fe(III) + Tr \rightleftharpoons Fe(III)Tr \qquad K_{Tr} = 10^{20} \ M^{-1}$$
$$Fe(III) + L \rightleftharpoons Fe(III)L \qquad K_L$$

and may calculate the ratio between the concentrations of Fe(III)Tr and Fe(III)L:

$$\frac{[Fe(III)Tr]}{[Fe(III)L]} = \frac{K_{Tr} \cdot [Tr]}{K_L \cdot [L]} \tag{13.2}$$

where [Tr] and [L] are concentrations of free transferrin and drug, respectively. If this is inserted into the expression for PMI we find:

$$PMI = \frac{K_L \cdot [L]}{K_{Tr} \cdot [Tr]} + 1 \tag{13.3}$$

In order for the drug to perturb the metal ion balance, the product $K_L \cdot [L]$ should be larger than $K_{Tr} \cdot [Tr]$. In the present example, the latter product is 10^{12} so if the stability of the drug–metal ion complex for example is $10^{10} \ M^{-1}$ the drug will play no role whatsoever in affecting the Fe(III) ion distribution in the plasma. Realistically, a concentration of a given pharmaceutical cannot exceed 1 mM. Thus, in this simplified example the iron(III) balance will only become perturbed if chelating agents with binding constants above 10^{15} are involved. Such drugs are known and used under certain circumstances (see Section 13.8.4).

For metal ions like calcium(II) which do not bind as strongly to chelates in the plasma (stability constants around $10^6\,M^{-1}$) the situation can be quite critical. Administrating drugs like tetracycline (Section 13.7.1) may affect the physiological calcium ion balance seriously.

13.5 CHELATE THERAPY

As demonstrated in Figure 13.2, inadequate supply of essential elements will lead to deficiency symptoms. However, the same elements will in excess be directly toxic irrespective of whether the excess is caused by insufficient excretion or extravagant intake. That heavy metals constitute a hazard to the health is well known. Both types of toxication can be treated by using antagonists (chelate therapy) which involves complex binding (sequestration) and transport of acutely poisonous elements by means of polydentate ligands (Table 13.4). When realizing the number of essential elements found in the organism, it is obvious that selectivity plays a vital role and thus constitutes a fundamental challenge in bioinorganic chemistry. Development of chelating pharmaceuticals that selectively sequester the undesired (heavy) metal ions becomes imperative; and here our knowledge of co-ordination chemistry becomes profitable. The most successful ligands demonstrate selectivity by (i) exclusive fitting to ions of definite size and charge; (ii) comprising donor atoms that prefer Lewis acids of certain hardness or softness (Section 13.4.2). Further, the chelates must (iii) form thermodynamically stable and kinetically inert co-ordination compounds (Section 13.4.1–13.4.5); and finally (iv) be able to excrete the undesired metal ion rapidly and effectively.

13.5.1 Synergistic chelate therapy

The purpose of chelate therapy is to couple proper sequestration with effective excretion; thus, combining several ligands is often exploited. In order to transfer a target metal across the membrane and out of the cell, the complex should be lipophilic and neutrally charged. Conversely, in the extracellular environment, it would be advantageous if the metal ion is co-ordinated in an electrically charged complex which is water soluble in order to be excreted through the kidneys. An example of synergistic chelate therapy is treatment of mercury(II) poisoning. Hg(II) ions will chelate strongly to the thiolate groups in BAL (Section 13.6.1) forming an electrically neutral compound. Since the complex is lipophilic, it is soluble in the membrane, and thus can be effectively conducted out of the cell by a

Table 13.4 Chelating ligands towards toxic metal ions

Ligand	Commercial or trivial name	Preferred metal ions
2,3-dimercapto-1-propanol	Dimercaprol (BAL)	$Hg^{2+}, As^{3+}, Sb^{3+}, Ni^{2+}$
D-β, β-dimethylcysteine	D-penicillamine, (D-PEN)	Cu^{2+}, Hg^{2+}
Ethylenediaminetetraacetic acid	EDTA	Ca^{2+}, Pb^{2+}
Desferrioxamine	DFO, desferral	Fe^{3+}, Al^{3+}

passive transport. Outside the cell, EDTA might sequester the Hg(II) ions in a charged Hg(II)EDTA^{2-} complex that may gently be excreted with the urine. Due to the high electrical charge, anionic forms of EDTA as such cannot pass the cell membrane. Another example of synergism is the enhanced elimination of iron when treatment with desferrioxamin is combined with addition of ascorbic acid.

13.6 SELECTED CHELATES

13.6.1 BAL

The first example of chelate therapy was performed during World War II when BAL (2,3-dimercapto-1-propanol; British Anti Lewisite (Figure 13.9)) was applied as antagonist against arsenic containing poison gas. BAL, being a very soft Lewis base, will preferentially co-ordinate to soft heavy metal ions. Thus, aside from As, the chelate will be highly efficient in treatment of mercury toxication. Today, however, BAL is exclusively utilized in connection with acute gold poisoning in patients undergoing treatment with gold containing pharmaceuticals (Section 13.8.6). BAL is a yellowish liquid with only limited solubility in water and with a very unpleasant odor. An advantage of BAL is its lipophilic character which facilitates transport into the cells. However, the drug itself is toxic and must be administered with great care.

A related chelate is unithiol (2,3-dimercaptopropanesulphonic acid) which is a derivative of BAL. This compound is water soluble and so are the stable heavy metal ion complexes. Unithiol may be used extracellularly in the treatment of acute toxication with the soft heavy metals like copper, lead, mercury, and cadmium.

13.6.2 D-penicillamine

The structure of D-penicillamine (D-PEN) is shown in Figure 13.9 where the three different donor groups should be noticed: Two hard donor atoms (amine-N and carboxylate-O) together with the soft thiolate ($-SH$) group. This makes the chelate a universal drug for both soft and hard Lewis acids but showing limited ion selectivity, however. D-PEN is water soluble and, in contrast to BAL, not inherently toxic. Nevertheless, the L-isomer is a vitamin-B$_6$ antagonist and thus harmful to the organism. D-PEN has found wide application and may in most cases replace BAL. It is often applied simultaneously with EDTA as in the treatment of lead poisoning and is also effective sequestering gold and mercury. Of particular interest is the administration of D-PEN to patients suffering from Wilson's disease (Section 13.8.6).

13.6.3 EDTA

Ethylenediaminetetraacetic acid (EDTA) (Figure 13.4), and its analogs are all excellent chelates sequestering most metal ions, but for this same reason not very

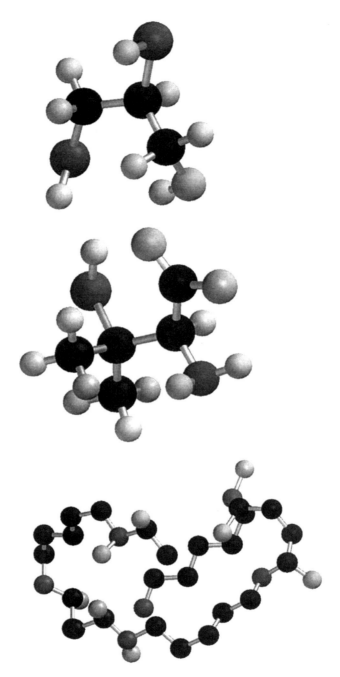

Figure 13.9 Selected ligands from Table 13.4. Structures of BAL (upper), D-PEN (center), and DFO (lower). Carbon atoms are black, oxygen light gray, nitrogen and sulfur dark gray. Hydrogen atoms (light) are only shown in the two former structures. The structure of EDTA is illustrated in Figure 13.4.

selective. EDTA co-ordinates preferentially to hard metal ions (Section 13.4.2) and due to the large chelate effect quite stable complexes are formed. EDTA is only slowly metabolized in the organism with a biological half-life of 1 h. Since EDTA is only inadequately absorbed from the gastrointestinal tract, it is usually administered by intravenous injections. But due to the low degree of selectivity the hazard of eliminating essential metal ions is high. Adding the drug as Na_2H_2EDTA, the serum concentration of calcium ions will be lowered (Section 13.4.6), possibly with severe muscle spasms as a result. Instead, the CaH_2EDTA salt is recommended, and in general the diet should be supplemented with essential metal ions during EDTA treatment.

13.6.4 Desferrioxamine

The siderophores are naturally occurring small molecule chelates secreted by many micro-organisms in order to extract iron from the surroundings. One important example of a siderophore is desferrioxamine (DFO, desferral) (Table 13.4 and Figure 13.9). The molecule is seen to contain a large amount of (hard) oxygen donor atoms which in an octahedral geometry render it highly specific towards iron(III), with a stability constant of not less than $10^{31}\,M^{-1}$ for the chelate. Other siderophores show stability constants for Fe(III) complexation up to $10^{50}\,M^{-1}$. The chelate is used in the treatment of acute iron poisoning and in certain cases of anaemia where iron is accumulated in liver and heart. The binding constants for the corresponding Fe(II) complexes are much smaller due to larger ionic radius and smaller charge of this ion, and release of iron can be induced simply by reduction of the Fe(III) ion. Since the co-ordination chemistry of Al^{3+} is quite similar to that of Fe^{3+}, DFO can also be used in cases of aluminum poisoning (Section 13.8.4). Incidentally, chelate formation also lies behind the body's strategy of producing fever in cases of infections. The higher temperature kills bacteria by reducing their ability to synthesize particular iron chelating ligands.

DFO and other siderophores have also been exploited as potential antimalarial chemotherapeutics. As free ligands they may block the iron metabolism, but the pharmacological prospects are not ideal (see Section 13.8.4).

13.7 DRUG–METAL ION INTERACTION

Many pharmaceuticals are inherently excellent chelates and may as such interact with metal ions, intra- as well as extracellularly. This interaction can be beneficial but also injurious. Favorable effects are seen where complex formation induces better uptake or transport of the drug while detrimental consequences occur if drug uptake is precluded. The effect is determined by a number of factors like charge, structure, and presence of hydrophobic or hydrophilic groups. The HSAB principle (Section 13.4.2) and knowledge of the chemistry of co-ordination compounds (Section 13.4.3) become useful in this context. Some examples are given in the following sections.

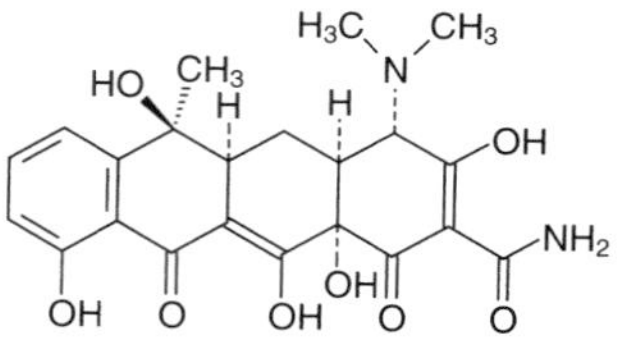

Figure 13.10 Drawing of the tetracycline molecule. Notice the abundance of oxygen atoms (hard bases).

13.7.1   Undesirable interactions

A well-known example of a harmful drug–metal ion interaction is inhibition of tetracycline uptake in the organism by calcium, zinc, and iron ions. The structure of the drug is shown in Figure 13.10, and it is seen that the molecule comprises a large number of (hard) donor atoms, first and foremost oxygen. Thus, it comes as no surprise that many hard metal ions will bind to this drug. Incidentally, the action of tetracycline seems to be related to its chelating ability to Mg^{2+} ions.

13.7.2   Beneficial interactions

Copper complexes with biological macromolecules will be treated in a later Section (13.8.6). But copper also co-ordinates to many pharmaceuticals and the anti-inflammatory effect of salicylic acid derivatives and also of other drugs involved in tissue repair seems to be related to Cu(II) chelation. The copper-containing enzyme lysyl oxidase catalyzes cross lacing of connective tissue, and copper ions are mobilized by co-ordination to smaller organic ligands. The same strategy of copper mobilization occurs with superoxide dismutase (Section 13.8.6), another important copper containing enzyme which catalyzes degradation of the superoxide radical, O_2^-:

$$2O_2^- + 2H^+ \rightarrow O_2 + H_2O_2$$

A Fe(II) chelate isolated from a *Streptomyces* fungus, bleomycin (Chapter 17) is exploited as an antitumour drug due to its ability to cleave DNA molecules (Section 13.8.4). A final important example of beneficial complex formation is related to zinc(II) ions. Zinc is found in the enzyme carbonic anhydrase which catalyzes the hydration of carbon dioxide (Section 13.8.7). Certain anti-epileptica, like acetazoleamide, co-ordinate to the zinc(II) ion directly in the enzyme and thus obstruct the catalytic transformation of carbon dioxide.

13.8   INORGANIC CHEMISTRY AND PHARMACEUTICALS

So far, the pharmaceutical industry has concentrated its effort mainly on developing drugs based upon organic chemistry and on natural products. However, the remaining part of the periodic table is manifesting itself with an ever increasing offering of diagnostics and genuine pharmaceuticals.

Table 13.5 Content of Na$^+$, K$^+$, and Cl$^-$ (concentrations in mM)

	Na$^+$	K$^+$	Cl$^-$
Sea water	460	10	550
Red blood cells	11	92	50
Blood plasma	160	10	100

13.8.1   Alkali metals

Sodium and potassium are found in large concentrations both in sea water and in the earth's crust. Thus, it is not surprising that all living organisms exploit these metal ions in relatively high quantities. In Table 13.5, some examples of Na$^+$, K$^+$, and Cl$^-$ (counter ion) content are presented.

The most important biological roles of sodium and potassium are (a) to stabilize cell membranes and enzymes by electrostatic effects and osmosis. Many biomolecules will thus denature when subjected to distilled water. Secondly, (b) these ions transmit electrical signals by diffusion through a certain concentration gradient.

Ions can be pumped actively across biological membranes against a concentration gradient, while the diffusion controlled concentration equilibrium proceeds passively through ion channels that are regulated chemically or electrostatically.

The most important difference between the chemistry of the individual alkali metals is due to their ionic radii and consequently the radius/charge ratio. Thus, the metal ions may possess individual functions in conjunction with specific ligands; the larger the radius the higher the co-ordination number becomes.

Lithium, sodium, and potassium exist in aqueous solution as labile hydrates (Section 13.4.3) which exchange water molecules extremely rapidly ($10^9 \, s^{-1}$ or faster). Many chelates form stable complexes with the alkali metals, such as EDTA. Lately, highly effective and specific ligands (ionophores) have been synthesized, like 'crown ethers' and 'cryptands'. Figure 13.11 shows a crown ether with a potassium ion attached.

In these compounds, the metal ions become co-ordinated to strategically positioned heteroatoms (O, N), and the size of the rings can be designed to adjust to certain metal ion radii. The biologically important aspect here is that the ion binds to heteroatoms on the inside of the macromolecule while the surface is more lipophilic. Consequently, such complexes will comfortably be transported across phospholipid double layers (5–6 nm) in biological membranes. Pharmacologically active natural products of this kind will function as antibiotics since they may transfer alkali metals in and out of the cells and thereby perturb the natural metal ion balance. Examples are valinomycin (Figure 13.12) and nonactin. The latter is, due to its size and number of binding centers, optimal for K$^+$ co-ordination (Table 13.6).

Another efficient method for controlled cation transport through lipid double layers involves incorporation of ionic channels in membranes. The gramicidins are relatively small peptides which have been used as antibiotics for more than 50 years. Dimers of the peptide form a tube that is 3 nm in length and with an inner diameter of about 0.4–0.5 nm. Thus, two dimers are needed to span inner to outer

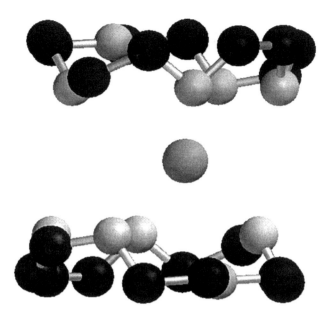

Figure 13.11 Crown ether with potassium. The potassium ion is seen squeezed in between the two ring systems and is co-ordinated to 8 oxygen atoms. Hydrogen atoms are not shown. Co-ordinates are taken from the Cambridge Crystallographic Data Centre.

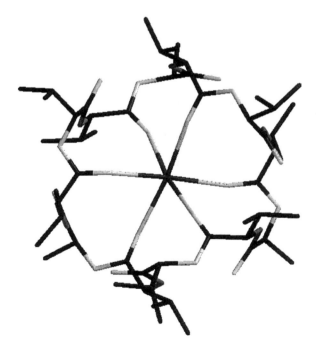

Figure 13.12 Potassium complex with valinomycin. Potassium is co-ordinated to 6 oxygen atoms. Co-ordinates are taken from the Cambridge Crystallographic Data Centre.

Table 13.6 Characteristic properties of alkali and alkaline earth metal ions

	Li^+	Na^+	K^+	Mg^{2+}	Ca^{2+}
Ionic radius (pm)	60	102	138	72	100
Co-ordination number	4	6	6–8	6	7–8
Preferred donor	oxygen	oxygen	oxygen	oxygen nitrogen phosphate	oxygen nitrogen

side of the membrane. The size of the hole restricts passage of ions to those with certain limited radii.

Lithium salts play a particular role in treatment of manic-depressive psychosis, and a large number of people take about 1 g of lithium carbonate each day. The effective plasma concentration is 1 mM while 2 mM exhibits toxic side effects, and already 3 mM is a lethal dose. The Li^+ ion has approximately the same radius as the Mg^{2+} ion, and both metal ions demonstrate high affinity phosphate binding. Lithium ions inhibit the enzymatic function of inositol monophosphatase thereby preventing release of phosphate from the active site. Inositol phosphatases are magnesium-dependent, and structural studies have shown that Li^+ may bind to one of the catalytic Mg(II) sites. Co-ordination of lithium ions to phosphate-containing messenger molecules could further perturb the *trans*-cellular communication which may be another rationale for its antipsychotic effect. Inositol phosphates are responsible for mobilizing calcium ions, and Li^+ will therefore influence the calcium ion level in cells, which makes it imperative to monitor the calcium concentration carefully in the patients during lithium treatment.

13.8.2 Alkaline earth metals

Among the essential metals, the magnesium ion, Mg^{2+}, has the smallest ionic radius which distinguishes it proficiently from Ca^{2+}. The high charge/radius ratio results in the Mg^{2+} ion being a particularly good Lewis acid with a preferred co-ordination number of 6. Binding (stability) constants for some representative complexes are given in Table 13.7.

Magnesium has an important role in stabilizing cell walls since it cross-laces the residing carboxylate and phosphate groups. The free magnesium ion concentration is typically 1 mM inside the cell. Deficiency in magnesium will induce accumulation of calcium ions as charge compensation intracellularly and eventually cause myospasms.

Table 13.7 Stability constants ($\log K$) of some typical Mg^{2+} and Ca^{2+} complexes at 25 °C and I = 0 M

	$\log K$	
	Mg^{2+}	Ca^{2+}
Acetate	1.3	1.1
EDTA	8.7	11
Glycine	3	1.5

Serious Mg^{2+} deficiency will result in mental and physical retardation, since magnesium is involved in the energy production (phosphate transport) and protein synthesis. The role of the magnesium ion seems to be essentially charge compensation for the negative charges of phosphate groups at pH 7. Mg^{2+} constitutes an essential part (prosthetic group) in a series of enzymes and in most cases phosphate seems to be involved. It is interesting to note that in spite of its great importance the concentration level of the magnesium(II) ion in the body is not controlled by some sophisticated physiological mechanism. It seems to be dictated solely by the solubility of the magnesium compounds with the anions present.

The calcium ion is probably the most important and ambidextrous of the essential metal ions in biology. The majority of this metal is found in the skeleton (about 1.0 kg in an adult person) while 10 g is engaged in a series of fundamental physiological processes from cell division and coagulation of blood to immune responses and muscle contraction. Deviations from the normal metabolism of the biominerals may lead to pathological effects, including deposition of calcium salts in blood vessels or in kidney stones. Also undesirable demineralization processes such as dental caries and bone resorption (osteoporosis) are commonly observed.

Contrary to magnesium, the concentration of Ca^{2+} inside the cell is vanishingly small, about 10^{-7} M, while the extracellular concentration is in the mM range. This requires very effective and specific calcium pumps in order to sustain this huge concentration gradient. Calcium is taken up in the small intestine bound to the active form of vitamin-D, in a yield of 50%. Excess of calcium is excreted through the kidneys.

Due to the larger size of the Ca^{2+} ion relative to that of Mg^{2+} (Table 13.6), calcium is often found attached to proteins with a co-ordination number of 7 or 8. Proteins with many acidic groups are particularly effective ligands for calcium ions, and a well-known example is parvalbumin (Figure 13.13) a protein located in smooth muscles. This protein is related to the extended family of the structurally flexible calmodulins which also co-ordinate to certain enzymes thereby activating them. Calmodulins are monomeric proteins consisting of a chain of 148 amino acids which are capable of binding up to four calcium ions. The 3D-structure was first determined for parvalbumin and termed the EF hand, where the letters E and F signify alpha helices. Another conformationally flexible class of calcium binding proteins, annexins, are important in cell regulation and blood coagulation.

Calcium ion release from storage proteins is the basis for the messenger function of Ca^{2+} ions which trigger liberation of a neurotransmitter, leading to opening of potassium ion channels. Calcium ion activation of phosphate transferring kinases should also be mentioned, due to its central role in muscle contraction and other Ca^{2+} controlled processes.

In association with membranes one finds some highly acidic calcium storage proteins called calsequestrines that bind up to 50 Ca^{2+} ions per molecule and release the metal ions through interactions with other macromolecules or by electrical impulses from nerve cells.

Barium sulphate (baryt) is used as X-ray contrasting agent and should as such not be confounded with barium carbonate which is dissolved in the acidic environment of the stomach. Ba^{2+} is highly toxic since it has an ionic radius similar to that of potassium and therefore will affect the cellular potassium transport.

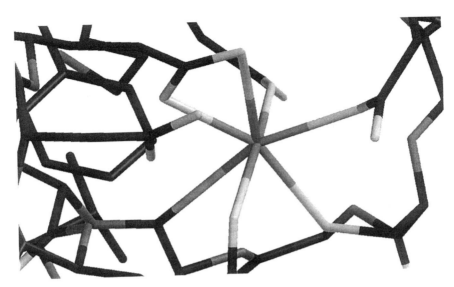

Figure 13.13 Molecular structure of parvalbumin. The metal ion center of parvalbumin. The calcium ion is shown seven-co-ordinated to peptide carbonyl and carboxylate oxygen atoms. A water molecule may further bind to the calcium ion. Co-ordinates are taken from the Protein Data Bank (1A75).

13.8.3   The chromium group

The chromate ion, CrO_4^{2-}, is carcinogenic but precisely why is not known. The ion shows resemblance to sulfate and indeed is carried inside the cell by the sulfate transporting system. In the cytoplasm, the chromate ion will react with sulfur-containing peptides like glutathione whereby Cr(VI) becomes reduced to Cr(V). In this oxidation state chromium reacts with DNA molecules, and oxidation of DNA is probably the reason for the mutagenic action.

Several decades ago, it was observed that vanadium(V) as the vanadate anion, VO_4^{3-}, could stimulate glucose uptake and glycogen synthesis. However, vanadate is too toxic for the human organism to be a useful insulin-mimetic. A new class of vanadium complexes have been synthesized with certain organic ligands and they seem to be less toxic to humans.

Cr(III) is, in contrast to Cr(VI), not carcinogenic. Indeed, it has been proposed that chromium in this oxidation state is of biological importance. It was earlier suggested that the glucose tolerance factor was a chromium(III) complex with nicotinamide and glutathione as ligands. This idea has now been abandoned, however. Still, it has been documented that diabetes mellitus can be affected in a positive manner by addition of Cr(III) compounds. The high level of chromium(III) in the plant, shepherd's bag, has been known and utilized by nature healers, but nowadays a water soluble chromium(III) nicotinamide complex is applied. The intrinsic problem with Cr(III) compounds is, as in the case of Fe(III), the inherently low solubility at pH 7. A tripicolinatochromium(III) complex is now marketed as a

Table 13.8 Distribution of group VIB metals in the earth's crust and in sea water (concentrations in ppm)

	Earth's crust	Sea water
Cr	100	$5 \cdot 10^{-4}$
Mo	1.5	0.01
W	1.5	$1 \cdot 10^{-4}$

nutritional supplement although its long-term biological effects on humans have not been fully characterized. The complex stimulates the activity of membrane spanning protein tyrosine kinases activated by insulin, but the mechanism is not fully understood and requires further examination.

There is no doubt about the importance of molybdenum being an essential trace element, which may derive from its relatively large abundance in sea water (Table 13.8). Mo is a constituent part of a series of enzymes all catalyzing biological oxidation- and reduction processes: N_2 reduction to NH_3 (nitrogen fixation); reduction of NO_3^- to NO_2^-; oxidation of SO_3^{2-} to SO_4^{2-}; oxidation of aldehydes to carboxylic acids; etc. All of these molybdenum-containing enzymes are exceedingly complex and contain other metal ions as well, often iron. The function of molybdenum is connected to its redox chemistry where, besides the stable Mo(VI) state, also complexes in the oxidation state (IV) have been characterized. Since molybdenum is generally found co-ordinated in poly-oxyanions, Mo is capable of mediating oxygen atom transfer as exemplified in some of the above processes. In Figure 13.14 is shown the prosthetic group in a Mo-containing enzyme, xanthine oxidase. Besides co-ordination to the protein by two thiolate side chains, Mo(VI) is also connected to two oxygen ligands.

Tungsten would seem to be precluded as an essential trace element. Nevertheless, some bacteria have been discovered that exploit W in the same manner as other species utilize Mo. It is interesting that both molybdate and tungstate oxyanions also demonstrate insulin-like effects.

13.8.4   Iron and cobalt

When oxygen, O_2, made its first appearance on the earthly scene about 2 billion years ago most of the living organisms probably perished. A few species survived by strictly isolating themselves in oxygen free pockets, becoming what nowadays would be labeled anaerobic organisms. New forms of life evolved, however, that were capable of exploiting the highly oxidizing property of dioxygen (aerobic organisms). Almost 20 times as much energy can be extracted from glucose in the presence of oxygen than in its absence. Thus, the need for oxygen transport as well as for the development of protective measures against undesirable redox processes (antioxidants) emerged.

Iron (together with copper) plays the leading role in all biological processes wherein oxygen turnover takes place. Iron(II) co-ordinates to a certain type of porphyrin and forms a complex labeled heme (Figure 13.15). Vertebrates utilize

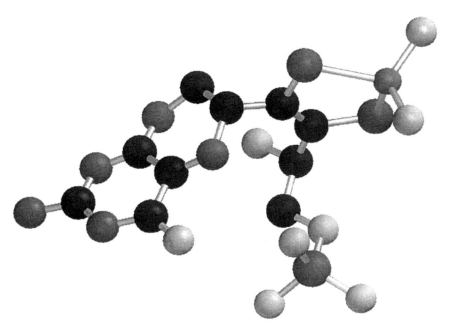

Figure 13.14 The prosthetic group in xanthine oxidase. The molybdenum ion is seen in the upper right corner co-ordinated in a tetrahedral arrangement to two thiolate sulfur atoms (dark gray) and two oxygen atoms (light gray). Co-ordinates are taken from the Protein Data Bank (1FIQ).

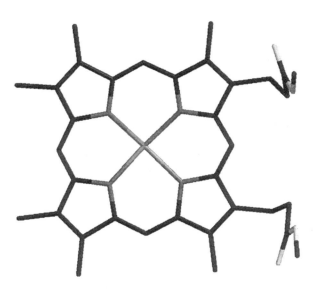

Figure 13.15 Heme. The heme prosthetic group consisting of an iron(II) ion complexed in a square planar geometry to four pyrrole nitrogen atoms of a substituted porphyrin ligand.

two such heme proteins for reversible O_2 transport and storage: Hemoglobin in red blood cells and myoglobin in muscle tissue. Anaemia results from insufficient dioxygen supply usually due to a low hemoglobin blood level. The oxygen molecule is co-ordinated axially to the heme group which contains a high spin (d^6) Fe(II) ion. The resulting oxo compound is, however, a low spin complex which stabilizes the Fe(II) state (Section 13.4.3) and thus prevents oxidation to Fe(III).

Cytochromes are heme proteins but here the shift between Fe(III) and Fe(II) is exploited in order to take up and deliver electrons. The reduction potentials extend over a huge range (+400 to −400 mV vs. the standard hydrogen electrode) which is brought about by exchanging the axial ligands. Anions stabilize Fe(III) and cause lowering of the standard potentials while co-ordination of aromatic and hydrophobic groups will cause an increase in the stability of the Fe(II) state.

Cytochromes are further part of the important respiration enzyme, cytochrome c oxidase which catalyzes the reduction of O_2 to H_2O. The enzyme activates and reduces 95% of the dioxygen we consume and couples exergonic O_2 reduction to endergonic proton pumping to drive ATP (adenosine triphosphate) synthesis. The organism is applying ATP for synthesizing important macromolecules (carbohydrates, proteins, lipids, etc.). There is now a rather good understanding of the reaction cycle of this large protein and the 3D-structure is also known with high precision.

Another significant heme enzyme is cytochrome P-450 which as a dioxygen activating metalloporphyrin catalyzes a series of important biological oxidation processes. Enzymatic monooxygenation reactions, e.g. the conversion of vitamin-D or transformation of drugs like morphine are examples of such processes. Unwanted reactions like epoxidation of benzene to produce carcinogenic derivatives or oxidation of nitrosamines to form reactive radicals are examples of a toxicological function of cytochrome P-450. An iron(V) oxo complex is the favored model for the activation of oxygen during the catalytic turnover.

Peroxidase and catalase are further illustrations of heme containing enzymes (antioxidants) which scavenge undesirable peroxides. There are also examples of other Fe-containing proteins which do not accommodate the heme group but where iron is co-ordinated in a cave-like complex together with sulfur. Some of these proteins possess a catalytic action and constitute part of redox enzymes.

Malaria is a devastating infectious disease killing close to 2 million children annually. The commonly used antimalarial therapy has become increasingly ineffective due to chloroquinone resistance. However, a new series of drugs based on tervalent metal ion co-ordination compounds like the ethylenediamine-*bis* [propylbenzylimino] Fe(III) complex exhibit highly selective activity, ironically particularly against chloroquinone resistant parasites. Heme, released from hemoglobin in the parasite, is very toxic to eukaryotic cells due to lysing of the membranes. In order to prevent this action the parasite polymerizes heme, but the above imino complexes inhibit this protective process thereby destroying the host.

Iron is the most abundant transition metal in biological chemistry, and transport and storage of this metal have been studied assiduously. The big challenge here is that Fe(II) easily becomes oxidized to Fe(III) and that the products formed generally are highly insoluble at pH 7. The solubility product of $Fe(OH)_3$ is thus 10^{-38} M^4 which implies that at neutral pH the concentration of Fe^{3+} is only 10^{-17} M, unless

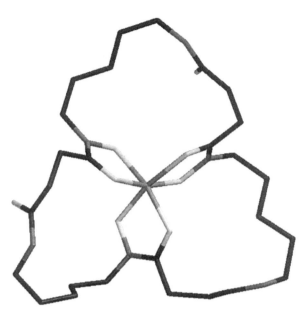

Figure 13.16 Structure of a siderophore. A siderophore iron(III) complex with hydroxamate groups (ferrioxamine). Fe(III) is co-ordinated to six oxygen atoms.

Fe(III) is sequestered to some chelate. Among the naturally occurring chelates we find the siderophores (Section 13.6.4). These compounds are either catecholates or hydroxamates (Figure 13.16) which form exceedingly stable complexes with Fe(III). The salmonella bacteria produce a siderophore which binds iron(III) with a stability constant of not less than 10^{50} M^{-1}. Another siderophore, desferrioxamine (Section 13.6.4) produced by the *Streptomyces* fungus is used in order to prevent iron poisoning in connection with blood transfusion. Pathogenic micro-organisms rely on a constant supply of iron, and therefore the availability of iron to bacteria invading the organism plays an important role in many diseases like cholera and tuberculosis where a decrease in iron content in the blood is invariably observed. The micro-organisms have to mobilize iron, but cannot exploit tightly bound iron in the blood serum. The heme–iron complex is very stable and iron can be liberated only by enzymatic degradation of the ligand. Effective iron scavenging chelates will thus act as potent antibiotics and naturally occurring iron complexing agents are therefore of great interest in medicine both as antibiotics and as drug delivery agents.

Iron as nutrient generally occurs by means of simple Fe(II) compounds although iron uptake is much more advantageous through the heme complex. Higher animals do not apply siderophores in the transport system but another protein called transferrin in which the metal ions are tightly bound to phenolate, carboxylate, and imidazole groups as well as to inorganic carbonate. Secured in this protein, Fe^{3+} is transferred into the cells where a concomitant hydrogen ion release takes place. Under these circumstances, the complex is much less stable and the iron(III) ions are released to the cytoplasm. Iron is immediately stored intracellularly (as FeO(OH) i.e. rust) in other non-heme proteins like ferritin and hemosiderin. The latter storage protein is particularly active during iron overload. When needed, iron ions are mobilized from ferritin by reduction of Fe(III) to Fe(II). Iron compounds are found in many redox processes including less desirable ones like free radical reactions. It is therefore of utmost importance that iron transport is carefully controlled. Chronic iron poisoning (hemochromatosis) usually originates from digestion of excess of the metal supplied from cooking utensils and results in corrosion of the gastrointestinal tract.

Other trivalent metal ions will also co-ordinate to transferrin, like Al(III) for instance. But since Al^{3+} cannot be reduced inside the cells, the process becomes irreversible and this is one rationale for the toxic effect of aluminium. Throughout the last decade it has been discussed whether aluminium is involved in Alzheimer's disease (see Chapter 10) where amyloid protein containing plaques concentrate in certain sections of the brain, e.g. the hippocampus. It has been demonstrated that Al^{3+} can cross link polynucleotides and that Alzheimer patients apparently have reduced transferrin activity. It also appears that exposure to aluminium in drinking water correlate with higher risk of attaining the disease. But this correlation does of course not necessarily mean causality, and a significant role of aluminium in the pathophysiology of Alzheimer's disease is unlikely.

Bleomycin (see Chapter 17) is an antitumor agent which is isolated from the *Streptomyces* fungus. Bleomycin couples to DNA with iron(II) ions co-ordinated to the peptide and, in the presence of dioxygen, a catalytic process is induced in which a phosphorous carbohydrate bond is broken. The mechanism is not fully comprehended but probably a Fe(V)-oxo compound is formed which may scavenge hydrogen atoms from the deoxyribose ring.

'Sodium nitroprusside', $Na_2[Fe(CN)_5NO]$ (Figure 13.17) is an active hypotensive agent used in treatment of heart infarct and in control of blood pressure during

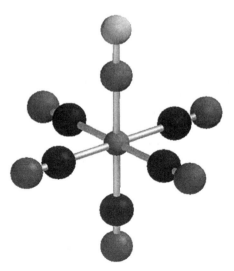

Figure 13.17 Nitroprusside. The 'nitroprusside' anion, $[FeCN_5NO]^{2-}$. The NO group is pointing upwards.

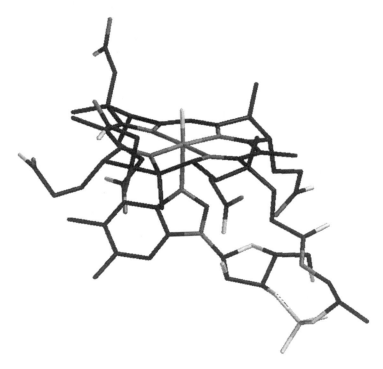

Figure 13.18 Coenzyme B$_{12}$. The prosthetic group in vitamin B$_{12}$. Besides co-ordinating to four corrin nitrogen atoms the cobalt(III) ion is also bound to an axial ligand, nitrogen from a benzimidazole group. Notice the vacant sixth position. This is the binding site for substrates. A phosphate group is seen in the lower right corner. Co-ordinates are taken from the Protein Data Bank (1CB7).

heart surgery. Release of NO causes relaxation of the muscles surrounding the blood vessels, probably by co-ordination of nitric oxide to an iron porphyrin receptor within the guanylate cyclase enzyme which converts guanine triphosphate to cyclic guanine monophosphate. NO is also synthesized in the human body in a process where an iron containing (heme) enzyme catalyzes oxidation of the amino acid, arginine, to nitric oxide.

The role of cobalt as essential trace element is confined to one function only, namely as the redox active metal ion in coenzyme-B$_{12}$ which contains a Co–C (adenosyl) bond. As early as in the 1920s, it was well established that pernicious anaemia could be cured with injections of extracts from liver samples, and trace element analysis demonstrated later that these extracts contained cobalt. A derivative of the co-enzyme, vitamin B$_{12}$, is the only essential cobalt compound known. One could term vitamin B$_{12}$ a natural drug since we cannot produce it ourselves. Co co-ordinates as Co^{3+} (low spin d^6) to a 15-membered corrin ring system reminiscent of the 16-membered porphyrin ring (compare Figure 13.15 with Figure 13.18), except that the ring has been diminished by one bond which coerces the ring system, in contrast to heme, to be non-planar.

The surprising observation upon examining the coenzyme-B_{12} structure is that one of the axial ligands can be an alkyl residue: $-C_nH_{2n+1}$. This is the only known example of a naturally occurring metal–carbon (metalloorganic) bond. The trivalent Co^{3+} ion in a low-spin d^6 hexaco-ordinated state becomes stabilized in a square planar geometry upon two electron reduction to Co^+ (d^8) (Section 13.4.3). The bond between cobalt and carbon is thus disrupted and the released ligand may be transferred to a substrate linked to the enzyme. With the coenzyme-B_{12} coupled to the right enzyme the rate of alkylation is accelerated up to 10^{10} times.

13.8.5 Platinum and ruthenium

The square planar 'cis-platinum' (cis-diamminedichloroplatinum(II); cisDDP) (Figure 13.19) is one of the most effective antitumor agents known. The detailed mechanism of its function is discussed in Chapter 17.

cisDDP is administered intravenously as an aqueous salt solution. Due to the large chloride ion concentration (~0.1 M) in the plasma the complex retains its composition and as an uncharged molecule it can diffuse (passively) across the cell membrane and enter the cell. However, here the chloride concentration is considerably smaller (~3 mM) and the complex is rapidly transformed into the cationic aqua complex, $[Pt(NH_3)_2(H_2O)_2]^{2+}$ (a thermodynamic effect). Since water molecules, as discussed in Section 13.4.5, have a lower trans-directing effect than ammonia they are easily substituted by other and better co-ordinating groups, e.g. base molecules like guanine from DNA. An equivalent complex can for steric reasons not be formed with the trans-isomer. In Figure 13.20, a model complex with two neighboring guanine bases is displayed. The co-ordination of platinum to guanosine in cis[Pt(NH_3)_2{d(pGpG)}] destroys the stacking of the bases and causes a sharp bend in the DNA helix structure (70–90° in contrast to the typical 10° in DNA).

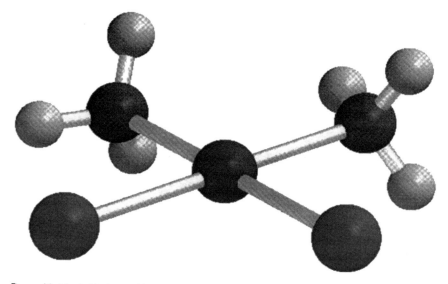

Figure 13.19 cis-Platinum. The square planar cis-diamminedichloroplatinum(II) complex.

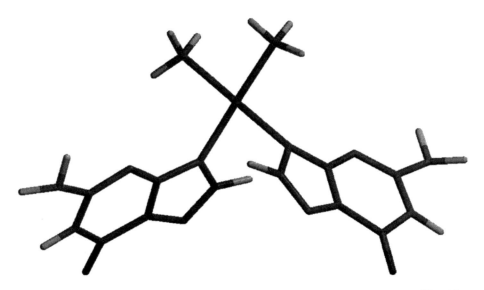

Figure 13.20 Platinum-DNA model complex. Square planar complex of platinum(II) with two ammine and two guanine ligands.

A pertinent question is now why the *cis*DDP drug (to some degree) selectively destroys tumor cells rather than normal healthy cells. Certain proteins have been isolated in human cells, 'high mobility group' proteins (HMG) which function as transcription factors. It has been observed that HMG proteins recognize and bind to the *cis*-platinum-DNA adduct. A consequence of such binding is inhibition of nucleotide excision which means that the adduct may block the *in vivo* repair in these cells. Apparently, the HMG proteins are expressed predominantly in tumor cells. This repair-shielding hypothesis would explain why tumor cells are particularly sensitive to *cis*-platinum. Figure 13.21 shows binding of HMG to DNA containing *cis*[Pt(NH$_3$)$_2${d(pGpG)}].

Tumor cells are known to contain a large concentration of transferrin receptors. This can be utilized in targeting strategies either by blocking iron uptake or for transfer and release of cytotoxic metals complexes inside the cells. Ruthenium(III) shows a very large affinity towards the imidazole side chain of histidine and by co-ordinating to one of the Fe(III) binding sites (His) in transferrin, Ru(III) is taken up by the cells. Ru(III) complexes with heterocyclic ligands like imidazole, indazole and bipyridine all show high activity against tumor metastases. Like for *cis*-platinum, aquation of the complex seems to be an important step. Ru(III) complexes are probably prodrugs which are reduced inside the cell to the more reactive Ru(II) species. The complexes bind to DNA, preferentially to N-7 of guanine bases.

13.8.6 Copper, silver, and gold

Copper and iron constitute the most important redox active transition metals in bioinorganic chemistry, and they seem to complement each other. Both

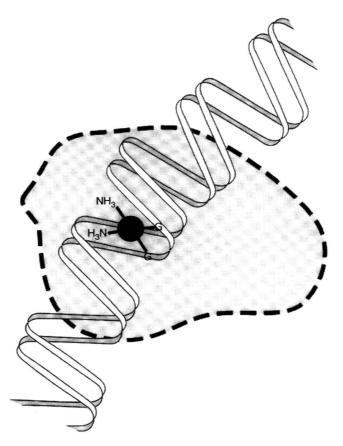

Figure 13.21 Binding of HMG to *cis*[Pt(NH₃)₂{d(pGpG)}]. Schematic drawing of how the high-mobility-group protein may bind to *cis*-platinum modified DNA.

copper- and iron proteins are involved in oxygen transport and charge transfer. But while the iron containing proteins and enzymes are always found intracellularly copper proteins and enzymes operate outside the cells. Molluscs (snails, clams, etc.) and arthropods (arachnids, crustaceans, etc.) utilize an extracellular copper protein, hemocyanin for oxygen transport, i.e. an analog to the intracellular iron containing heme protein, hemoglobin.

In humans, most copper is found in the brain and in heart and liver. The high metabolic rate of these organs requires relative large concentrations of copper containing enzymes, some of which are presented below. Not surprisingly, copper deficiency leads to brain diseases and anaemia.

Copper is also found in many oxygenating enzymes, i.e. proteins which catalyze the incorporation of oxygen into organic substrates. An important example is dopamine-β-hydroxylase which catalyzes an insertion of oxygen into the β-carbon of the side chain of dopamine to produce norepinephrine. This enzyme contains

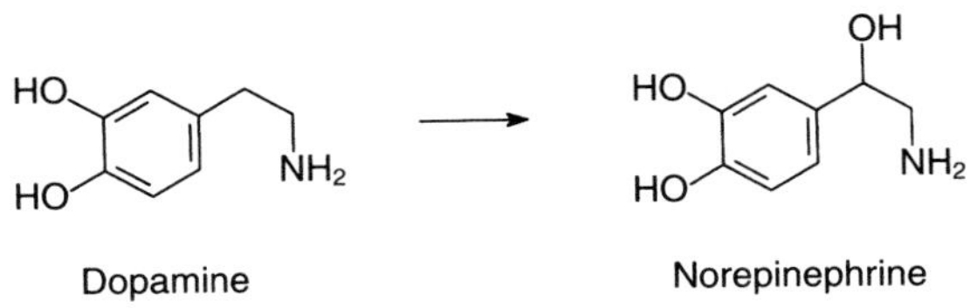

Figure 13.22 Dopamine-β-hydroxylase oxygenation of dopamine (left) to norepinephrine (right). The reducing substrate, ascorbate, reduces both Cu(II) ions to Cu(I) in the enzyme, one of which then binds to the oxidizing substrate, O_2.

one pair of Cu(II) ions per active center. Ascorbate reduces the copper(II) ions to Cu^+ which bind O_2 whereupon the hydroxylation takes place (Figure 13.22). The two copper ions in this enzyme are at least 0.4 nm apart and hence catalysis is unlikely to involve a binuclear copper center. Instead a model has been proposed in which the two copper ions perform different functions; one copper is involved in electron transfer from ascorbate while the other binds dioxygen and performs the substrate hydroxylation. Another member of this class of proteins, peptidyl-α-amidase catalyzes the conversion of C-terminal glycine extended peptides to their bioactive amidated forms, and hence is responsible for the biosynthesis of essential neuropeptide hormones like vasopressin and oxytocin.

Copper is also integrated into the so-called oxidases that catalyze the reduction of dioxygen to water. Here we find the very important enzyme, cytochrome *c* oxidase which besides two Fe-heme groups include three copper ions in two distinct centers. This enzyme has already been discussed in Section 13.8.4. Many other oxidases exclusively contain copper and often in functional groups of 4 metal ions at a time. Ceruloplasmin is a 130 kDa multicopper oxidase which is widely distributed in vertebrates. It occurs in plasma and plays an important role in iron homeostasis. Other functions include its participation in antioxidant defence and in processes related to metabolism of copper, biogenic amines, and nitric oxide. Its main physiological function seems to be the ferroxidase activity, and inherited mutations or targeted disruption of the ceruloplasmin gene leads to impaired iron efflux from cells. Oxidation of Fe(II) released from cells and its subsequent incorporation into apotransferrin is the mechanism wherby ceruloplasmin is involved in mediating iron from cellular stores.

The human variant of the antioxidant enzyme, superoxide dismutase, contains both copper and zinc (13.7.2). The toxic superoxide anion, O_2^-, is sometimes deliberately produced by organisms for particular objectives. Thus, some phagocytes which are part of the immune system in higher organisms produce large quantities of superoxide together with peroxide and hypochlorite by means of oxidases in order to kill invading micro-organisms. In unfortunate cases this protection system may fail giving rise to certain autoimmune diseases like rheumatoid arthritis. Under these circumstances superoxide dismutase is administered as an anti-inflammatory pharmaceutical. The same therapy is consistently applied during open heart surgery in order to protect the tissue against oxidative attack by the superoxide radical. Also the process of aging and neurodegenerative diseases like amylotropic lateral sclerosis have been linked to O_2^- production.

A large group of electron transfer proteins is found in which a single copper ion is co-ordinated per molecule. They partake in e.g. the photosynthesis and in the bacterial respiration system.

Copper is a potent poison for any cell and thus proteins of the metallothionein type (Section 13.8.7) exist which will transport excessive copper ions out of the cells. Due to the delicate balance between plethora and deficiency of copper a tight control of uptake and excretion of this metal is needed. Excess of copper leads to copper accumulation in liver and brain which untreated leads to severe damage of these organs and results in early death (Wilson's disease). Therapy with powerful copper chelates like d-penicillamine (Section 13.6.2) can keep the copper concentration on a suitable level. Deficiency in copper is just as serious since it leads to grave mental and physical illnesses (e.g. Menkes' disease). Like in Wilson's disease it involves a hereditary dysfunction in copper metabolism. The gene is localized on the X chromosome and both the intact and the defect gene have been cloned. The corresponding Cu-containing ATPase has been shown to posses a large content of cysteines which tightly bind the soft Cu(I) ions.

Certain copper complexes also exhibit antitumor activities. The compounds should be uncharged (lipophilic) and co-ordination compounds between Cu(II) and phenanthroline, thiosemicarbazone and salicylic acid derivatives have proven effective in treatment of certain forms of leukemia.

The term 'prions' is used to describe proteins involved in certain neuro-degenerative maladies like the Creutzfeld–Jacob disease. In the primary sequence of a prion protein an octapeptide sequence ProHisGlyGlyGlyTrpGlyGln, repeated up to 10 times in certain pathologies has been identified. These octapeptides are gaining much attention as potential copper co-ordination sites, as this copper binding may induce conformational changes/oligomerization, responsible for the pathological forms of the prions.

Silver is of little interest in a bioinorganic context except that many silver(I) compounds can be used as effective antibacterial drugs, like silver sulfadiazene which is used clinically in ointments as an antimicrobial agent in instances of severe burns. Also silver nitrate has been applied in dilute solutions in cases of eye infections due to its antiseptic property. Small concentrations (<1%) of silver nitrate show low toxicity.

Gold, on the other hand, has been applied in certain contexts during history. Already the ancient Chinese several thousand years ago produced an elixir containing colloidal gold which should ensure eternal life. The benefit of this treatment has never been fully documented, however. Nevertheless, gold(I) compounds are currently the only class of drugs known to halt the progression of rheumatoid arthritis. Initially, gold compounds like gold sulfide and gold thiomalate were painfully administered as intramuscular injections. Later it was discovered that triethylphosphinegold(I) tetra-O-acetylthioglucose (auranofin, Figure 13.23) was equally effective and could be administered orally. As is seen, in this drug gold is co-ordinated as Au(I) to sulfur- and phosphorous containing ligands.

The mode of action of gold(I) compounds is still not explained satisfactorily. As an extremely soft metal ion Au(I) shows a large affinity towards soft bases like sulfur (thiolates) and phosphorous (phosphines) while the affinity towards

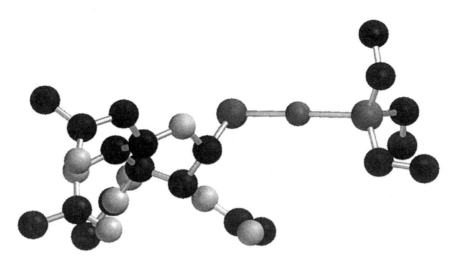

Figure 13.23 Auranofin. Gold(I) is co-ordinated linearly to a phosphine group (right) and a thiolate (left).

oxygen- and nitrogen containing ligands is small. Most Au(I) complexes have a co-ordination number of two and with a linear geometry. The Au(I) co-ordination in auranofin is shown in Figure 13.23. Several explanations have been propounded for the mechanism of gold(I) compounds in treatment of rheumatoid arthritis. In this context, it is interesting to note that the copper level is directly related to the extent of the disease. This has lead to proposals that anti-arthritic drugs like D-PEN and auranofin operate by affecting the center of co-ordination for copper ions, like the one found in human serum albumin. Albumin is the most abundant protein in plasma, with an approximate concentration ~0.6 mM. It consists of a single polypeptide chain including 585 amino acids one of which, in position 34, is a cysteine with a free thiolate side chain. As demonstrated by NMR studies, auranofin co-ordinates to this site and induces a conformational change in the protein. This affects the copper binding center in albumin (imidazole from a histidine group) whereby the copper homeostasis becomes perturbed. It has been suggested that the damage of the joints due to tissue inflammation is the result of lipid oxidation caused by free radicals such as O_2^-. This notion provides a link from gold to copper. Yet, in another hypothesis gold(I) complexes are suggested to inhibit formation of undesired antibodies in the collagen region.

It seems like the soft Lewis base, cyanide, plays a significant role in gold metabolism since patients who are in auranofin treatment excrete $[Au(CN)_2]^-$ in the urine. Cyanide ions are natural metabolites in the human organism and are formed by oxidation of thiocyanate by means of the myeloperoxidase enzyme. The dicyanoaurate(I) complex in itself possesses an anti-arthritic function and might be the proper active component. Thus, the ligand in auranofin (and in analogous gold(I) preparations) might just serve as binding and transport agent. The cyano complex has also been reported to exhibit anticancer and anti-HIV activity.

Gold-based pharmaceuticals unfortunately possess unpleasant side effects which include allergic reactions as well as gastrointestinal and renal problems. These side effects may be linked to the production of gold(III) metabolites which are strongly oxidizing. Patients with gold-related dermatitis exhibit an intense reaction to Au(III) exposure but not to Au(I). Strong oxidants as peroxide and hypochlorite, the latter synthesized *in vivo* from chloride by the myeloperoxidase enzyme in phagocytic cells, oxidize gold(I) to gold(III). Thus, a better understanding of the mechanism of gold preparations is indeed needed in order to produce more effective and less toxic gold-based drugs.

13.8.7   Zinc, cadmium, and mercury

Zinc is involved in a large number of biological processes and today more than 200 proteins containing Zn^{2+} are known. Among these, many essential enzymes are found which catalyze the transformation or degradation of proteins, nucleic acids, lipids, etc. Besides, the zinc ion stabilizes many different proteins like insulin. Thus, it is not very surprising that zinc deficiency will lead to severe pathological effects. The recommended daily intake of zinc is $\sim$15 mg (Table 13.1) only half of which is absorbed. Although food generally contains sufficient zinc to maintain this level, zinc deficiency occurs, producing effects like poor appetite, growth retardation, and skin lesions to mention but a few. The most affected enzymes are alkaline phosphatase and carboxypeptidase.

There is no ligand stabilization energy associated with the d^{10} Zn^{2+} ion which makes the metal ion quite tolerant to severe distortions of the preferred tetrahedral co-ordination. An important reason for cadmium, mercury, and lead poisoning is the ability of these ions to substitute for zinc in vital enzymes. The chemical advantage of zinc is first and foremost the high ionization potential of Zn^{2+} that makes it an excellent Lewis acid under physiological conditions at pH $\sim$7. When a substrate co-ordinates to Zn(II) in an enzyme, it becomes polarized and this includes both water, peptides, esters, and other molecules. The zinc ion thus manifests similar catalytic effect as strong acids, only at neutral pH. The pK_a value of a water molecule bound to zinc in an enzyme is typically less than 7.

Carbonic anhydrase is an enzyme which catalyzes the hydrolysis of CO_2:

$$CO_2 + H_2O \rightleftharpoons H^+ + HCO_3^-$$

and is of fundamental significance in respiration. The catalytic process occurs 10^7 times faster in the presence of the zinc enzyme compared with the uncatalyzed reaction. The process is delineated in Figure 13.24. Certain anti-epileptic pharmaceuticals like acetazil amide co-ordinate, as described earlier, directly to the zinc(II)

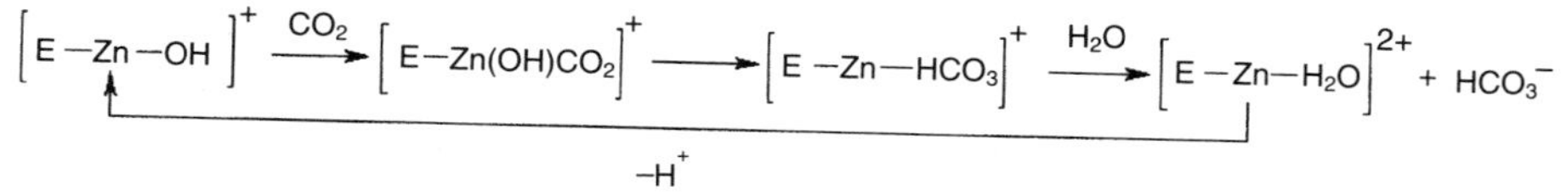

Figure 13.24 Function of carbonic anhydrase.

ion in the active center of the enzyme and thus obstructs the catalytic transformation of carbon dioxide. With accumulation of CO_2 in the blood stream pH drops, and it has been suggested that this perturbs the GABA concentration in brain cells, either by increasing the GABA synthesis or by blocking the process of degradation (see Chapter 9).

In the same manner zinc-containing enzymes do for example catalyze cleaving of peptides (carboxypeptidase) and transformation of alcohols into aldehydes (alcohol dehydrogenase). Primary and secondary alcohols are rapidly and reversibly oxidized to aldehydes and ketones, respectively, by alcohol dehydrogenase, which is therefore responsible for the large concentrations of acetaldehyde accumulating after oxidation of ethanol and leading to effects ranging from the 'hangover' syndrome to liver damages. The process involves NAD^+ dependent oxidation of the alcohol and is thus a redox reaction. The zinc(II) ion being redox inactive serves to bind and activate the substrate.

Collagenases, in which zinc is co-ordinated to three histidine ligands are essential for development of the embryo and for wound healing. Zinc dependent tissue-dissolving enzymes are also involved in degradation of amyloid proteins in AD (see Chapter 10). Another interesting aspect related to zinc containing proteases is snake toxin which contains enzymes that effectively dissolve connective tissue and inhibit blood clotting. These toxins, however, completely loose their effect by sequestration of the metal ion. Neurotoxins produced by the tetanus and botulinum bacteria also contain zinc dependent proteases which specifically destroy synaptic membrane proteins.

Insulin consists of two relatively short peptide chains, and in the pancreas the hormone is stored in different hexamer modifications which besides calcium contain two or four zinc ions. Insulin is mobilized by reversible removal of zinc ions by chelating agents. While Zn^{2+} only plays a structural role here, thiolate co-ordinated Zn(II) is found in the DNA repair protein where it recognizes mutagenic methylated forms of guanine bases and removes the methyl group.

A relatively new field involving zinc bioinorganic chemistry is the so-called zinc fingers, small proteins which recognize DNA base sequences and thereby contribute to regulation of the genetic transcription. The reason for their name, zinc fingers, is obvious as shown in Figure 13.25. Zinc(II) is co-ordinated in a tetrahedral geometry to two thiolates (from cysteine) and two imidazoles (from histidine) in the protein while neighboring amino acid residues (the fingers) protrude into the DNA molecule where they couple specifically to DNA base pairs by wrapping closely around the double stranded DNA, featuring several protein/base pair contacts and thus securing multiple recognition. Zinc co-ordination to thiolate cysteines has also been observed in proteins with repair function as well as in nucleic acid binding proteins of the HIV retrovirus.

Cadmium exhibits many chemical similarities to zinc and therefore binds to the same proteins. Cadmium, however, being a 'softer' Class b metal (Section 13.4.2) co-ordinates with higher affinity to sulfur containing amino acid residues. But since the Cd^{2+} ion is a much poorer Lewis acid than Zn^{2+}, cadmium incorporation into enzymes will impede any catalytic action. Thereby cadmium becomes significantly more poisonous than e.g. lead. Cadmium is absorbed through the food particularly from animal organs and from mushrooms. Certain small cysteine rich proteins,

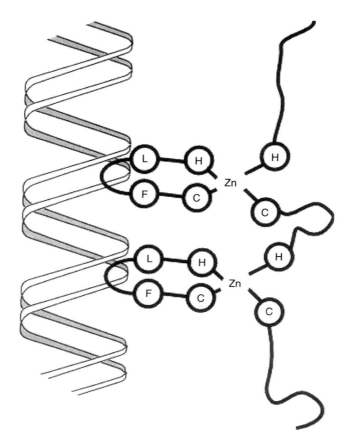

Figure 13.25 Zinc fingers. Zn(II) is co-ordinated to two cysteine (C) thiolates and two histidine (H) imidazoles in a tetrahedral geometry. Neighboring hydrophobic amino acids, leucine (L) and phenylalanine (F) form contact with DNA bases.

called metallothionein (Figure 13.26), are found in liver and kidneys. These proteins bind Cd^{2+}, Hg^{2+}, and Cu^+ (the soft metal ions) with very high affinity and thus serve in detoxication.

Mercury is even more toxic than cadmium due to the high solubility of the Hg^{2+} salts at physiological pH. Besides, metal organic mercury(II) compounds are easily formed (e.g. CH_3Hg^+, methyl mercury) which as chlorides are soluble in biological membranes and comfortably penetrate into the cells. Organic mercury compounds may be produced by bio-alkylation, i.e. the process catalyzed by vitamin B_{12} (Section 13.8.4). Cadmium and mercury compounds should under no circumstances be exposed to the environment, and notwithstanding the possible industrial usefulness, these metal ions should be operated in minimum amount and with great care.

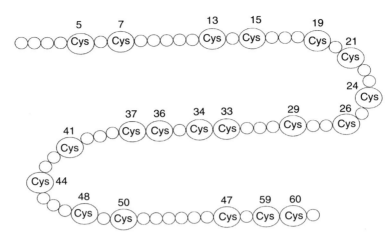

Figure 13.26 Metallothionein. Amino acid sequence of the metallothionein protein. Notice that approximately 1/3 of the amino acids are cysteine residues which will bind avidly to soft heavy metal ions.

13.8.8 Antimony and bismuth

As seen in Figure 13.1, arsenic might be an essential trace element while antimony and bismuth are not. However, the latter two elements have been applied in medicine for centuries. The early arsenic drugs developed by P. Ehrlich have already been mentioned (Section 13.1.2). As with arsenic the lower oxidation state of antimony(III) is the most toxic one, and only Sb(V) is used in pharmaceuticals. Presently, drugs based on antimony(V) complexes with polyhydroxy (carbohydrate) ligands are applied against diseases caused by certain parasites. Although the mechanism of action is not fully understood there are strong indications that Sb(V) is transferred to the particular site of attack where it becomes reduced to the more toxic Sb(III) which then destroys the parasite.

Bismuth compounds have been used extensively in treatment of gastrointestinal diseases. Due to the rather strong oxidizing properties of Bi(V), only drugs based on the 'softer' bismuth(III) ion are used, however. A potent antiulcer pharmaceutical is a colloidal Bi(III) citrate complex. Again, the mechanism of action is poorly understood, but polymers of the compound might be deposited in the ulcer wound forming a protective coating.

Some bismuth(III) complexes with sulfur containing ligands show high activity against the *Heliobacter pylori* bacteria. In this case inhibition of the nickel(II) containing enzyme, urease, that catalyzes the degradation of urea into carbon dioxide and ammonia, seems a plausible rationale for the antibacterial action. The ammonia produced from urea will neutralize the environment of the bacteria and help them to survive under the acidic conditions of the gastric lumen and mucosa (pH ~ 2). The antiulcer effect of the Bi(III) thiolate complexes is higher than for the thiolates alone, indicating that bismuth is more than just delivering the sulfur containing ligand to the target. A noteworthy feature of the complex

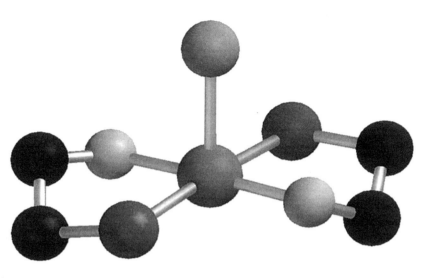

Figure 13.27 Bismuth antiulcer complex. Bismuth(III) complex with two chelating 2-mercapto-ethanol ligands and an axial chloride ion. Sulfur atoms are dark gray, oxygen atoms are light gray and carbon atoms black. Hydrogen atoms are not shown. The sixth position is occupied by an electron lone pair.

(Figure 13.27) is the position of a lone pair on one side of the bismuth co-ordination sphere. This may have an important bearing on the inhibitory function of the compound.

13.9   CONCLUDING REMARKS

As has hopefully come out of this chapter, the inorganic chemistry plays an increasingly important role in modern drug development. There are more than 25 elements with unambiguous importance for biological processes and in future pharmacology research, studies of uptake, metabolism, and excretion of these elements ought to be included. Besides, many compounds with other elements in the periodic table possess potential possibilities in development of biologically active complexes. In many cases, it will be possible to control metabolism of essential metal ions by means of organic pharmaceuticals since an intimate synergism exists between the function of inorganic elements and organic compounds of the body. As is well established, metal ions control some of the fundamental biochemical processes such as DNA and RNA replication, and many enzymes hereby hold a key position as pharmaceutical targets. A large need for development of new methods and strategies exists for testing inorganic compounds, and new techniques are further needed in modern pharmacological experimentation with inorganic molecules all the way from analytical tools to examination of co-ordination compounds in intact biological material. A larger emphasis should be put on kinetics rather than stability of inorganic compounds, since the most interesting biological processes, more often than not, take place rapidly and far from equilibrium. Hereby, a new and exciting field of research with a variety of challenges has opened in bioinorganic chemistry.

FURTHER READING

Cotton, F.A., Wilkinson, G. and Gaus, P.L. (1995) *Basic Inorganic Chemistry*. New York: J. Wiley.

Guo, Z. and Sadler, P.J. (2000) Medicinal inorganic chemistry. *Adv. Inorg. Chem.*, **49**, 183–306.

Kaim, W. and Schwederski, B. (1994) *Bioinorganic Chemistry: Inorganic Elements in the Chemistry of Life*. New York: J. Wiley.

Lippard, S.J. and Berg, J.M. (1994) *Principles of Bioinorganic Chemistry*. Mill Valley, California: University Science Books.

Sadler, P.J. (1991) Inorganic chemistry and drug design. *Adv. Inorg. Chem.*, **36**, 1–48.

Williams, R.J.P. and Frausto da Silva, J.J.R. (1996) *The Natural Selection of the Chemical Elements. The Environment and Life's Chemistry*. Oxford: Clarendon Press.

Chapter 14

Design and application of prodrugs

Claus S. Larsen and Jesper Østergaard

14.1 THE PRODRUG CONCEPT

14.1.1 Definition

As a result of rational drug design or the employment of combinatorial chemistry in combination with high throughput screening, a huge number of novel active molecules emerges. However, many such potential leads exhibiting high affinities towards a variety of molecular targets (i.e. receptors, enzymes, etc.) are, *per se*, prevented from becoming real drug candidates due to their inherent physico-chemical properties. This being based on the fact that only seldomly an active agent with optimal structural configuration for eliciting the desired therapeutic response at the target site possesses the best molecular form and properties for its delivery to the site of ultimate action (see Section 14.1.2).

There are several approaches that potentially can be taken in dealing with poor drug delivery characteristics. It is possible to circumvent some drug delivery problems by dosage form design. A second approach is to make a new drug analog of the original drug. In this approach, entirely new molecules exhibiting the desired physicochemical properties are designed; but changes in the pharmacological profile, as compared to the original drug, may be the outcome resulting in the demand for further expensive and time consuming biological testing. Often poor delivery characteristics of potential drug candidates are efficiently overcome by exploitation of bioreversible chemical derivatization or in other words the prodrug approach.

Prodrug design comprises an area of drug research devoted to optimization of drug delivery where the pharmacologically inactive prodrug requires trans-formation within the body in order to release the active drug. This approach has many advantages. First, the changes in physicochemical properties and the pharmacological profile of the drug are transient since the well-characterized parent drug molecule is regenerated from the prodrug *in vivo*. Second, introduction of a number of chemical transient changes in the drug molecule is possible allowing prodrug derivatives with a broad spectrum of physicochemical properties to be synthesized. The prodrug approach can be illustrated as shown in Figure 14.1. In this example, a drug molecule exhibits poor membrane permeability due to suboptimal physicochemical properties. By covalent attachment of a pro-moiety (or transport-moiety) to the active compound, a prodrug is formed, which overcomes the barrier for the clinical use of the drug. Once past the barrier, ideally, the

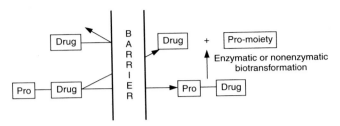

Figure 14.1 Schematic illustration of the prodrug concept.

prodrug undergoes quantitative chemical or enzymatic conversion to the parent compound (and a nontoxic transport-moiety). Prodrug formation can thus be considered as a means to mask temporarily undesirable physicochemical properties of the parent molecule.

14.1.2   Barriers to drug action

Administration of a prodrug is one of the avenues when attempting to control drug delivery and generate predictable drug concentration vs. time profiles at specific drug receptors. The rationale behind the prodrug approach is that the prodrug is capable of overcoming one or more of the barriers to drug delivery more efficiently than the parent drug. Some of the potential barriers related to the pharmaceutical and pharmacokinetic phase, respectively, are depicted in Scheme 14.1. The former phase comprises (i) incorporation of a potential drug entity into a convenient drug delivery system or a dosage form; and (ii) release of the active from the formulation whereas the pharmacokinetic phase embraces the absorption, distribution, metabolism, and excretion of the drug.

Major drug formulation barriers resulting from the physicochemical properties of the drug include

- Poor aqueous solubility
    - preventing the drug from being administered in form of injectables
    - giving rise to dissolution rate-limited (and variable) oral bioavailability
- Low lipophilicity
    - limiting the design of lipid-based formulations
- Chemical instability
    - preventing the drug from being incorporated into adequate dosage forms

In the pharmacokinetic phase, major barriers limiting the therapeutic value of an active agent, are

- Incomplete absorption across biological membranes such as the gastro-intestinal mucosa and the blood–brain barrier
- Low and variable bioavailability due to extensive first-pass metabolism

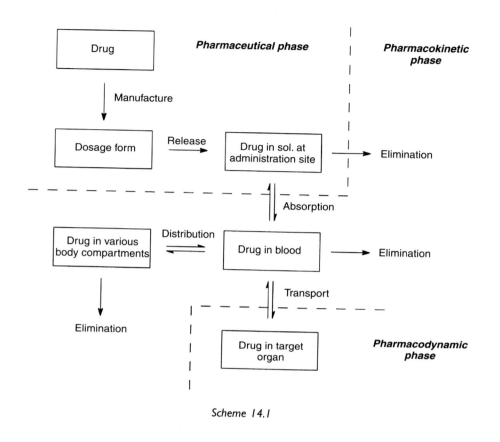

Scheme 14.1

- Too rapid absorption or excretion when a longer duration of action is desired
- Lack of site-specificity

14.1.3 Prodrug design in an industrial setting

An application for marketing authorization of a new chemical entity (NCE) is granted on basis of adequate demonstration of the quality, safety and efficacy of the drug. This comprehensive documentation comprises a compilation of the results obtained from a large number of multifaceted activities many of which are interrelated in such a manner that delay in one area may influence the momentum of other activities significantly. In order to minimize the time to marketed drug, it is therefore important to select the lead candidate early in the development process. A prerequisite for selecting the right candidate is that the appropriate amount of information is available at this decision point. Traditionally, lead selection has been based almost exclusively on target activities with little attention paid to the physicochemical and pharmacokinetic behavior of the potential leads.

In recent years, however, preliminary data related to the latter two areas have been included in the selection criteria.

The regulatory authorities consider a prodrug of a lead as a NCE. Thus, already performed studies (for example toxicity studies) using such a lead have to be repeated in case the prodrug is to be introduced in the development programme. From the above, proper exploitation of the prodrug approach appears most realistic if prodrug design constitutes, at least partly, an integral part of the drug design process. Attempts to identify suitable prodrug derivatives to improving drug therapy are obvious when recognized that the physicochemical characteristics of a highly interesting lead compound constitute an impediment to further development. In addition, utilization of prodrug design should also be considered in relation to (i) development of two or more dosage forms of the drug candidate; (ii) improved competitiveness of the drug in the marketplace accomplished by optimization of parameters like bioavailability or pharmacokinetic profile; and (iii) strategies in the areas of patent life time and product life circle management.

14.2   CHOICE AND FUNCTION OF THE PRO-MOIETY

Drug candidates may possess a variety of functional groups available for bioreversible chemical derivatization (see Section 14.3). Simple prodrug derivatives are obtained by direct attachment of a functional group of the pro-moiety to a functional group of the active agent. The types of sufficiently labile drug pro-moiety linkages formed in this way are limited for each chemical functional group as for example a carboxyl group. On the other hand, within a particular type of prodrug linkage bioreversible derivatives of a drug candidate such as carboxylic acid esters exhibiting significantly different properties might be designed dependently on the transport-moieties chosen (Figure 14.2). Thus, the desired rate and mechanism of cleavage of the prodrug bond might be accomplished by selection of an appropriate transport-moiety. In addition, the chemical nature of the applied pro-moiety influences the physicochemical and pharmacokinetic characteristics of the designed

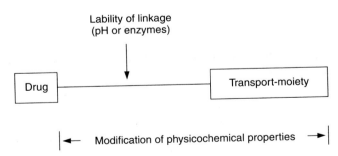

Figure 14.2 Function of transport-moiety to provide control of lability of prodrug bond and to optimize physicochemical properties.

prodrug as outlined below. Rational prodrug design, therefore, consists of three basic steps:

(1) Identification of the drug delivery problem
(2) Identification of the physicochemical properties required for maximum efficacy or delivery
(3) Selection of a transport-moiety providing a prodrug derivative exhibiting the proper physicochemical characteristics and which can be cleaved in the desired biological compartment

14.2.1   Cleavability of the prodrug bond

A basal prerequisite for the prodrug approach to be useful in solving drug delivery problems is the availability of chemical derivative types satisfying the prodrug requirements, the most prominent of these being reconversion of the prodrug to the parent drug *in vivo*. This prodrug–drug conversion process may take place before absorption, after entrance into the systemic circulation or at the specific site of drug action in the body, all dependent upon the specific goal for which the prodrug is designed. Whereas prodrugs designed to overcome solubility problems in formulating intravenous (i.v.) injectables should be converted immediately after i.v. administration, the rate of conversion should be lower in case a prodrug is aimed at providing a sustained drug action through rate-limiting cleavage of the prodrug bond.

Conversion or activation of prodrugs to the parent drug molecules in the body is the result of enzyme-mediated cleavage or pH-dependent hydrolysis of the established prodrug linkage. Within a homologous series of derivatives of the same drug (for example different carboxylic acid esters) the chemical nature of the pro-moiety may give rise to both electronic and steric effects influencing the lability of the prodrug bond. Prediction of chemical reactivity through substituent effects is often possible from empirical linear free energy relationships (LFERs). In the present context simple LFERs considered are linear correlations of the general form

$$\log k_x = \log k_H + \rho \sigma_x \tag{14.1}$$

where k_H is the rate constant for hydrolysis of the prodrug derivative possessing a hydrogen atom at the substitution site, and k_x refers to the rate constant for the derivative in which the hydrogen atom at the substitution site has been replaced by the substituent X. The substituent constant σ_x refers to the electronic (or steric) effect of the substituent. While the substituent constant is a parameter which in essence is dictated by the chemical nature of the substituent, the reaction constant ρ varies with the type of reaction and external conditions such as the solvent. In other words ρ is a quantitative measure of the sensitivity of the given reaction to polar or steric substituent effects. In rational prodrug design facile identification of suitable pro-moieties providing feasible chemical lability of the prodrug linkage is often possible from such linear correlations established by using tabulated values of, for example, Hammett's or Taft's polar substituent constants (reflecting electronic

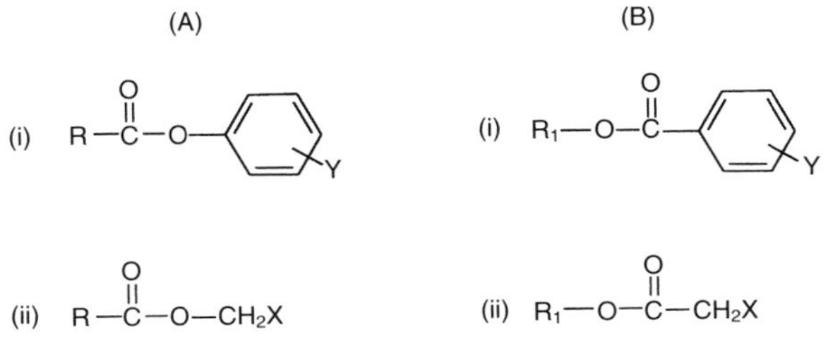

(A)

(B)

(i)   R—C(=O)—O—⟨aromatic ring⟩—Y

(i)   R₁—O—C(=O)—⟨aromatic ring⟩—Y

(ii)   R—C(=O)—O—CH₂X

(ii)   R₁—O—C(=O)—CH₂X

Figure 14.3 Types of ester derivatives: (A) Drug containing a carboxylic acid group; and (B) Drug containing a hydroxy functional group.

effects resulting from substitution in aromatic and aliphatic structures, respectively) and Charton's steric parameters.

For drug substances containing a carboxyl group, ester derivatives can be obtained from aliphatic alcohols and phenol type compounds (Figure 14.3A). Similarly, if the drug possesses an OH-group, different types of ester derivatives might be synthesized (Figure 14.3B). Neutral or alkaline hydrolysis of ester functions are facilitated by low electron density at the carbonyl carbon atom. Such an electron deficiency at the reaction site is accomplished by introducing an electronegative substituent in (i) the *meta-* or *para-*position of the aromatic ring (substituent Y) or (ii) aliphatic structures (substituent X). The majority of prodrugs to be activated by non-enzymatic processes is characterized by a high chemical instability at physiological pH (7.4) while preferably exhibiting a higher stability at lower pH. As will be discussed below an example of such prodrug types is *N*-Mannich bases (Section 14.3.2.1). A serious drawback of prodrugs requiring chemical (non-enzymatic) release of the active agent is the inherent lability of the compounds, raising some stability issues at least in cases of liquid dosage forms. In particular situations, such formulation problems have been overcome by using a more sophisticated approach involving double prodrugs where use is made of an enzymatic release mechanism prior to the spontaneous reaction (Section 14.3.1).

Prodrugs might be designed to be cleaved by action of enzymes to ensure fast regeneration of the drug once the barrier to efficient drug delivery has been overcome. In addition, site-specific drug delivery through site-specific prodrug activation may be accomplished exploiting that a target tissue contains specific enzymes or high concentrations of particular enzymes relative to non-target tissues (Section 14.4.2.2). Although examples of drug substances regenerated from their prodrugs by biochemical reductive or oxidative processes are available, the most common prodrugs are those requiring a hydrolytic cleavage mediated by hydrolases such as esterases and lipases. Rates of enzyme hydrolysis can to some degree be described as a function of some combination of electronic, steric, and hydrophobic parameters. However, application of LFERs to reactions catalyzed by hydrolytic enzymes appears less straightforward. For example, while the chemical reactivity of ester derivatives is readily predictable on basis of the steric and electronic properties of the substituents in both the acyl and alcohol moieties, this does not apply for enzyme-facilitated hydrolysis. In general, steric effects alter non-enzymatic and enzymatic ester hydrolysis rates in the same direction. For enzymatic ester hydrolysis, the hydrophilic property and charge of the ester may play a major role and consequently non-enzymatic hydrolysis cannot be used as a reliable guide to enzyme-catalyzed reactions. Thus, initial assessment of the susceptibility of prodrug candidates to undergo enzyme-mediated cleavage might be achieved by measurement of the stability of the derivatives after incubation in plasma or a homogenate from liver, intestine, skin or cornea, dependent on the intended route of administration of the prodrug. To this end, it should be emphasized that enzyme capacities might be subject to significant interspecies variation. For example, esters are usually hydrolyzed markedly faster in rat plasma than in human plasma whereas dog plasma often is less efficient than human plasma.

The influence of chemical structure on the chemical and enzymatic lability of a homologous series of potential prodrug candidates can be illustrated by the data obtained (Table 14.1) for various esters of the model drug compound benzoic acid. The rate of hydroxide ion-catalyzed hydrolysis of these esters is primarily determined by the polar (electronic) effects exhibited by the alcohol moieties of the esters since the steric effects in these portions can be considered to be almost constant due to the presence of a methylene group connected to oxygen in all the derivatives. Omitting the rate data for compound 8, where intramolecular catalysis by the carboxylate anion occurs, and compound 11, the hydrolysis rates of these esters are correlated by the following expression

$$\log k_{OH} = 0.54\sigma^* + 0.74 \quad (n = 16; \ r = 0.962) \tag{14.2}$$

Table 14.1 Rate data for the alkaline and enzymatic hydrolysis of various benzoic acid esters at 37 °C

Compound	R	σ^* for R	k_{OH} (M^{-1} min^{-1})	80% Human plasma	
				k(min^{-1})	$t_{1/2}$ (min)
1	H	0.49	13.6	6.4×10^{-3}	108
2	CH_3	0.00	6.59	3.3×10^{-3}	210
3	C_2H_5	−0.10	5.52	1.5×10^{-2}	46
4	C_3H_7	−0.12	4.50	1.7×10^{-2}	40
5	C_4H_9	−0.25	5.33	2.9×10^{-2}	24
6	C_6H_5	0.75	13.0	3.7×10^{-2}	19
7	$CH_2C_6H_5$	0.27	4.63	4.7×10^{-2}	15
8	$(C=O)O^-$	−1.06	6.28	$<10^{-4}$	$>100\,h$
9	$(C=O)OCH_3$	2.00	70.1	2.0×10^{-1}	3.5
10	$(C=O)OC_2H_5$	2.26	60.3	4.4×10^{-2}	16
11	$(C=O)CH_2C_6H_5$	–	55.7	2.7×10^{-1}	2.6
12	$(C=O)NH_2$	1.68	69.9	1.7×10^{-2}	40
13	$(C=O)N(CH_3)_2$	1.94	19.2	>5.0	$<8\,s$
14	SCH_3	1.56	24.4	3.1×10^{-2}	22
15	$(S=O)CH_3$	2.88	274	5.9×10^{-1}	1.2
16	$(O=S=O)CH_3$	3.68	592	5.8×10^{-1}	1.2
17	$CH_2N(CH_3)_2$	0.49	9.83	>8.0	$<5\,s$
18	$CH_2N(CH_3)_3^+$	1.90	95.1	>8.0	$<5\,s$

where k_{OH} is the 2nd order rate constant for specific base catalysis of hydrolysis ($M^{-1} min^{-1}$) and the Taft polar substituent constant σ^* refers to R in RCH_2OH for the alcohols. This LFER may be useful for prediction of the reactivity of a benzoate ester derivative solely on basis of the σ^* value of the appropriate alcohol substituent. A large number of σ^* values are compiled in the literature. The variation of rate of hydrolysis can also be accounted for in terms of the different stabilities of the leaving alcohol groups as expressed by the pK_a values of the alcohols.

In contrast, the plasma-catalyzed hydrolysis (pH 7.4) of the esters cannot be correlated in the same manner. It is apparent that by increasing the chain length in the alkyl esters, the enzymatic reactivity increases except when going from methyl to ethyl. The N,N-dimethylglycolamide ester 13 is seen to be cleaved extremely fast in human plasma although being chemically highly stable. The rapid rate of hydrolysis of compound 13 has been attributed to a pseudocholinesterase present in plasma. The protonated esters 17 and 18 are also cleaved very rapidly in plasma in contrast to the benzoylglycolic acid (compound 8). The high resistance of the latter derivative towards enzymatic hydrolysis is most likely caused by its negative charge at physiological pH due to the observation that various other esters with an ionized carboxylate group such as hemisuccinate esters are poor substrates for hydrolytic plasma enzymes.

14.2.2 Modification of physicochemical properties

Prodrug design has been used to improve the performance of drugs by overcoming various barriers to drug delivery (Section 14.1.2). In most cases, this has been accomplished by formation of prodrug derivatives altering the basic physicochemical characteristics of a drug substance which in addition to chemical stability encompasses (i) lipophilicity; and (ii) aqueous solubility. The fraction of a drug which reaches the receptor for therapeutic response is largely governed by dissolution and transport processes. These processes are primarily dependent on the latter two fundamental physicochemical properties. Due to this fact several more or less successful attempts to create tools for estimating aqueous solubility and lipophilicity of prodrugs have been made as outlined in the following sections.

14.2.2.1 Lipophilicity

Probably the most successful application of bioreversible derivatization is in the area of improving the passive drug transport across various biological membranes. In general, the transport rate is usually enhanced by attachment of a hydrophobic group to a drug substance, e.g. by formation of a more lipophilic derivative. Initially, the rate of diffusion across the membrane will increase exponentially with increasing lipophilicity of prodrug derivatives of a given compound. At higher lipophilicities, the transport rate levels off reaching a maximum value. Since an increase in lipophilicity, with a few exceptions, is accompanied by a comparable or greater decrease in aqueous solubility further increment in lipophilicity will ultimately result in a decrease in the flux over the membrane due to poor aqueous solubility. Thus, it is apparent that both solubility and lipophilicity constitute the most important factors in passive drug absorption. Drugs, which are too polar or hydrophilic often exhibit poor transport properties, whereas those that are too non-polar or lipophilic frequently have low bioavailability as a consequence of insufficient aqueous solubility. Although being the subject of some debate as to which *in vitro* partitioning system best mimics biological membranes, lipophilicity most often is expressed by the *n*-octanol-water partition coefficient (P_{oct}) given as the ratio of the activities (or in dilute solution the concentrations) of the solute in the two phases at equilibrium. A $\log P_{oct}$ value of 1 expresses that the solute concentration in the octanol phase, at equilibrium, is ten times higher than in the aqueous phase. However, the equilibrium constant *per se* does not give insight into the absolute magnitude of the concentration of a solute in the two respective phases. Therefore, two compounds having the same P_{oct} value may vary with respect to membrane transport properties since significant difference in size of intermolecular cohesive forces of the two substances (for example hydrogen bonding) will result in different absolute affinities for the two almost immiscible phases. The optimal balance between aqueous solubility and $\log P_{oct}$ to ensure good absorption depends on the nature of the biomembrane and the volume of the aqueous phase adjacent to the membrane. If dissolution phenomena are not rate-limiting, a $\log P_{oct}$ of about 2 appears optimal for gastrointestinal absorption.

In the area of parenteral oil depot formulations the prodrug approach has been extensively exploited to generate prodrug derivatives with feasible lipophilicities (see Section 14.4.3). For this type of formulations the rate of prodrug release from the oil vehicle, and thus the duration of action, is at least partly dictated by the partition coefficient of the entity between the oil and the tissue fluid after intramuscular (i.m.) injection.

Since many drugs are either weak acids or bases or salts hereof, dissociation constitutes a factor in determining absorbability. It is generally accepted that the unionized and thus most lipophilic form of an acidic or basic drug is absorbed far more efficiently than the ionic species. Assuming that partitioning only takes place for unionized species, the partition coefficient of a weak acid at a given pH can be expressed by

$$P_{pH} = P_{HA} f_{HA} \tag{14.3}$$

where P_{HA} is the intrinsic partition coefficient of the weak acid and f_{HA} is the fraction of the undissociated acid at the particular pH value ($f_{HA} = [H^+]/[H^+] + K_a$). Equation 14.3 can also be written in the form

$$\log P_{pH} = \log P_{HA} - \log (1 + 10^{(pH-pK_a)}) \tag{14.4}$$

where K_a is ionization constant of the acid. The analogous expression for a weak base is

$$\log P_{pH} = \log P_B - \log (1 + 10^{(pK_a-pH)}) \tag{14.5}$$

where P_B is the intrinsic partition coefficient of the weak base.

Partition coefficients of chemical entities can be predicted reasonably well by several group contribution approaches. In prodrug design, the lipophilicity (expressed as the *n*-octanol-water partition coefficient) of members of a homologous series of derivatives are generally estimated with acceptable accuracy by using tabulated values of the Hansch substituent constant Π_X defined as

$$\Pi_X = \log P_{RX} - \log P_{RH} \tag{14.6}$$

where P_{RX} is the partition coefficient for the derivative RX which is obtained from the derivative RH by substitution of a hydrogen atom with the group or atom X.

14.2.2.2   Solubility

In spite of the great importance of aqueous solubility in the pharmaceutical and other applied chemical disciplines, it is a very poorly understood phenomenon. There are no generally useful guidelines for estimating the solubility of a drug substance in water based on consideration of its structure and physicochemical properties. One reason for the lack of predictability of the solubility of crystalline compounds is that it is not a simple equilibrium, but it rather consists of a combination of equilibria.

Intermolecular interactions in the crystalline state constitute important factors in determining the aqueous solubility of a drug, due to their influence on the thermodynamic activity of the solid drug. The melting point (*MP*) and the thermodynamic activity of a drug in its solid phase are two distinct parameters, but are related to a certain degree. Both properties have been used as indicators of the strength of interactions in the crystalline phase. Quantitative relationships between molecular structure and melting point are generally not found. Qualitatively, melting points within a series of structurally similar compounds increase with increasing molecular weight (*MW*), compactness, rigidity, and symmetry, and the number of polar, particularly hydrogen bonding, groups in the molecule. Thus, for closely related series of compounds linear correlations in melting points have occasionally been observed although linearity of such correlations cannot be accounted for thermodynamically.

Although based on many assumptions and approximations a rough estimate of the ideal solubility of non-electrolytes at 25 °C from chemical structure and *MP* (in Celcius degrees) is provided by the expression

$$\log X_{id} = -\frac{\Delta S_f}{2.303\, R\, 298.15}(MP - 25) \tag{14.7}$$

where $\log X_{id}$ is the logarithm of the mole fraction solubility, ΔS_f is the entropy of fusion and R refers to the gas constant. Assuming that $\Delta S_f = 13.5\,\mathrm{cal\ K^{-1}\ mol^{-1}}$ for rigid molecules equation (14.7) might be written

$$\log X_{id} = -0.0099(MP - 25) \tag{14.8}$$

revealing an apparent linearity between ideal solubility and *MP*. The anti-epileptic agent phenytoin (**14.1**) is a high melting, weakly acidic, and sparingly water-soluble drug. Phenytoin exhibits poor oral bioavailability after administration in various dosage forms. In order to disrupt the major intermolecular interactions in the crystal lattice responsible for the undesired physicochemical properties, a series of 3-acyloxymethyl derivatives of phenytoin (**14.2a–j**) was synthesized. The derivatives

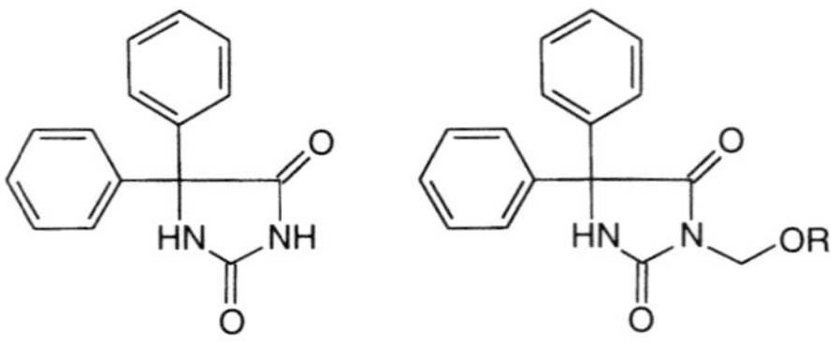

(14.2a)	R= (C=O)CH₃
(14.2b)	R= (C=O)C₂H₅
(14.2c)	R= (C=O)C₃H₇
(14.2d)	R= (C=O)C₄H₉
(14.2e)	R= (C=O)C(CH₃)₃
(14.2f)	R= (C=O)C₅H₁₁
(14.2g)	R= (C=O)C₆H₁₃
(14.2h)	R= (C=O)C₇H₁₅
(14.2i)	R= (C=O)C₈H₁₇
(14.2j)	R= (C=O)C₉H₁₉

Scheme 14.2

were reasonable soluble in various metabolizable glycerol esters such as tributyrin and triolein allowing the prodrugs to be incorporated in soft gelatine capsules. The prodrug 3-pentanoyloxymethyl-5,5-diphenylhydantoin (**14.2f**) when administered in tributyrin gave superior oral phenytoin bioavailability in rats when compared to sodium phenytoin administered as an aqueous solution. Some physicochemical data for the derivatives are presented in Table 14.2. As seen from Figure 14.4 a reasonable linearity between the logarithm of molar solubility of the prodrug derivatives in ethyl oleate and their *MPs* was established implying that crystal lattice energy differences, as indicated by *MP* behavior, appear to influence the solubility of the esters in this organic solvent.

The approach represented by equations (14.7) and (14.8) has been extended to provide approximate predictions of aqueous solubility of non-electrolytes. The real solubility of crystalline drugs involves the consideration of the aqueous activity coefficient as well as the ideal solubility. In this case, a relationship between molar aqueous solubility (*S*) (25 °C), and the partition coefficient P_{oct} and the *MP* might be established according to the semi-empirical expression

$$\log S \cong -a \log P_{oct} - b\, MP + c \tag{14.9}$$

Table 14.2 Melting point (*MP*), molecular weight (*MW*), and molar solubility (*S*) at 25 °C of various esters of 3-hydroxymethyl-5,5-diphenylhydantoin in ethyl oleate. **14.2a–j** refer to the chemical structures presented in Scheme 14.2

Compound	MP (°C)	MW	$10^3 \times S(M)$
14.2a	158–159	324.3	4.63
14.2b	172–174	338.4	5.02
14.2c	134–135	352.4	13.1
14.2d	89–92	366.4	111.4
14.2e	134–135	366.4	25.9
14.2f	107–108	380.4	52.3
14.2g	87–88	394.5	74.5
14.2h	67.5–68.0	408.5	257.0
14.2i	78.5–80.0	422.5	129.0
14.2j	56–57	436.5	281.8

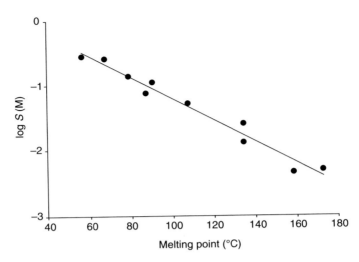

Figure 14.4 Plot of the logarithm of the molar solubility S of various 3-acyloxymethyl-5,5-diphenylhydantoins in ethyl oleate at 25 °C against their melting points.

where a, b and c are constants varying slightly depending on the basic chemical structure of the series of compounds investigated. For rigid and short molecules $\Delta S_f = 13.5 \, \text{cal} \, \text{K}^{-1} \, \text{mol}^{-1}$ and equation (14.9) becomes

$$\log S \cong -1 \log P_{oct} - 0.01 \, MP + 1.05 \tag{14.10}$$

In attempt to improve the therapeutic value of the anticancer agent 5-fluorouracil (5-FU) (**14.3**) several prodrug types have been evaluated. Among these, various N_1- and N_3-monosubstituted bioreversible derivatives of 5-FU have been investigated (Scheme 14.3). The physicochemical characterization of the derivatives included determination of MP, S, and P_{oct} with the latter two parameters determined for the undissociated forms of the derivatives. By multiple-regression analysis of the parameters of this series of 5-FU derivatives, covering a considerable range of MPs, $\log P$, and $\log S$ values, the following relationship between the parameters were found

$$\log S = -0.98 \, (\pm 0.13) \log P - 0.009 \, (\pm 0.002) \, MP + 0.12 \, (\pm 0.33)$$
$$(n = 15; \quad r = 0.914) \tag{14.11}$$

which is in surprisingly good agreement with the theoretical correlation given by equation (14.10). Although semi-empirical of nature such relationships may be valuable for the prediction of aqueous solubilities of congeneric series of prodrug derivatives from the knowledge of the MP and P_{oct}, the latter being easily estimated *a priori* by group contribution approaches.

Aqueous solubility limitations are critical for the development of parenteral and oral drug products. For poorly soluble non-electrolytes the prodrug approach

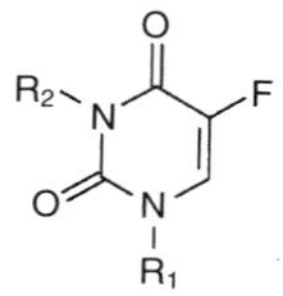

(14.3)

Compound:

5-Fluorouracil (5-FU) **(14.3)**	$R_1 = H$	$R_2 = H$
1-acyloxymethyl-5-FU	$R_1 = CH_2O-acyl$	$R_2 = H$
3-acyloxymethyl-5-FU	$R_1 = H$	$R_2 = CH_2O-acyl$
3-acyl-5-FU	$R_1 = H$	$R_2 = acyl$
3-alkoxycarbonyl-5-FU	$R_1 = H$	$R_2 = (C=O)O-alkyl$
3-aryloxycarbonyl-5-FU	$R_1 = H$	$R_2 = (C=O)O-aryl$
1-alkylcarbamoyl-5-FU	$R_1 = (C=O)N-alkyl$	$R_2 = H$

Scheme 14.3

has been applied to circumvent solubility problems by using transport-moieties possessing an ionizable functional group, e.g. phosphate esters, amino acid esters and hemiesters of dicarboxylic acids (see Section 14.4.3), allowing various salts of such prodrug derivatives to be formed. In spite of the fact that salt formation is routinely employed, quantitative relationships between chemical structure and physicochemical properties of salts are virtually non-existing. In qualitative terms, however, it is recognized that increased compactness, symmetry, and rigidity of the ions would be expected to decrease escape tendencies of the salts. Likewise, it is generally observed that increasing lipophilicity of the counterion decreases water solubility. In thermodynamic terms the molar free energy change when a salt is dissolved in water, ΔG_{sol} can be expressed as

$$\Delta G_{sol} = \Delta G_+ + \Delta G_- - \Delta G_{lattice} \tag{14.12}$$

where ΔG_+, ΔG_-, and $\Delta G_{lattice}$ are the energies of hydration of the cation, hydration of the anion, and the crystal lattice energy, respectively. Consequently, the solubility will depend on which terms, the hydration energies or the lattice energy, are most sensitive to changes in structure. In optimization of aqueous solubility by prodrug design both of the latter two parameters therefore have to be taken into consideration. Significant increase in aqueous solubility has been achieved via simple bioreversible modifications which result in disruption of the crystal lattice. To this end, the use of the prodrug approach can be illustrated by considering the antiviral agent vidarabine (**14.4**). The poor aqueous solubility of the drug substance (0.0018 M) at 25 °C is most likely caused by strong intermolecular hydrogen bonding in the crystalline state as reflected in its *MP* (260 °C). The significantly enhanced solubility of the 5′-formate ester (**14.5**), corresponding to approximately 0.12 M (25 °C), has been attributed to disruption of the strong intermolecular interactions in the crystal as judged by the decrease in *MP* of the derivative

$$(14.4) \quad R = H$$

$$(14.5) \quad R = \overset{\overset{\displaystyle O}{\|}}{C} - H$$

(175 °C). Thus, a 60-fold increase in solubility is the result of incorporation of the small, polar formyl group in **14.4**. The 5'-formate ester prodrug is rapidly hydrolyzed in human blood with a half-life of 6–8 min, and it appears to be a useful parenteral delivery form of vidarabine, although the solution stability is rather limited.

14.2.3   Macromolecular transport vectors

Most drug candidates have *MWs* of about 200–500 dalton. A bioreversible derivative obtained by covalent attachment of a pro-moiety of similar size to such therapeutic agents can be referred to as a low molecular weight prodrug. In ophthalmic drug delivery, for example, where the active agent only has to pass one biological barrier (cornea) before reaching the target area, it is possible by proper selection of the transport-moiety to synthesize prodrug derivatives endowed with feasible membrane transport properties and *in vivo* labilities. In case the target site only can be reached after transport via the systemic circulation the *in vivo* fate of the drug is affected by drug distribution, protein binding, tissue storage, and excretion, not to mention the enormous range of metabolic reactions that drugs may undergo. The latter processes are also influenced by the physicochemical properties of the drug or prodrug derivative, however in a less predicitive manner limiting the use of the low molecular weight prodrug approach to optimize systemic site-specific drug delivery or drug targeting (Section 14.4.2). Drug targeting is especially attractive for highly toxic compounds and for drugs having a narrow therapeutic window. In its simplest sense, targeted drug delivery is achieved by enhancing drug availability at the target or response site while minimizing its availability at other sites, especially those that manifest toxicity.

The chemotherapeutic utility of macromolecular prodrugs, in which a drug is attached to a macromolecule through a bioreversible linkage, to provide drug targeting has been the focus of intense research for decades. Although an account on low molecular weight prodrugs is the subject of the present chapter, a brief description of the potential utility of the macromolecular prodrug approach is given below. The rationale behind this approach is that the transport properties of the macromolecular prodrug should be dictated predominantly by the macromolecular transport vector. In the field of cancer, chemotherapy design

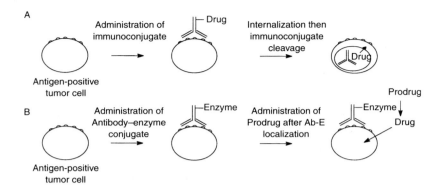

Figure 14.5 (A) Simplified scheme of the site-directed drug delivery to and activation of a monoclonal antibody-drug conjugate in a tumor cell; (B) simplified scheme of the site-specific activation of a prodrug at a tumor cell using the ADEPT concept.

of macromolecular prodrugs has received considerable interest since anticancer agents tend to be highly toxic and their effectiveness limited by a very small therapeutic ratio. Thus, macromolecular conjugates obtained by a bioreversible attachment of anticancer agents to a wide array of macromolecules endowed with intrinsic target receptor affinities such as monoclonal antibodies (mAB) and hormones have been evaluated *in vitro* and *in vivo* (Figure 14.5). Despite the tremendous efforts devoted to the design of parenteral site-specific soluble macromolecular drug carrier systems, the current level of success has been rather disappointing. There are at least three major reasons for this: (i) the multitude of physiological barriers the macromolecular prodrug has to fight against on its way from the administration site to the ultimate target of the drug entity; (ii) the task of accomplishing the correct timing of the events leading to optimal drug action, e.g. selective regeneration and suitable maintenance of the active agent at the target site; and (iii) potential immunogenicity and loss of the intrinsic receptor affinity upon covalent linkage of the cytotoxic agent to the macromolecular transport vector.

An interesting principle bearing some resemblance to antibody-based macro-molecular prodrugs is the so-called ADEPT concept (antibody-directed enzyme prodrug therapy) (Figure 14.5). In the ADEPT approach, an enzyme, which catalyzes the conversion of a low molecular weight prodrug to the active cytotoxic drug, is covalently linked to a monoclonal antibody that binds antigen preferentially expressed on the surface of tumor cells, or in tumor interstitium. In the first step, the mAB-enzyme complex is administered and accumulates at the tumor site. Enough time is allowed for clearance of the complex from normal (non-target) tissue before the prodrug of the anticancer agent is administered. This leads to enzyme-catalyzed regeneration of the cytotoxic parent drug specifically at the tumor site. Although drawbacks to the use of the ADEPT approach are similar to those mentioned above for antibody-based macromolecular prodrugs, the concept appears potentially attractive due to the possibility of using enzymes which have catalytic properties different from those of any endogenous enzyme.

Besides drug targeting, other important objectives may be achieved by using soluble macromolecular prodrugs, including:

(1) Stabilization of the therapeutic agent
(2) Enhancement of drug solubility
(3) Improvement of circulation life time
(4) Extended duration of action

The latter objectives may be obtained by employing biodegradable macromolecular pro-moieties without any apparent specificity for discrete cell-surface receptors encompassing proteins, polypeptides, polysaccharides as well as synthetic polymers. The composition of such macromolecular prodrugs can be created in a more or less sophisticated way as evident from the schematic presentation given in Figure 14.6. Prodrug derivatives, in which the drug is linked directly to the macromolecular backbone, may act as a depot releasing the active agent in a predictable manner. In most cases, regeneration rates of the parent drug are exclusively governed by pH-dependent hydrolysis due to the bulky polymer matrix rendering the hydrolytic center inaccessible to enzymatic attack.

Intercalation of a spacer arm between the drug and the carrier may serve three purposes. First, the terminal functional group of the spacer arm can be varied, thus allowing covalent drug fixation to be established through a variety of chemical bonds. Second, steric hindrance of enzyme activation of the liganded drug might be circumvented by augmenting the distance between the drug and the carrier backbone. By proper selection of the spacer arm encompassing both the length and the chemical structure, and the spacer to drug bond, a localized effect may be obtained in case the spacer-drug link is designed to be cleaved selectively by enzymes secreted extracellularly by the target pathological cells. Third, sequentially labile macromolecular prodrugs can be constructed in such a way that the pH-dependent hydrolysis only liberates the spacer-drug derivative, i.e. the corresponding low molecular weight prodrug. After parenteral administration, the macromolecular derivative might

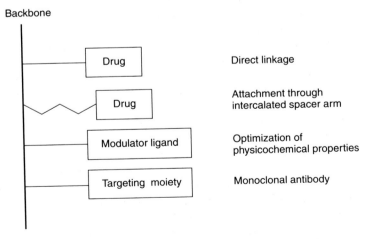

Figure 14.6 Schematic presentation of possible macromolecular prodrug structures.

therefore act as a depot releasing the low molecular weight prodrug, which after extravasation or diffusion from the injection site is activated at the diseased tissue.

The disposition and persistance of the macromolecular conjugate might be altered or improved by employing different types of ligands. Linkage of, *per se*, inactive chemical entities to the polymeric carrier can modify the overall physicochemical characteristics of the derivatives resulting in for example a diminished liver uptake. Of a more speculative utility is the incorporation of a target specific moiety in order to guide the prodrug selectively to the target area.

14.3   BIOREVERSIBLE DERIVATIVES FOR VARIOUS FUNCTIONAL GROUPS

The most common type of prodrugs are esters derived from hydroxy or carboxyl groups present in the parent drug molecules. In a number of cases, however, other strategies are required, since the drug to be modified does not contain such groups readily amenable to esterification. Therefore, bioreversible derivatives of a variety of functional groups have been investigated in the design of potentially useful prodrug types, some of which are presented in Table 14.3. An outline of the more commonly used types of derivatives is given in the following sections.

Table 14.3 Prodrug forms of various functional groups in drug substances

Functional group	Prodrug form	
-COOH	$-\overset{\overset{O}{\|\|}}{C}-OR$	Esters
	$-\overset{\overset{O}{\|\|}}{C}-O-\overset{\overset{R_1}{\|}}{C}H-O-\overset{\overset{O}{\|\|}}{C}-R_2$	α-Acyloxyalkyl esters
	$-\overset{\overset{O}{\|\|}}{C}-NHR$	Amides
-OH	$-O-\overset{\overset{O}{\|\|}}{C}-R$	Esters
	$-O-\overset{\overset{O}{\|\|}}{C}-OR$	Carbonate esters
	$-O-\overset{\overset{O}{\|\|}}{P}\underset{\diagdown OH}{\diagup OH}$	Phosphate esters
	$-OR$	Ethers
	$-O-\overset{\overset{R_1}{\|}}{C}H-O-\overset{\overset{O}{\|\|}}{C}-R_2$	α-Acyloxyalkyl ethers
-SH	$-S-\overset{\overset{O}{\|\|}}{C}-R$	Thioesters

Functional group	Structure	Name
$>C=O$	$-S-CH(R_1)-O-\overset{O}{\overset{\|}{C}}-R_2$	α-Acyloxyalkyl thioethers
	$-S-S-R$	Disulphides
	$-\overset{OR_1}{\underset{OR_2}{\overset{\|}{\underset{\|}{C}}}}-$	Ketals
	$>C=N-R$	Imines
	$>C-O-\overset{O}{\overset{\|}{C}}-R$	Enol esters
	(ring) C–O–N	Oxazolidines
	(ring) C–S–N	Thiazolidines
$-NH_2$	$-NH-\overset{O}{\overset{\|}{C}}-R$	Amides
	$-NH-\overset{O}{\overset{\|}{C}}-O-R$	Carbamates
	$-N=\overset{R_1}{\underset{R_2}{C}}$	Imines
	$-NH-\overset{R}{\underset{\|}{C}}=\overset{R_1}{\underset{\|}{C}}-R_2$	Enamines
	$-NH-CH_2-\overset{R_1}{\underset{\|}{N}}-\overset{O}{\overset{\|}{C}}-R_2$	N-Mannich bases
	$-NH-\overset{O}{\overset{\|}{C}}-O-\overset{R_1}{\underset{\|}{CH}}-O-\overset{O}{\overset{\|}{C}}-R_2$	N-Acyloxyalkoxycarbonyl derivatives
$\overset{\diagdown}{\underset{\diagup}{-N}}$	$\overset{\diagdown}{\underset{\diagup}{-N}}\overset{+}{}-\overset{R_1}{\underset{\|}{CH}}-O-\overset{O}{\overset{\|}{C}}-R_2$	N-Acyloxyalkyl derivatives
$R_1-\overset{O}{\overset{\|}{C}}-OR_2$	$R-SO_2N=\overset{R_1}{\underset{O-R_2}{C}}$	N-Sulphonyl imidates
$-SO_2NH_2$	$-SO_2NH-CH_2O-R$	N-Sulphonyl imidates
NH-Acidic group	$-\overset{O}{\overset{\|}{C}}-\overset{R}{\underset{\|}{N}}-CH_2-N\overset{R_1}{\underset{R_2}{}}$	N-Mannich bases
e.g. $-\overset{O}{\overset{\|}{C}}-\overset{R}{\underset{\|}{HN}}$	$-\overset{O}{\overset{\|}{C}}-\overset{R}{\underset{\|}{N}}-CH_2OH$	N-Methyols
or heterocyclic amine	$-\overset{O}{\overset{\|}{C}}-\overset{R}{\underset{\|}{N}}-\overset{R_1}{\underset{\|}{CH}}-O-\overset{O}{\overset{\|}{C}}-R_2$	N-Acyloxyalkyl derivatives

14.3.1   Esters as prodrugs for compounds containing carboxyl or hydroxy groups

The popularity of using esters as a prodrug type for drugs containing carboxyl or hydroxy functions (or thiol groups) stems primarily from the fact that the organism is rich in enzymes capable of hydrolyzing ester bonds. The distribution of esterases is ubiquitous and several types are found in the blood, liver, and other organs or tissues. In addition, by appropriate esterification it is possible to obtain derivatives with almost any desirable aqueous solubility or lipophilicity as well as *in vivo* lability, the latter being dictated by electronic and steric factors (Section 14.2.1). Accordingly, a significant number of carboxylic acid drugs and drugs containing alcohol groups have been modified for a multitude of reasons employing the ester prodrug approach. Examples of applications of the latter prodrug type are found in Section 14.4.

The pH-dependent rate of hydrolysis of simple ester derivatives *in vitro* can often be described by the general rate equation

$$k_{obs} = k_{H^+} a_{H^+} + k_o + k_{OH^-} a_{OH^-}$$

(14.13)

where k_{obs} is the observed pH-dependent pseudo-1st order rate constant for hydrolytic cleavage of the ester bond, and k_{H^+} and k_{OH^-} represent the 2nd order rate constants for specific acid and base catalysis, respectively. k_o is the apparent 1st order rate constant for the spontaneous degradation. a_{H^+} and a_{OH^-} refer to the hydrogen and hydroxide ion activity, respectively. Plots of $\log k_{obs}$ against pH yield the characteristic U-shaped pH-rate profile or a V-shaped profile in case the contribution of the spontaneous reaction to k_{obs} becomes insignificant. Although differing with respect to stability in aqueous solution the chemical instability of ester derivatives may be high and aqueous dosage forms can therefore be difficult to formulate. In attempt to improve the aqueous solubility of metronidazole (**14.6**), the solubility of which is about 1% w/v, eight amino acid esters of the drug were prepared and evaluated for their feasibility as water-soluble parenteral delivery forms of metronidazole. As seen from Table 14.4 the ester prodrugs exhibit poor stability in aqueous buffer pH 7.4 (37 °C). Even at lower pH the esters are too unstable to be formulated as a ready-to-use injection formulation. Table 14.4 also illustrates that the rate of regeneration of **14.6** from the prodrugs mediated by plasma enzymes depends strongly on the chemical structure of the pro-moiety. For further information about different ester types introduced to improve the aqueous solubility of drugs containing a hydroxy group (Drug-OH) see Section 14.4.3.

Not only steric effects within the alcohol portion have influence on the enzymatic hydrolysis of esters. Enzyme-mediated hydrolysis might also be highly sensitive to steric hindrance caused by the acyl portion. In penicillins, for example, the environment around the carboxyl group is sterically hindered, and simple aliphatic

(14.6)

Table 14.4 Half-lives for the hydrolysis of various amino acid esters of metronidazole (**14.6**) in 80% human plasma (pH 7.4) and 0.05 M phosphate buffer (pH 7.40) at 37 °C

Ester	$t_{1/2}$ *in human plasma* (min)	$t_{1/2}$ *in buffer* (min)
N,N-dimethylglycinate	12	250
Glycinate	41	115
N-Propylglycinate	8	90
3-Aminopropionate	207	315
3-Dimethylaminopropionate	46	52
3-Dimethylaminobutyrate	334	580
4-Morpholinoacetate	30	1880
4-Methyl-1-piperazinoacetate	523	1720

or aromatic esters are not sufficiently labile *in vivo* to function as prodrugs. This shortcoming can be overcome by preparing a double ester prodrug type, acyloxyalkyl or alkoxycarbonyloxyalkyl esters, in which the terminal ester group is accessible to enzymatic cleavage. The first step in regeneration of the parent drug from this type of esters is enzyme-catalyzed hydrolysis of the terminal ester bond with the formation of a highly unstable α-hydroxyalkyl ester which rapidly dissociates by a spontaneous reaction to yield the parent acidic drug and an aldehyde (Scheme 14.4). By a similar mechanism, alkoxycarbonyloxyalkyl esters (containing a terminal carbonate ester function) release an alcohol, carbon dioxide and an aldehyde upon hydrolysis. Double prodrugs might be the result of chemical structures different from the above mentioned double esters and refer, in general, to prodrugs where activation of the drug is initiated by enzymatic cleavage of a terminal functional group under formation of an unstable intermediate which undergoes a fast, spontaneous rearrangement to the active agent.

The applicability of α-acyloxyalkyl esters as biologically reversible transport forms has also been extended to include the phosphate group, phosphonic acids and phosphinic acids. An example is compound **14.7**, an angiotensin converting enzyme (ACE) inhibitor, where the phosphinic acid group has been *O*-α-acyloxy-alkylated to yield fosenopril (**14.8**) which is better absorbed orally than the parent active compound as a consequence of its greater lipophilicity.

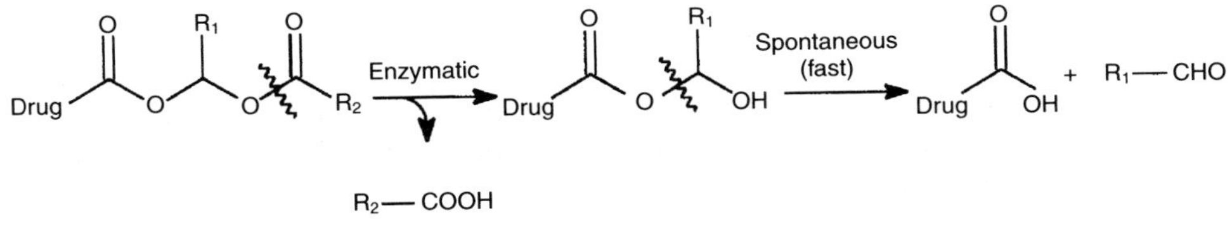

Scheme 14.4

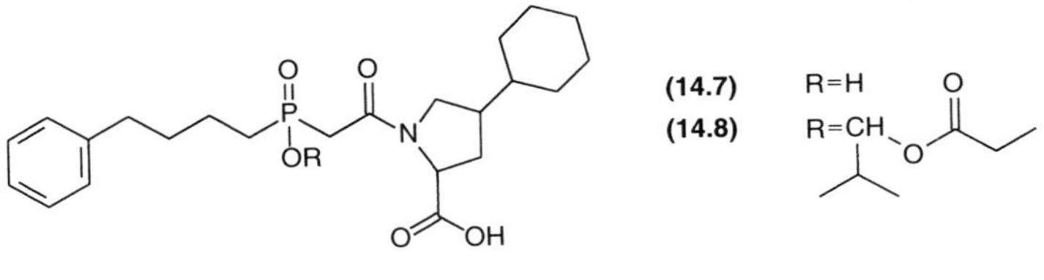

(14.7) R=H
(14.8) R=CH

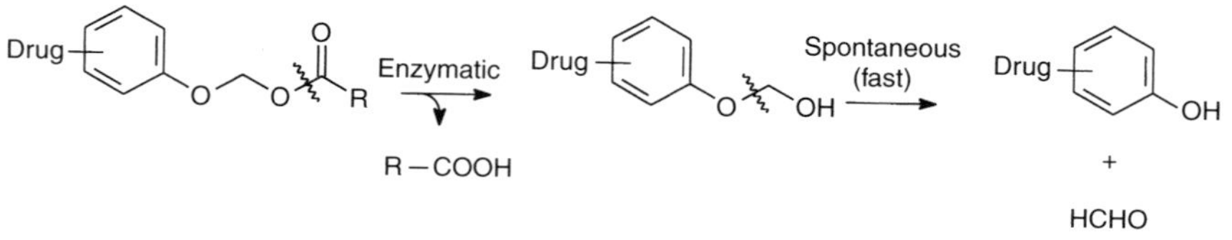

Scheme 14.5

O-α-Acyloxyalkyl ethers may constitute a useful prodrug type for compounds containing a phenol group. Such derivatives are hydrolyzed by a sequential reaction involving formation of an unstable hemiacetal intermediate (Scheme 14.5). Like normal phenol esters, they are susceptible to enzymatic hydrolysis by e.g. human plasma enzymes. This type of ethers are, however, more stable against hydroxide ion-catalyzed hydrolysis than phenolate esters, a feature which makes them potentially more favorable in prodrug design.

14.3.2   Prodrugs for amides, imides and other NH-acidic compounds

14.3.2.1   N-Mannich bases

N-Mannich bases can function as prodrug candidates for NH-acidic compounds like various amides, imides, and hydantoins as well as for aliphatic and aromatic amines (see Section 14.3.3.3). They are generally formed by reacting an NH-acidic compound with formaldehyde, or, in very rare cases, other aldehydes and a primary or secondary aliphatic or aromatic amine (Scheme 14.6).

N-Mannich bases are readily hydrolyzed in aqueous solution. The rate of hydrolysis usually increases with increasing pH resulting in a sigmoidal (S-shaped) pH-rate profile. The shape of the pH-rate profile can be accounted for by assuming spontaneous decomposition of the free N-Mannich base (B) and the protonated form (BH$^+$). The expression of the pH-dependent pseudo-1st order rate constant (k_{obs}) is

$$k_{obs} = k_1 f_B + k_2 f_{BH^+} = k_1 \left(\frac{K_a}{a_{H^+} + K_a} \right) + k_2 \left(\frac{a_{H^+}}{a_{H^+} + K_a} \right) \tag{14.14}$$

where f_B and f_{BH^+} are the fractions of the N-Mannich species on basic and acidic form, respectively. K_a is the apparent ionization constant for the protonated N-Mannich base, and k_1 and k_2 represent the 1st order rate constants for the spontaneous degradation of B and BH$^+$, respectively.

The reaction mechanism proposed for the decomposition involves as rate-limiting step an unimolecular N–C bond cleavage with formation of an amide (or imide) anion and an immonium cation. In subsequent fast steps, a solvent molecule

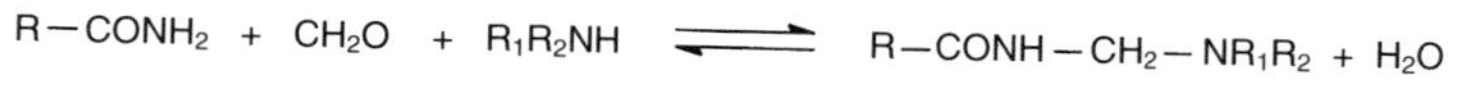

$$R-CONH_2 + CH_2O + R_1R_2NH \rightleftharpoons R-CONH-CH_2-NR_1R_2 + H_2O$$

Scheme 14.6

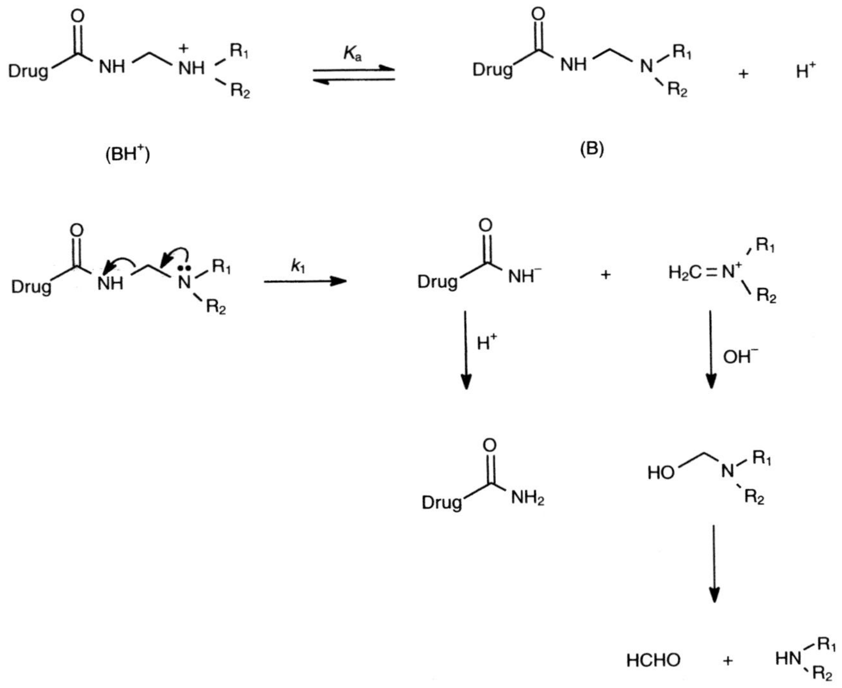

Scheme 14.7

transfers a proton to the anion and a hydroxide ion to the immonium ion, giving methylolamin which rapidly dissociates to formaldehyde and amine (Scheme 14.7). The structural effects on the decomposition rate of N-Mannich bases derived from carboxamides, sulphonamides or imides, and aliphatic or aromatic amines involve (i) steric effects; (ii) basicity of the amine component; and (iii) acidity of the amide component. The effect of these factors are most pronounced with respect to the rate constant k_1 and, accordingly, to the degradation rate in weakly acidic to basic aqueous solution. The rates of hydrolysis of unprotonated N-Mannich bases are accelerated strongly by (i) increasing steric effects within the amine substituent; (ii) increasing basicity of the amine component; and (iii) increasing acidity of the parent amide-type compound. For some N-Mannich bases of benzamide and various amines the rate constant k_1 can be expressed by the following equation

$$\log k_1 = 2.30v - 3.50 \quad (k_1 \text{ in min}^{-1};\ 37\,^\circ\text{C}) \tag{14.15}$$

where v is Charton's steric substituent constant for alkyl amino groups. The marked influence of the steric effect on k_1 is evident from comparison of the k_1 values for benzamide N-Mannich bases of diethylamine (0.52 min^{-1}) and ethylamine (0.0084 min^{-1}).

For amines having the same steric properties but differing in basicity, the rate constants k_1 for degradation of the respective N-Mannich bases increase almost

10-fold with an increase of unity of the pK_a of the amines. Further, the reactivity of this prodrug type increases strongly with increasing acidity of the parent amide-type compound. Thus, for N-Mannich bases derived from morpholine the following relationship has been observed

$$\log k_1 = -1.15\,pK_a + 13.9 \quad (k_1 \text{ in min}^{-1};\ 37\,^{\circ}C) \tag{14.16}$$

where pK_a refers to the ionization constant for the parent amide-type compound. For benzamide, for example, pK_a is about 14.5. From the above it appears that by suitable selection of the amine component, it should be possible to obtain prodrugs of a given amide-type drug varying significantly with respect to *in vivo* lability. Furthermore, other physicochemical properties such as aqueous solubility, dissolution rate, and lipophilicity can be modified for the parent drug compound.

Transformation of an amide into an N-Mannich base introduces a readily ionizable amino function which may allow the preparation of derivatives with greatly enhanced water solubility at slightly acidic pH values where, fortunately, the stability often is sufficiently high. The concept of N-Mannich base formation of NH-acidic compounds to yield more soluble prodrugs has been utilized in the case of clinically used rolitetracycline (**14.10**). This water-soluble N-Mannich base of tetracycline and pyrrolidine is decomposed quantitatively to tetracycline (**14.9**) in neutral aqueous solution, the half-life being 40 min at pH 7.4 and 37 °C. Breakdown of this prodrug is not catalyzed by enzymes, a feature generally observed for N-Mannich bases.

Several biologically active peptides have been identified, including small peptides consisting of only two amino acids. The clinical utility of such chemical entities is, however, seriously hampered by substantial delivery problems. Peptides are highly polar compounds and do not easily pass biological membranes by passive diffusion. In addition, they suffer from considerable metabolic lability. An α-aminoamide moiety is found in many peptides, and a potentially useful and broadly applicable prodrug type for this group may be 4-imidazolidinones formed by reacting such peptides with ketones or aldehydes (Scheme 14.8). Such imidazolidinyl peptides, which may be regarded as cyclic N-Mannich bases, undergo a complete hydrolysis in the pH range 1–10 with maximum rates normally occurring at pH > 4.

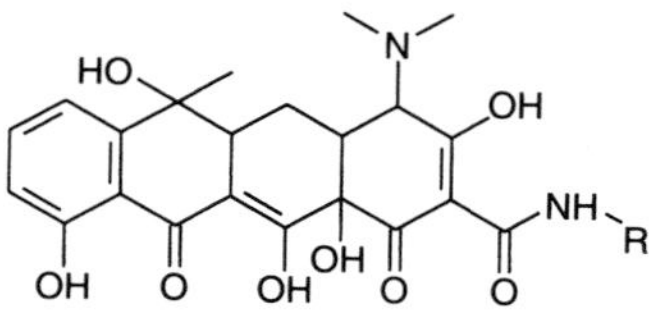

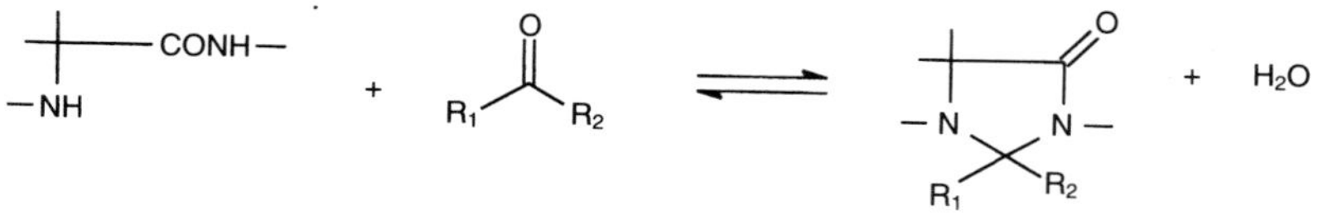

Scheme 14.8

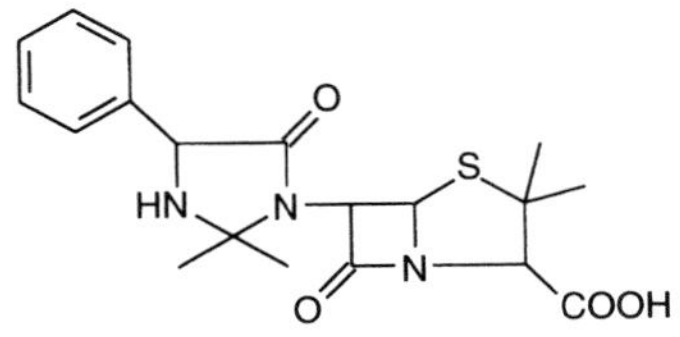

(14.11)

Another example of cyclic *N*-Mannich base-type prodrugs is clinically used hetacillin (**14.11**) which is formed by condensation of ampicillin with acetone. The prodrug is readily hydrolyzed to yield the active ampicillin and acetone, $t_{1/2}$ being 15–20 min at pH 4–8 (35 °C). An advantage of hetacillin is its higher stability in concentrated aqueous solutions compared to ampicillin sodium, which undergoes a facile intermolecular aminolysis by attack of the side-chain amino group in one molecule on the β-lactam moiety of a second molecule.

14.3.2.2   *N-α-acyloxyalkyl derivatives*

N-α-acyloxyalkylation is a commonly used approach to provide prodrugs of various secondary amides, imides, hydantoins, uracils, and tertiary or *N*-heterocyclic amines. By variation of the acyl portion of this type of derivatives it is possible to control the rate of regeneration of the parent drug and to obtain prodrugs with varying physicochemical properties. Whereas, the derivatives which can be referred to as double prodrugs, exhibit reasonable stability in aqueous solution *in vitro* comparable to that of other esters, they are in general rapidly cleaved *in vivo* by virtue of enzyme-mediated hydrolysis. The activation of the parent NH-acidic compound is accomplished by a two-step reaction (Scheme 14.9). The enzymatic cleavage of the ester bond results in the formation of an intermediate *N-α*-hydroxyalkyl derivative which instantaneously decomposes to yield the parent NH-acidic compound and the corresponding aldehyde. Thus, the rate of drug formation is solely dependent on the rate of the initial ester cleavage which as previously mentioned can be controlled by predominantly steric factors.

N-α-acyloxymethylation is most commonly employed, providing derivatives from which formaldehyde is released from the *N*-hydroxymethyl intermediate. In this case, instantaneous decomposition of the formed intermediate requires that the pK_a of the NH-acidic agent is lower than about 10.5 as evident from the established linear relationship between the rate of hydrolysis (expressed in terms

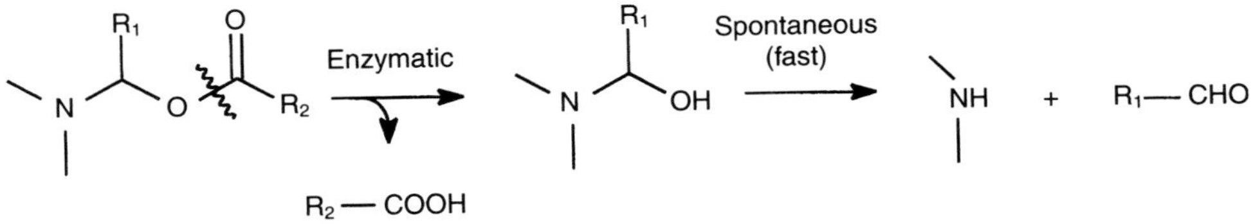

Scheme 14.9

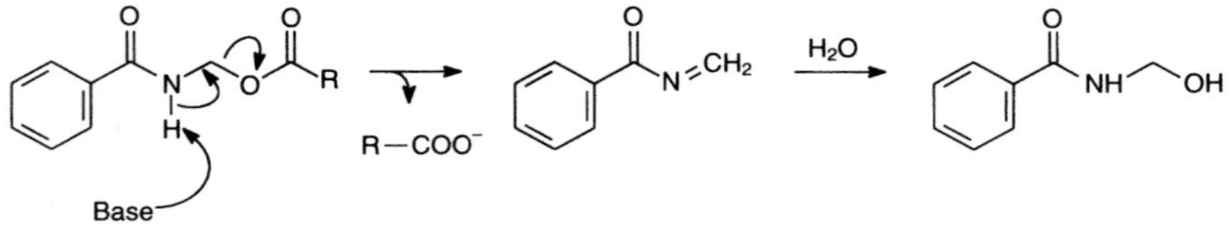

Scheme 14.10

of the half-life) at pH 7.4 of such *N*-hydroxymethyl derivatives and the pK_a of the parent NH-acidic chemical entity

$$\log t_{1/2} = 0.77 pK_a - 8.34 \quad (t_{1/2} \text{ in min; } 37\,^\circ C) \qquad (14.17)$$

However, by using other aldehydes than formaldehyde, the *N*-α-alkylol intermediates thus formed would be more unstable than the *N*-methylol analog, hence expanding the applicability of *N*-α-acyloxyalkylation to NH-acidic drugs possessing pK_a values above 11. It should be emphasized that *N*-α-acyloxyalkylation of NH-acidic compounds like primary amides, carbamates, and sulphonamides is not feasible due to the *in vitro* instability of the derivatives. The latter type of derivatives is extremely unstable in aqueous solution decomposing by an elimination–addition mechanism involving a reactive *N*-acylimine intermediate as illustrated in Scheme 14.10 for *N*-α-acyloxymethyl derivatives of benzamide. In similar derivatives derived from secondary amides the nitrogen atom has no hydrogen attached, and the formation of an *N*-acylimine by a base-catalyzed process is thereby not possible.

14.3.2.3   *N-acyl derivatives*

N-acylation of amide- and imide-type compounds may be a useful prodrug approach in some particular cases. In assessing *N*-acylated amides or imides as potential prodrugs it is important to consider the possibility of drug regeneration afforded by enzyme-catalyzed hydrolysis. Thus, N_3-acetyl-5-fluorouracil (**14.12**) and N_1-ethoxycarbonyl-5-fluorouracil (**14.13**) hydrolyze with half-lives of 40 and 550 min, respectively, at pH 7.4 and 37 °C. In 80% human plasma, however, half-lives of about 2–4 min have been observed. As a result of their altered physicochemical properties and easy bioconversion, these prodrug derivatives of 5-FU have shown improved ocular and rectal absorption as compared to the parent drug.

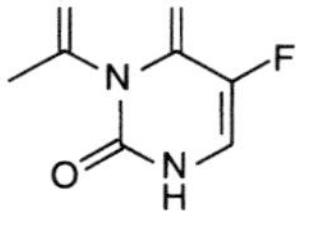

(14.12) 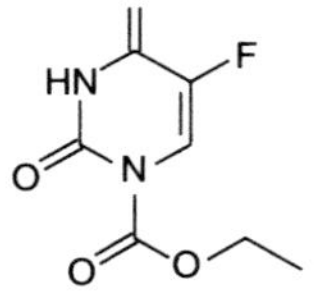   (14.13)

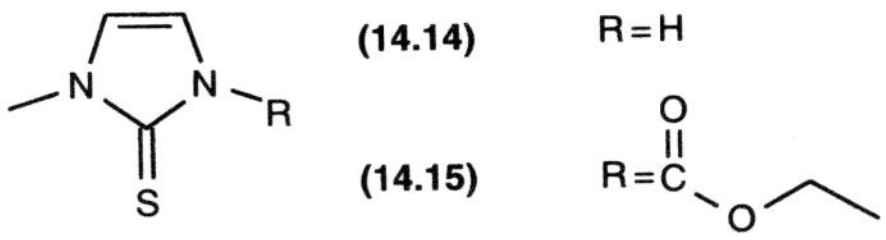

(14.14)   R = H

(14.15)   R = C (=O) O— (ethyl)

Carbimazole (**14.15**) is a widely used prodrug of the antithyroid methimazole (**14.14**). In the presence of serum enzymes, the ethoxycarbonyl group is rapidly cleaved.

14.3.3 Prodrugs for amines

14.3.3.1 Amides

In prodrug design, *N*-acylation of amines to yield amides has been used only to a limited extent due to the relatively high stability of amides *in vivo*. However, certain activated amides are sufficiently chemically labile including the *N*-L-isoleucyl derivative of dopamine and the *N*-glycyl derivative midodrin (**14.17**) which is an orally absorbable prodrug of compound (**14.16**).

14.3.3.2 N-acyloxyalkoxycarbonyl derivatives

The utility of carbamates as prodrug derivatives for amines (R−NH−(C=O)−OR$_1$) is limited due to the general resistance of carbamates to undergo enzymatic cleavage *in vivo*. By introduction of an enzymatically labile ester function in the carbamate structure it is, however, possible to circumvent this problem. Thus, *N*-acyloxyalkoxycarbonyl derivatives of primary and secondary amines may be readily transformed to the parent amine *in vivo*. Enzymatic hydrolysis of the ester moiety in such derivatives leads to an unstable hydroxyalkoxycarbonyl intermediate which spontaneously decomposes into the parent amine via a labile carbamic acid (Scheme 14.11). Such acyloxyalkyl carbamates may be promising biolabile

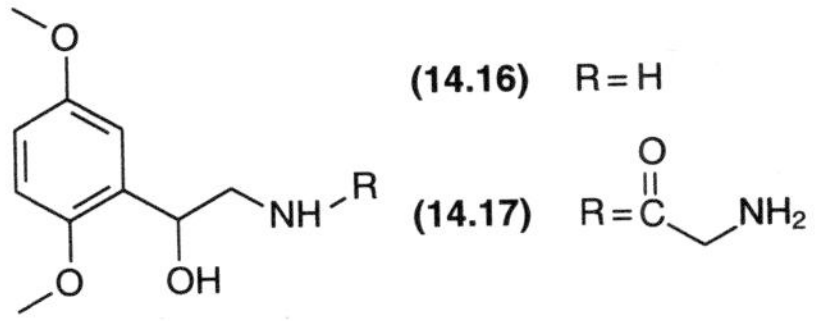

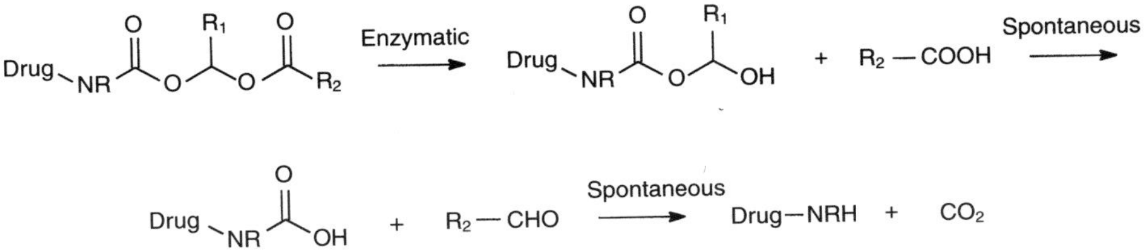

(14.16)   R = H

(14.17)   R = C(=O) NH$_2$

Scheme 14.11

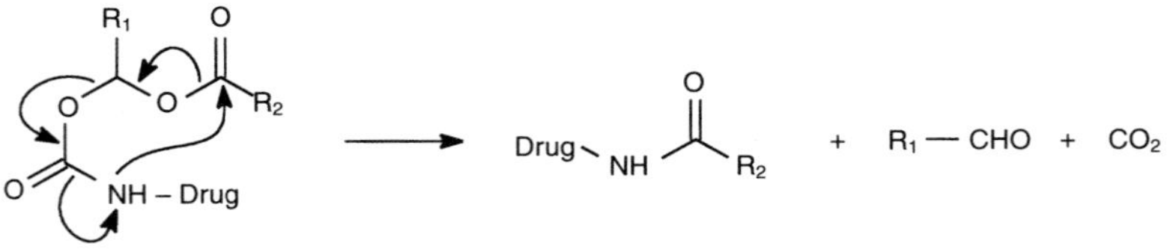

Scheme 14.12

prodrugs for amino functional drugs since they are neutral compounds and combine a high stability in aqueous solution with a high susceptibility to undergo enzymatic reconversion to the active agent initiated by hydrolysis of the terminal ester function. In case of primary amines, it should be noticed that an intramolecular acyl transfer reaction, leading to the formation of a stable *N*-acylated parent amine (Scheme 14.12), may compete with the reaction sequence presented in Scheme 14.11 at physiological pH and thus diminish the amount of amine regenerated. Such intramolecular *N*-acylation is structurally impossible in derivatives obtained from secondary amines.

14.3.3.3 N-Mannich bases

Besides being considered as a potential approach of derivatizing amide-type drugs (see Section 14.3.2.1), *N*-Mannich base formation can also be thought as a means of forming prodrugs of primary and secondary amines in which case the amide-type component constitutes the transport-moiety. By *N*-Mannich base formation, the pK_a value of the corresponding acid of the amine component is lowered by about 3 units. Thus, compared to the parent amines the derivatives are much less protonated at physiological pH, resulting in enhanced biomembrane-passage ability. This expectation of increased lipophilicity has been confirmed for e.g. the *N*-Mannich base derived from benzamide and phenylpropanolamine (α-(1-aminoethyl)benzylalcohol). The partition coefficient of the derivative between *n*-octanol and phosphate buffer pH 7.4 is about 100-times higher than that of the parent amine. By benzamidomethylation, the pK_a of phenylpropanolamine decreases from 9.4 to 6.2 revealing that the derivative is predominantly unprotonated at pH 7.4, a major contributing factor to the enhanced *P* value of the latter compound.

The availability of biologically acceptable amide-type pro-moieties affording an appropriate cleavage rate of a *N*-Mannich base of a given amine at pH 7.4 is limited. In search for useful candidates, it has been found that *N*-Mannich bases of salicyl-amide (**14.20**) and different aliphatic amines including amino acids show an unexpectedly high cleavage rate at neutral pH, thus indicating the utility of this transport group (Scheme 14.13). Although the salicylamide *N*-Mannich bases are more stable in weakly acidic solution (pH 2–5) than at pH 7.4, a drawback to the use of this prodrug type still is its limited *in vitro* stability. Improved stability may be achieved by further derivatization of the latter type of *N*-Mannich bases under formation of double prodrugs. Since the hydroxy group is responsible for the high reactivity of these derivatives, presumably through intramolecular catalysis, protection of this

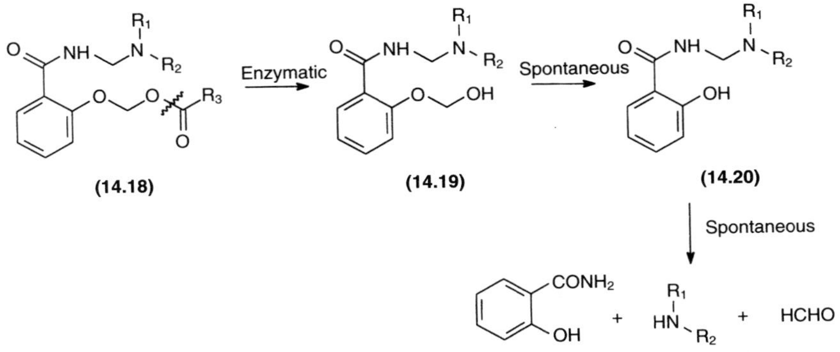

Scheme 14.13

group can afford derivatives exhibiting enhanced *in vitro* stability. This is actually achievable by acyloxymethylation of the phenolic hydroxy group. The *O*-acyloxy-methyl derivative (**14.18**) is significantly more stable than (**14.20**) in the pH range 2–8. In the presence of human plasma, the ester group is rapidly hydrolyzed by virtue of enzymatic catalysis yielding (**14.19**) which spontaneously degrades to (**14.20**) (Scheme 14.13). In addition to providing an *in vitro* stabilizing effect, the concept of *O*-acyloxymethylation makes it possible to obtain prodrug derivatives of a given amine possessing varying physicochemical properties of importance for drug delivery, such as water solubility and lipophilicity. This can simply be effected by selection of an appropriate acyloxymethyl group (varying the R_3 group).

14.3.4 Prodrugs for compounds containing carbonyl groups

Despite the existence of a fairly large number of drugs containing a carbonyl group only a few bioreversible derivatives have been explored for molecules containing an aldehydic or ketonic functional group. Potential prodrug types include Schiff bases, oximes and enol esters, however, only oxazolidines and thiazolidines are briefly considered in the following section.

14.3.4.1 Oxazolidines and thiazolidines

In addition to constituting a possible approach of derivatizing β-aminoalcohols (see Section 14.3.6), oxazolidine formation can also be thought as a means of achieving prodrugs of aldehydes and ketones in which case the β-aminoalcohol component acts as the transport-moiety (Scheme 14.14). In considering oxazo-lidines as prodrug candidates for carbonyl-containing chemical entities, their weakly basic character (pKa 5–7) may be advantageous since such derivatives are protonated at acidic pH and may thus exhibit a desired aqueous solubility at low pH.

Thiazolidines have been applied as prodrug derivatives for various steroids containing a 3-carbonyl group to improve their topical anti-inflammatory activity. Thiazolidines (spirothiazolidines) of hydrocortisone and hydrocortisone 21-acetate

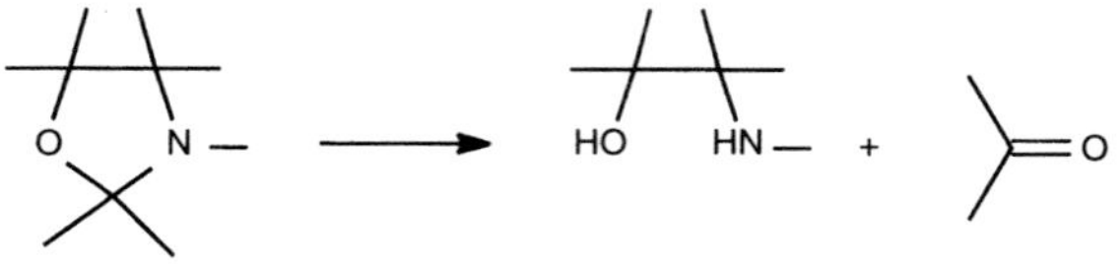

Scheme 14.14

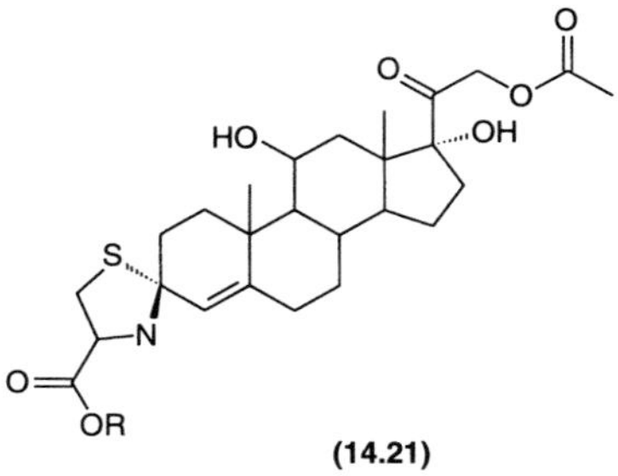

(14.21)

(**14.21**), prepared with cysteine esters or related β-aminothiols, have been shown to be readily converted to the parent corticosteroids at conditions similar to those prevailing in the skin, thus meeting the requirement for a prodrug. Thiazolidine ring opening proceeds by a spontaneous S_N1 cleavage of the carbon–sulphur bond to give a Schiff base intermediate which then is hydrolyzed. In particular, cysteine derivatives may be attractive as pro-moieties due to release of cysteine as a by-product. Also, the carboxyl group of cysteine is easily esterifiable, thus providing a convenient method for changing the lipophilicity/hydrophilicity of the spirothiazolidine prodrugs.

14.3.5 Drug activation from intramolecular cyclization reactions

14.3.5.1 Ring-opened derivatives as prodrugs for cyclic drugs

Pilocarpine (**14.22**) is used as a typical miotic agent for controlling the elevated intraocular pressure associated with glaucoma. Its ocular bioavailability is low and the duration of action is short, thereby necessitating frequent dosing corresponding to 3–6 times a day. This leads to transient peaks and valleys in pilocarpine concentration in the eye, which in turn result in dose-related ocular side effects such as myopia and miosis. There is, therefore, a high incidence of patient non-compliance, which has been suspected to be responsible for inadequate pressure control and deterioration of vision. A useful prodrug of pilocarpine should (i) exhibit a higher lipophilicity than pilocarpine in order to enable an efficient corneal membrane transport; (ii) possess adequate solubility and stability for formulation as eyedrops; (iii) be converted to the active within cornea or once the membrane has been passed; and (iv) lead to a controlled release and hence prolonged duration of action of pilocarpine.

Pilocarpic acid esters may be promising prodrug candidates with the above mentioned desired attributes. A series of alkyl and aralkyl esters of pilocarpic acid (**14.23**)

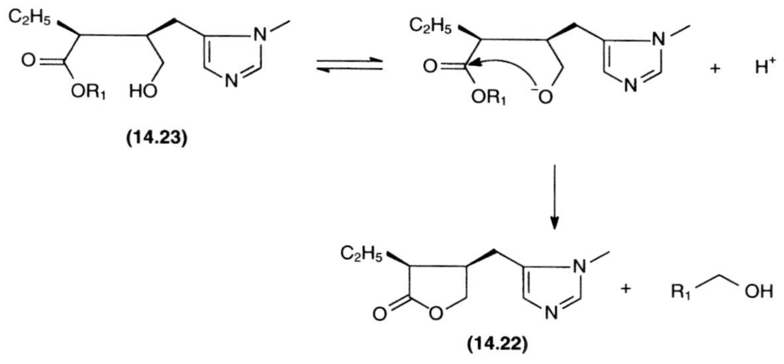

Scheme 14.15

has been shown to function as prodrugs of pilocarpine both *in vitro* and *in vivo*. In aqueous solution, the esters undergo quantitative and apparent specific base-catalyzed lactonization to pilocarpine (Scheme 14.15). As appears from the rate data shown in Table 14.5, the various esters differ greatly in their rates of cyclization, the variation being fully accounted for in terms of polar effects exerted by the alcohol portion of the esters. An LFER was found between the logarithm of half-time of pilocarpine formation (pH 7.4; 37 °C) and the Taft polar substituent constant σ^*, the latter referring to R in RCH_2OH for the alcohols according to the expression

$$\log t_{1/2} = -1.44\sigma^* + 2.73 \ (t_{1/2} \text{ in min}) \ (n = 9; \ r = 0.998) \tag{14.18}$$

It is apparent that by appropriate variation of the alcohol portion of the esters, there are possibilities to vary and predict the rate of ring closure and hence to

Table 14.5 Rate data for the conversion of pilocarpic acid monoesters to pilocarpine in aqueous solution (37 °C), Tafts polar substituent constant σ^* refering to R in the alcohols RCH_2OH, and partition coefficients for the compounds

Compound	R	σ^* for R	$t_{1/2}^a$ (min)	$\log P^b$
Pilocarpine				−0.15
Pilocarpic acid esters:				
Methyl	H	0.49	95	0.07
Ethyl	CH_3	0.00	510	0.58
Butyl	$CH_2CH_2CH_3$	−0.12	820	1.58
Hexyl	$(CH_2)_4CH_3$	−0.23	1105	2.56
Benzyl	C_6H_5	0.75	50	1.82
4-Chlorobenzyl	C_6H_4-4-Cl	0.87	30	2.54
4-Methylbenzyl	C_6H_4-4-CH_3	0.59	77	2.31
4-tert-butylbenzyl	C_6H_4-4-$C(CH_3)_3$	0.52	87	3.52
Phenetyl	CH_2-C_6H_5	0.27	227	2.16

Notes
a Half-live of lactonization at pH 7.40.
b Logarithm of the partition coefficients between octanol and 0.05 M phosphate buffer solution at pH 7.40.

control and modify the rate of pilocarpine generation. Likewise, by proper selection of the alcohol moiety it is possible to confer a wide range of lipophilicities on the prodrug derivatives (Table 14.5).

The rate of cyclization of the monoesters to yield pilocarpine increases proportionally with the hydroxide ion concentration in the pH range 3.5–10. The main drawback of these derivatives is their limited solution stability, making it difficult to prepare ready-to-use solutions with a not too low pH and an acceptable shelf-life. This problem can, however, be totally overcome by blocking the free hydroxy group in the monoesters by further esterification. The double esters (**14.24**) or double prodrugs thus obtained are highly stable in aqueous solution even at pH 6–7 (predicted shelf-lives exceeding 5 years at 25 °C). In addition these, double prodrugs are subject to facile enzymatic hydrolysis at the *O*-acyl bond. In human plasma or rabbit eye tissue homogenate, pilocarpine is formed from the double prodrugs in quantitative amounts through a sequential process (Scheme 14.16). Besides solving the stability problem of the monoester derivatives, the pilocarpic acid diesters were found to possess even better ocular delivery characteristics including enhanced absorption and longer lasting pilocarpine activity. Although highly lipophilic at pH 7.4, the basic character of the imidazole moiety in the compounds (pK$_a$ about 7) allows for the preparation of sufficiently water-soluble salts, e.g. nitrates or fumarates.

Similar ring-opened double prodrugs are peptide derivatives of 2-aminobenzophenones (**14.25**) which may be water-soluble prodrugs of diazepam and related slightly soluble 1,4-benzodiazepines, suitable for parenteral administration. The derivatives are stable *in vitro*, but are cleaved *in vivo* by aminopeptidases with formation of a 2-aminoacetamidobenzophenone (**14.26**) which subsequently undergoes a spontaneous cyclization to the corresponding benzodiazepine (**14.27**) (Scheme 14.17).

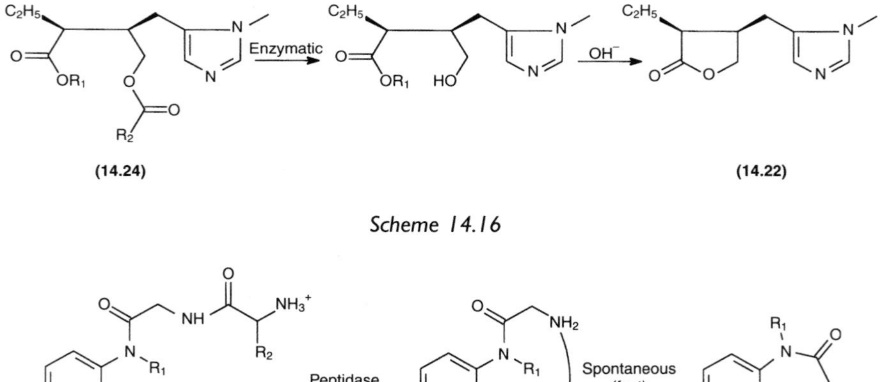

(14.24)   (14.22)

Scheme 14.16

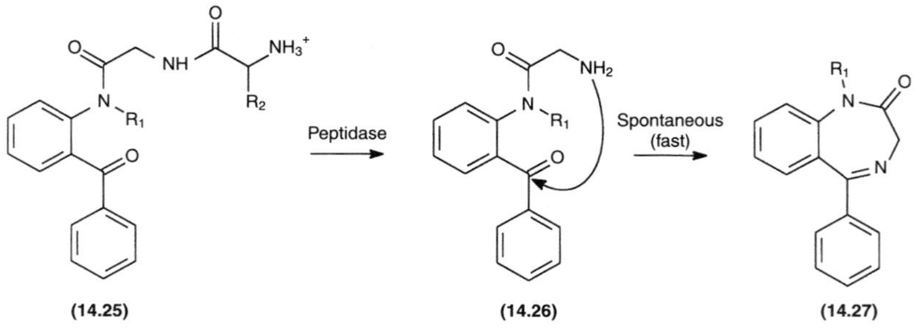

(14.25)   (14.26)   (14.27)

Scheme 14.17

The rate of *in vivo* hydrolysis of the peptide linkage depends markedly upon the L-amino acid attached to the 2-aminoacetamidobenzophenone where peptide derivatives from Phe and Lys are cleaved much faster than those from Gly and Glu. Whereas the benzophenone derived from diazepam cyclizes almost immediately, that of demethyldiazepam shows a half-life of conversion of 15 min at pH 7.4 and 37 °C.

14.3.5.2   *Drug release facilitated by intramolecular cyclization reactions*

Many bioreversible derivates rely on enzymatic hydrolysis of the prodrug bond for achievement of useful regeneration rates of the active agent. However, these conditions are not always attainable or may be subject to considerable inter- or intra-species variability. A prodrug strategy to overcome this problem takes advantage of facile intramolecular cyclization reactions where a latent nucleophile is unmasked by different biological or chemical triggering mechanisms that in turn initiate the cyclization reaction to release the parent drug (Figure 14.7). Generally, intramolecular nucleophilic catalysis is favored by formation of five- or six-membered cyclic transition states. In addition to the character of the nucleophile and the type of carboxylic acid derivative, the rate of an intramolecular reaction is dependent on the degrees of freedom of the intercalated alkyl chain. Thus, steric factors resulting in less flexible molecules may lead to increased reaction rates.

Alkylaminoethyl carbamate prodrugs (**14.28**) have been developed using a terminal free amino group as a nucleophile to facilitate the release of the melanocytotoxic agent 4-hydroxyanisole (**14.29**) (Scheme 14.18). These prodrugs were developed to release the parent drug in a non-enzymatic fashion and, therefore, to avoid the potential variation in release rates due to variable enzyme activities among individuals. At pH 7.4 (37 °C) the most labile prodrug ($R_1=CH_3$, $R_2=CH_3$) released the drug with a half-life of 36 min. In comparison, the related derivative only differing by an extension of the carbon chain between the two nitrogen atoms to 3 methylenes was much less reactive exhibiting a $t_{1/2}$ of 942 min.

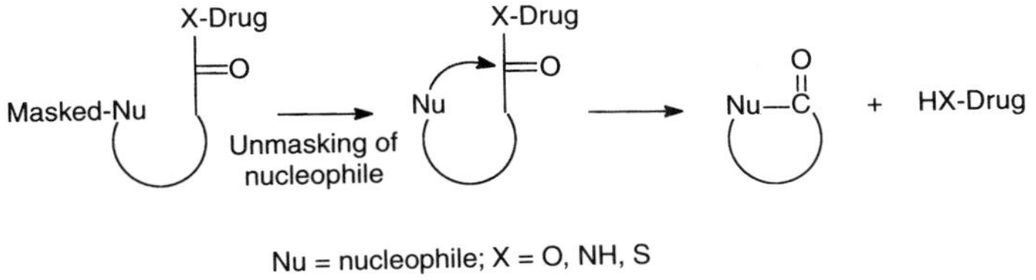

Nu = nucleophile; X = O, NH, S

Figure 14.7 Prodrug strategy that takes advantage of intramolecular cyclization reactions.

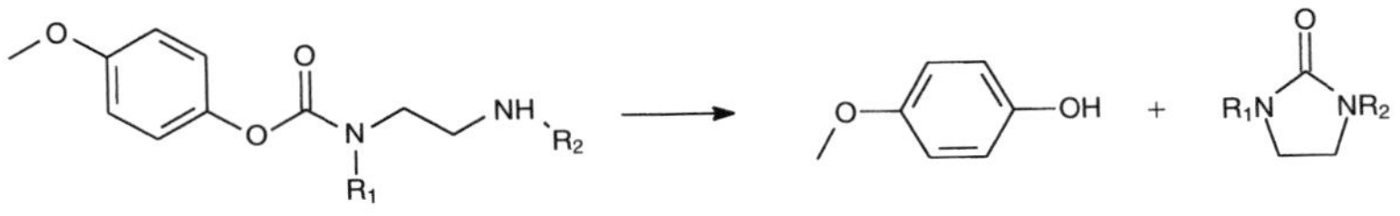

(14.28)   (14.29)

Scheme 14.18

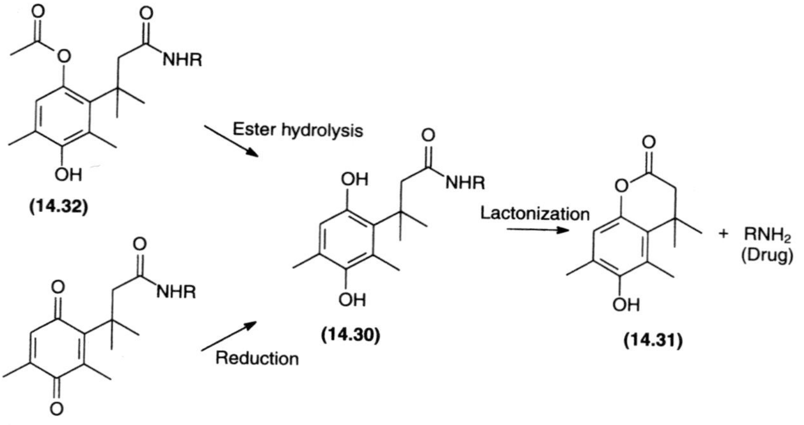

Scheme 14.19

The chemically highly reactive phenolamide derivative **14.30** can function as a prodrug for an amine drug. The intramolecular lactonization reaction, affording the parent amine drug and the lactone (**14.31**), proceeds with a half-life of about 1 min at physiological pH and temperature. The reactivity of this compound is attributed to the presence of the 'trimethyl lock' (methyl groups in positions 3, 3 and 6'). The half-life is, however, too short for practical use. In order to transform (**14.30**) into a chemically more stable and yet enzymatically labile prodrug the double prodrugs (**14.32**) and (**14.33**) have been developed. The parent amine is regenerated via a two-step process. The initial enzymatic step may be catalyzed by esterases or reductive mechanisms, the ester portion in (**14.32**) and the quinone portion in (**14.33**) being transformed to (**14.30**), respectively, followed by the nonenzymatic lactonization (Scheme 14.19).

14.3.6 Cyclic prodrugs involving two functional groups of the drug

Bioreversible cyclization of the peptide backbone may constitute a promising approach in small peptide drug delivery. Backbone cyclization caps the C- and N-terminal functionalities and may result in conformationally restricted cyclic peptides possessing a higher stability toward proteolysis as compared to their corresponding linear peptides. Further advantages of this cyclization strategy can be reduction in charge of the peptide, creation of solution structures that may allow for intramolecular hydrogen bonding and reduction in hydrodynamic volume. The latter characteristics may all add to improved membrane transport properties of such cyclized derivatives. Methodologies reported for linking the N-terminal amino group to the C-terminal carboxyl group include the use of (i) an acyloxyalkoxy pro-moiety (**14.34**); (ii) a 3-(2'-hydroxy-4',6'-dimethylphenyl)-3,3-dimethylpropionic acid pro-moiety (**14.35**); and (iii) a coumaric acid pro-moiety (**14.36**) (Figure 14.8).

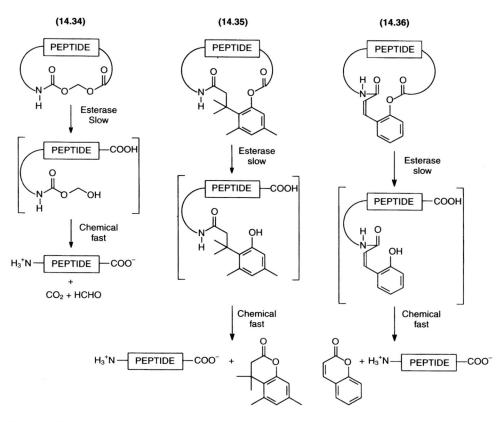

Figure 14.8 Proposed pathway of conversion of acyloxyalkoxy-based cyclic prodrugs (**14.34**), 3-(2'-hydroxy-4',6'-dimethylphenyl)-3,3-dimethyl-propanoic acid-based cyclic prodrugs (**14.35**), and coumaric acid-based cyclic prodrugs (**14.36**) to the parent peptide in esterase containing media.

Using a model hexapeptide, H-Trp-Ala-Gly-Gly-Asp-Ala-OH, cyclic prodrugs have been obtained by employing the above methodologies (i) and (ii). These derivatives were designed to be susceptible to esterase metabolism (slow step) leading to a series of consecutive chemical reactions by which the linear peptide was regenerated. In aqueous buffer at pH 7.4 (37 °C) both prodrugs degraded quantitatively to the hexapeptide. Hydrolysis of the cyclic derivatives proceeded much faster in human blood than in the buffer solution. *In vitro* transport studies (Caco-2 cells) have revealed that in comparison with the hexapeptide, both cyclic prodrugs showed at least a 70-fold higher capacity of permeating this cell culture model of the intestinal mucosa.

Oxazolidines (see Section 14.3.4.1) can be prodrug candidates for the β-amino-alcohol function which is present in several drugs, e.g. various sympathomimetic amines and β-blockers. By varying the carbonyl moiety, oxazolidines exhibiting different stabilities can be obtained. Thus, the following half-lives of hydrolysis of

(14.37)

various (–)-ephedrine oxazolidines (**14.37**) have been found at pH 7.4 and 37 °C: 5 min (benzaldehyde), 5 sec (salicylaldehyde), 30 min (pivaldehyde), and 6 min (cyclohexanone).

14.4   APPLICATIONS OF THE PRODRUG APPROACH

The prodrug approach has been successfully applied to a wide variety of drugs. Most applications have aimed at (i) enhancing biomembrane transport and bioavailability; (ii) increasing site-specificity; and (iii) improving drug formulation.

14.4.1   Biomembrane passage and bioavailability

Therapeutic agents have to permeate one or more biological membrane(s) in order to reach the target site. Although drugs are administered by a number of quite different routes, this section primarily deals with the use of prodrug design to solve delivery problems related to some of the most widely used routes of administration, e.g. oral, dermal and ocular drug delivery.

14.4.1.1   Oral absorption

For orally administered drugs one major challenge of reaching their sites of action is that they have to cross the intestinal epithelial cells to enter the systemic circulation. Poor transport properties may lead to low bioavailability which may also result from low water solubility, low stability in the gastrointestinal juices or extensive first-pass metabolism.

   Well-known examples of transiently increasing the lipophilicity to enhance absorption of polar drugs by prodrug modification include various ampicillin derivatives. Being zwitterionic in the pH range of the gastrointestinal tract, ampicillin (**14.38**) possesses a low lipophilicity and the absorption fraction after oral administration amounts to about 30%. Altering the polarity of the penicillin by esterification of the free carboxyl group to form the prodrugs pivampicillin (**14.39**) and bacampicillin (**14.40**) has proven successful, resulting in essentially complete absorption of (**14.38**). During or after entering into the systemic circulation, these prodrugs are cleaved by enzymes to yield the active antibiotic. A discussion of the mechanism of cleavage of such double ester prodrugs is given in Section 14.3.1. Recently, it has been realized that some orally administered peptidomimetic drugs are absorbed through the intestinal peptide transport systems. One of these transport systems accepts various β-lactam antibiotics, including ampicillin, and acts as

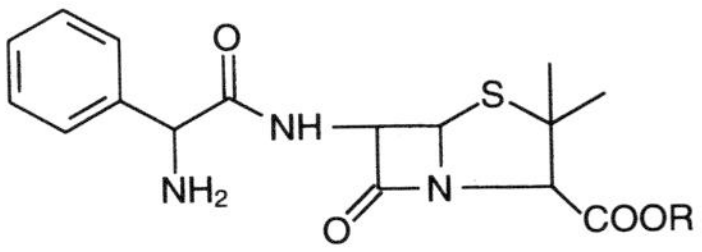

(14.38) R = H

(14.39) R = CH$_2$

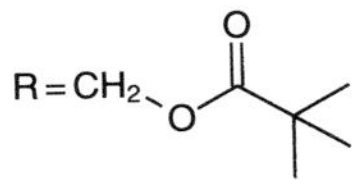

(14.40) R = CH

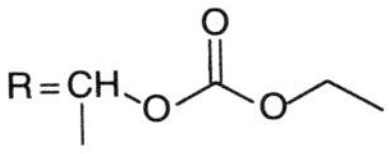

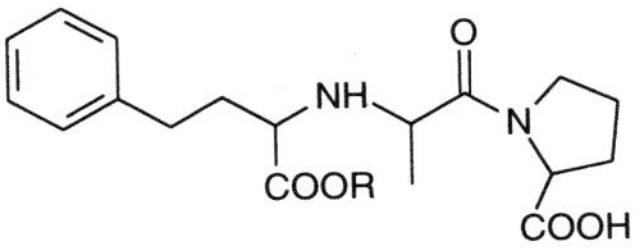

(14.41) R = H
(14.42) R = C$_2$H$_5$

a carrier for their absorption. The enhanced lipophilicity of the ampicillin pro-drugs favors passive membrane transport but the improved bioavailability could also reflect that the ester derivatives are better substrates for the carrier system than ampicillin. Also various peptidic ACE inhibitors like enalapril (14.42) are substrates for peptide transport systems. Enalapril is the ethyl ester of the active acid (14.41). Although the ethyl ester is much better absorbed than the active acid, it is rather slowly cleaved in the organism by liver hydrolases.

The intestinal peptide transport systems have been a key target for prodrug approaches. According to this approach, prodrugs appropriately designed in the form of di- or tripeptide analogs (the di- or tripeptide constituting the 'functionally based' pro-moiety) can be absorbed across the intestinal brush border membrane via a peptide transport system. The prodrug may be targeted to the epithelial membrane and hydrolyzed on the apical surface of the epithelium prior to absorption by the transporter or may be absorbed intact and hydrolyzed intracellularly by peptidases or esterases prior to exit from the cell. A dipeptidyl prodrug derivative of L-α-methyldopa, L-α-methyldopa-L-phenylalanine (14.43) has been prepared. This prodrug displayed up to 20 times increase in intestinal permeability compared to the parent compound in *in situ* single pass rat intestinal perfusion studies. Experiments have shown the occurrence of hydrolysis of the prodrug in intestinal cell homogenates, suggesting liberation of the parent compound after intestinal uptake.

Several drugs show poor and variable oral absorption characteristics as a result of insufficient water solubility (less than about 0.1% w/v) leading to dissolution rate-limited absorption. An example of a prodrug used to increase the aqueous solubility and to improve dissolution behavior is the water-soluble dipotassium salt of clorazepate (14.44) which is marketed as a prodrug of the slightly soluble

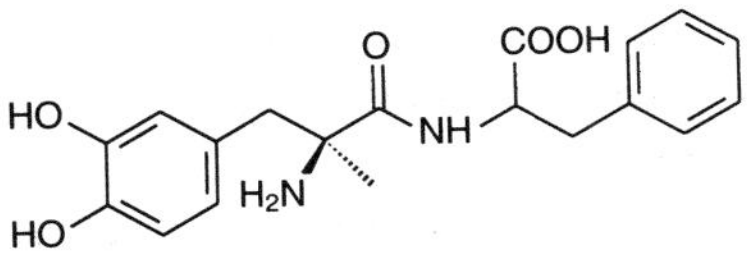

(14.43)

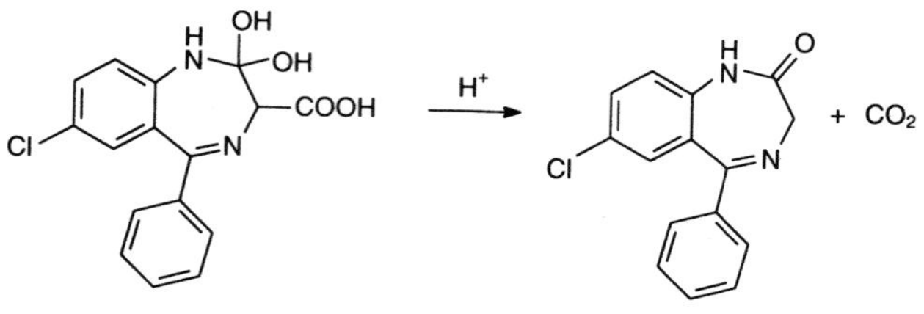

(14.44)   **(14.45)**

Scheme 14.20

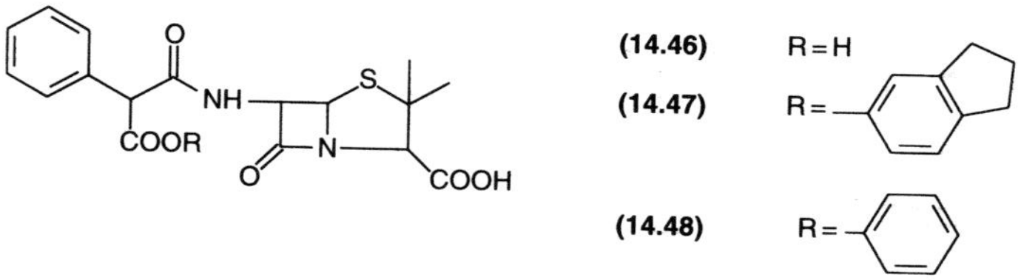

(14.46)   R = H

(14.47)   R =

(14.48)   R =

demethyldiazepam (**14.45**). In acidic solution clorazepate spontaneously decarboxylates to the parent drug constituting the form absorbed (Scheme 14.20). Prodrug strategies to enhance aqueous solubility is further dealt with in Section 14.4.3.

The poor gastrointestinal absorption of carbenicillin (**14.46**) is due to acid-catalyzed degradation of the drug in the stomach as well as to its strongly polar character. By bioreversible esterification of the side-chain carboxyl group, the more acid-stable and lipophilic derivatives carindacillin (**14.47**) and carfecillin (**14.48**) are obtained. Following absorption carbenicillin is released in the blood by enzymatic hydrolysis of these clinically used prodrugs.

14.4.1.2   Dermal absorption

The potential of various prodrug types to enhance the delivery of drugs through the skin (transdermal delivery) and into the skin (dermal delivery) have been investigated. Most drugs diffuse poorly through the skin, in particular through stratum corneum, because of unfavorable physicochemical properties. Several studies have demonstrated biphasic solubility as being an important determinant of the flux across the skin, i.e. in order to diffuse readily through the skin a compound should possess adequate water as well as lipid solubility. This can often be achieved by the prodrug approach and, in fact, the dermal delivery of several drug molecules such as steroids, antiviral, and antipsoriasis agents have been improved by this approach.

Levonorgestrel (**14.49**) is a very potent, lipophilic contraceptive drug which is very poorly soluble in water (1μg/ml at 25°C), and does not permeate through the skin at a sufficient rate. Two carbonate ester prodrugs containing hydroxy functional groups in the alkyl portion of the pro-moiety **14.50** and **14.51** were synthesized. Although the prodrugs were more soluble in aqueous ethanol than the parent steroid, their $\log P_{oct}$ values were close to that of levonorgestrel indicating that the

(14.49)   R = H
(14.50)   R = (C=O)OCH₂CH(OH)CH₂OH
(14.51)   R = (C=O)O(CH₂)₄CH(OH)CH₂OH

(14.52)   R = H
(14.53)   R = CH₂O(C=O)CH₃
(14.54)   R = CH₂O(C=O)CH(CH₃)₂

octanol solubility of the esters also exceeded that of the steroid. Thus, the carbonate ester prodrugs (**14.50**) and (**14.51**) exhibit greater biphasic solubility than levonorgestrel and were found to enhance the transdermal delivery of total levonorgestrel 30 and 15 times, respectively.

Nalidixic acid (**14.52**) is a relatively high melting solid which is poorly soluble in water and isopropyl myristate, but has shown some promise in the topical treatment of psoriasis. By esterifying the carboxyl group by *O*-acyloxymethylation, prodrug derivatives **14.53** and **14.54** being both more lipid- and water-soluble have been obtained. Diffusion studies *in vitro* using human skin have shown that the isobutyryloxymethyl derivative affords a 5–6 fold enhanced delivery of nalidixic acid from both polar and non-polar vehicles relative to application of nalidixic acid itself.

14.4.1.3 *Ocular absorption*

A major problem in ocular therapeutics is the attainment of an optimal drug concentration at the site of action. The difficulty is largely due to the fact that all of the existing drugs, many of which were originally developed for systemic use, lack the physicochemical properties for overcoming the severe constraints imposed by the eye on drug absorption. These constraints include precorneal factors that rapidly remove the drug from the conjunctival sac where it is applied and a well-designed corneal structure that restricts the passage of drug molecules. The net result is that less than 10%, and often 1% or less, of the instilled dose is ocularly absorbed. Corneal drug penetration is inefficient owing to a mismatch of the physicochemical properties of the drug with those of the cornea. Optimal $\log P_{oct}$ values of 2–3 for transcellular corneal drug permeation have been suggested. This observation has formed the basis for bioreversible modification of hydrophilic ophthalmic drugs, the first of which was epinephrine. Since then, several other ophthalmic drugs have been investigated for prodrug derivatization including timolol, pilocarpine, and terbutaline.

Epinephrine (**14.55**) has long been used for the treatment of glaucoma although its corneal absorption is poor because of its high polarity and rapid metabolic destruction. Originally, epinephrine solutions were manufactured with a pH of about 3.5 due to the high instability of the ophthalmic agent in aqueous solution.

(14.55)   **(14.56)**   **(14.57)**

Optimum stability is observed in the pH range 3–4. In addition to acid-catalyzed racemization, epinephrine is extremely sensitive to oxidation, a reaction which is base-catalyzed. Even at low pH levels, oxidation occurs rapidly and such formulations exhibited short shelf-lives. Later, it was observed that such ophthalmic solutions could be stabilized by incorporation of boric acid which forms a 1:1 complex (**14.56**) with epinephrine thereby masking the labile *ortho*-diphenol structure. In the presence of the antioxidant sodium bisulfite this complex was much less sensitive to oxidation allowing the preparation of a reasonably stable ophthalmic solution with a pH close to 7.

  Thus, two problems – ocular irritation and instability in solution – were solved by this formulation approach. However, bioavailability of (**14.55**) from the latter formulation type was still very poor. The development of the prodrug, dipivefrin (**14.57**) has lead to a markedly improved ocular delivery of epinephrine. This dipivalate ester prodrug is much more lipophilic than epinephrine and esterification of the phenolic hydroxy groups gives rise to a derivative exhibiting significantly better chemical and metabolic stability than the parent drug. These properties coupled with a sufficiently high susceptibility to undergo enzymatic hydrolysis in the eye during and after absorption are responsible for the approximately 20 times higher antiglaucoma activity of dipivefrin in comparison with parent epinephrine upon local administration in humans. In addition, undesirable cardiotoxic side effects due to epinephrine absorption from the tear duct overflow are diminished because lower doses of the prodrug can be used.

14.4.1.4   Prevention of first-pass metabolism

Extensive presystemic metabolism may exclude a pharmacologically interesting lead candidate, intended for the oral route, from further development due to formation of unwanted metabolites and variable bioavailability. This metabolic inactivation of chemical entities may take place in the intestinal lumen, at the brush border of the intestinal cells, in the mucosal cells lining the gastrointestinal tract, the liver, or the lung. Although liver first-pass metabolism is avoided by using alternative routes of administration such as the sublingual and transdermal route, oral administration is most convenient and generally preferred for most drug substances.

  The prodrug approach may be useful in reducing or circumventing first-pass metabolism where the obvious approach is to transiently mask the metabolic labile

(14.58) R = H

(14.59) R = C(=O)—(phenyl with H₂N)

(14.60) R = C(=O)—(phenyl with HO)

(14.61) R = C(=O)—(phenyl)

functionalities in the drug molecule. The latter approach, however, requires regeneration of the drug after the prodrug has entered the systemic circulation. Many drugs containing phenolic hydroxy groups undergo extensive first-pass metabolism. Rapid inactivation of such drugs (e.g. morphine, isoprenaline, naltrexone, and various steroids) is the result of sulphate conjugation, glucuronidation or methylation of the phenolic moieties. By masking the metabolizable phenol group of the opioid antagonist naltrexone (**14.58**) in the form of the anthranilate ester (**14.59**) and the salicylate ester (**14.60**), prodrugs with significantly enhanced oral bioavailability have been obtained. Oral administration of (**14.59**) and (**14.60**) to dogs resulted in a bioavailability of the parent drug of 49 and 31%, respectively. In comparison, the bioavailability of naltrexone was about 1% whereas the unsubstituted benzoate ester (**14.61**) did not improve the absorption fraction. Hydrolysis data revealed that the esters (**14.59**) and (**14.60**) are more stable toward enzymatic hydrolysis than the benzoate ester, indicating that these esters survive presystemic hydrolysis to a greater extent.

Orally administered drugs can gain access to the systemic circulation via two separate and functionally distinct absorption pathways – the portal blood and the intestinal lymphatics, with the former representing the major absorption path for the vast majority of orally administered drugs. The intestinal lymphatics are a specialized absorption and transport pathway for lipids and highly lipophilic compounds ($\log P > 5$–6). Drug delivery opportunities associated with intestinal lymphatics include the bypass of hepatic first-pass metabolism after oral dosing. The overall lipophilicity of the drug or prodrug constitutes the major factor governing the extent of lymphatic absorption. Two approaches have been explored for achieving sufficiently lipophilic, bioreversible derivatives encompassing the formation of simple ester derivatives and the design of prodrugs involving 'functionally based' pro-moieties. The latter approach to enhance lymphatic absorption has arisen from an understanding of the processes associated with the absorption and subsequent intracellular processing of absorbed lipid digestion products. Intestinal lymphatic delivery of a variety of glyceride prodrugs have been investigated in which the drug has been conjugated to either mono- or diglycerides.

Testosterone (**14.62**) undergoes almost quantitative first-pass metabolism after oral administration. Various depot injectables consisting of esters of testosterone dissolved in vegetable oils are available for the treatment of androgen deficiency syndromes. In addition, an oral formulation containing testosterone undecanoate (**14.63**) is marketed. It has been shown that the latter highly lipophilic ester is almost exclusively transported via the intestinal lymphatics. Oral bioavailability of testosterone after administration of (**14.62**) and (**14.63**) to humans of 3.6 and 6.8%,

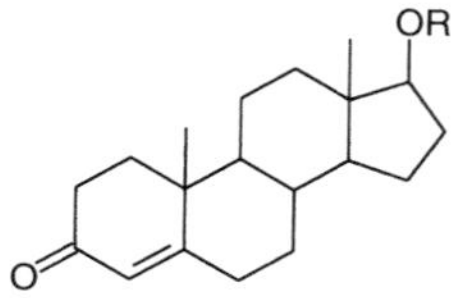

(14.62)   R = H

(14.63)   R = (C=O)C$_{10}$H$_{21}$

respectively, have been found in a comparative bioavailability study. The far from quantitative absorption of the ester prodrug might reflect that the ester is partly hydrolyzed in the intestinal lumen or might be due to a limited transport capacity of the gastrointestinal lymphatics.

An alternative way to protect a phenolic moiety against presystemic metabolism is to prepare an ester derivative endowed with a built-in esterase inhibiting function. In this case, the prodrug can diminish its own rate of hydrolysis, and thereby pass intact through the gut wall and liver. This strategy has been employed for the bronchodilator agent terbutaline (14.67). N,N-disubstituted carbamate esters are generally very stable against both chemical and enzymatic hydrolysis and have, in addition, esterase-inhibiting properties. The prodrug bambuterol (14.64) was found to possess these properties, being a potent inhibitor of pseudocholinesterase. Upon oral administration most of the dose given reaches the systemic circulation in intact form. Reconversion to parent terbutaline proceeds through consecutive reactions involving an initial enzyme-mediated oxidation to give N-hydroxymethyl carbamates (14.65), which subsequently are decomposed spontaneously to formaldehyde and N-monomethyl carbamates (14.66). The latter derivative is hydrolyzed by virtue of pseudocholinesterase (Scheme 14.21). This enzyme is selectively inhibited by bambuterol. Thus, the prodrug inhibits its own

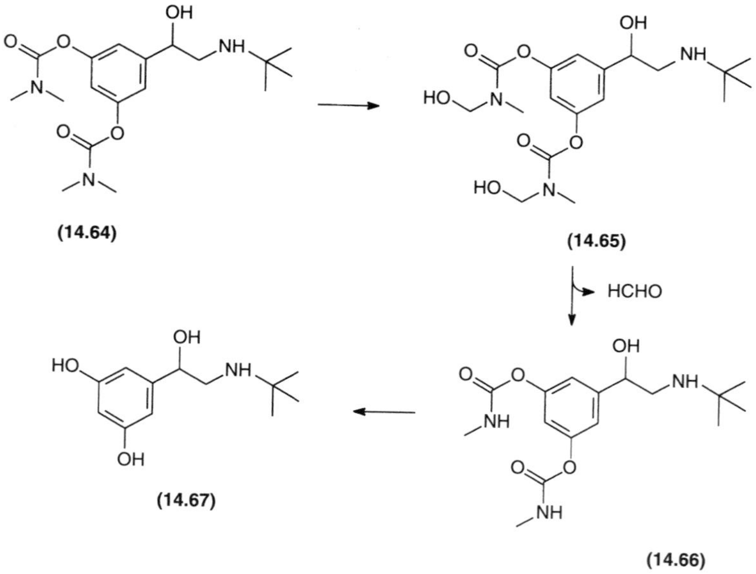

Scheme 14.21

hydrolysis resulting in a slow formation of the active drug. In addition to these desirable gains in bioavailability and duration of action, bambuterol affords enhanced delivery of the parent drug to its site of action, the lungs, with concomitant reduction of side effects due to lower plasma levels of free terbutaline.

14.4.2   Site-specific drug delivery

Although the concept of targeted or site-specific drug delivery has been evolving for quite some time, the routine attainment of targeted delivery is still one of the most elusive pharmaceutical challenges. Site-specific drug delivery might be achieved by site-directed drug delivery or site-specific bioactivation. The former concept relates to design of prodrugs that afford an increased or selective transport of the parent drug to the site of action. Site-directed delivery can further be divided into localized site-directed and systemic site-directed drug delivery. The objective of the second approach is to accomplish bioreversible derivatives that are distributed throughout the organism but undergo bioactivation only in the vicinity of the target area. In the following, examples will be given to illustrate the possible utilization of these principles to achieve drug targeting.

14.4.2.1   Site-directed drug delivery

Up to now, successful site-directed drug delivery has been achieved in the field of localized drug delivery where the prodrug is applied directly to the target organ which is the case in dermal and ocular delivery (see Sections 14.4.1.2 and 14.4.1.3).

Compared to localized drug delivery, systemic site-directed delivery constitutes a much more difficult task (see also Section 14.2.3), since the drug has to be transported via the systemic circulation to the desired organ or tissue, passing various complex and not easily predictable barriers on the way. Besides various attempts to accomplish drug targeting in cancer chemotherapy, an interesting approach to obtain site-directed delivery to the brain has been investigated. The drug (D), which is aimed to be delivered to the brain, is coupled to a quaternary carrier (i.e. N-methylnicotinic acid) $(QC)^+$ to yield $D-QC^+$ which is reduced to the neutral, lipophilic dihydro form (dihydrotrigonelline) (D-DHC) (Scheme 14.22). After administration, this compound is distributed throughout the body including the brain. D-DHC is then enzymatically oxidized back to the original quaternary

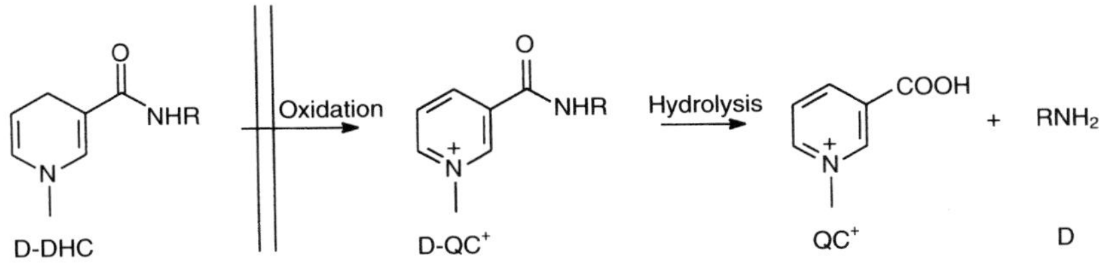

Scheme 14.22

entity (D-QC)$^+$. The latter hydrophilic compound is prevented from passing through the blood–brain barrier. Thus, the ionic form is trapped in the brain and undergoes slow enzymatic cleavage releasing the active agent. Because of the facile elimination of D-QC$^+$ from the circulation only small amounts of the free drug are released in the blood. This concept has been applied to several drugs including dopamine, phenytoin, and penicillins.

14.4.2.2 Site-specific bioactivation

Quantitative or qualitative differences between the target site and non-target sites might be exploited in prodrug design to activate or release the active agent in the vicinity of the target area. Differences in pH or more often in enzyme levels have founded the platform for synthesis of bioreversible derivatives which after the distribution phase are selectively activated in the desired organ within the body.

Site-specific activation can be exemplified by the action of the antiviral agent acyclovir (**14.68**) where the herpesvirus encoded enzyme, pyrimidine deoxynucleoside (thymidine) kinase, is responsible for converting acyclovir to its phosphate monoester (Figure 14.9). Subsequently, cellular enzymes catalyze the formation of the di- and triphosphorylated species, the latter substance being the active one. The triester formation takes place to a much greater extent in the herpes-infected cells. Thus, acyclovir displays a high therapeutic activity against herpesvirus and very low toxicity against uninfected host cells. The selectivity of action is manifested in the fact that a 3000-fold higher concentration of acyclovir is needed to inhibit uninfected cell multiplication.

An example of pH-dependent bioactivation relates to the action of the anti-ulcer drug omeprazole (**14.69**). The drug is an effective inhibitor of gastric acid secretion by inhibiting the gastric H$^+$, K$^+$-ATPase. This enzyme is responsible for the gastric acid production and is located in the secretory membranes of the parietal cells. Omeprazole is, *per se*, inactive but requires transformation within the acidic compartment of the parietal cells into the active inhibitor, a cyclic sulfenamide (**14.70**). This intermediate reacts with thiol groups in the enzyme forming a disulphide complex (**14.71**) thereby inactivating the enzyme

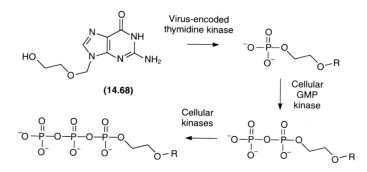

Figure 14.9 Bioconversion of antiviral agent acyclovir (**14.68**), to the pharmacologically active triphosphate ester.

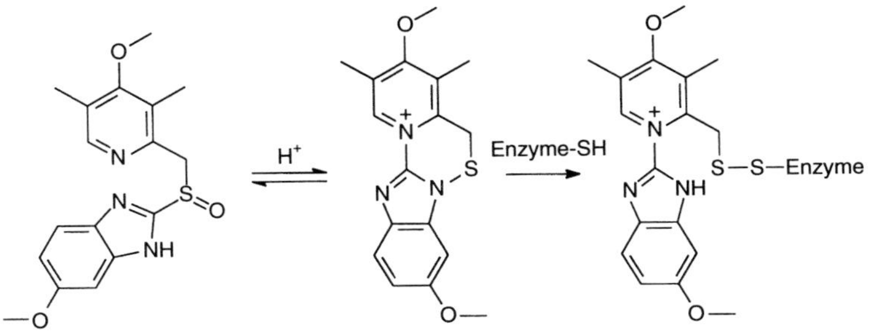

(14.69)   (14.70)   (14.71)

Scheme 14.23

(Scheme 14.23). A combination of factors, therefore, contributes to the specific action of omeprazole:

(1) Omeprazole is a weak base (pK$_a$ of the pyridine nitrogen is 4.0) and the drug concentrates in acidic compartments, i.e. in the parietal cells, which have the lowest pH of the cells in the body
(2) The low pH value of the parietal cells initiates the conversion of omeprazole into the active inhibitor in the vicinity of the target enzyme
(3) The active inhibitor is a permanent cation with limited possibilities to permeate the membranes of the parietal and other cells, and thus will be retained at its site of action
(4) At physiological pH 7.4 omeprazole has good stability and only modest conversion to the active species occurs

There are various colonic disorders warranting delivery of effective amounts of drug compounds selectively to the diseased site. The ability of the gut microflora to hydrolyze different chemical bonds has formed the basis for design of several prodrug types. The prodrug sulfasalazine (**14.72**) has long been used in the management of colon inflammatory disorders like ulcerative colitis. After passage through the small intestine the active species, 5-aminosalicylic acid (5-ASA) (**14.74**), is released from the prodrug after cleavage of the azo-bond by action of azo-reductases secreted from colonic bacteria. However, disadvantages of sulfasalazine therapy include absorption of intact prodrug from the small intestine and systemic adverse reactions. A more elegant prodrug of 5-ASA, olsalazine (**14.73**), has been developed, consisting of two 5-ASA molecules linked together by an azo-bond (Scheme 14.24). The latter twin prodrug releases two molecules of 5-ASA in the colon and due to its highly polar nature only negligible amounts are absorbed from the small intestine.

The examples cited in the last two sections illustrates the utility of the prodrug concept to achieve site-specific drug delivery. For the design of prodrugs directed

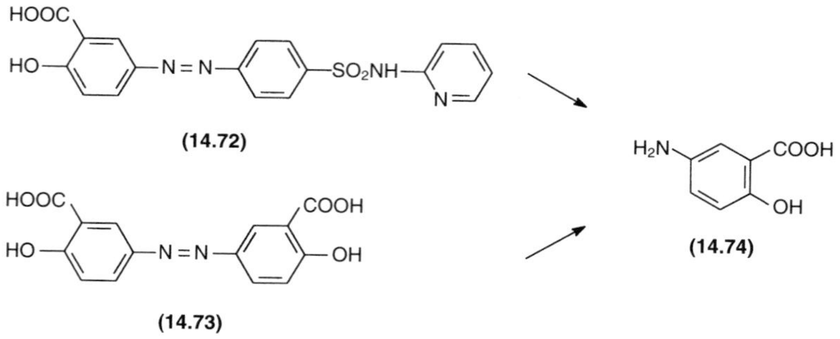

(14.72)

(14.73)

(14.74)

Scheme 14.24

selectively to their site of action, the following basal criteria must be taken into consideration:

(1) The prodrug should be able to reach the site of action
(2) The prodrug should be converted efficiently to the drug at the site of action
(3) The parent active should to some extent be retained or trapped at the target site for a sufficient period of time to exert its effect

The reason why attempts to promote site-specific drug delivery via prodrugs have failed in many cases, is that not all criteria have been met.

14.4.3   Improvement of drug formulation

Successful development of a drug candidate includes the design of dosage forms exhibiting suitable shelf-lives. Despite the fact that solid oral dosage forms are the most used types of formulations, the chemical kinetics of drug degradation in the solid state is far from fully understood. For a drug which is susceptible to hydrolysis it is primarily moisture in the dosage form that causes its instability. In this case, stability problems might be circumvented by using a poorly soluble prodrug derivative or salt. Changing the properties of a drug in the crystalline state by bioreversible derivatization may also lead to improved *in vitro* stability. Dinoprostone (prostaglandin E_2, PGE_2) (**14.75**) is a crystalline solid (mp 63 °C), stable at room temperature for only a short period of time, but liquefies and decomposes rapidly after a few months. As other β-ketols, PGE_2 is easily dehydrated under formation of prostaglandin A_2. Based on the assumption that the decomposition rate was

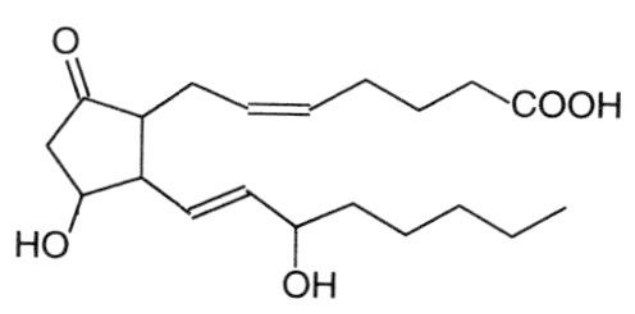

(14.75)

related to the crystalline interaction energy, a series of *para*-substituted phenyl esters of PGE$_2$ was synthesized. Storage of these higher melting esters at room temperature for up to 30 months revealed no detectable deterioration.

Intramuscular oil depot injections are available for long-term administration of antipsychotics and a number of steroids. The principal role of depot neuroleptic therapy is to ensure patient compliance. Oily injections are marketed for steroid hormones exhibiting low and variable oral bioavailability due to extensive first-pass metabolism in the gastrointestinal tract and the liver. Pharmacokinetic studies have demonstrated that the rate of release of chemical entities from oil solutions is, at least partly, related to the pH-dependent oil vehicle–water distribution coefficient. The prodrug approach has successfully been applied on a variety of drugs to design derivatives, most often in the form of ester derivatives, possessing suitable lipophilicities and thereby desired durations of action. After i.m. administration the prodrugs are slowly released from the injection site. Reconversion to the parent drug may take place in the tissue fluid at the injection site or in the blood. The rate of prodrug liberation from the oil vehicle decreases with increasing lipophilicity of the derivatives. In case of the neuroleptic agent, fluphenazine (**14.76**) duration of action is 6–8 h after intramuscular injection. In contrast, the more lipophilic enanthate ester **14.77** and decanoate ester **14.78** show a duration of action of 1–2 and 3–4 weeks, respectively, following i.m. injection in a sesame oil vehicle. Similar long-acting fatty acid ester prodrugs of various other clinically used neuroleptics such as flupenthixol, zuclopenthixol and haloperidol are available. Clinically, depot neuroleptics possess several advantages over short-acting oral forms including enhanced patient compliance, reduced relapse and rehospitalization rate, and reduced daily dose.

Several steroids are also frequently used in the form of long-acting prodrugs. Thus, for testosterone (**14.62**) the following esters have been used in oil solutions or suspensions: cypionate (**14.79**), isocaproate, valerate, phenylpropionate, enanthate and undecanoate.

The greatest utility of the prodrug approach in solving pharmaceutical formulation problems is probably to modify the aqueous solubility of drugs. Whereas poorly water-soluble bioreversible derivatives, such as the palmitate esters of

(**14.76**)   R = H
(**14.77**)   R = (C=O)C$_6$H$_{13}$
(**14.78**)   R = (C=O)C$_9$H$_{19}$

(**14.79**)

chloramphenicol and clindamycin, have been designed to mask the bitter taste of the parent antibacterial agents, the prodrug approach has mainly been used to increase the water solubility of drugs, thereby allowing convenient solution formulations for intravenous and ophthalmic use to be prepared (see also Section 14.2.2.2).

Ester formation has long been recognized as an effective way to enhance the aqueous solubility of drugs containing a hydroxy functional group (Drug-OH). Water-soluble derivatives might be obtained from dicarboxylic acid hemiesters (notably hemisuccinates), sulphate esters, phosphate esters, α-amino or related short-chained aliphatic amino acid esters, and aminomethylbenzoate esters. These types of esters should ideally provide high water solubility at the pH of optimum stability, sufficient stability in aqueous solution, i.e. shelf-lives above 2 years, combined with a rapid and quantitative conversion to the parent drug _in vivo_. Hemisuccinate esters do, however, possess limited solution stability and, in addition, they exhibit a slow and incomplete conversion _in vivo_ to the parent agent. This has been reported for esters of various corticosteroids, chloramphenicol, and metronidazole. Sulphate esters are, in contrast, rather stable in solution, but an impediment to their use might be a high resistance to enzymatic hydrolysis. In general, phosphate ester sodium salts are freely soluble in water and they exhibit a reasonable stability in aqueous solution. The susceptibility of phosphate ester prodrugs to undergo enzyme-mediated hydrolysis may, however, vary dependent on the chemical nature of the parent drug. Whereas α-amino or related short-chained aliphatic amino acid esters might be cleaved by plasma hydrolases, such derivatives are prevented from being employed in ready-to-use aqueous formulations due to their limited solution stability. The major reason for the high instability of the latter ester type in aqueous solution at pH values affording their favorable water solubility (pH 3–5) is the strongly electron-withdrawing effect of the protonated amino group which activates the ester linkage towards hydroxide ion attack. In particular cases, facilitation of hydrolysis may additionally arise from intramolecular catalysis by the terminal amino group. An effective and simple means to avoid the hydrolysis facilitating effect of the amino group and yet retain a rapid rate of enzymatic ester hydrolysis is to incorporate a phenyl group between the ester moiety and the amino group. In this case intramolecular catalytic reactions of the amino group is no longer possible due to steric hindrance. Such _N_-substituted 3- or 4-aminomethyl benzoate esters have been found to be readily soluble in water at weakly acidic pH values and to possess a high stability in such solutions in combination with a feasible susceptibility towards enzymatic cleavage. Thus, the 4-(morpholinomethyl)benzoate ester (**14.80**) of metronidazole possesses a predicted shelf-life of more than 10 years in aqueous solution pH 4 and 25 °C.

(**14.80**)

Table 14.6 Examples of water-soluble prodrug derivatives of drugs containing a hydroxy group (Drug-OH) and their chemical and enzymatic reactivity

Prodrug derivatives		Stability in solution	Enzymatic lability
Hemisuccinates	Drug$-$O$-\overset{\overset{O}{\|}}{C}-CH_2CH_2$ $-\overset{\overset{O}{\|}}{C}-O^-$	Limited	Limited
Sulphates	Drug$-$O$-$SO$_3^-$	High	Low
Phosphates	Drug$-$O$-$PO$_3^{2-}$	High	High/Limited
α-Amino acid esters	Drug$-$O$-\overset{\overset{O}{\|}}{C}-\overset{\overset{R}{\|}}{C}H-NH_3^+$	Limited	High
Dialkylaminoacetates	Drug$-$O$-\overset{\overset{O}{\|}}{C}-CH_2-\overset{\overset{R_1}{\|}}{\underset{\underset{R_2}{\|}}{^+NH}}$	Limited	High
Aminomethyl benzoate esters*	Drug$-$O$-\overset{\overset{O}{\|}}{C}-$⟨benzene⟩$-CH_2-\overset{\overset{R_1}{\|}}{\underset{\underset{R_2}{\|}}{^+NH}}$	High	High

Note
*3 or 4 position.

In human plasma, the half-life of the prodrug is less than 1 min. The stability characteristics of the ester types dealt with above are summarized in Table 14.6.

A novel prodrug approach for improving the water solubility of poorly soluble drugs containing a tertiary amine group relates to the formation of N-phosphonooxymethyl derivatives which can be considered as double prodrugs since regeneration of the parent amine initially requires phosphatase catalyzed hydrolysis of the phosphate ester bond. The resulting hydroxymethyl intermediate undergoes spontaneous degradation releasing the parent amine and formaldehyde (Scheme 14.25). The prodrug derivative (14.81) obtained from N-phosphonooxymethylation of the tricyclic dibenzoxazepine antipsychotic agent loxapine (14.82) showed a more than 15 000-fold improvement in solubility at pH 7.4 relative to loxapine and the predicted shelf-life of an aqueous formulation was about 2 years.

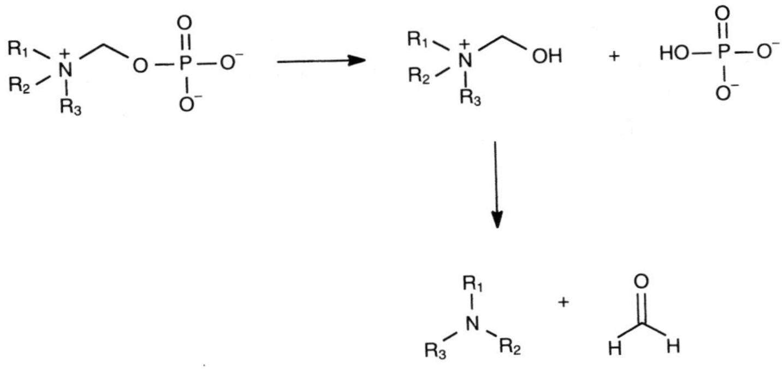

Scheme 14.25

(14.81)   (14.82)

Following i.v. administration to beagle dogs the prodrug was found to be rapidly and quantitatively converted to the parent drug.

FURTHER READING

Bagshawe, K. (Theme ed.) (1996) Enzyme-prodrug therapy. *Adv. Drug Delivery Rev.*, **22**, 265–376.

Bundgaard, H. (ed.) (1985) *Design of Prodrugs*. Amsterdam: Elsevier.

Bundgaard, H. (1989) The double prodrug concept and its applications. *Adv. Drug Delivery Rev.*, **3**, 39–65.

Larsen, C. (1989) Dextran prodrugs – structure and stability in relation to therapeutic activity. *Adv. Drug Delivery Rev.*, **3**, 103–154.

Oliyai, R. and Stella, V.J. (1993) Prodrugs of peptides and proteins for improved formulation and delivery. *Ann. Rev. Pharmacol. Toxicol.*, **32**, 521–544.

Sloan, K.B. (ed.) (1992) *Prodrugs, Topical and Ocular Drug Delivery*. New York: Marcel Dekker Inc.

Soyez, H., Schacht, E. and Vanderkerken, S. (1996) The crucial role of spacer groups in macromolecular prodrug design. *Adv. Drug Delivery Rev.*, **21**, 81–106.

Stella, V.J. (Theme ed.) (1996) Low molecular weight prodrugs. *Adv. Drug Delivery Rev.*, **19**, 1–330.

Stella, V.J., Mikkelsen, T.J. and Pipkin, J.D. (1980) Prodrugs: the control of drug delivery via bioreversible chemical modifications. In *Drug Delivery Systems, Characteristics and Biomedical Applications*, edited by R.L. Juliano, pp. 112–176. New York: Oxford University Press.

Yang, C.Y., Dantzig, A.H. and Pidgeon, C. (1999) Intestinal peptide transport systems and oral drug availability. *Pharm. Res.*, **16**, 1331–1343.

Chapter 15

Peptides and peptidomimetics

Kristina Luthman and Uli Hacksell

15.1 INTRODUCTION

A large number of endogenous peptides have been isolated and characterized (Table 15.1). These peptides are involved in a wide range of important physiological processes both centrally and peripherally. Drug intervention with the formation, breakdown or receptor interaction of peptides might provide therapeutic opportunities. The most well-known drug that interacts with peptide receptors is morphine. It was isolated from opium in 1803. However, whereas its analgesic efficacy and other CNS effects were discovered already in the nineteenth century, the fact that morphine interacts with receptors for opiate peptides was verified only relatively recently. Currently, numerous drug discovery efforts are focussed on processes involving peptides and intense research and development efforts during the past 30 years have provided important peptide interacting drugs such as captopril and losartan.

15.1.1 Peptide structure

Already in 1902, Hofmeister and Fischer independently reported that peptides consist of amino acids (Table 15.2) linked via amide bonds (peptide bonds). A peptide have a chain length between 2 and 50 amino acids whereas proteins include more than 50 amino acids. The different properties of the individual amino acids together with the amino acid sequence (the primary structure) determine the physico-chemical properties of the peptides. All amino acids except glycine are chiral (Figure 15.1). In Nature, the L-configuration is predominating but peptides from micro-organisms and some opioid peptides isolated from the skin of amphibians also contain D-amino acids.

Most peptides are flexible and frequently adopt a large number of conformations in solution. This flexibility is caused by the rotation about single bonds within each amino acid. The torsions in the backbone of particular interest for peptide over-all conformations are the ψ, ϕ and ω angles (Figure 15.2). Many combinations of ψ and ϕ angles are disallowed because of unfavorable steric interactions. The relationship between the ψ, ϕ and energy is often visualized in Ramachandran maps in which the approximate areas of allowed ψ/ϕ angles can be identified. Short peptides exist in a multitude of conformations in solution whereas longer peptides may adopt stable secondary structures such as α-helices, β-sheets and turns.

Table 15.1 Some important endogenous peptides

Peptide	Amino acid sequence
Angiotensin I (Ang I)	DRVYIHPFHL
Angiotensin II (Ang II)	DRVYIHPF
Arginine vasopressin (AVP)	CYFQNCPRG-NH$_2$
Bradykinin	RPPGFSPFR
Cholecystokinin (CCK-33)	CGNLSTCMLGTYTQDFNKFHTFPQTAIGVGAP-NH$_2$
Dynorphin B	YGGFLRRIRPKLKWDNQ
Endomorphin I	YPWF-NH$_2$
Endomorphin II	YPFF-NH$_2$
β-Endorphin	YGGFMTSEKSQTPLVTLFKNAIIKNAYKKGQ
Endothelin (ET-1)	CSCSSLMDKECVYFCHLDIIW
(Leu)Enkephalin	YGGFL
(Met)Enkephalin	YGGFM
Galanin	GWTLNSAGYLLGPHAIDNHRSFHDKYGLA-NH$_2$
Gastrin	pEGPWLEEEEEAY(SO$_3$H)GYGWMDF-NH$_2$
Gastrin releasing peptide	APVSVGGGTVLAKMYPRGNHWAVGHLM-NH$_2$
Ghrelin	GSS(OOCn-C$_7$H$_{15}$)FLSPEHQKAQQRKESKKPPAKLQPR
Gonadotropin-releasing hormone (Gn-RH)	pEHWSYGLRPG-NH$_2$
Neurokinin A (NKA)	HKTDSFVGLM-NH$_2$
Neurokinin B (NKB)	DMHDFFVGLM-NH$_2$
Neuropeptide Y (NPY)	YPSKPDNGPEDAPAEDMARYYSALRHYINLITRQRY-NH$_2$
Neurotensin (NT)	pELYQNKPRRPYIL
Oxytocin	CYIQNCPLG-NH$_2$
Somatostatin (SST)	AGCKNFFWKTFTSC
Substance P (SP)	RPKPQQFFGLM-NH$_2$
Thyrotropin-releasing hormone (TRH)	pEHP-NH$_2$
Vasoactive intestinal peptide (VIP)	HSDAVFTDNYTRLRKQMAVKKYLNSILN-NH$_2$

Table 15.2 The chemical name of the 20 common amino acids and their 3 and 1 letter codes

Alanine	Ala	A	Leucine	Leu	L
Arginine	Arg	R	Lysine	Lys	K
Asparagine	Asn	N	Methionine	Met	M
Aspartic acid	Asp	D	Phenylalanine	Phe	F
Cystein	Cys	C	Proline	Pro	P
Glutamic acid	Glu	E	Serine	Ser	S
Glutamine	Gln	Q	Threonine	Thr	T
Glycine	Gly	G	Tryptophan	Trp	W
Histidine	His	H	Tyrosine	Tyr	Y
Isoleucine	Ile	I	Valine	Val	V

15.1.2   Solid phase peptide synthesis

A major milestone in peptide chemistry was achieved in 1953 with the isolation, characterization and synthesis of the peptides oxytocin and vasopressin

Figure 15.1 Structures of L- and D-amino acids.

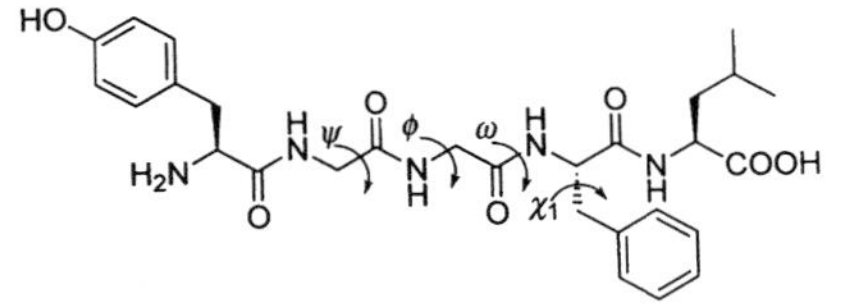

Tyrosyl-glycyl-glycyl-phenylalanyl-leucine (Leu-Enkephalin)

Tyr-Gly-Gly-Phe-Leu (YGGFL)

Figure 15.2 Structures of Leu-enkephalin. Also shown are the ψ, ϕ, ω and χ torsion angles.

(*J. Am. Chem. Soc.*, 1953, 75, 4879 and 4880). Another major step in the synthesis of biologically active peptides and peptide analogs was the introduction of the solid phase synthetic method by Merrifield in 1963 (*J. Am. Chem. Soc.*, 1963, 85, 2149). In this method, the peptide is synthesized from the C-terminal to the N-terminal end (Figure 15.3). The C-terminal amino acid is linked to an insoluble polystyrene based polymer and the peptide is then conveniently synthesized by sequential coupling of properly protected amino acids. The most commonly used N-terminal protecting groups are the base labile 9-fluorenylmethoxycarbonyl (Fmoc) and the acid labile *tert*-butoxycarbonyl (Boc) moieties. The carboxylic acid function has to be activated before coupling. Protecting groups and coupling reagents are improved continuously.

The synthesized peptide is cleaved from the polymer resin and fully deprotected by HF- or TFA-treatment. The synthesis may be performed either by using single amino acid couplings or the fragment condensation technique. The latter strategy is mainly used in the synthesis of longer peptide and small proteins, but also in the synthesis of modified peptides using non-peptidic building blocks.

The peptide synthesis of today has been automated. Although the synthesis of a peptide is trivial a considerable amount of time has to be spent on its purification, usually using reversed phase HPLC or electrophoresis techniques. Synthesized peptides are characterized by amino acid analysis, mass spectrometry, and NMR-spectroscopy. Sequence analyses can be performed by Edman degradation and mass spectrometry (FAB-MS and MS-MS). Production of endogenous peptides and proteins may also be achieved using genetic engineering techniques.

15.1.3   Biosynthesis of peptides

Peptide precursors are biosynthesized on the ribosome as higher molecular forms (prepropeptides) (Figure 15.4). During the transport through the endoplasmatic reticulum to the Golgi apparatus, an N-terminal signal peptide of 20–30 amino

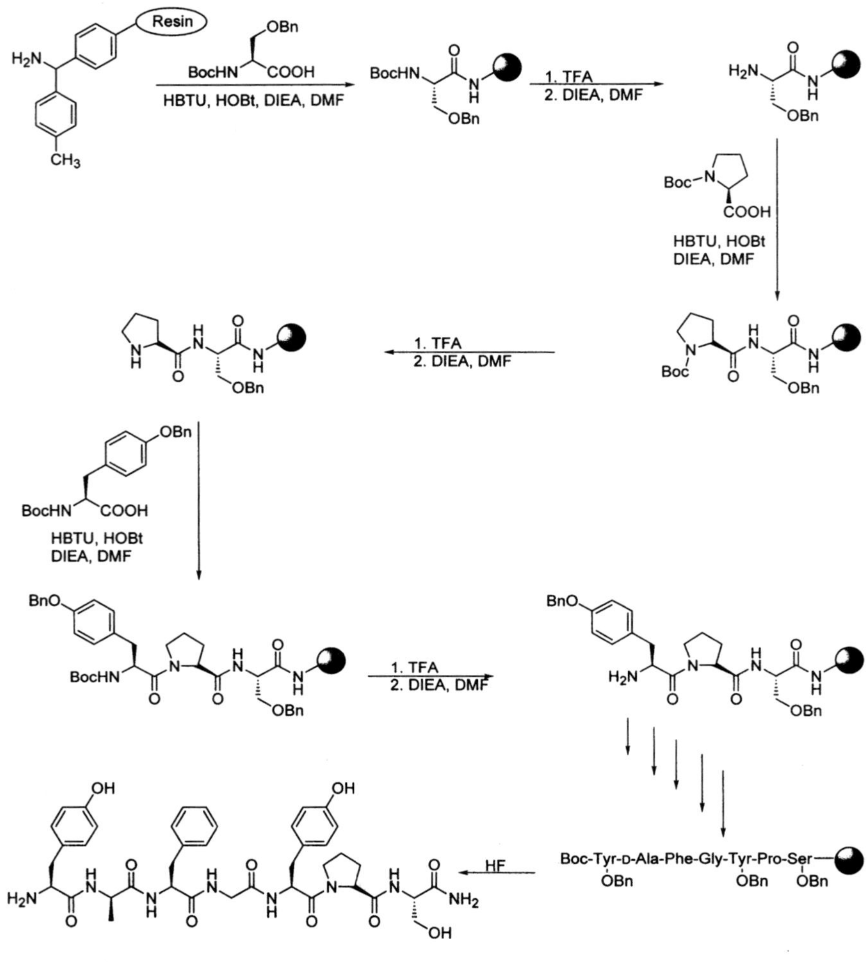

Figure 15.3 Solid phase synthesis of the amphibian heptapeptide dermorphin. HBTU: 2-(1*H*-benzotriazol-1-yl)-1,1,3,3-tetramethyluronium hexafluorophosphate; HOBt: 1-hydroxybenzotriazole; DIEA: diisopropylethylamine; DMF: dimethylformamide; TFA: trifluoroacetic acid; •: polystyrene resin with a specific spacer for synthesis of C-terminal amidated peptides.

acids is cleaved off to generate the propeptide. This cleavage is catalyzed by specific peptidases. The propeptides are further processed to their active forms and structural modifications like acetylation, glycosylation, sulphation, phosphorylation, or C-terminal amidation may occur. The peptides are stored in synaptic vesicles and are released into the environment by appropriate stimuli. The peptides act mainly as neurotransmitters, neuromodulators, and hormones, thus influencing a series of vital functions such as metabolism, immune defence, digestion, respiration, sens-

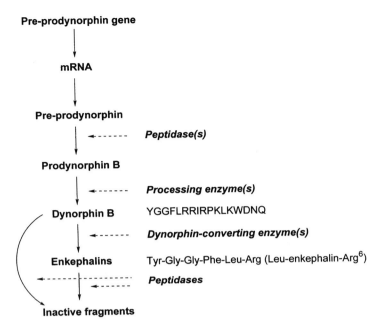

Figure 15.4 Flowchart showing the biosynthesis of dynorphin B and its breakdown.

itivity to pain, reproduction, behavior and electrolyte levels. The breakdown of a peptide *in vivo* is frequently less specific than that of small molecular transmitters since it involves peptidases of low specificity. The peptide fragments formed on peptide degradation may be inactive or display biological activity; e.g. dynorphin B produces the potent hexapeptide Leu-enkephalin-Arg[6] on degradation.

Some endogenous peptides such as the amyloid precursor protein (APP) which is believed to be responsible for the neurodegeneration in Alzheimer's disease, are quite toxic. The membrane anchored APP can be cleaved by β- and γ-secretases to form a 42-amino acid peptide called amyloid β peptide (Aβ) (Figure 15.5). This peptide is quite hydrophobic and is prone to nucleation and fibril formation. The Aβ-production ultimately leads to amyloid plaque formation in the brain of Alzheimer patients. The β-secretase cleavage of APP is considered the rate-limiting step in the Aβ-synthesis and an intense search for inhibitors of this enzyme is ongoing.

15.1.4 Peptide–G-protein coupled receptor interactions

Many peptide receptors belong to the GPCR super family. Frequently only a small number of amino acids (4–8) are responsible for the recognition and activation of the GPCR (the 'message' part). These important amino acids can be identified by amino acid substitutions which lead to pronounced changes in the biological response. The part of the peptide not directly involved in the binding to the GPCR (the 'address' part) serves to fix the important amino acids in a

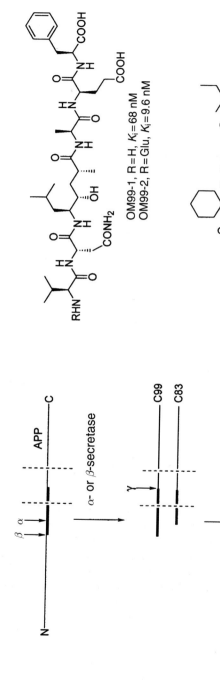

OM99-1, R=H, K_i=68 nM
OM99-2, R=Glu, K_i=9.6 nM

IC_{50}=4 μM

Figure 15.5 Schematic representation of the Aβ-formation from amyloid precursor protein (APP) by β- and γ-secretase cleavage (left). Dotted lines represent the lipid bilayer. Pseudopeptides with inhibitory activity towards γ-secretase (right).

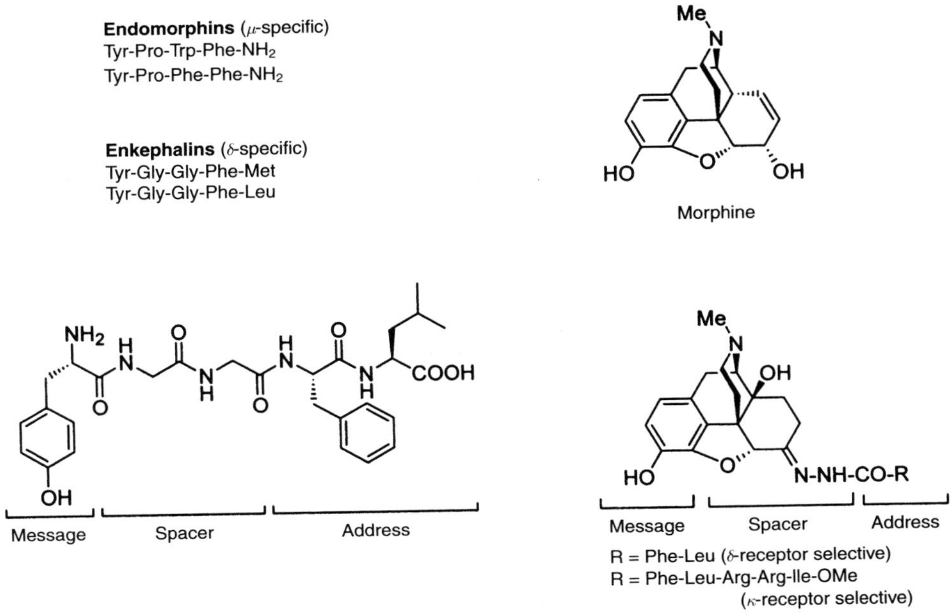
Endomorphins (μ-specific)
Tyr-Pro-Trp-Phe-NH2
Tyr-Pro-Phe-Phe-NH2
Enkephalins (δ-specific)
Tyr-Gly-Gly-Phe-Met
Tyr-Gly-Gly-Phe-Leu
Me
N
HO
O
OH
Morphine
NH2
H
N
O
COOH
OH
Message
Spacer
Address
Me
N
OH
HO
O
N-NH-CO-R
Message
Spacer
Address
R = Phe-Leu (δ-receptor selective)
R = Phe-Leu-Arg-Arg-Ile-OMe
(κ-receptor selective)

Figure 15.6 Structural relationship between the endomorphins, enkephalins and the peptidomimetic morphine. Also illustrated is the concept of message and address parts of peptides.

proper spatial arrangement and confers additional affinity and selectivity for the receptor. The concept of address and message parts in enkephalin is illustrated in Figure 15.6.

15.2 STRATEGIES FOR PEPTIDOMIMETIC DRUG DISCOVERY

The peptide receptors and the enzymes involved in the biosynthesis and degradation of peptides have become attractive targets in drug discovery research. Most biologically active peptides display receptor affinities (K_D) in the nM–pM range (10^{-9}–10^{-12} M). However, peptides are rarely useful as drugs due to their (i) low oral bioavailability; (ii) rapid degradation by endogenous peptidases; (iii) rapid excretion through liver and kidneys; and (iv) side effects due to their interaction with several different receptors (lack of selectivity). Hence, current research in the field mainly deals with the challenging task of circumventing these limitations; orally effective and metabolically stable analogs of peptidic hormones, neurotransmitters, and neuromodulators are needed and could lead to drugs with useful pharmacological/therapeutical profiles. These compounds are often referred to as 'peptidemimetics' or 'peptidomimetics'.

According to Morgan and Gainor, peptidomimetics can be defined as 'structures which serve as appropriate substitutes for peptides in interaction with receptors and enzymes. The mimics must possess not only affinity but also efficacy or substrate function'. The most well-known peptidomimetic is probably morphine which acts as an agonist on opiate receptors (Figure 15.6). The research on peptidomimetics deals with peptides and proteins as lead compounds for the discovery of other classes of compounds through a variety of research strategies. Since peptide–receptor antagonists/inverse agonists or enzyme inhibitors do not interact with receptors in the same way as the endogenous peptide they should not be regarded as peptidomimetics. However, all ligands for peptide receptors or peptide degrading enzymes are termed peptidomimetics in the current literature.

In general, a successfully designed peptidomimetic should be metabolically stable, have good (preferably oral) bioavailability, have high receptor affinity and selectivity, and should produce a minimum of side effects. However, today it is not known how to rationally convert (*de novo*) a peptide into a non-peptide while maintaining the biological activity. There is no strategy which guarantees the discovery of ligands with high affinity, efficacy, and specificity. In general, the discovery of novel ligands for peptide receptors has not been based on a thorough understanding of the key-intermolecular interactions. Instead, receptor-based random screening has been the most rewarding method. Below follows an outline of different strategies used in the development of peptidomimetics.

15.2.1   Design of peptidomimetics

A design process which is based on the primary structure of a peptide and on insight into its biological activity may be used for the development of peptido-mimetics. Such a process requires a close collaboration between specialists from the areas of synthetic chemistry, NMR-spectroscopy, crystallography, molecular modeling, and biology. In 1980, Farmer described how to convert a peptide into a peptidomimetic. He defined a set of rules (The Farmer's rules) for this process:

1   'The design of nonpeptidic analogs of a bioactive peptide should start from the simplest conceivable structures that might possibly have a peptidomimetic activity.' Large parts of the peptide can be removed without loss of activity and determinations of the smallest active fragment can be performed by a stepwise cleavage of amino acids from both the N- and the C-terminal ends of the natural peptide. Hydrophobic residues are usually important for receptor binding but polar residues are likely to be important for intrinsic activity.
2   'A nonpeptidic analog of a bioactive peptide should not occupy space outside that believed to be occupied by the peptide itself.' In addition, the functional groups should be maintained during the first stages of the conversion of a peptide into a non-peptide.
3   'Conformational flexibility should be maximized until lead activity is discovered in a nonpeptidic structure.' At least some conformational flexibility should be retained in the first set of mimetic compounds. Potency and selectivity may then be improved by introduction of conformational constraints.

4   'The design of nonpeptidic peptidomimetics should rely heavily on mimicking the topology of backbone peptide bonds, especially where there are regular secondary structures.' Analogs of secondary structures such as α-helices or β-sheets are unlikely to exhibit selectivity. Analogs mimicking tertiary structures should be more useful.

Experimental studies of designed drugs should be performed continuously during the design process and should provide information on pharmacodynamic as well as pharmacokinetic parameters such as biological activity, absorption, first-pass metabolism, CNS-penetration (if important), and water solubility. In addition, structure–activity relationships should be deduced. Several examples are available in the literature which demonstrate that Farmer's rules can successfully be employed.

15.2.1.1   Amino acid manipulations

Following the identification of the smallest active fragment of a peptide the role of each amino acid should be determined. Initially, a systematic replacement of the side chains with methyl groups, i.e. exchange of one amino acids at the time for alanine (Ala scan), can be performed. This should allow the identification of side chains of importance either for the receptor interaction or for folding of the peptide into its bioactive conformation. Phenylalanine scans indicate the role of hydrophobicity in special parts on the peptide. A systematic replacement of L-amino acids with D-amino acids or proline scans may be informative in the initial exploration of structural requirements for receptor recognition and binding. A more elaborate strategy may also involve the systematic introduction of conformational constraints by, e.g. N- or α-methylations (the conformational flexibility of the modified peptide should change dramatically due to the limited rotation around the ψ/ϕ bonds). Several unnatural amino acids in which the physico-chemical parameters differ from the natural amino acids, have been synthesized. Selected examples are shown in Figure 15.7. The common feature of these structures is the conformationally constrained side chains. The amino acids Tic and Aib are frequently used as replacements for Phe and Ala, respectively.

15.2.1.2   Peptide backbone modifications

In large peptides, the backbone mainly serves as a structural matrix. The conformation of the backbone positions the side chains in defined spatial positions which allow optimal interactions with the enzyme or receptor protein. The amide bonds themselves may also be of importance for binding to enzymes and receptors. Several amide bond isosteres have been designed, synthesized and introduced into peptide analogs. These fragments are mainly used to enhance the stability towards protease degradation but may also be useful tools in studies of structural mimicry. An appropriate amide bond replacement should, e.g. exhibit similar geometrical, conformational, electrostatical, and hydrogen bonding properties as the amide bond itself. Although a large number of amide isosteres are known 'a convincing imitation of the amide bond in the ground state has not yet been achieved' according to Giannis and Kolter. Some examples of amide isosteres are shown in Figure 15.8.

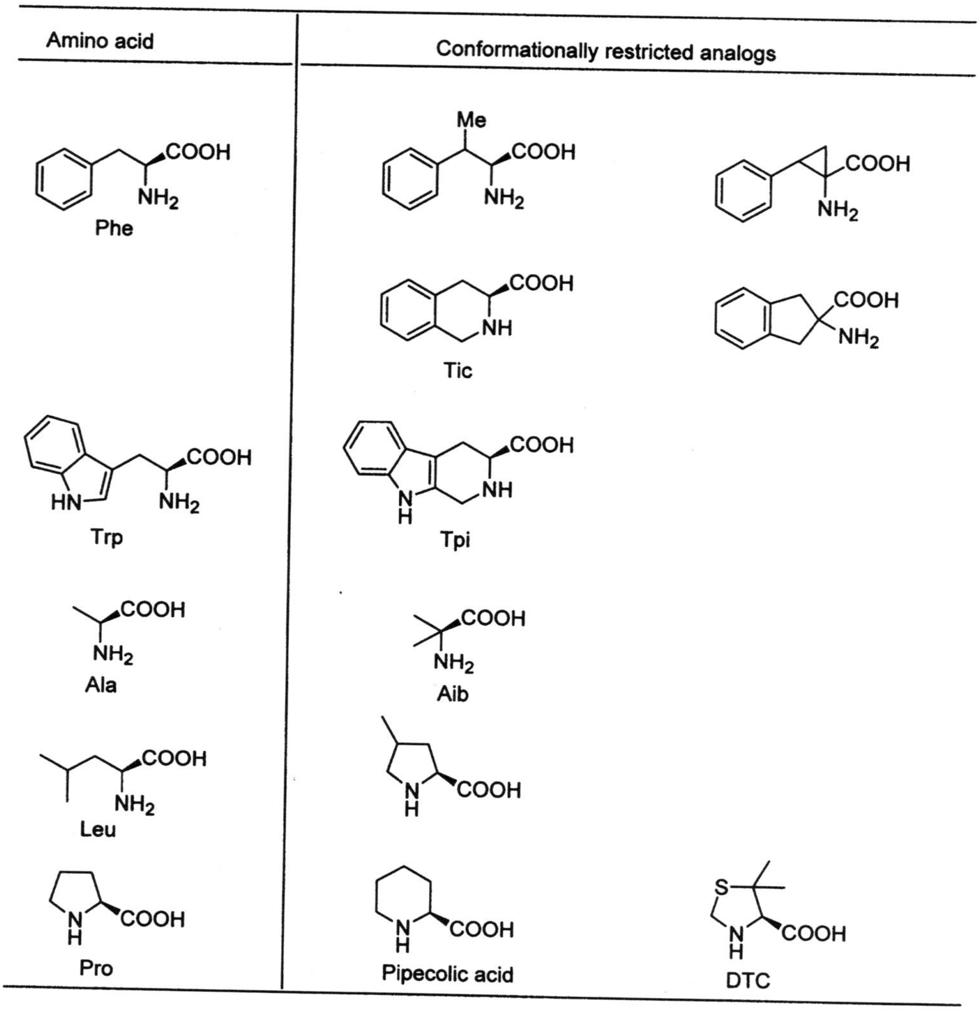

Figure 15.7 Some unnatural amino acids which impose conformational constraints when introduced in peptides.

Retro-inverse isosteres not only reverse the direction of the peptide but also have the L-amino acids exchanged for D-amino acids. Incorporation of a retro-inverse isostere results in a pseudopeptide with a similar topology as the native peptide, however, it is no longer sensitive to peptidase degradation.

15.2.1.3 Di(oligo)peptidomimetics

Replacement of larger structural moieties with di- or tripeptidomimetic structures are of interest since these modified peptides bridge the gap between peptide

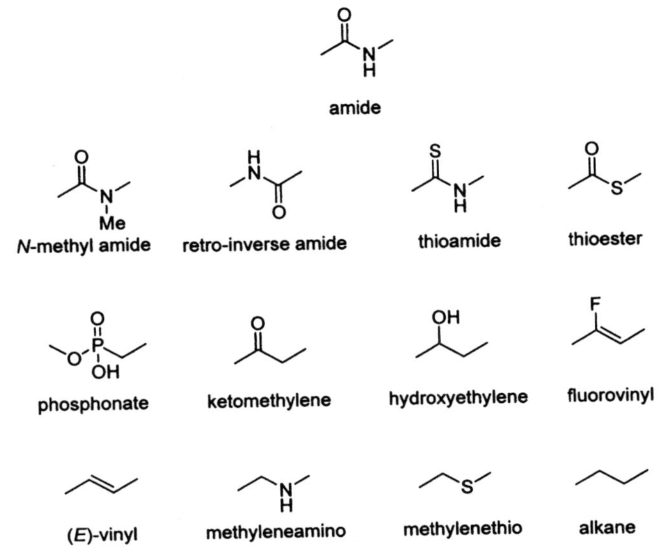

amide

N-methyl amide   retro-inverse amide   thioamide   thioester

phosphonate   ketomethylene   hydroxyethylene   fluorovinyl

(E)-vinyl   methyleneamino   methylenethio   alkane

Figure 15.8 Some amide isosteres.

analogs and non-peptidic structures. Several lactams have been synthesized as bridging elements to stabilize certain backbone conformations. These mimetic structures are based on side chain to side chain, or side chain to backbone cyclizations (Figure 15.9). Mimetic moieties involving the peptide bond, such as azole-derived mimetics, have also been successfully used as dipeptide replacements. It should be noted, however, that the incorporation of a specific di(oligo)-peptidomimetic moiety into different peptides may affect the biological activity differently.

15.2.1.4   Local or global conformational constraints

The bioactive conformation of a peptide is the conformation recognized by and/or interacting with the binding domain(s) of a receptor or enzyme. Unfortunately, the bioactive conformation of a peptide may be poorly populated in the absence of the receptor and, consequently, it may be quite different from conformations observed by e.g. NMR-spectroscopy or X-ray crystallography. Molecular mechanics calculations and molecular dynamics studies of isolated peptides have also been performed in attempts to deduce the bioactive conformations of peptides but, in general, these studies are non-informative. Recently, computational studies have been performed in which the peptide has been allowed to interact with the receptor structure. However, bioactive conformations are probably best deduced by use of conformationally restricted mimetics.

Introduction of conformational constraints aims to stabilize either local or global conformations. Local conformational constraints could include the replacement

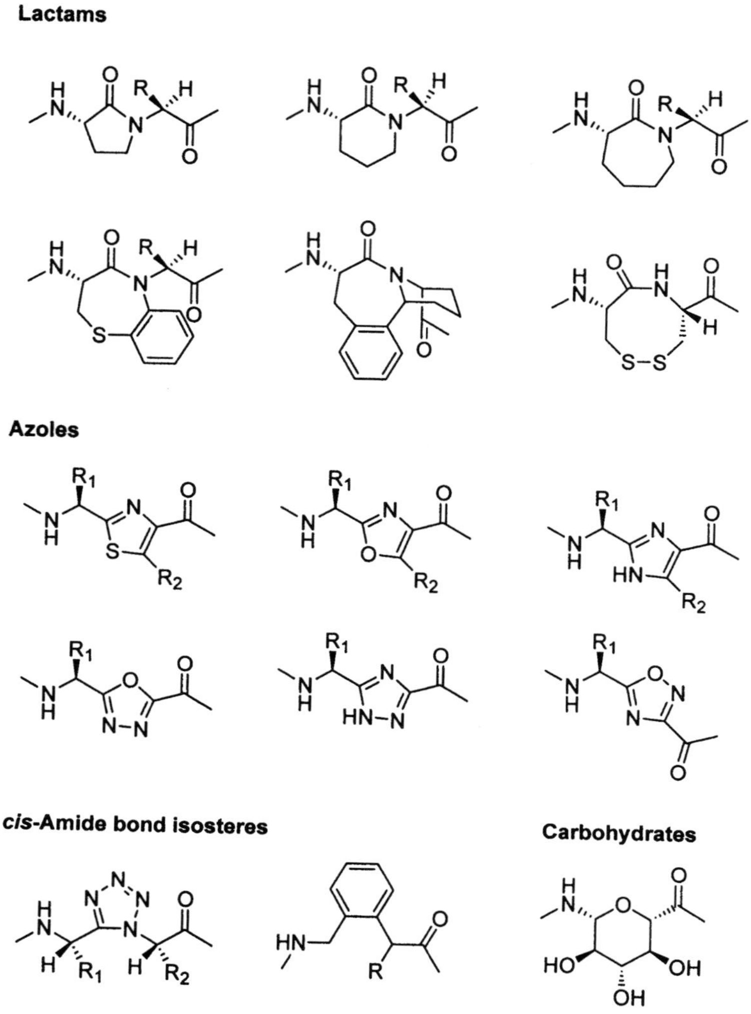

Lactams

Azoles

cis-Amide bond isosteres   **Carbohydrates**

Figure 15.9 Some dipeptidomimetics.

of the amide moiety by isosteres (methylamino, ketomethylene, inverse amide, etc.) and introduction of amino acid residues/mimics which restrict the conformational flexibility. A disadvantage with these approaches is that the introduction of local constraints may have unpredicted effects on the over-all conformational equilibrium. Global constraints may involve cyclic disulfide bridges. Alternatively, side chains not involved in the receptor recognition/interaction could be connected by cyclization. Backbone to backbone cyclizations provide another type of global conformational constraints (Figure 15.10).

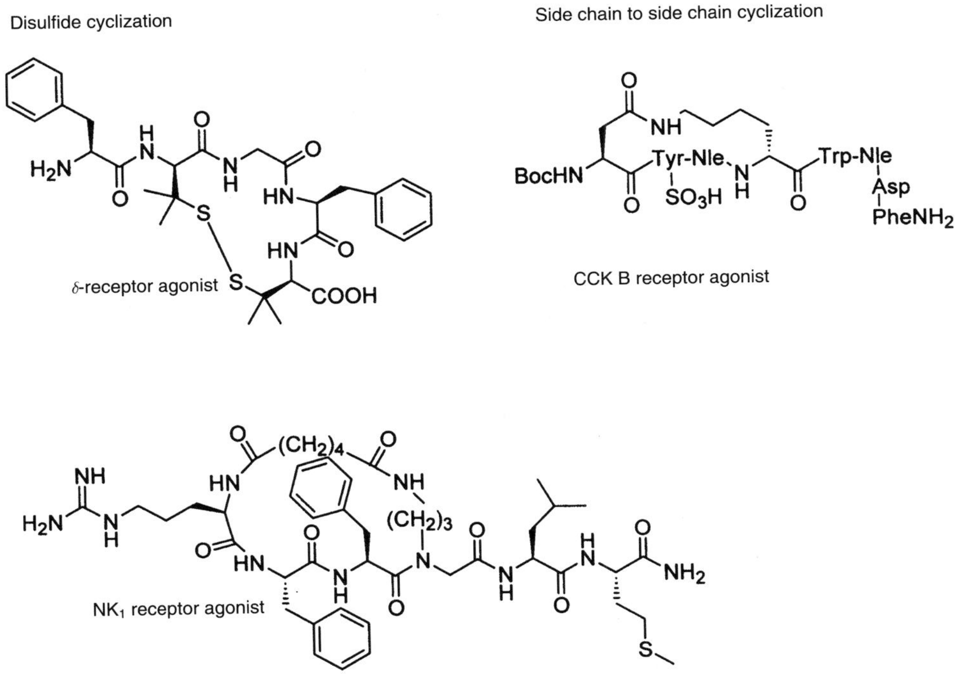

Figure 15.10 Some peptides which have been cyclized to restrict global conformational mobility.

15.2.1.5 *Mimics of peptide secondary structures*

There are three classes of secondary structure elements of a peptide: (1) α-helices; (2) β-sheets; and (3) turns and loops. A secondary structure mimetic is a structural moiety that, when incorporated into a peptide, forces the peptide to adopt a specific conformation.

15.2.1.6 *β- and γ-turn mimetics*

Turns and loops are important conformational characteristics of peptides and proteins. A β-turn is formed from four amino acids and is stabilized by a hydrogen bond between the first and the third amino acid. A γ-turn is formed in a similar way from three amino acids (Figure 15.11). Large numbers of turn mimetics have been designed and synthesized but most have resulted in inactivity when incorporated into peptides. A selection of turn mimetics are shown in Figure 15.11.

15.2.1.7 *α-helix and β-sheet mimetics*

α-Helix and β-sheet motifs are well characterized structural features of peptides and proteins. Some examples of α-helix initiators and β-sheet inducers are shown in Figure 15.12.

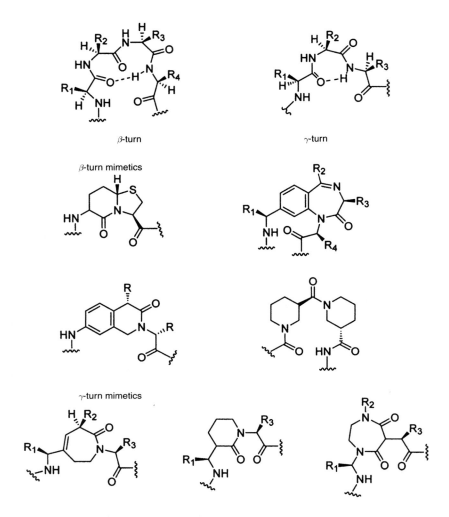

Figure 15.11 The structures of β- and γ-turns (top). Also shown are some β- and γ-turn mimetics.

15.2.1.8 Scaffold mimetics

Topological constraints may also provide information about the bioactive conformation; important amino acid side chains are positioned in proper relative positions onto a molecular template (scaffold), i.e. in agreement with the bioactive topology. The optimal molecular scaffold appears to be a highly functionalized small (5–7-membered) ring of defined stereochemistry. In Figure 15.13, some interesting scaffold mimetics are shown.

The strategies described above are empirical and time consuming. Novel combinatorial chemistry techniques that permit the controlled synthesis of peptide

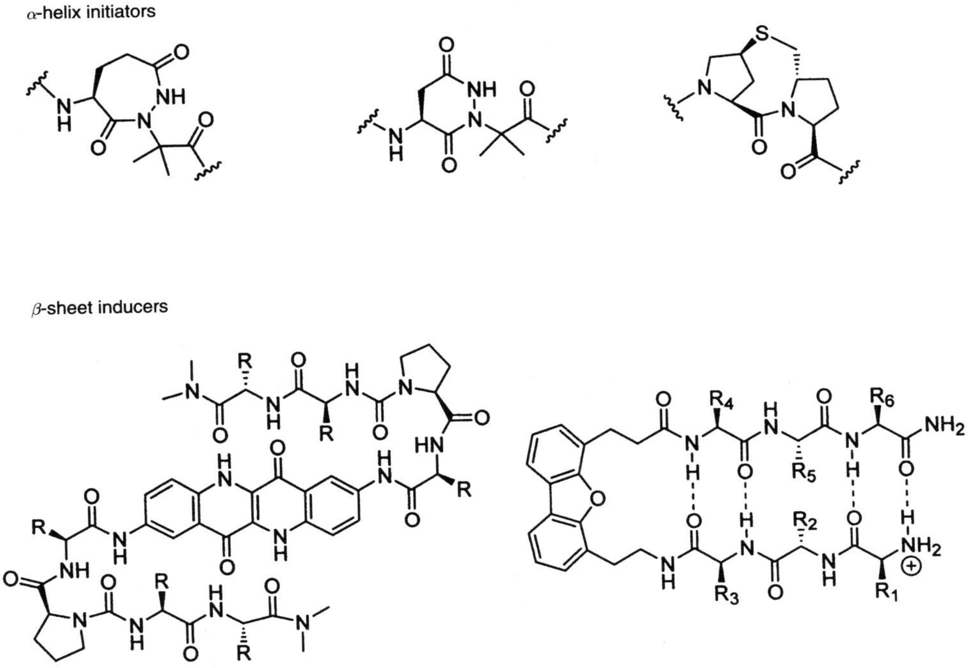

α-helix initiators

β-sheet inducers

Figure 15.12 Structures mimicking various aspects of peptide secondary structure.

libraries in which various mimetic moieties are introduced would probably lead to a more efficient research process.

15.2.2 Discovery of peptidomimetics using receptor/ enzyme-based screening

Extensive efforts have been put into peptide–receptor-based screening of small molecules, natural products, or microbial broths. Although identified leads may show quite weak affinity structural optimization may improve both affinity and selectivity. Most frequently, receptor antagonists have been discovered by this approach. However, in recent years, an increased number of peptide receptor agonist have been identified. The main reason for this trend is believed to be the use of functionalized assays in high throughput screening.

Access to the detailed structure of the binding site of a peptide receptor or enzyme active site would make it possible to use structure-based design technology in attempts to generate efficient agonists/substrates or antagonists/inhibitors. Unfortunately, our knowledge about the structure of ligand binding sites on receptors is very limited. However, structures of several active sites of enzymes have been obtained. In addition, their mechanisms of action have been deduced and this information can also be used efficiently in the lead optimization process as

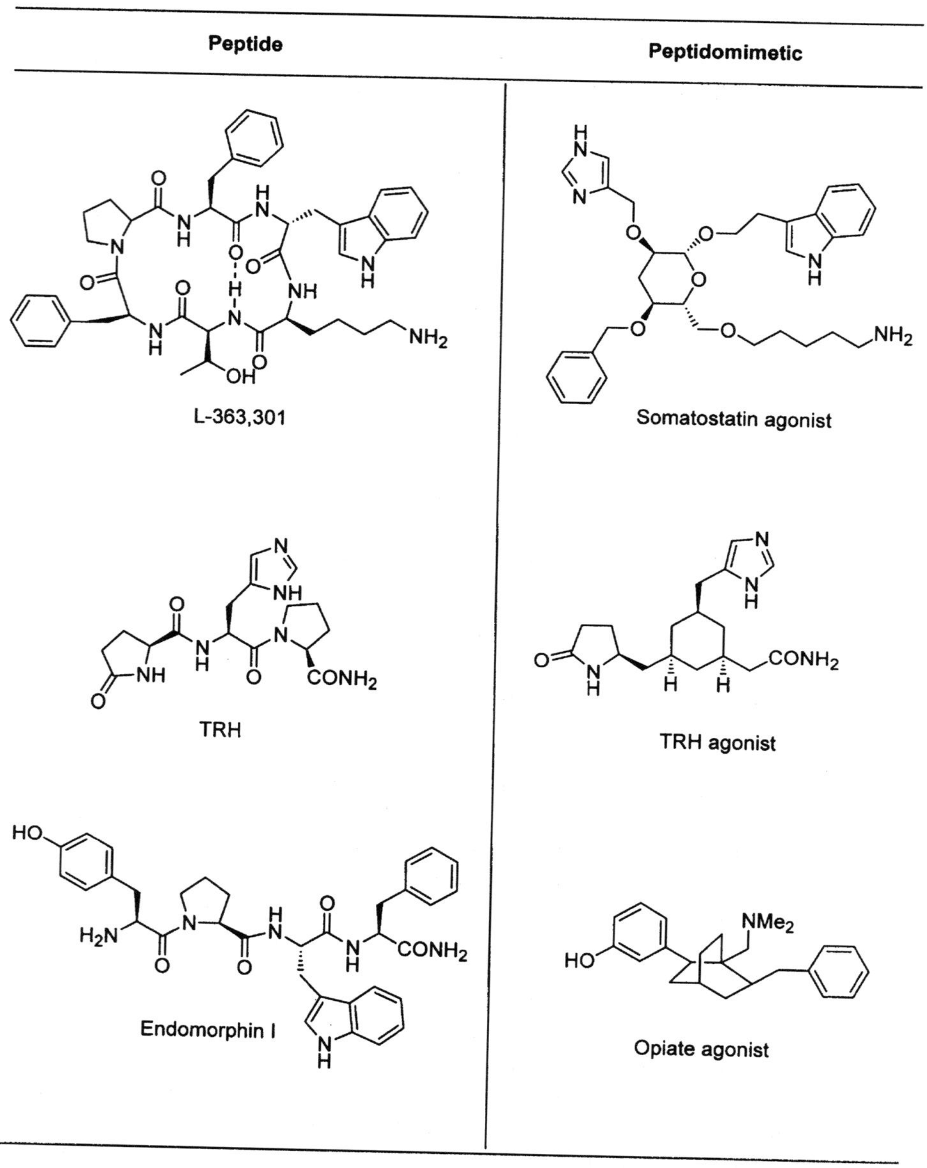

Peptide	Peptidomimetic

L-363,301

Somatostatin agonist

TRH

TRH agonist

Endomorphin I

Opiate agonist

Figure 15.13 Some examples of scaffold-based peptidomimetics.

exemplified by the discovery of the ACE inhibitors (Figure 15.14). In the following sections several examples will be given of peptidomimetics developed after design-based optimization of lead compounds identified in screening programs. Examples of agonists developed from antagonist structures will be given, e.g. angiotensin II, cholesystokinin, bradykinin and arginine vasopressin receptor agonists.

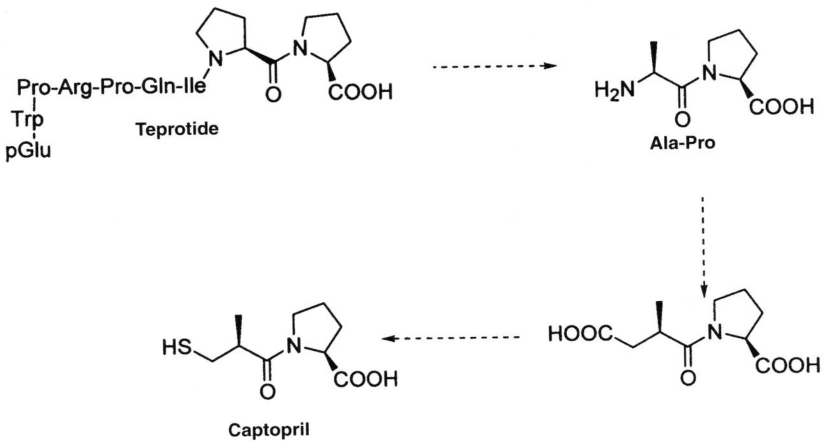

Figure 15.14 The process leading to the discovery of captopril.

15.2.2.1 Angiotensin converting enzyme (ACE) inhibitors and angiotensin II receptor ligands

The ACE-inhibitors were discovered using the nonapeptide teprotide, that was isolated from snake venom, as the molecular lead (Figure 15.14). The optimization of the lead started from the weak inhibitor Ala-Pro, a modified C-terminal fragment of teprotide. The ACE is known to be a metalloprotease with a Zn^{2+} ion in the active site and a carboxylic acid group was introduced to increase the co-ordination of the inhibitor to the enzyme. The successful result of this modification led to the replacement of the carboxylic acid group by a thiol function which co-ordinates even stronger to Zn. The resulting compound, captopril, has been used as an orally active antihypertensive drug for several years.

An early example of discovery of non-peptidic peptide–receptor ligands by receptor-based screening followed by design-based optimization is provided by the angiotensin II receptor (AT_1) antagonist DuP753 (Losartan, Figure 15.15) that was developed from S-8308 which also contains an imidazole moiety. The design was carried out using computer modeling and it has been suggested that the side chains of amino acids Tyr, Ile, and Phe in AngII are mimicked correctly by DuP753. Recently, also AT_1 receptor agonists e.g. L-162,313 and L-162,782 were discovered in screening programs for antagonists (Figure 15.15). Interestingly, the structural similarities between the novel agonists and antagonists are profound, L-162,782 and L-162,389 differ only in one methyl group (Figure 15.15).

15.2.2.2 Cholecystokinin (CCK) receptor ligands

Another early example of discovery of non-peptidic peptide–receptor ligands is provided by the cholecystokinin (CCK) receptor antagonists MK-329 and L-365,260 (Figure 15.16) that were developed from Asperlicin. The CCK-receptor affinity of Asperlicin was discovered by screening. These antagonists contain the

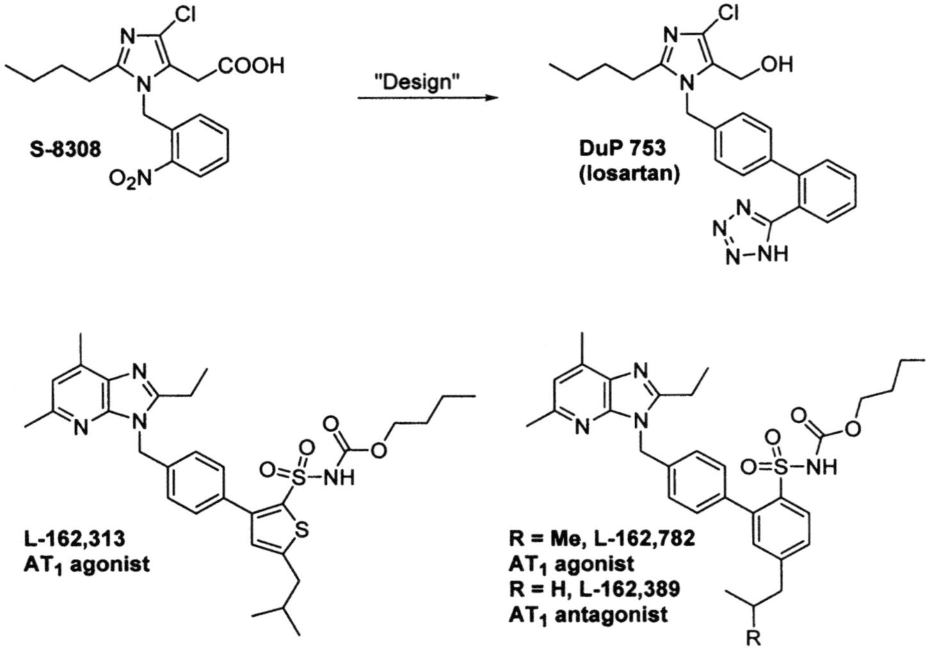

Figure 15.15 The AT$_1$-receptor antagonist DuP753 was developed from S-8308. Recently structurally related non-peptidic agonists were also discovered.

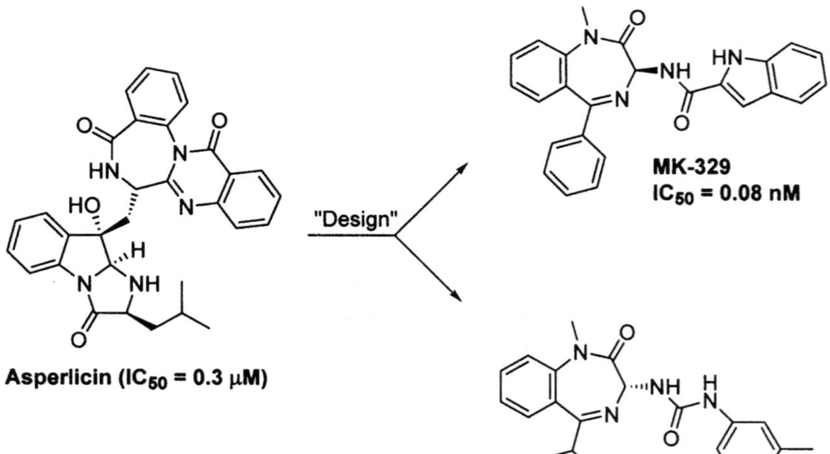

Figure 15.16 Peptide receptor ligands from receptor-based screening. Two CCK antagonists have been developed from asperlicin.

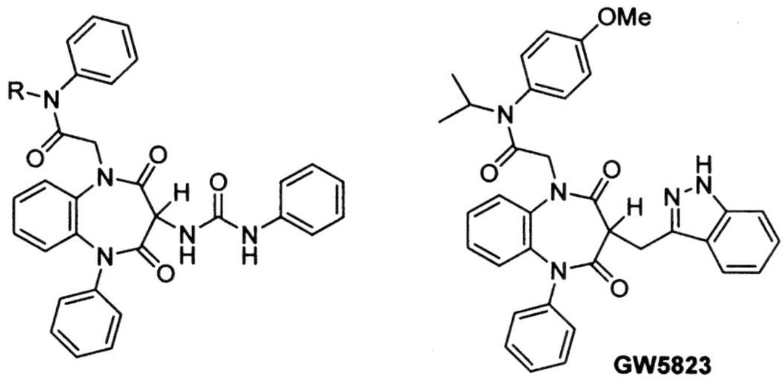

R=Me (antagonist)
R=iPr (CCK-A agonist)

GW5823
Orally active CCK-A selective agonist
(IC_{50} = 23 nM)

Figure 15.17 CCK-A receptor agonists based on the 1,5-benzodiazepine framework. The successful use of the 'agonist trigger' is shown.

1,4-benzodiazepine structure. The benzodiazepine moiety is also present in many other non-peptidic peptide–receptor ligands and has been termed a 'privileged structure' for peptide receptor affinity.

The term 'agonist trigger' was coined during the development of CCK receptor agonists containing a 1,5-benzodiazepin framework (Figure 15.17). The agonist/antagonist activity could be modulated by the N^1-anilinoacetamido moiety, an N^1-methyl group gave antagonist activity whereas an isopropyl group gave agonist activity. The successful use of a combination of information obtained from Asperlicin and the agonistic effect triggered by an isopropyl group lead to the development of the first orally active CCK-A selective agonist GW5823 (Figure 15.17).

15.2.2.3 *Arginine Vasopressin (AVP) receptor ligands*

Recently a series of arginine vasopressin (AVP) V_2 receptor agonists based on the benzazepin skeleton was discovered. The design of agonists was based on a lead structure obtained by analysis of metabolites from antagonists, such as tolvaptan (Figure 15.18). A large series of compounds were synthesized with high affinity for the V_2 receptor but with varying functional activities. The agonist effect was determined as percentage of maximal cAMP accumulation. The V_2-receptor agonist activity is severely restricted by the size of the P1 region of the receptor and even small structural changes in this region could lead to drastic differences in agonist action. Therefore, it was hypothesized that this region contains an activation cavity. The P2 binding region seems to be important for the affinity. Some agonist structures are shown in Figure 15.18.

15.2.2.4 *Bradykinin receptor ligands*

The structural similarities between agonists and antagonists at peptide receptors can also be illustrated by ligands for the bradykinin B_2-receptor. Agonists at the

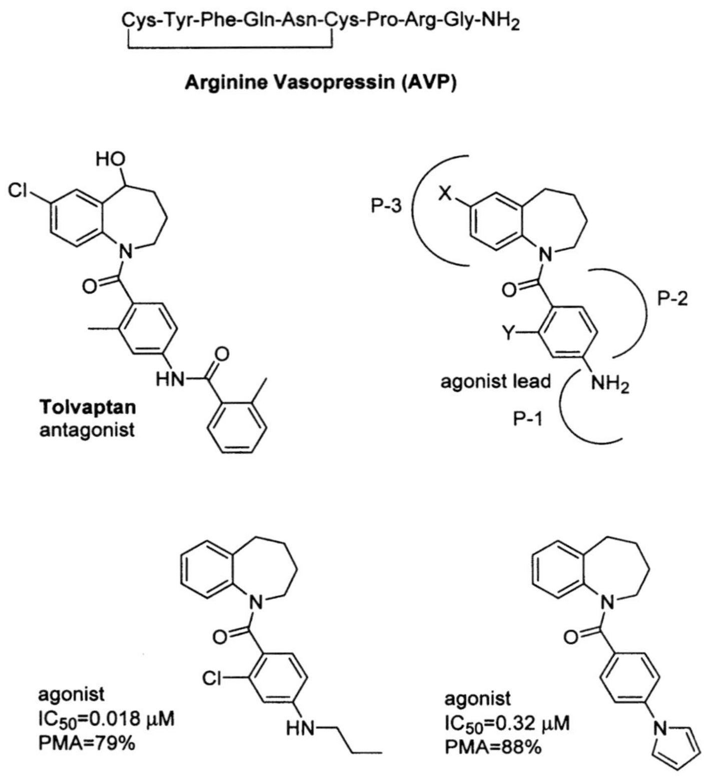

Cys-Tyr-Phe-Gln-Asn-Cys-Pro-Arg-Gly-NH$_2$

Arginine Vasopressin (AVP)

Figure 15.18 Design of novel non-peptidic AVP agonists based on the benzazepine skeleton. PMA = percentage of maximal cAMP accumulation at a concentration of 1 μM. The P-1, P-2 and P-3 binding regions are also shown.

B$_2$-receptor are expected to be important e.g. in hypertension, and several peptidic agonists are known. The first non-peptidic B$_2$-agonist FR190997 was recently identified among a large series of bradykinin-receptor antagonists (Figure 15.19).

15.2.2.5   Mimetics of growth hormone regulating peptides

Growth hormone release is regulated by different peptides such as growth hormone releasing hormone (GH-RH), growth hormone secretagogues (GHS), and somatostatin. It was not until recently the endogenous ligand for the GHS receptor was identified to be the 28 amino acid peptide ghrelin. Ghrelin is a linear peptide containing an *n*-octanoyl modification on Ser3. Several non-peptidic agonists at the GHS-receptor(s) has been identified, they exhibit a large structural diversity (Figure 15.20).

Growth hormone release is negatively regulated by somatostatin activation of the sst$_2$-receptor subtype. Somatostatin regulates also the release of other hormones such as glucagon, insulin and gastrin, the different functional activities being regulated by activation of different sst-receptor subtypes. Non-peptidic subtype

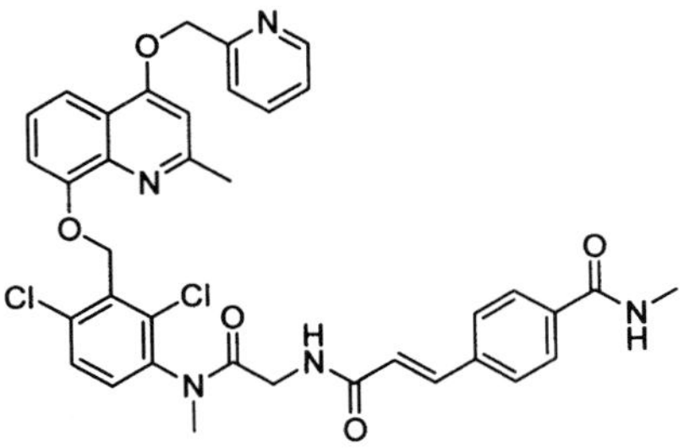

FR190997

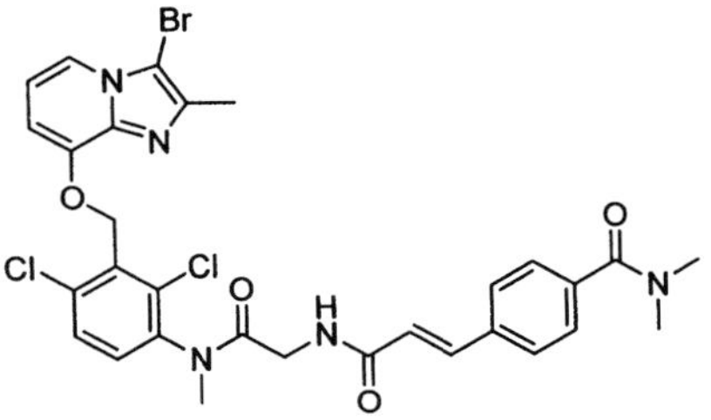

FR167344

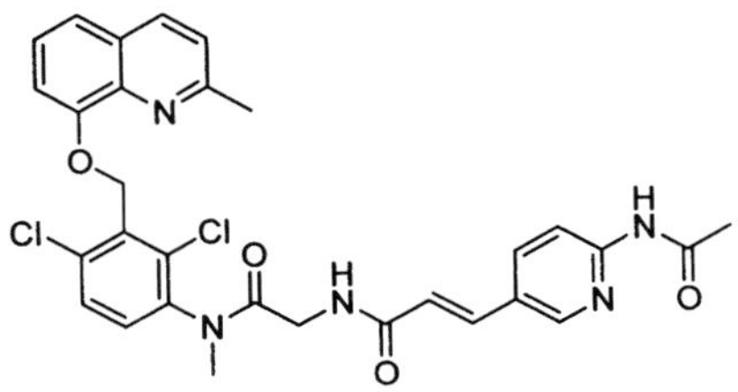

FR173657

Figure 15.19 The bradykinin B_2-receptor agonist FR190997 and some structurally related antagonists.

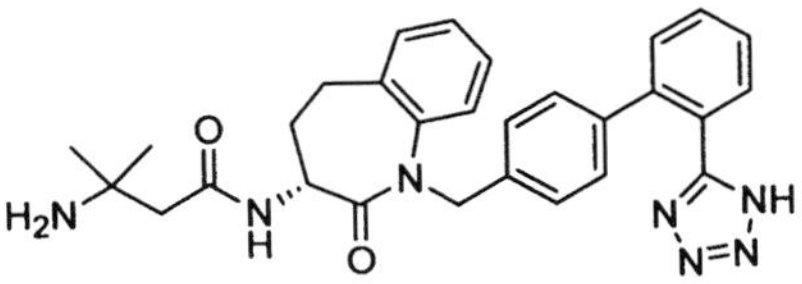

L-692,429

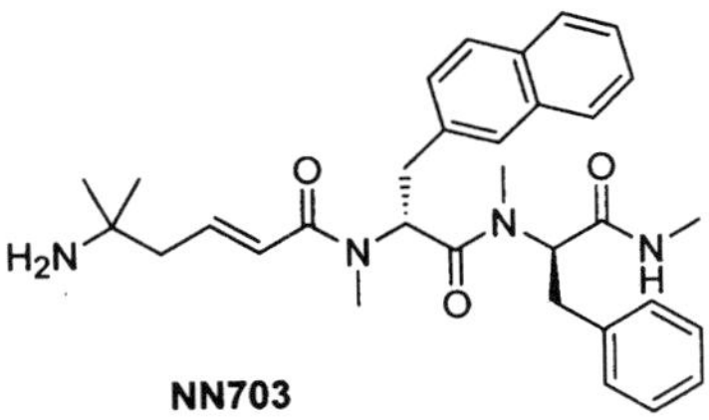

NN703

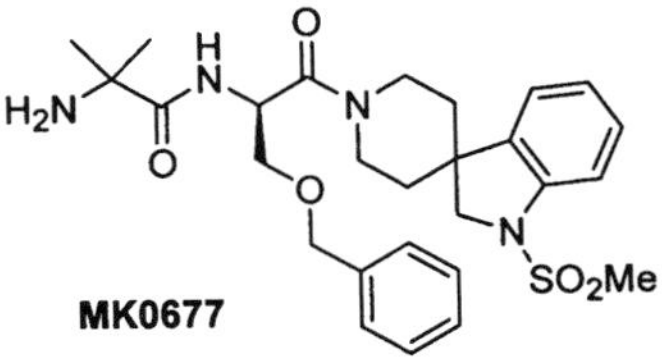

MK0677

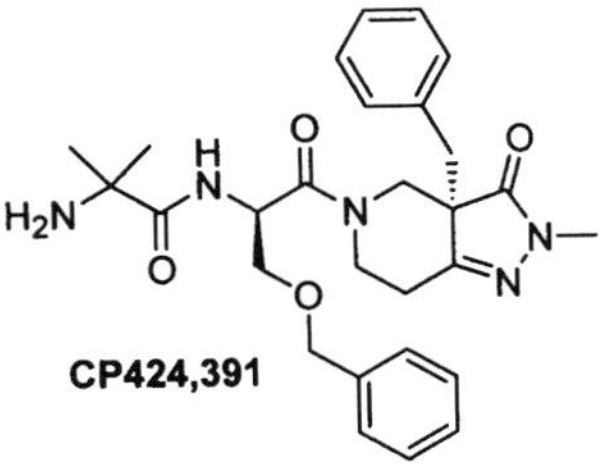

CP424,391

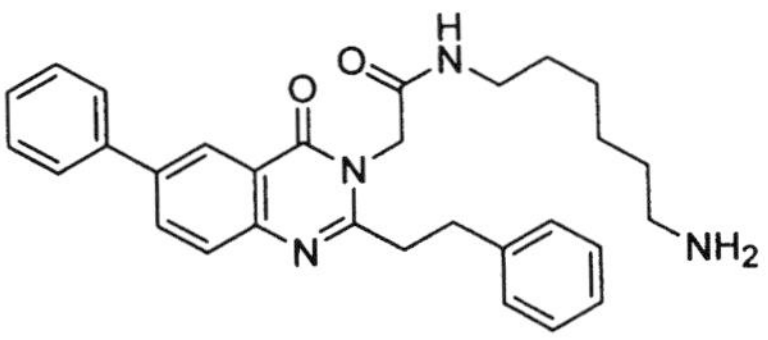

Figure 15.20 Some non-peptidic GHS-receptor agonists.

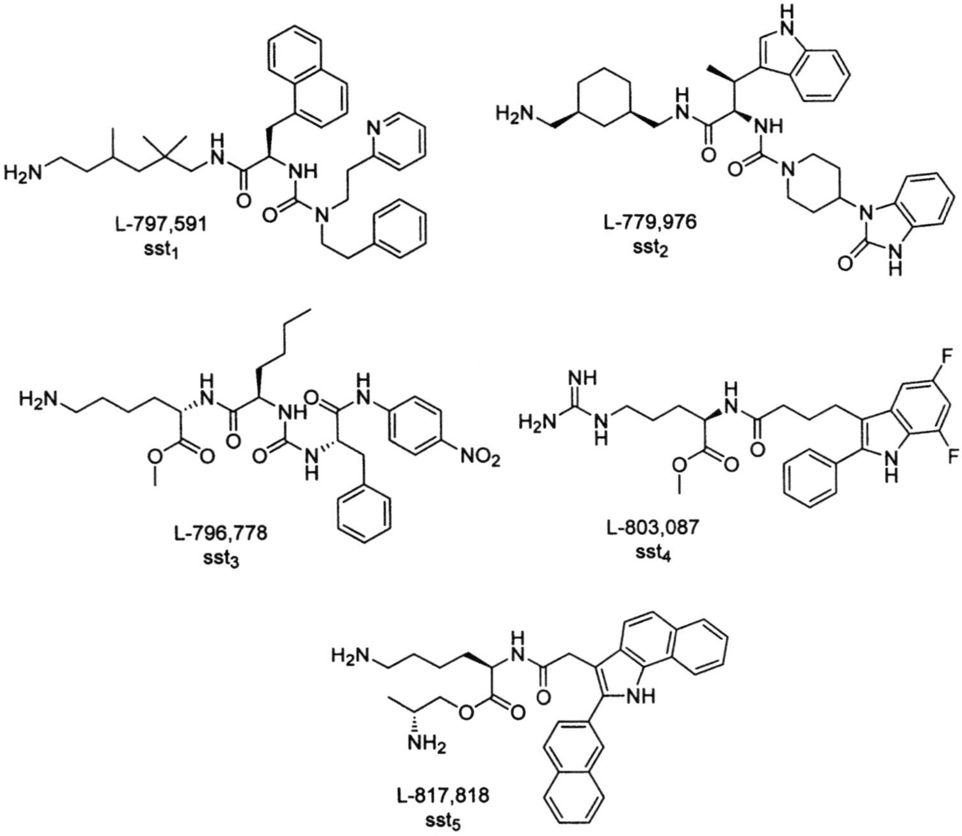

Figure 15.21 Subtype specific somatostatin receptor agonists have been identified by a combination of combinatorial chemistry and molecular modeling.

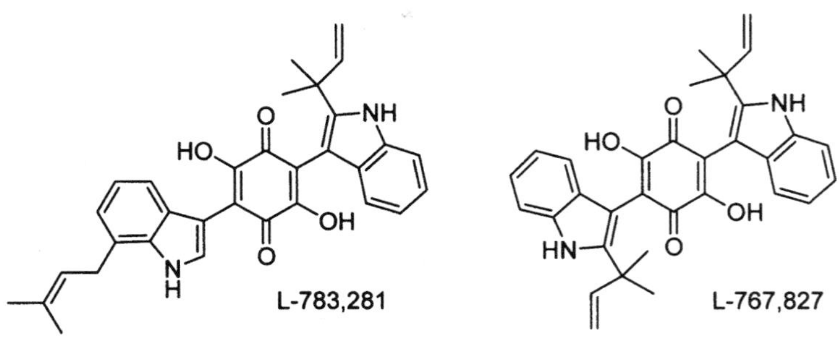

Figure 15.22 Recently discovered small molecule insulin mimetics.

receptor specific agonists have been identified by a combination of combinatorial chemistry and molecular modeling using the cyclic hexapeptide somatostatin agonist (L-363,377) as a lead (Figure 15.21).

15.2.2.6 Small molecule insulin mimetics

Recently non-peptide small molecule insulin mimetics were discovered. The quinone derivative L-783,281, isolated from a fungal extract, showed potent anti-diabetic activity. Interestingly, the mimetic has been shown to bind to a different binding site on the insulin receptor than insulin itself. The structurally related compound hinulliquinone (L-767,827) also showed activity in the antidiabetic assay, however this symmetrical molecule was a 100 times less potent than L-783,281 (Figure 15.22).

FURTHER READING

Adang, A.E.P., Hermkens, P.H.H., Linders, J.T.M., Ottenheijm, H.C.J. and van Staveren, C.J. (1994) Case histories of peptidomimetics: progression from peptide to drugs. *Recl. Trav. Chim. Pays-Bas*, **113**, 63–78.

Aquino, C.J., Armour, D.R., Berman, J.M., Birkemo, L.S., Carr, R.A.E., Croom, D.K., Dezube, M., Dougherty, Jr., R.W., Ervin, G.N., Grizzle, M.K., Head, J.E., Hirst, G.C., James, M.K., Johnson, M.F., Miller, L.J., Queen, K.L., Rimele, T.J., Smith, D.N. and Sugg, E.E. (1996) Discovery of 1,5-benzodiazepines with peripheral cholecystokinin (CCK-A) receptor agonist activity. 1. Optimization of the agonist 'trigger'. *J. Med. Chem.*, **39**, 562–569.

Aramori, I., Zenkoh, J., Morikawa, N., Asano, M., Hatori, C., Sawai, H., Kayakiri, H., Satoh, S., Inoue, T., Abe, Y., Sawada, Y., Mizutani, T., Inamura, N., Nakahara, K., Kojo, H., Oku, T. and Notsu, Y. (1997) Nonpeptide mimic of bradykinin with long-acting properties at the bradykinin B$_2$ receptor. *Mol. Pharmacol.*, **52**, 16–20.

Bednarek, M.A., Feighner, S.D., Pong, S.-S., Kulju McKee, K., Hreniuk, D.L., Silva, M.V., Warren, V.A., Howard, A.D., van der Ploeg, L.H.Y. and Heck, J.V. (2000) Structure–function studies on the new growth hormone-releasing peptide, ghrelin: minimal sequence of ghrelin necessary for activation of growth hormone secretagogue receptor 1a. *J. Med. Chem.*, **43**, 4370–4376.

Beeley, N.R.A. (2000) Can peptides be mimicked? *Drug Discovery Today*, **5**, 354–363.

Bélanger, P.C. and Dufresne, C. (1986) Preparation of exo-6-benzyl-exo-2-(m-hydroxy-phenyl)-1-dimethylaminomethylbicyclo[2.2.2]octane. A non-peptide mimic of enkephalins. *Can. J. Chem.*, **64**, 1514–1520.

Benz, H. (1994) The role of solid-phase fragment condensation (SPFC) in peptide synthesis. *Synthesis*, 337–358.

Berts, W. and Luthman, K. (1999) Synthesis of a complete series of C-4 fluorinated Phe-Gly mimetics. *Tetrahedron*, **55**, 13819–13830.

Borg, S., Estenne-Bouhtou, G., Luthman, K., Csöregh, I., Hesselink, W. and Hacksell, U. (1995) Synthesis of 1,2,4-oxadiazole, 1,3,4-oxadiazole, and 1,2,4-triazole-derived dipeptidomimetics. *J. Org. Chem.*, **60**, 3112–3120.

Borg, S., Vollinga, R.C., Labarre, M., Payza, K., Terenius, L. and Luthman, K. (1999) Design, synthesis, and evaluation of Phe-Gly mimetics: heterocyclic building blocks for pseudopeptides. *J. Med. Chem.*, **42**, 4331–4342.

Boyle, S., Guard, S., Higginbottom, M., Horwell, D.C., Howson, W., McKnight, A.T., Martin, K., Pritchard, M.C., O'Toole, J., Raphy, J., Rees, D.C., Roberts, E., Watling, K.J.,

Woodruff, G.N. and Hughes, J. (1994) Rational design of high affinity tachykinin NK₁ receptor antagonists. *Bioorg. Med. Chem.*, **2**, 357–370.

Chorev, M. and Goodman, M. (1993) A dozen years of retro-inverso peptidomimetics. *Acc. Chem. Res.*, **26**, 266–273.

Chung, Y.J., Christianson, L.A., Stanger, H.E., Powell, D.R. and Gellman, S.H. (1998) A β-peptide reverse turn that promotes hairpin formation. *J. Am. Chem. Soc.*, **120**, 10555–10556.

de Tullio, P., Delarge, J. and Pirotte, B. (1999) Recent advances in the chemistry of cholecystokinin receptor ligands (agonists and antagonists). *Curr. Med. Chem.*, **6**, 433–455.

Duncia, J.V., Carini, D.J., Chiu, A.T, Johnson, A.L., Price, W.A., Wong, P.C., Wexler, R.R. and Timmermans, P.B.M.W.M. (1992) The discovery of DuP753, a potent, orally active nonpeptide angiotensin II receptor antagonist. *Med. Res. Rev.*, **12**, 149–191.

Evans, B.E., Bock, M.G., Rittle, K.E., DiPardo, R.M., Whitter, W.L., Veber, D.F., Anderson, P.S. and Freidinger, R.M. (1986) Design of potent, orally effective, nonpeptidal antagonists of the peptide hormone cholecystokinin. *Proc. Natl. Acad. Sci. USA*, **83**, 4918–4922.

Farmer, P.S. (1980) Bridging the gap between bioactive peptides and nonpeptides: some perspectives in design. *Drug Design*, Vol. X, pp. 119–143.

Gallop, M.A., Barrett, R.W., Dower, W.J., Fodor, S.P.A. and Gordon, E.M. (1994) Applications of combinatorial technologies to drug discovery. 1. Background and peptide combinatorial libraries. *J. Med. Chem.*, **37**, 1233–1251.

Gante, J. (1994) Peptidomimetics – tailored enzyme inhibitors. *Angew. Chem. Int. Ed. Engl.*, **33**, 1699–1720.

Giannis, A. and Kolter, T. (1993) Peptidomimetics for receptor ligands – Discovery, development, and medical perspectives. *Angew. Chem. Int. Ed. Engl.*, **32**, 1244–1267.

Gilon, C., Halle, D., Chorev, M., Selinger, Z. and Byk, G. (1991) Backbone cyclization: a new method for conferring conformational constraint on peptides. *Biopolymers*, **31**, 745–750.

Golic Grdadolnik, S., Mierke, D.F., Byk, G., Zeltser, I., Gilon, C. and Kessler, H. (1994) Comparison of the conformation of active and nonactive backbone cyclic analogs of substance P as a tool to elucidate features of the bioactive conformation: NMR and molecular dynamics in DMSO and water. *J. Med. Chem.*, **37**, 2145–2152.

Gordon, E.M., Barrett, R.W., Dower, W.J., Fodor, S.P.A. and Gallop, M.A. (1994) Applications of combinatorial technologies to drug discovery. 2. Combinatorial organic synthesis, library screening strategies, and future directions. *J. Med. Chem.*, **37**, 1385–1401.

Ghosh, A.K., Shin, D., Downs, D., Koelsch, G., Lin, X., Ermolieff, J. and Tang J. (2000) Design of potent inhibitors for human brain memapsin 2 (β-secretase). *J. Am. Chem. Soc.*, **122**, 3522–3523.

Graf von Roedern, E. and Kessler, H. (1994) A sugar amino acid as a novel peptidomimetic. *Angew. Chem. Int. Ed. Engl.*, **33**, 687–689.

Henke, B.R., Aquino, C.J., Birkemo, L.S., Croom, D.K., Dougherty, Jr., R.W., Ervin, G.N., Grizzle, M.K., Hirst, G.C., James, M.K., Johnson, M.F., Queen, K.L., Sherrill, R.G., Sugg, E.E., Suh, E.M., Szewczyk, J.W., Unwalla, R.J., Yingling, J. and Willson, T.M. (1997) Optimization of 3-(1*H*-indazol-3-ylmethyl)-1,5-benzodiazepines as potent, orally active CCK-A agonists. *J. Med. Chem.*, **40**, 2706–2725.

Hirschmann, R. (1991) Medicinal chemistry in the golden age of biology: lessons from steroid and peptide research. *Angew. Chem. Int. Ed. Engl.*, **30**, 1278–1301.

Hirschmann, R., Nicolaou, K.C., Pietranico, S., Leahy, E.M., Salvino, J., Arison, B., Cichy, M.A., Spoors, P.G., Shakespeare, W.C., Sprengler, P.A., Hamley, P., Smith III, A.B., Reisine, T., Raynor, K., Maechler, L., Donaldson, C., Vale, W., Freidinger, R.M., Cascieri, M.R. and Strader, C.D. (1993) *De novo* design and synthesis of somatostatin non-peptide peptidomimetics utilizing β-D-glucose as a novel scaffolding. *J. Am. Chem. Soc.*, **115**, 12550–12568.

Hirschmann, R., Hynes, Jr., J., Cichy-Knight, M.A., van Rijn, R.D., Sprengeler, P.A., Spoors, P.G., Shakespeare, W.C., Pietranico-Cole, S., Barbosa, J., Liu, J., Yao, W., Rohrer, S. and Smith, A.B., III. (1998) Modulation of receptor and receptor subtype affinities using diastereomeric and enantiomeric monosaccharide scaffolds as a means to structural and biological diversity. A new route to ether synthesis. *J. Med. Chem.*, **41**, 1382–1391.

Hirst, G.C., Aquino, C., Birkemo, L., Croom, D.K., Dezube, M., Dougherty, Jr., R.W., Ervin, G.N., Grizzle, M.K., Henke, B., James, M.K., Johnson, M.F., Momtahen, T., Queen, K.L., Sherrill, R.G., Szewczyk, J., Willson, T.M. and Sugg, E.E. (1996) Discovery of 1,5-benzodiazepines with peripheral cholecystokinin (CCK-A) receptor activity (II). Optimization of the C3 amino substituent. *J. Med. Chem.*, **39**, 5236–5245.

Hong, L., Koelsch, G., Lin, X., Wu, S., Terzyan, S., Ghosh, A.K., Zhang, X.C. and Tang, J. (2000) Structure of the protease domain of memapsin 2 (β-secretase) complexed with inhibitor. *Science*, **290**, 150–153.

Houghten, R.A. (1985) General method for the rapid solid-phase synthesis of large numbers of peptides: specificity of antigen–antibody interaction at the level of individual amino acids. *Proc. Natl. Acad. Sci. USA*, **82**, 5131–5135.

Houghten, R.A., Pinilla, C., Blondelle, S.E., Appel, J.R., Dooley, C.T. and Cuervo, J.H. (1991) Generation and use of synthetic peptide combinatorial libraries for basic research and drug discovery. *Nature*, **354**, 84–86.

Howson, W. (1995) Rational design of tachykinin receptor antagonists. *Drug News Perspect.*, **8**, 97–103.

Hruby, V.J. (1982) Conformational restrictions of biologically active peptides via amino acid side chain groups. *Life Sci.*, **31**, 189–199.

Hruby, V.J., Al-Obeidi, F. and Kazmierski, W. (1990) Emerging approaches in the molecular design of receptor-selective peptide ligands: conformational, topographical and dynamic considerations. *Biochem. J.*, **268**, 249–262.

Hruby, V.J. (1993) Conformational and topographical considerations in the design of biologically active peptides. *Biopolymers*, **33**, 1073–1082.

Hruby, V.J. and Balse, P.M. (2000) Conformational and topographical considerations in designing agonist peptidomimetics from peptide leads. *Current Med. Chem.*, **7**, 945–970.

Humphrey, J.M. and Chamberlin, A.R. (1997) Chemical synthesis of natural product peptides: coupling methods for the incorporation of noncoded amino acids into peptides. *Chem. Rev.*, **97**, 2243–2266.

Höllt, V. (1986) Opioid peptide processing and receptor selectivity. *Ann. Rev. Pharmacol. Toxicol.*, **26**, 59–77.

Hölzemann, G. (1991) Peptide conformation mimetics part 1 and 2. *Kontakte (Darmstadt)*, 3–12, 55–63.

Kahn, M. (1993) Peptide secondary structure mimetics: recent advances and future challenges. *Synlett*, 821–826.

Kalindjian, S.B., Dunstone, D.J., Low, C.M.R., Pether, M.J., Roberts, S.P., Tozer, M.J., Watt, G.F. and Shankley, N.P. (2001) Nonpeptide cholecystokinin-2 receptor agonists. *J. Med. Chem.* **44**, 1125–1133.

Kazmierski, W.M. (ed.) (1999) *Methods Mol. Med.*, **23**(Peptidomimetics Protocols). Totowa, New Jersey, USA: Humana Press.

Kessler, H. (1982) Conformation and biological activity of cyclic peptides. *Angew. Chem. Int. Ed. Engl.*, **21**, 512–523.

Kim, H.-O. and Kahn, M. (2000). A merger of rational drug design and combinatorial chemistry: development and application of peptide secondary structure mimetics. *Combinatorial Chemistry & High Throughput Screening*, **3**, 167–183.

Kivlighn, S.D., Huckle, W.R., Zingaro, G.J., Rivero, R.A., Lotti, V.J., Chang, R.S.L., Schorn, T.W., Kevin, N., Johnson, Jr., R.G., Greelee, W.J. and Siegl, P.K.S (1995) Discovery of L-162,313: a nonpeptide that mimics the biological actions of angiotensin II. *Am. J. Physiol.*, R820–R823.

Kojima, M., Hosoda, H., Date, Y., Nakazato, M., Matsuo, H. and Kangawa, K. (1999) Ghrelin is a growth-hormone-releasing acylated peptide from stomach. *Nature*, **402**, 656–660.

Kondo, K., Ogawa, H., Shinohara, T., Kurimura, M., Tanada, Y., Kan, K., Yamashita, H., Nakamura, S., Hirano, T., Yamamura, Y., Mori, T., Tominaga, M. and Itai, A. (2000) Novel design of nonpeptide AVP V$_2$ receptor agonists: structural requirements for an agonist having 1-(4-aminobenzoyl)-2,3,4,5-tetrahydro-1*H*-1-benzazepin as a template. *J. Med. Chem.*, **43**, 4388–4397.

Kreil, G. (1994) Peptides containing a D-amino acid from frogs and molluscs. *J. Biol. Chem.*, **269**, 10967–10970.

Liao, S., Alfaro-Lopez, J., Shenderovich, M.D., Hosohata, K., Lin, J., Li, X., Stropova, D., Davis, P., Jernigan, K.A., Porreca, F., Yamamura, H.I. and Hruby, V.J. (1998) *De novo* design, synthesis, and biological activities of high-affinity and selective non-peptide agonists of the δ-opioid receptor. *J. Med. Chem.*, **41**, 4767–4776.

Liskamp, R.M.J. (1994) Conformationally restricted amino acids and dipeptides, (non)peptidomimetics and secondary structure mimetics. *Recl. Trav. Chim. Pays-Bas*, **113**, 1–19.

Moore, C.L., Leatherwood, D.D., Diehl, T.S., Selkoe, D.J. and Wolfe, M.S. (2000) Difluoro ketone peptidomimetics suggest a large S1 pocket for Alzheimer's γ-secretase: implications for inhibitor design. *J. Med. Chem.*, **43**, 3434–3442.

Morgan, B.A. and Gainor, J.A. (1989) Approaches to the discovery of non-peptide ligands for peptide receptors and peptidases. *Ann. Rep. Med. Chem.*, **24**, 243–252.

Olson, G.L., Bolin, D.R., Bonner, M.P., Bös, M., Cook, C.M., Fry, D.C., Graves, B.J., Hatada, M., Hill, D.E., Kahn, M., Madison, V.S., Rusiecki, V.K., Sarabu, R., Sepinwall, J., Vincent, G.P. and Voss, M.E. (1993) Concepts and progress in the development of peptide mimetics. *J. Med. Chem.*, **36**, 3039–3049.

Olson, G.L., Cheung, H.-C., Chiang, E., Madison, V.S., Sepinwall, J., Vincent, G.P., Winokur, A. and Gary, K.A. (1995) Peptide mimetics of thyrotropin-releasing hormone based on a cyclohexane framework: design, synthesis, and cognition-enhancing properties. *J. Med. Chem.*, **38**, 2866–2879.

Ostresh, J.M., Husar, G.M., Blondelle, S.E., Dörner, B., Weber, P.A. and Houghten, R.A. (1994) 'Libraries from libraries': Chemical transformation of combinatorial libraries to extend the range and repertoire of chemical diversity. *Proc. Natl. Acad. Sci. USA*, **91**, 11138–11142.

Ramachandran, G.N. and Sasisekharan, V. (1968) Conformation of polypeptides and proteins. *Adv. Prot. Chem.*, **23**, 283–437.

Rist, B., Entzeroth, M. and Beck-Sickinger, A.G. (1998) From micromolar to nanomolar affinity: a systematic approach to identify the binding site of CGRP at the human calcitonin gene-related peptide 1 receptor. *J. Med. Chem.*, **41**, 117–123.

Rohrer, S.P., Birzin, E.T., Mosley, R.T., Berk, S.C., Hutchins, S.M., Shen, D.-M., Xiong, Y., Hayes, E.C., Parmar, R.M., Foor, F., Mitra, S.W., Degrado, S.J., Shu, M., Klopp, J.M., Cai, S.-J., Blake, A., Chan, W.W.S., Pasternak, A., Yang, L., Patchett, A.A., Smith, R.G., Chapman, K.T. and Schaeffer, J.M. (1998) Rapid identification of subtype-selective agonists of the somatostatin receptor through combinatorial chemistry. *Science*, **282**, 737–740.

Saulitis, J., Mierke, D.F., Byk, G., Gilon, C. and Kessler, H. (1992) Conformation of cyclic analogues of substance P: NMR and molecular dynamics in dimethyl sulfoxide. *J. Am. Chem. Soc.*, **114**, 4818–4827.

Schmidhammer, H. (1998) Opioid receptor antagonists. *Prog. Med. Chem.*, **35**, 83–132.

Schulz, G.E. and Schirmer, R.H. (1979) *Principles of Protein Structure*. New York: Springer-Verlag.

Schmidt, B., Lindman, S., Tong, W., Lindeberg, G., Gogoll, A., Lai, Z., Thörnwall, M., Synnergren, B., Nilsson, A., Welch, C.J., Sohtell, M., Westerlund, C., Nyberg, F., Karlén, A. and Hallberg, A. (1997) Design, synthesis and biological activities of four angiotensin II receptor ligands with γ-turn mimetics replacing amino acid residues 3–5. *J. Med. Chem.*, **40**, 903–919.

Schmitz, R. (1985) Friedrich Wilhelm Sertürner and the discovery of morphine. *Pharmacy in History*, **27**, 61–74.

Spatola, A.F. (1983) Peptide backbone modifications: a structure–activity analysis of peptides containing amide bond surrogates, conformational constraints, and related backbone replacements. In *Chemistry and Biochemistry of Amino Acids, Peptides, and Proteins*, Vol. VII, edited by B. Weinstein, pp. 267–357, New York: Marcel Dekker.

Toniolo, C. (1990) Conformationally restricted peptides through short-range cyclizations. *Int. J. Peptide Protein Res.*, **35**, 287–300.

Wiley, R.A. and Rich, D.H. (1993) Peptidomimetics derived from natural products. *Med. Res. Rev.*, **13**, 327–384.

Zhang, B., Salituro, G., Szalkowski, D., Li, Z., Zhang, Y., Royo, I., Vilella, D., Diez, M.T., Pelaez, F., Ruby, C., Kendall, R.L., Mao, X., Griffin, P., Calaycay, J., Zierath, J.R., Heck, J.V., Smith, R.G. and Moller, D.E. (1999) Discovery of small molecule insulin mimetic with antidiabetic activity in mice. *Science*, **284**, 974–977.

Chapter 16

Classical antiviral agents and design of new antiviral agents

Piet Herdewijn and Erik de Clercq

16.1 CLASSICAL ANTIVIRAL AGENTS

16.1.1 Introduction

More than 50 years have elapsed since the discovery of the first antiviral agents, i.e. methisazone and 5-iodo-2′-deoxyuridine. In contrast to the evolution in other fields, the antiviral chemotherapy has evolved very slowly at the start. The reasons therefore are multiple:

- close association between the replicative cycle of the virus and the metabolism of the cell;
- the intracellular location of the virus;
- viruses possess considerable fewer virus-associated or -encoded enzymes than bacteria;
- effective vaccines have been developed for the prevention of some severe viral infections; and
- antiviral research is a high-risk enterprise for industry.

However, the interest in antiviral chemotherapy has been boosted considerably since the identification, now more than 15 years ago, of HIV (human immuno deficiency virus) as the causative agent of the acquired immune deficiency syndrome (AIDS).

Viral infections can vary from mild and transient to severe and irreversible, and occasionally lead to death. Viral infections can cause chronic degenerative disease and are also implicated in various forms of cancer in man. Many viral infections, even if not life-threatening, have an important socio-economic impact.

The classical antiviral agents that are, at present, used in the clinic have all evolved from random screening and serendipity. The rational design of antivirals is a relatively new approach and has mainly been used in the anti-HIV field and more recently in the anti-HCV (hepatitis C virus) field. All antiviral agents depend for their activity on interactions with the virus-encoded enzymes. Progress in the molecular biology of viral–host interaction has uncovered new targets for antiviral chemotherapy, and thus, compounds with a different chemical structure. In the first part of this chapter, an overview is given of classical antiviral agents. In the second part, more recent developments in antiviral drug design are summarized.

(16.1)
5'-Iodo-2'-deoxyuridine

(16.2)
Thymidine

(16.3)
Zidovudine

5-Iodo-2′-deoxyuridine (IdUrd, IDU) (**16.1**) has a structure that is very similar to that of the natural nucleoside thymidine (**16.2**). The van der Waals radius of an iodo group is somewhat larger than that of a methyl group, and the pKa of 5-iodouracil, the 6-membered heterocyclic unit of 16.1, is about 1.5 units lower than that of thymine, the corresponding heterocyclic unit of 16.2. This results from the inductive effect of the iodo group in the 5-position. These slight differences are apparently sufficient for IdUrd to become a rather selective antiviral agent. W.H. Prusoff synthesized IdUrd first in 1959 by iodination of 2′-deoxyuridine with iodine/nitric acid. IdUrd is active against the multiplication of *Herpes simplex* virus type 1 (HSV-1), *Herpes simplex* virus type 2 (HSV-2) and vaccinia virus (VV) *in vitro* and has proven efficacious in the treatment of herpes eye infections (i.e. herpetic keratitis). Its toxicity, however, does not allow systemic use.

Also there is a great resemblance in the structures of thymidine and 3′-azido-3′-deoxythymidine (zidovudine, AZT) (**16.3**). Here, the 3′-position is substituted with an azido group. This compound was the first to be approved by the FDA for the treatment of AIDS patients. J.P. Horwitz synthesized it first in 1964 starting from thymidine. Also, the modes of action of IdUrd and zidovudine are quite similar. They have to be metabolized intracellularly to their 5′-triphosphate derivatives and these triphosphates then interact with (viral) DNA synthesis.

These two nucleoside analogs (IDU and AZT), which resemble very well their natural counterpart, have had a tremendous impact on antiviral research. IDU has long been a model compound for the design of new and more selective antiherpes agents. The advent of AIDS, the identification of a retrovirus as the causative agent of the disease and the observation that its replication can be blocked by simple nucleosides, gave an important incentive to the search for new antiviral agents.

In this chapter, we will see how selectivity can be obtained by interference with virus-specific targets. The identification of specific, virus-encoded, enzymes has proved the key step in the design of new antiviral compounds.

In the design of new nucleoside analogs, targeted at viral DNA synthesis, the discovery of HPMPC [(S)-1-(3-hydroxy-2-phosphonylmethoxypropyl)cytosine] (**16.4**) and PMPA [(R)-9-(2-phosphonylmethoxypropyl)adenine] (**16.5**) as potent inhibitors of CMV (cytomegalo virus) and HIV, respectively, could be considered as important progress. Their antiviral activity clearly indicates that mimicking nucleoside metabolites, e.g. nucleoside monophosphates, can overcome at least

(16.4)   (16.5)

the first step of intracellular phosphorylation. It also proves that such phosphonate analogs can be taken up by the cell sufficiently well to exhibit their antiviral action. This brings us one step nearer to the target (viral DNA) site.

Nucleosides are naturally occurring molecules, which play a crucial role in cell multiplication and function. As a consequence, cells contain a whole battery of enzymes for the anabolism and catabolism of nucleosides. All of these enzymes are potential targets for the action of the modified nucleosides, and this can lead to premature death of the cell. Especially the interaction of the inhibitor with normal cellular DNA may be hazardous in that it could lead to mutagenicity, carcinogenicity or teratogenicity. Moreover, good *in vitro* antiviral activity not necessarily predicts equivalent *in vivo* activity. These considerations make the design of new nucleoside antivirals both a difficult and challenging task.

16.1.2   Base-modified pyrimidine nucleosides as antiherpes agents

The intracellular metabolism and mode of action of IdUrd (**16.1**) can be presented as follows (Scheme 16.1):

IdUrd can be phosphorylated by both cellular and virus-encoded thymidine kinases (i). However, IdUrd is phosphorylated more efficiently by the HSV-encoded thymidine kinase than by the cellular thymidine kinase, which explains its (modest) selectivity as an antiherpes agent. IdUrd 5'-monophosphate is then phosphorylated to the diphosphate (ii) and triphosphate (iii). IdUrd can be incorporated in both cellular and viral DNA. This incorporation impairs the subsequent transcription and replication processes and is believed to be the major reason for the activity and toxicity of IdUrd. As also evident from the above reaction scheme (Scheme 16.1), IdUrd (**16.1**) is a substrate for thymidine phosphorylase (iv) and for thymidylate synthase (v). Both processes lead to deactivation (of IdUrd). Together with the feedback inhibition of the phosphorylated products on the regulatory enzymes of nucleotide biosynthesis, the general biochemical reaction scheme as depicted for IdUrd also holds for most other pyrimidine nucleoside analogs, and could explain their antiviral activity and toxicity.

A crucial enzyme in the anabolism of pyrimidine 2'-deoxynucleosides is the thymidine kinase, which phosphorylates the nucleoside to its 5'-monophosphate derivative. Some herpes viruses (i.e. HSV-1, HSV-2) and also *Varicella-zoster* virus

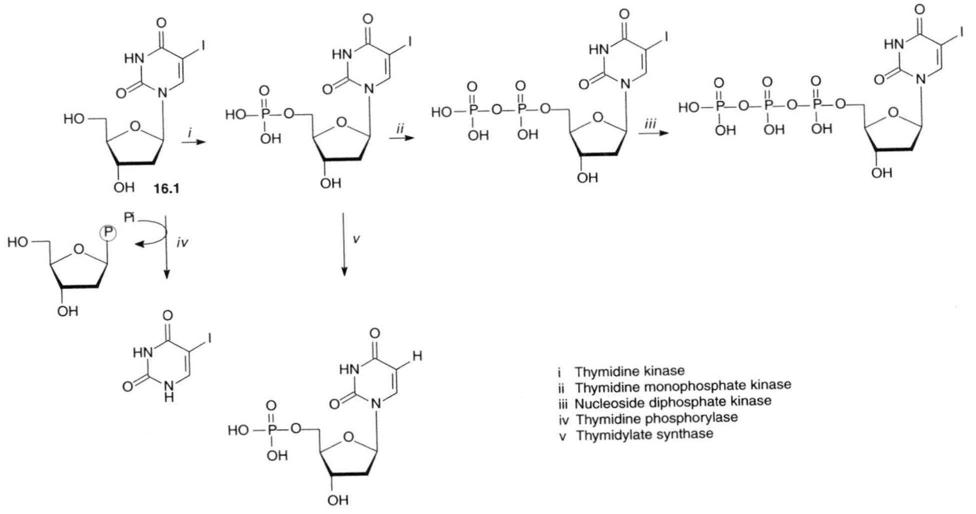

Scheme 16.1

i   Thymidine kinase
ii Thymidine monophosphate kinase
iii Nucleoside diphosphate kinase
iv Thymidine phosphorylase
v   Thymidylate synthase

(VZV) encode for their own thymidine kinase. Introduction of a substituent in the 5-position of the pyrimidine ring has led to compounds with higher affinity for the virus-encoded enzyme than for the cellular enzyme, and thus greater selectivity as antiviral agents. Pertinent examples of this 'second' generation of antiviral compounds are 5-ethyl-2'-deoxyuridine (EtdUrd) (**16.6**) and, even more so, 5-(*E*)-bromovinyl-2'-deoxyuridine (BVdUrd, BVDU) (**16.7**).

There is a marked difference in the phosphorylation capacity of the thymidine kinases of different herpes viruses. While the HSV-1-encoded thymidine kinase is capable of converting BVdUrd to its 5'-monophosphate and further onto its 5'-diphosphate, the HSV-2-encoded thymidine kinase is unable to further phosphorylate BVdUrd monophosphate onto its diphosphate. This differential behavior in phosphorylation may explain the differences found in the activity of BVdUrd against HSV-1 and HSV-2. The mode of binding of BVdUrd to the HSV-1 thymidine kinase has been determined (Figure 16.1). The 3-NH and 4-CO groups of the pyrimidine moiety interact with Gln-125. The bulky 5-substituent occupies a pocket available in the neighborhood of residues Trp-88, Tyr-132, Arg-163 and Ala-167. A change in conformation of one residue (Tyr-132) is needed for accommodation of the bromovinyl group. The binding mode of the deoxyribose moiety of BVdUrd is similar to that of dThd.

The BVdUrd and EtdUrd can also be incorporated into DNA. Because of the specific phosphorylation of EtdUrd and BVdUrd by the virus-infected cells, only the virus-infected cells that have allowed phosphorylation of the compounds will be sensitive to their eventual antiviral action (following incorporation into DNA).

The BVdUrd is superior in potency to any other antiherpes agent against both HSV-1 and VZV infections, i.e. it is 1000-fold more active *in vitro* against VZV than acyclovir, the most commonly used drug for the treatment of VZV infections. The VZV is responsible for primary (varicella or chickenpox) and recurrent (zoster and

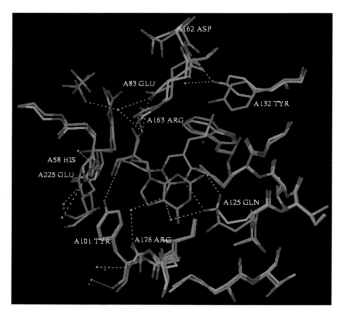

(16.6)   (16.7)   (16.8)   (16.9)

Figure 16.1 Binding of BrvdUrd and acyclovir (**16.11**) in the active site of the thymidine kinase (TK) of *Herpes simplex* virus type 1. The pyrimidine moiety of BrvdUrd has an orientation different from that of the guanine moiety of acyclovir. Intermolecular hydrogen bonding is shown for the TK/BrvdUrd complex.

shingles) infections, following reactivation of the virus. BVdUrd (brivudin) is currently the most potent antiviral agent on the market for the treatment of VZV infections.

The IdUrd monophosphate can be dehalogenated by thymidylate synthase to give dUrd monophosphate (Scheme 16.1), which is the natural substrate for the enzyme. Thymidylate synthase is responsible for the conversion of dUrd monophosphate to dThd monophosphate using N^5, N^{10}-methylenetetrahydrofolic acid as methyl donor. This is the key enzyme in the *de novo* biosynthesis of the dThd metabolites (Scheme 16.2).

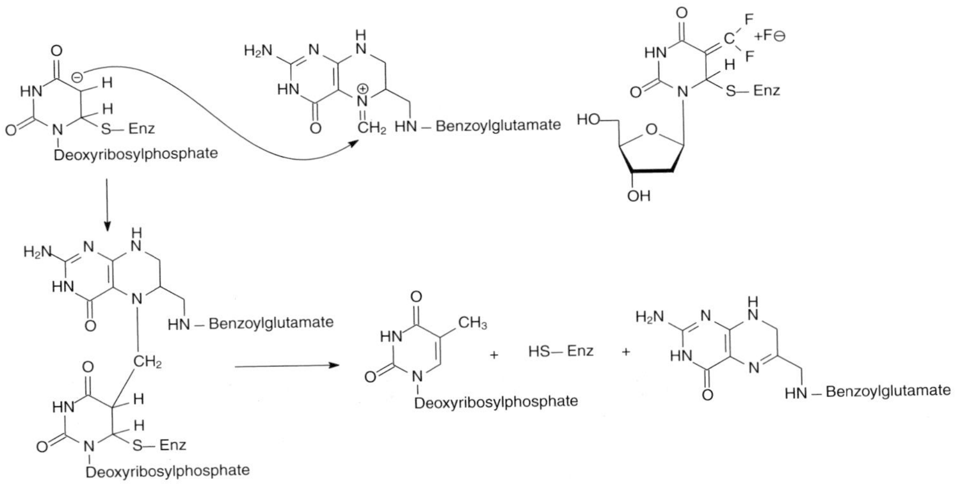

Scheme 16.2

When the iodo group of IdUrd (**16.1**) is replaced by a strong electron with-drawing substituent (X), which forms a stable C–X bond, the compound could inhibit thymidylate synthase without functioning as a substrate. This is the case for 5-fluoro-2′-deoxyuridine (**16.8**) and 5-trifluoromethyl-2′-deoxyuridine (**16.9**). The pK_a of 5-fluorouracil is 8.04, as compared to 7.35 for 5-trifluoromethyluracil and 9.94 for thymine, the 6-membered heterocyclic unit containing a methyl group in the 5-position. While 5-fluorouracil is used in cancer chemotherapy, 5-trifluoromethyl-2′-deoxyuridine (F_3dThd, TFT) (**16.9**) is used for the topical treatment of herpetic keratitis.

F_3dThd (**16.9**) is phosphorylated by viral and cellular kinases to the mono-phosphate and further to the di- and triphosphate. Here again, phosphorylation is more efficient in HSV-infected than uninfected cells. Incorporation into DNA occurs and could contribute to the antiviral activity of F_3dThd. However, F_3dThd owes its antiviral activity mainly to the inhibition of thymidylate synthase. The mode of action of F_3dThd can be explained by assuming a nucleophilic attack of the enzyme at the 6-position of the heterocyclic base, which leads to the generation of a reactive difluoromethylene at the 5-position (Scheme 16.2). This enzyme is an interesting target for those viruses, which do not encode for a functional thymidine kinase. These viruses must rely on the *de novo* biosynthesis of dThd monophosphate starting from *N*-carbamoylaspartate to form the necessary quant-ities of dThd triphosphate that are needed for their own DNA synthesis.

16.1.3 Sugar-modified purine nucleosides

9-(β-D-Arabinofuranosyl)adenine (ara-A) (**16.10**) is a naturally occurring nucleo-side, which was synthesized 8 years before it was isolated. Ara-A is an antiviral agent with a multiple mode of action. Theoretically, drugs that have multiple modes of action are most likely to avoid drug-virus resistance but, they may also have the highest risk for toxic side effects. The relative role of the different actions in the overall antiviral activity of ara-A is not well known. Ara-A is phosphorylated to its monophosphate and further to its di- and triphosphate. This triphosphate inhibits DNA polymerases, which could explain the activity of ara-A against DNA viruses. Ara-A can also be incorporated into both host cell DNA and viral DNA. Furthermore, ara-A inhibits methyltransferase reactions presumably through inhibition of S-adenosylhomocysteine hydrolase and accumulation of S-adenosylhomocysteine. The latter acts as a product inhibitor of transmethylation reactions such as those involved in the maturation of viral mRNA. Ara-A has been used for the treatment of HSV-1 encephalitis and *Herpes zoster* in immunocompromised patients, but is now surpassed by acyclovir for this purpose. A major disadvantage of ara-A is that it is promptly deaminated *in vivo* by adenosine deaminase, converting the amino group into an oxo group. The resulting hypoxanthine analog has markedly reduced antiviral activity as compared to ara-A.

The search for inhibitors of the adenosine deamination reaction has led to the discovery at the Wellcome Research Laboratories of 9-(2-hydroxyethoxymethyl) guanine (acyclovir) (**16.11**) as an antiviral agent. This compound, whose action is surprisingly similar to that of the aforementioned pyrimidine nucleoside analogs, has oriented research in the direction of the acyclic nucleoside analogs. This research has yielded a number of active congeners, i.e. 9-(1,3-dihydroxy-2-propoxymethyl)guanine (ganciclovir) (**16.12**) and penciclovir (**16.13**). As of today, acyclovir has remained the 'gold' standard for the treatment of HSV infections, whereas ganciclovir is used in the treatment of CMV infections, and both penciclovir (as its prodrug form, famciclovir) and acyclovir (as its prodrug form, valaciclovir) for the treatment of VZV infections.

All of these compounds can be considered as analogs of 2′-deoxyguanosine or carbocyclic 2′-deoxyguanosine (*vide infra*) from which the 2′-carbon (ganciclovir, penciclovir) or both the 2′- and 3′-carbons (acyclovir) have been deleted. The antiviral activity of acyclovir was discovered by accident, whereas ganciclovir (**16.12**) was the result of a structure–activity design starting from acyclovir as the model compound. From a structural viewpoint, ganciclovir is more closely related to 2′-deoxyguanosine than is acyclovir.

The antiviral activity of acyclovir (**16.11**) can be explained by the same biochemical reaction scheme as presented for IdUrd (Scheme 16.1). There are, however, subtle differences that explain the greater selectivity of acyclovir. Acyclovir is phosphorylated to its monophosphate by a virus-specific thymidine/deoxycytidine kinase, which actually recognizes acyclovir as a deoxycytidine analog. Viruses, which encode for such an enzyme (HSV-1, HSV-2, VZV, but not CMV) are susceptible to the antiviral action of acyclovir. Although the natural substrates for this enzyme are pyrimidine nucleosides, it apparently accepts purine derivatives as substrates. The structure of the complex of HSV-1 thymidine kinase with acyclovir, ganciclovir and penciclovir has been determined by X-ray crystallography. The guanine moiety of all three compounds lay in a similar location, with hydrogen bond pairing being made with Gln-125 via the 1-NH and 6-CO groups (Figure 16.1). In uninfected cells, phosphorylation occurs to a limited extent. The monophosphate of acyclovir is phosphorylated to the diphosphate by GMP kinase and further to its triphosphate by various cellular enzymes. The triphosphate of

(16.10)
Ara-A

(16.11)
Acyclovir

(16.12)
Ganciclovir

(16.13)
Penciclovir

acyclovir is a competitive inhibitor of dGTP for the viral DNA polymerase and can also function as a substrate resulting in the incorporation of acyclovir into DNA and chain termination. Acyclovir is given orally or intravenously in the treatment of HSV and VZV infections, and topically in the treatment of HSV infections (i.e. herpetic keratitis and herpes labialis). For oral use, acyclovir, because of its limited oral bioavailability is now substituted by its oral prodrug form, valaciclovir.

As compared to acyclovir, ganciclovir (16.12) is more easily phosphorylated in CMV-infected cells by the virus-encoded (UL 97) protein kinase and its triphosphate has a five-fold greater affinity than ACV (acyclovir) triphosphate for CMV DNA polymerase. Ganciclovir can be incorporated both internally and at the 3'-terminal end of DNA. Ganciclovir is active against HSV-1, HSV-2, VZV, CMV and EBV. It is fairly toxic for the bone marrow (neutropenia). Its clinical use is restricted to the treatment of CMV infections in immunocompromised patients.

Penciclovir (16.13) has the same antiviral spectrum as acyclovir. As compared to acyclovir, penciclovir leads to higher triphosphate concentrations in virus-infected cells and its antiviral activity persists for a longer time after removal of the compound. In fact, after removal of acyclovir, antiviral activity rapidly disappears. Not only penciclovir, but also BVdUrd (16.7) and ganciclovir (16.12) show persistent antiviral activity after the drugs have been removed from the medium. This is due to the greater stability of their triphosphates as compared to that of acyclovir triphosphate.

16.1.4 Ribavirin

In contrast with the preceding compounds, ribavirin (16.14) has a broad spectrum activity against RNA and DNA viruses both *in vitro* and *in vivo*. R.K. Robins first synthesized ribavirin. The structural requirements for the broad-spectrum antiviral activity of ribavirin are very stringent. The compound shows its greatest potency against myxo (influenza) and paramyxo (respiratory syncytial) virus infections. Ribavirin also shows activity against some hemorrhagic fever viruses such as Lassa, Machupo, Pichinde, Rift Valley and Hantaviruses. Therapeutic efficacy has been demonstrated with ribavirin, given as a small-particle aerosol, in infants suffering from respiratory syncytial virus (RSV) infection. The compound has been approved for the treatment of RSV infections, as well as human hepatitis C virus (HCV) infections, for the latter only in combination with interferons.

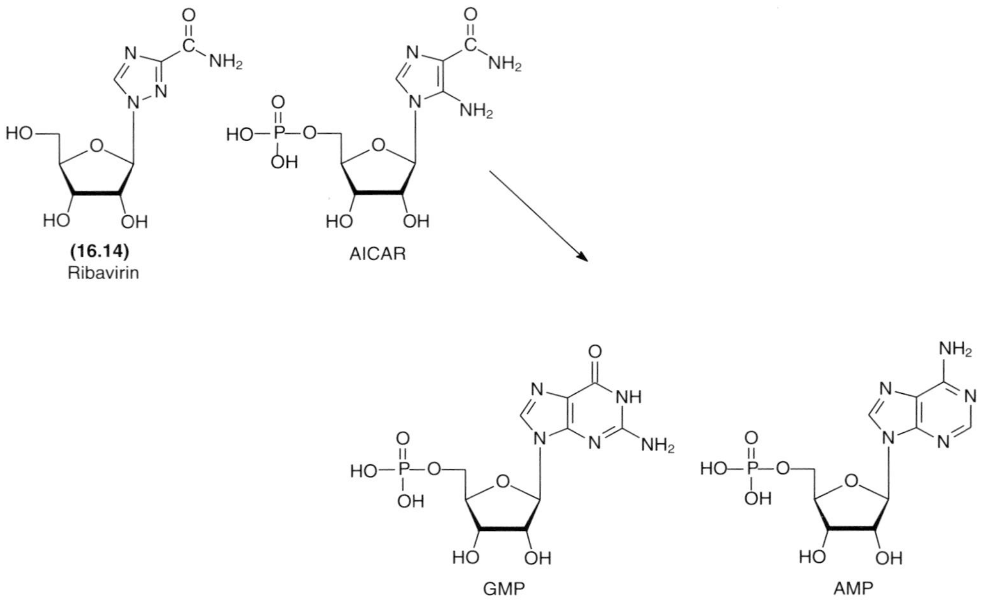

Scheme 16.3

The mode of action of ribavirin is multipronged and may also vary from one virus to another. Ribavirin (5′-monophosphate) can be considered as an analog of AICAR (Scheme 16.3) which is a precursor of both AMP and GMP.

As has been elucidated by X-ray crystallography studies, there is a nice resemblence between ribavirin and guanosine; by rotating the amide group, also good resemblence is found between ribavirin and adenosine (Scheme 16.3).

16.1.5 Compounds which inhibit the replication of the human immunodeficiency virus (HIV)

Human immunodeficiency virus is a retrovirus, which means that, once it has infected the cell, its genomic RNA is transcribed to proviral DNA by a virus-specific enzyme (the RT). This enzyme has a broader substrate specificity than cellular DNA polymerases, and has since long been recognized as a target for antiviral chemotherapy. Here, the task to design specific antiviral agents is somewhat more difficult than for herpes viruses, since HIV does not encode for a virus-specific kinase which could confine the metabolism of the nucleoside analogs to the virus-infected cells.

Fifteen compounds have now been approved for the treatment of HIV infection from which zidovudine (**16.3**) was the first one. Nine of them are targeted at the viral RT and the other six are targeted at the viral protease. Among the reverse transcriptase inhibitors, six are nucleoside analogs (zidovudine (**16.3**)) didanosine (**16.15**), zalcitabine (**16.16**), stavudine (**16.17**), lamivudine (**16.18**), abacavir (**16.19**). These dideoxynucleoside analogs must be phosphorylated through

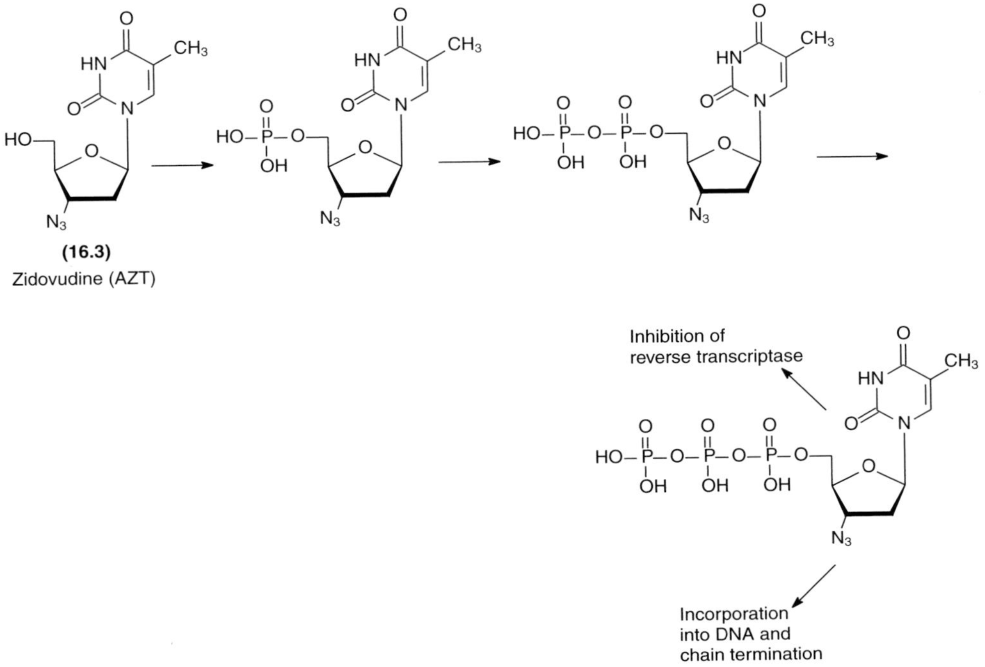

(16.3)
Zidovudine (AZT)

Inhibition of
reverse transcriptase

Incorporation
into DNA and
chain termination

Scheme 16.4

three consecutive kinase reactions to the triphosphate form before they can interact as competitive inhibitors with respect to the natural substrates at the RT. The intracellular metabolism of dideoxynucleosides is dependent on the type of compound, the type of cell and the anabolic state of the cells.

Zidovudine is phosphorylated by the cellular thymidine kinase to its 5′-monophosphate (Scheme 16.4). This 5′-monophosphate is then phosphorylated to the di- and triphosphate by thymidylate kinase and, subsequently, nucleoside-5′-diphosphate kinase, respectively. As the efficiency of conversion of zidovudine-5′-monophosphate to its diphosphate by thymidylate kinase is much lower than the efficiency of phosphorylation of the natural substrate, zidovudine-5′-monophosphate accumulates in the cells. In its triphosphate form, AZT is a more efficient inhibitor of the RT than of the cellular DNA polymerases. The AZT is incorporated into DNA and functions as a chain terminator.

The active metabolite of didanosine (**16.15**) is dideoxyadenosine-5′-triphosphate. Didanosine is first converted to dideoxyinosine-5′-monophosphate. Through a sequential action of adenylosuccinate synthetase and lyase, dideoxyadenosine-5′-monophosphate is formed which is further converted to the above mentioned triphosphate. Stavudine (**16.17**) is less efficiently phosphorylated to its 5′-monophosphate than zidovudine but readily proceeds from its monophosphate onto its di- and triphosphate so that equivalent levels of the active metabolites (5′-triphosphates) are attained into the cells. Zalcitabine (**16.16**), lamivudine (**16.18**) and

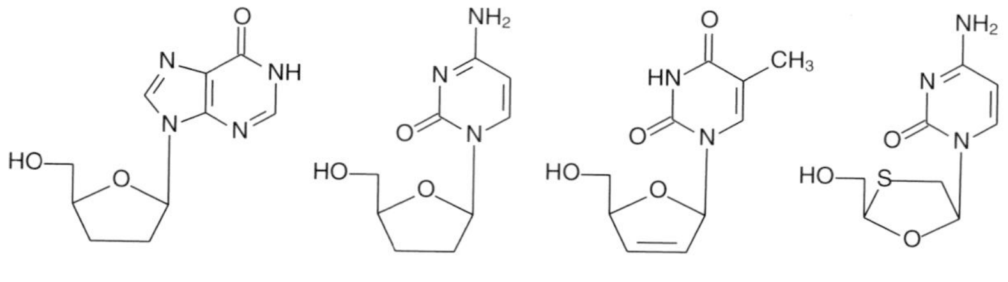

(16.15)
Didanosine

(16.16)
Zalcitabine

(16.17)
Stavudine

(16.18)
Lamivudine

abacavir (**16.19**) are also converted intracellularly to their active triphosphates. All these triphosphates inhibit DNA polymerase α, β and γ to a lesser extent than RT and, once incorporated, all these nucleosides function as chain terminators. As a rule, the relative ability of the dideoxynucleoside analogs to generate 5′-triphosphates intracellularly is of greater importance in determining the eventual capacity to block HIV replication than the relative abilities of the resultant triphosphates to inhibit the viral RT.

Abacavir is phosphorylated by adenosine phosphotransferase to abacavir monophosphate, which is then converted by a cytosolic deaminase to carbovir monophosphate before being further processed to the di- and triphosphate of carbovir (the guanine analog of abacavir) (scheme 16.5). This intracellular activation pathway enables abacavir to overcome the pharmacokinetic and toxicological deficiencies of carbovir while maintaining potent and selective anti-HIV activity.

The NNRTIs nevirapine (**16.20**), delavirdine (**16.21**) and efavirenz (**16.22**) block the HIV-1 RT reaction through interaction with an allosterically located, non-substrate binding 'pocket' site. This binding pocket is located at about 10 Å distance from the substrate-binding site. The binding of an NNRTI and NRTI (nucleoside reverse transcriptase inhibitor) to the RT is a co-operative process, and this might explain the synergistic effect of both types of inhibitors when used in combination.

Several studies have revealed a common mode of binding for the different NNRTIs with their target site at the HIV-1 RT. The NNRTIs cause a repositioning of the three-stranded β-sheet in the p66 subunit (containing the catalytic aspartic acid

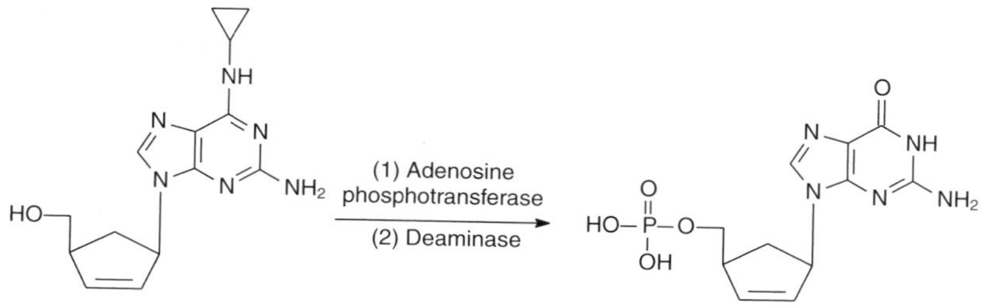

(16.19)
Abacavir

(1) Adenosine phosphotransferase
(2) Deaminase

Carbovir 5′-O-monophosphate

Scheme 16.5

(16.20)
Nevirapine

(16.21)
Delavirdine

(16.22)
Efavirenz

residues 110, 185 and 186). This suggests that the NNRTIs inhibit HIV-1 RT by locking the active catalytic site in an inactive conformation. As an example, the binding of delavirdine to HIV-1 RT is described (Figure 16.2). Delavirdine is hydrogen-bonded to the main chain of Lys-103 and extensively interact with Pro-236 by hydrophobic contacts. Part of delavirdine protrudes into the solvent creating a channel between Pro-236 and the polypeptide segments 225–226 and 105–106.

The HIV protease inhibitors [saquinavir (**16.23**), ritonavir (**16.24**), indinavir (**16.25**) (Figure 16.3), nelfinavir (**16.26**), amprenavir (**16.27**) and lopinavir (**16.28**) prevent the cleavage of the gag and gag-pol precursor polyproteins to the functional proteins (p17, p24, p7, p6, p2, p1, protease, RT, integrase), thus arresting maturation

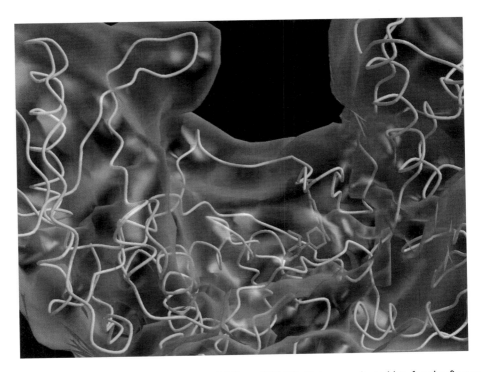

Figure 16.2 Mode of binding of delavirdine (**16.21**) to HIV RT. Colors used are blue for the fingers, yellow for the palm, red for the thumb domain and gray for the rest.

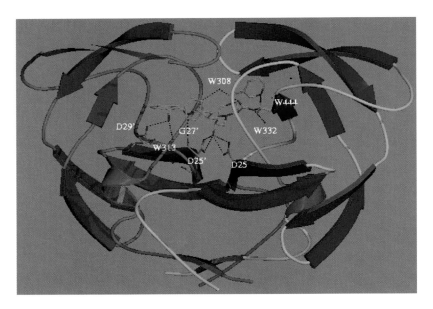

Figure 16.3 Structure of HIV-1 protease in complex with indinavir (**16.25**).

(16.23)
Saquinavir

(16.24)
Ritonavir

(16.25)
Indinavir

(16.26)
Nelfinavir

(16.27)
Amprenavir

(16.28)
Lopinavir

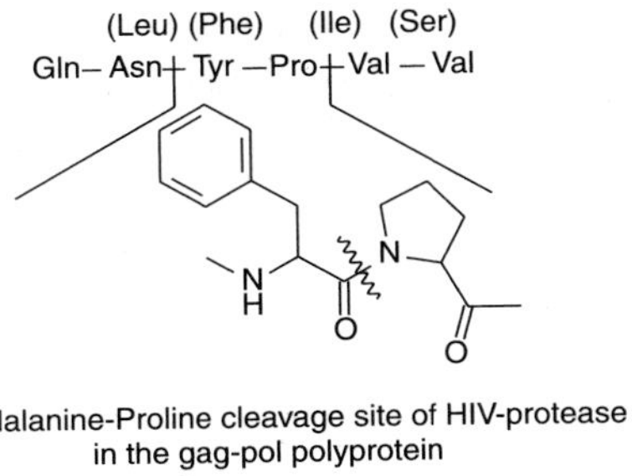

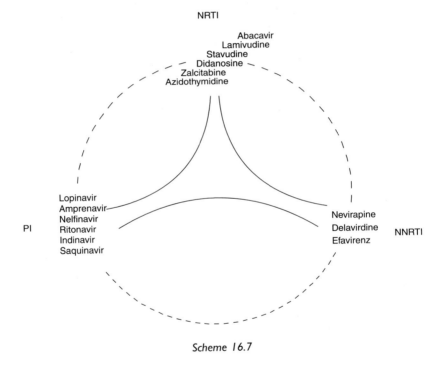

Phenylalanine-Proline cleavage site of HIV-protease
in the gag-pol polyprotein

Scheme 16.6

Scheme 16.7

and thereby blocking infectivity of the nascent virions. The HIV protease inhibitors have been tailored after the target peptidic linkage in the gag and gag-pol polyproteins that need to be cleaved by the viral protease, i.e. the phenylalanine-proline sequence at positions 167 and 168 of the gag-pol polyprotein.

All protease inhibitors that are currently licensed for the treatment of HIV infection, are peptidomimetics where the carbonyl group of the peptide bond is substituted by an hydroxyethylene group (Scheme 16.6).

Synergistic anti-HIV activity is observed when NRTIs are combined with other NRTIs or NNRTIs or with protease inhibitors (PIs). This treatment regimen allows the individual compounds to be used at lower doses and, in preventing virus break-through, they also prevent the virus from becoming resistant to the compounds.

Combination of NRTIs, NNRTIs and PIs (Scheme 16.7) have been found to decrease HIV viral load, to increase CD4 count and to decrease mortality and delay disease progression, particularly in AIDS patients with advanced immune suppression. When initiated during early asymptomatic HIV infection, highly active anti-retroviral therapy (HAART) initiates rapid reversal of disease-induced T-cell activation, while preserving pretherapy levels of immune function, suggesting that therapeutic benefit may be gained from early aggressive anti-HIV chemotherapy.

16.2   DESIGN OF NEW ANTIVIRAL AGENTS

16.2.1   Nucleoside prodrugs

The activity of a compound *in vivo* is highly dependent on the formulation in which the compound is presented. Active research is focused on developing prodrugs with optimal bioavailability. Apart from the classical approach of using esters as prodrugs, other approaches are based on the knowledge of the different enzymes involved in nucleoside metabolism. One of the oldest examples in the nucleoside field is the use of ara-A 5'-monophosphate (**16.29**) (Scheme 16.8). Ara-A has a very low solubility in water (approximately 0.5 mg/ml). Administration of ara-A by infusion requires large volumes (2 liter for an adult person). The greater solubility of ara-A monophosphate permits the use of smaller infusion volumes.

Another enzyme which has proved valuable in the prodrug design is xanthine oxidase. Guanine nucleosides are very insoluble in water because of the strong intermolecular associations through hydrogen bonds and stacking between the base moieties. As a consequence, compounds such as acyclovir (**16.11**) are quite insoluble in body fluids. The 6-deoxy analog of acyclovir (desiclovir) (**16.31**) is more soluble and is metabolized *in vivo* by xanthine oxidase to acyclovir. When administered orally, 6-deoxyacyclovir gives the same blood levels of acyclovir as those obtained with intravenous acyclovir. An analogous approach has also proved successful for ganciclovir (**16.12**). The diacetyl derivative of the 6-deoxy analog of ganciclovir (**16.30**) gives peak plasma concentrations after 1 h which are tenfold higher than those detected following an equivalent oral dose of ganciclovir. This prodrug (**16.30**) has been given the name of famciclovir, which has been launched for the systemic (i.e. oral) treatment of HSV and VZV infections.

Abacavir (**16.19**) is another example of a prodrug form of a purine nucleoside. This compound is intracellularly activated to (−)-carbovir triphosphate, as mentioned above.

The therapeutic armarmentarium of acyclic anti-HSV and anti-VZV nucleosides has been extended to the L-valyl ester of acyclovir (valaciclovir) (**16.32**). This drug is a prodrug of acyclovir, and has been developed because of the low oral bioavailability of the parent compound. It is used for the systemic (i.e. oral) treatment of HSV and VZV infections. Valaciclovir is absorbed through a stereospecific transporter of the intestine cells and is rapidly hydrolyzed upon absorption, yielding acyclovir.

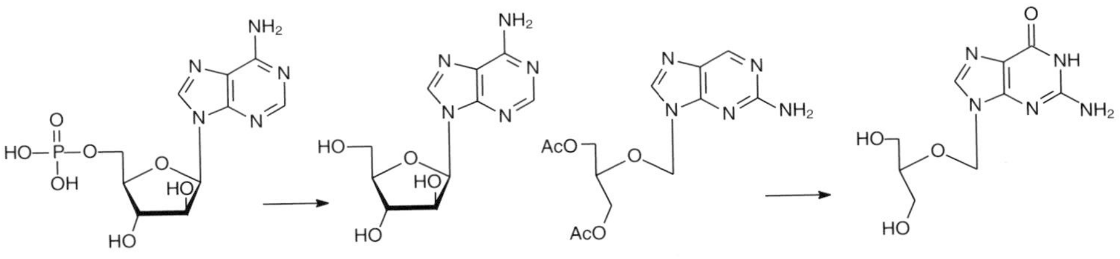

(16.29) **(16.10)** **(16.30)** **(16.12)**

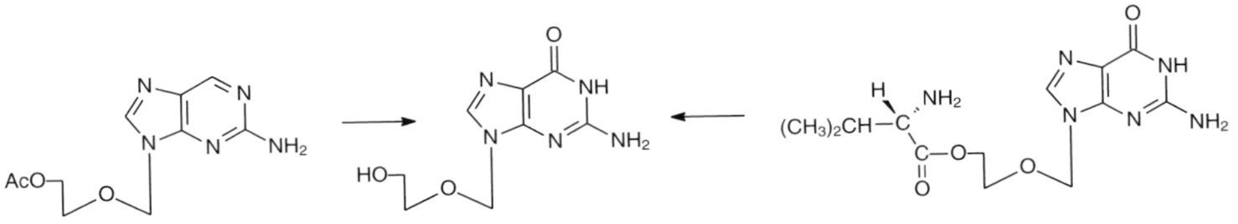

(16.31) **(16.11)** **(16.32)**

Scheme 16.8

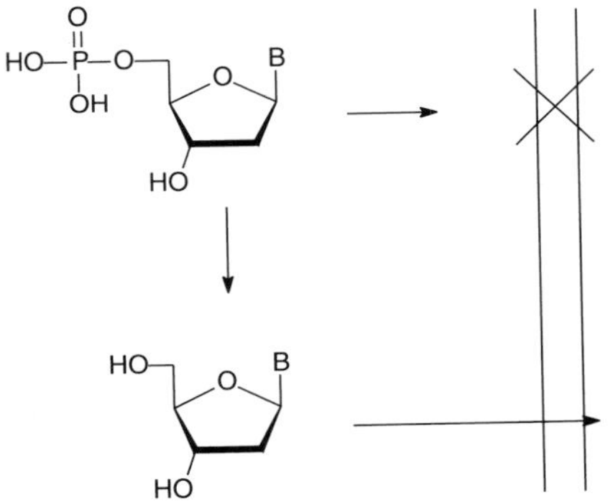

Scheme 16.9

16.2.2 Analogs of 5′-monophosphates and nucleotide prodrugs

As most, if not all, nucleosides need to be phosphorylated to exert their antiviral activity, an interesting approach would be based upon the use of the phosphorylated derivatives themselves.

The main problem associated with this approach, however, is that the phosphorylated derivatives are as such not taken up by cells (Scheme 16.9). Furthermore, 5′-*O*-phosphates of nucleosides are easily dephosphorylated by esterases which thereby release the parent nucleosides.

The cyclic monophosphate of ganciclovir (**16.33**), however, is taken up intact by the cell and opened intracellularly to the (*S*)-enantiomer of ganciclovir monophosphate (Scheme 16.10), which is then further phosphorylated to the triphosphate.

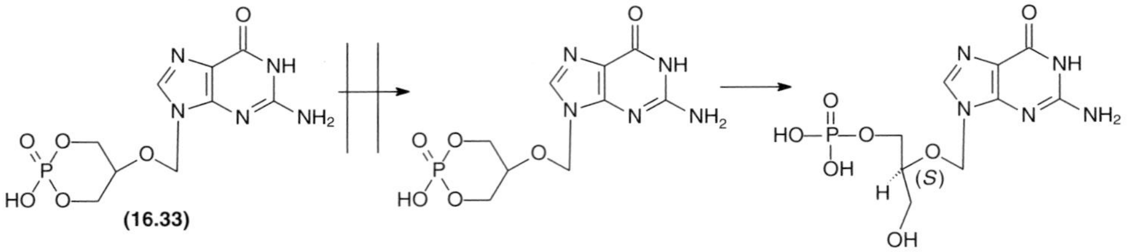

Scheme 16.10

This compound (2'-norcGMP) (**16.33**) shows a broad-spectrum activity against DNA viruses (i.e. HSV-1, HSV-2, CMV, VZV and also against TK⁻ HSV strains) *in vitro*. It is also effective orally and topically in preventing orofacial HSV-1 infection and genital HSV-2 infection in mice.

Because the first phosphorylation by nucleoside kinase is the rate-limiting step in the metabolic activation of most anti-HIV dideoxy nucleoside analogs, several prodrug strategies have been designed to bypass the nucleoside kinase step. These 'masked' nucleotides can penetrate cells and deliver the nucleoside 5'-monophosphate intracellularly. For example, the stavudine-MP prodrug (**16.34**) containing an ester at the phosphate moiety and a methyl ester of alanine linked to the phosphate through a phosphoramidate linkage, showed anti-HIV activity superior to that of stavudine (**16.17**) and, in contrast to stavudine, proved also active against HIV in thymidine kinase-deficient cells. Following intracellular uptake, the stavudine-MP triester gives rise to the formation of stavudine-MP, stavudine-DP and stavudine-TP and also to a new metabolite, alaninyl stavudine-MP, which could be considered as an intracellular depot form of stavudine and/or stavudine-MP.

A logic pursuit of this approach has led to the development of the nucleoside phosphonate derivatives. In designing such compounds, one should take into account that a glycosidic bond is *a priori* sensitive to chemical and enzymatic degradation, whereas an alkylated purine or pyrimidine base should not have this problem. Thus, a new series of purine and pyrimidine derivatives with an aliphatic side chain and a phosphonate group attached to it was developed. The first compound of this series, (*S*)-HPMPA or (*S*)-9-(3-hydroxy-2-phosphonylmethoxy-propyl)adenine (**16.35**) was conceived after another acyclic nucleoside, (*S*)-DHPA or (*S*)-9-(2,3-dihydroxypropyl)adenine (**16.36**), that had been synthesized earlier

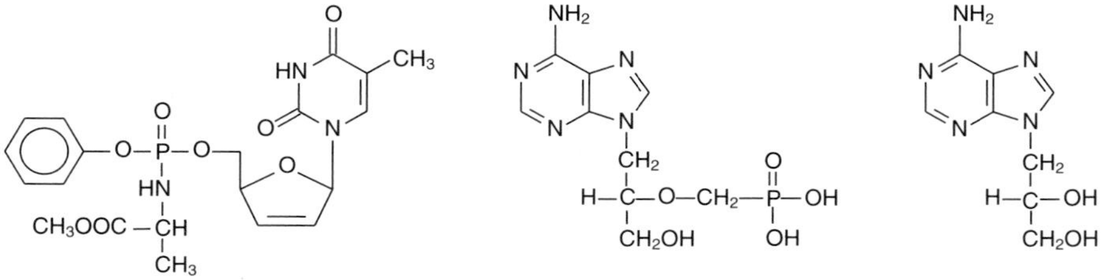

(**16.34**)

(**16.35**)
(*S*)-HPMPA

(**16.36**)
(*S*)-DHPA

and shown to inhibit the multiplication of several DNA viruses (i.e. vaccinia virus) and RNA viruses (i.e. vesicular stomatitis virus) *in vitro*.

(S)-HPMPA (**16.35**) has broad-spectrum activity against DNA viruses (i.e. HSV-1, TK⁻ HSV-1, HSV-2, VZV, TK⁻ VZV, CMV, EBV, pox- and adenoviruses). The most interesting features of this compound are, on the one hand, that it is stable against metabolic degradation but is capable of penetrating cells, thus circumventing the need for phosphorylation by dThd kinase (or other nucleoside kinases). Within the cell, (S)-HPMPA is further phosphorylated by cellular enzymes (i.e. AMP kinase and/or PRPP synthetase) to its diphosphoryl derivative. (S)-HPMPA inhibits viral DNA synthesis at a concentration which is several orders of magnitude lower than the concentration required for inhibition of cellular DNA synthesis. Three compounds, derived from (S)-HPMPA, show even more interesting activity: PMEA (adefovir) (**16.37**) and (S)-HPMPC (cidofovir) (**16.4**) and PMPA (tenofovir) (**16.5**). As PMEA (**16.37**) and PMPA (**16.5**) are not sufficiently bioavailable by the oral route, they are administered in their oral prodrug forms: *bis*(POM)PMEA (**16.38**) and *bis*(POC)PMPA (**16.39**), respectively (Scheme 16.11).

Cidofovir (HPMPC) (**16.4**) is active against herpes, adeno, polyoma, papilloma and pox viruses. Cidofovir delays progression of CMV retinitis in patients with AIDS. It has been formally licensed for this indication. Cidofovir also holds great promise for the treatment of various papilloma virus-associated lesions. The antiviral activity spectrum of adefovir is unique in that it encompasses both retroviruses and hepadnaviruses as well as herpes viruses. It could be used for the treatment of HIV and HBV infections as well as for the prophylaxis of herpes virus infections and is now primarily pursued, as its oral prodrug form (adefovir

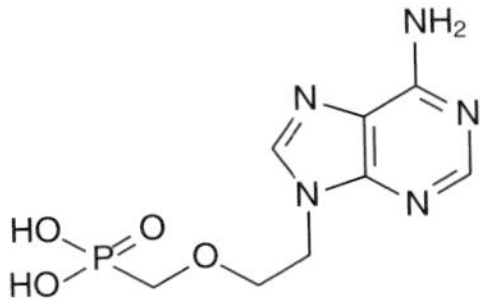

(16.37)

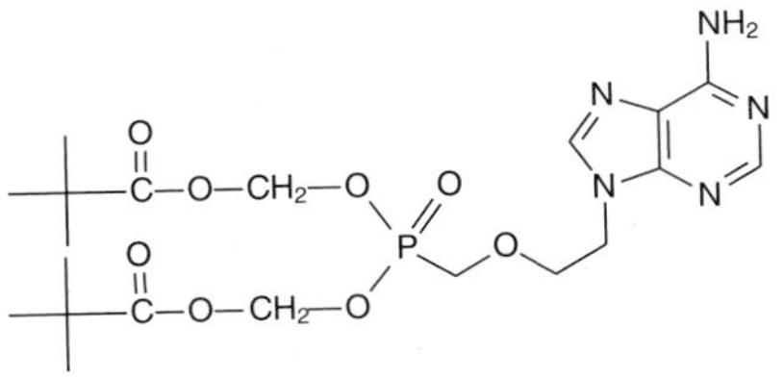

(16.38)

bis(pivaloyloxymethyl)-
9-(2-phosphonomethoxyethyl)adenine

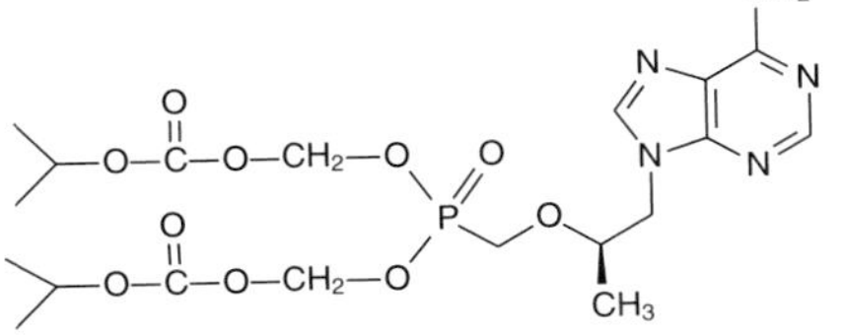

(16.39)

bis[(isopropoxycarbonyl)oxymethyl]-
(R)-9-(2-phosphonomethoxypropyl)adenine

Scheme 16.11

dipivoxil or bis (POM)PMEA) for the treatment of HBV infections. The activity of PMPA is confined to retroviruses and hepadnaviruses. It is pursued in its oral prodrug form (tenofovir disoxoproxil or bis(POC)PMPA), for the treatment of HIV infections.

The main advantage of the acyclic nucleoside phosphonates over the 'classical' nucleoside analogs is their prolonged antiviral action, which allows infrequent dosing, i.e. once daily for the oral formulation of adefovir and tenofovir; once weekly for intravenous or intralesional cidofovir; once daily for cidofovir if applied topically as eyedrops or gel.

16.2.3   Nucleosides with the non-natural L-configuration

All nucleosides described in the previous sections, except for **16.18** (lamivudine), possess the D-configuration. Until recently, it was generally accepted that nucleosides belonging to the L-series would not be accepted as substrates for enzymes and, thus, not active. Surprising results, however, were obtained with these 'mirror-image' nucleosides.

Dideoxycytidine (**16.16**) is very active against HIV (EC_{50}:0.01 µM), but is also quite toxic (CC_{50}:10 µM). CC_{50} is defined as the concentration required to reduce cell growth by 50%. Its L-isomer (**16.40**) is slightly less active against HIV (EC_{50}:0.02 µM) but has markedly lower toxicity (CC_{50}:100 µM). This difference has also been observed with 3'-thia-2',3'-dideoxycytidine. The activity (EC_{50}) and toxicity (CC_{50}) of the compound with the 'natural' (+)-structure is 0.25 µM and 1 µM, respectively. The 'unnatural' (−)-isomer (**16.18**) is as active (0.2 µM) but less toxic (>100 µM). A striking characteristic of **16.40** and **16.18** and of their 5-fluorinated congeners (**16.41**) and (**16.42**) is that they are not only active against HIV but also HBV, which extends their potential use to the treatment of this latter disease. It has been suggested that the low toxicity of the L-series is due to the fact that these non-natural compounds are not transported into mitochondria. Part of the toxicity of the anti-HIV nucleosides zidovudine, zalcitabine and didanosine could be attributed to the inhibition of mitochondrial DNA synthesis.

16.2.4   Non-nucleoside antivirals outside the anti-HIV field

Numerous non-nucleoside compounds have been described that show *in vitro* antiviral activity against a wide variety of viruses. Some of these compounds have been marketed. Already in the fifties, methisazone (**16.43**) was mentioned for

(16.40) X = H
(16.41) X = F

(16.18) X = H
(16.42) X = F

prophylactic use against smallpox and therapeutic use against the complications of vaccinia virus vaccination.

Amantadine (**16.44**) and rimantadine (**16.45**) target the influenza A virus M2 protein, a membrane protein that is essential to virus replication. They are used in the prophylaxis and early treatment of influenza A virus infections; in this regard rimantadine is as efficacious as amantadine and less prone to toxic side effects (i.e. for the CNS). Phosphonoformic acid (PFA) (**16.46**) has been pursued for the treatment of CMV infections (particularly retinitis) in immunocompromised patients, as an alternative to ganciclovir (**16.12**) treatment, and for the treatment of TK⁻ HSV infections, also in immunocompromised patients, following resistance development to acyclovir (**16.11**).

Haemagglutinin and neuraminidase are glycoproteins that occur on the surface of influenza virus and they interact with receptors which contain terminal neuraminic acid residues. Neuraminidase destroys receptors recognized by haemagglutinin by cleaving the α-ketosidic bond linking a terminal neuraminic acid residue to the adjacent oligosaccharide moiety. One of the effects of neuraminidase inhibitors is that virions stay attached to the membrane of infected cells and to each other and virus spread is inhibited. Neuraminidase is a tetramer composed of a cytoplasmic tail, a transmembrane domain, a stalk region, and a globular head. The residues forming the active site are highly conserved among all A and B influenza viruses. Reversible competitive neuraminidase inhibitors, zanamivir (**16.47**), oseltamivir (**16.48**) and RWJ-270201 (**16.49**), inhibit replication of both influenza A and B viruses. Zanamivir is delivered by inhalation because of its low oral bioavailability whereas oseltamivir is administered orally. Early treatment with either drug reduces the severity and duration of influenza symptoms.

Interferons have been proposed for the treatment of several viral infections, i.e. due to rhinovirus, influenza virus, herpes viruses, papilloma virus, adenovirus, hepatitis B virus, hepatitis C virus and others, but their usefulness has remained

(16.43)   (16.44)   (16.45)   (16.46)

(16.47)   (16.48)   (16.49)
Zanamivir   Oseltamivir   RWJ-270201

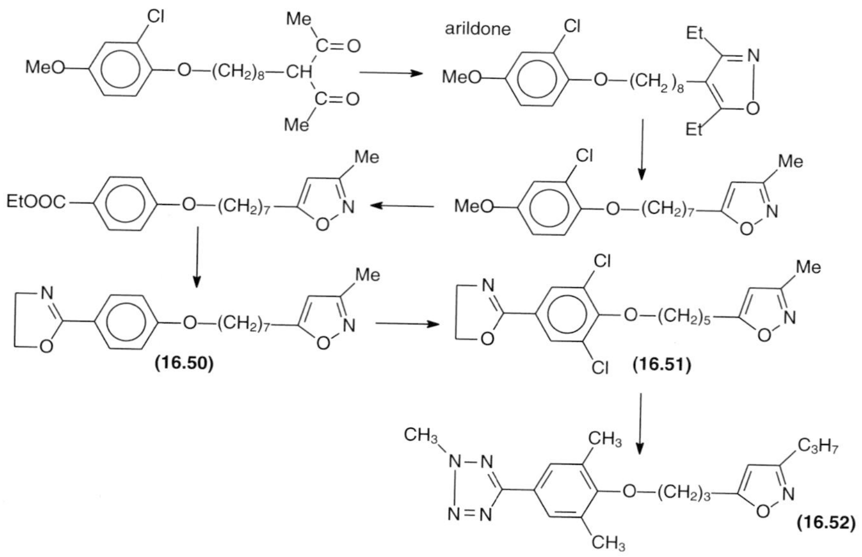

Scheme 16.12

controversial. Disoxaril (**16.50**) and its 4-methyloxazoline analog exhibit broad-spectrum activity both against rhinoviruses and enteroviruses. These compounds are derived from arildone, a compound which is quite active against poliovirus but only marginally active against rhinoviruses. Systematic variation of the substituents on the phenyl ring and introduction of different heterocyclic rings on the 'other side' has led to the discovery of disoxaril (**16.50**) as a potent antirhinovirus compound (Scheme 16.12).

These compounds specifically bind to the viral capsid and inhibit uncoating of the viral RNA. The interaction of these compounds with the viral capsid protein VP1 of rhinovirus-14 has been studied by X-ray crystallography. These compounds fit into a specific hydrophobic pocket, which corresponds to the cell receptor binding site and interacts with domains 1 and 2 of ICAM-1 (Figure 16.4). Elucidation of the mode of action of the compounds at the molecular level may lead to compounds with greater activity and selectivity. Following this lead, an analog of disoxaril, WIN 54954 (**16.51**) was shown to be more effective than disoxaril. However, due to the acid lability, the oxazoline ring, these molecules only have a short half-life. New analogs with a tetrazole ring such as **16.52** were, therefore, designed. These molecules likewise demonstrate a broad-spectrum activity against human rhinoviruses at $\pm 0.02\,\mu M$.

A problem in the development of antirhinovirus compounds is the number of different serotypes (>100). Given the relative harmlessness of the common cold infection, any candidate drug has to be absolutely free of toxic side effects to be acceptable for clinical use. Nevertheless, a good antirhinovirus compound will be of great value because of the socio-economic impact of this disease. The problem with the above mentioned compounds is that they do not demonstrate a significant

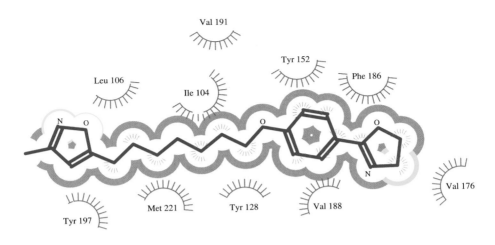

Figure 16.4 Interaction of compound **16.50** with the capsid VPI of rhinovirus-14.

16.53
Pleconaril

clinical effect against the infection if administered after the onset of symptoms. However, they are able to reduce the symptoms of the infection when used prophylactically (i.e. disoxaril (**16.50**) and WIN 54954 (**16.51**) against human Coxsackie A21 virus infection).

Pleconaril (**16.53**) is a metabolically stable capsid-function inhibitor with an oral bioavailability of 70%. It is a broad-spectrum antiviral showing potent antienterovirus and antirhinovirus activity. The integration of pleconaril into the capsid of picornaviruses prevents the virus from attaching to cellular receptors and from uncoating. Pleconaril has been shown to have clinical benefits and a favorable safety profile.

16.2.5 New developments in the anti-HIV-field

The replicative cycle of HIV-1 offers a wealth of potential targets for antiviral agents. The currently used anti-HIV agents interact with either the RT or viral protease. The most important alternative targets together with an example of an inhibitor are given in Table 16.1.

A great variety of polyanionic compounds have been described to block HIV replication through interference with virus adsorption to the cell surface. They are

Table 16.1 Targets in the replicative cycle of HIV-1 and potential inhibitory agents

Target	Potential anti-HIV agent
Viral adsorption through binding to the viral envelope glycoprotein gp120	Polysulfates or -sulfonates
Viral entry through blockade of the viral co-receptors CXCR4 or CCR5	Bicyclams
Virus-cell fusion, through binding to the viral glycoprotein gp41	T-20 peptide
Viral assembly and disassembly, through NCp7 zinc-finger-targeted agents	DIBA
Proviral DNA integration through integrase inhibitors	L-chicoric acid
Viral mRNA transcription, through inhibitors of the transcription process.	Fluoroquinolone K-12

assumed to exert their anti-HIV activity by shielding off the positively charged sites in the V3 loop of the viral envelope glycoprotein (gp120), which is necessary for virus attachment to the cell surface heparan sulphate (the primary binding site to the CD4 receptor of the CD4$^+$ cells). The major role of polysulfate or sulfonate compounds in the management of HIV infections may reside in the prevention of sexual transmission of HIV infection, as these compounds, if applied as a vaginal formulation, may successfully block HIV infection through both virus-to-cell and cell-to-cell contact.

To enter cells, following binding with the CD4 receptor, the HIV-1 particles must interact with the CXCR4 co-receptor or CCR5 co-receptor. CXCR4 is the co-receptor for X4 HIV-1 strains that infect T-cells, and CCR5 is the co-receptor for R5 HIV-1 strains that infect macrophages. These receptors normally act as receptors for chemokines. The bicyclams are highly potent and selective inhibitors of HIV-1 and HIV-2 replication. They bind to the CXCR4 receptor, which is a co-receptor for HIV entry into T-cells. The activity spectrum of bicyclam is restricted to those HIV variants (T-tropic) that use the CXCR4 receptor for entering the cells. The most potent compound is AMD 3329 (**16.54**), with an EC_{50} value against HIV-1 and HIV-2 replication of 0.8 and 1.6 nM respectively, which is about three- to five-fold lower than the EC_{50} of AMD 3100 (**16.55**). In Phase I clinical trial, **16.55** is well tolerated following single 15 min i.v. injection of doses of 10, 20, 40 and 80 μg/kg.

The interaction of the HIV-1 envelope glycoprotein gp120 with the co-receptor CXCR4 or CCR5, respectively, is followed by a spring-loaded action of the viral glycoprotein gp41, that then anchors into the target cell membrane. This initiates the fusion of the two lipid bilayers, that of the viral envelope with that of the cellular plasma membrane. T-20 is a synthetic, 36-amino acid peptide corresponding to residues 127–162 of the ectodomain of gp41. T-20 was selected after a specific domain predictive of α-helical secondary structure. T-20 afforded 100% blockade of virus-mediated cell–cell fusion at concentrations ranging from 1 to 10 ng/ml. An initial clinical trial has been carried out with T-20 in 16 HIV-infected adults. At 100 mg twice daily, T-20 achieved by 15 day a 1.5- to 2.0-fold reduction in

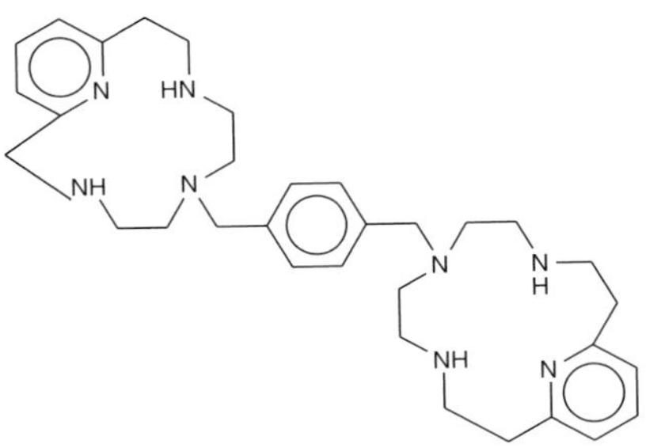

(16.54)

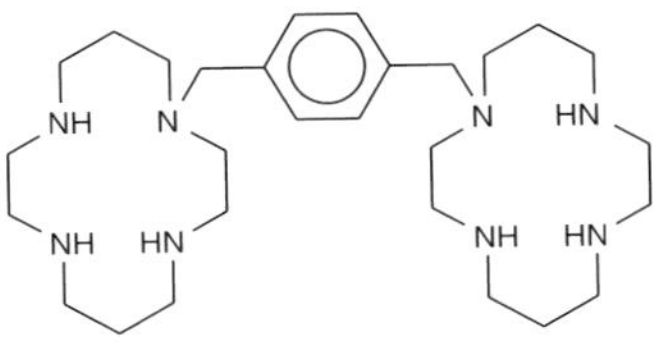

(16.55)

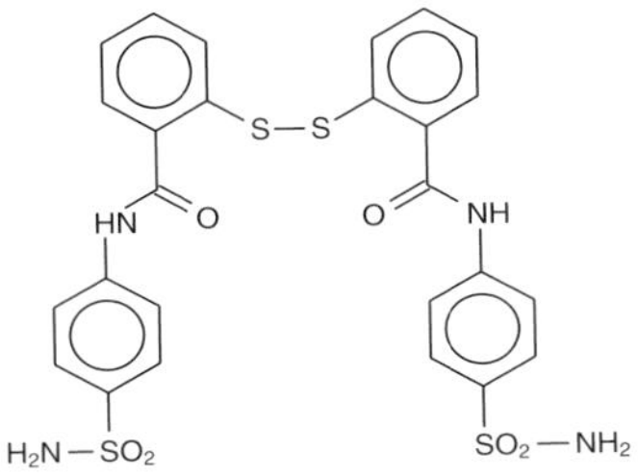

(16.56)

plasma HIV RNA. In a preliminary study, 1000-fold suppression of HIV-1 RNA was maintained for 20 weeks, no evidence of genotypic resistance to T-20 was observed, and no anti-T-20 antibodies were detected after 28 weeks of administration of T-20.

The two zinc fingers in the nucleocapsid (NCp7) protein comprise the proposed molecular target for zinc-releasing compounds such as the 2,2′-dithiobisbenzamide-1 (DIBA) (**16.56**). This compound can interfere with both early (uncoating, disassembly) and late phases (packing, assembly) of retrovirus replication. Its effect at the late phase (assembly) would result in abnormal processing of the gag precursor, due to the formation of intermolecular cross-links among the zinc fingers of adjacent NCp7 molecules and the release of non-infectious virus particles. The DIBA is able to enter intact virions, and the cross-linkage of NCp7 in virions correlates with loss of infectivity and decreased proviral DNA synthesis during acute infection.

Retrovirus integration requires at least two viral components, the retroviral enzyme integrase, and *cis*-acting sequences at the retroviral DNA termini U3 and U5 ends of the long terminal repeats (LTRs). Since HIV, like other retroviruses, cannot replicate without integration into a host chromosome, integrase has been considered as an attractive therapeutic target. A well documented HIV integrase inhibitor is L-chicoric acid (**16.57**). Integrase was identified as the molecular target for the action of L-chicoric acid when a single amino acid substitution in the integrase made the corresponding HIV-1 mutant resistant to L-chicoric acid.

(16.57)

(16.58)

(16.59)

However, it has been demonstrated that this diacid owes its anti-HIV activity in cell culture primarily to an interaction with the viral envelope gp120 and, consequently, inhibition of virus adsorption. Meanwhile, diketo acid (DKA) (**16.58**) derivatives have been identified as 'genuine' intergrase inhibitors that owe their anti-HIV activity in cell culture to integrase inhibition.

At the transcription level, HIV gene expression may be inhibited by compounds that interact with cellular factors that bind to the LTR promoter and that are needed for basal level transcription, such as the NF-κB inhibitors. Greater specificity, however, can be expected from those compounds that specifically inhibit the transactivation of the HIV LTR promoter by the viral Tat protein. Tat may be important, not only for translocation but also for nuclear localization and *trans*-activation, and thus targeting of the Tat basic domain may provide great scope for therapeutic intervention in HIV-1 infection. A number of compounds have been reported to inhibit HIV-1 replication through interference with the transcription process, e.g. the fluoroquinolones. The inhibitory effects of the fluoroquinolones on the HIV-1 LTR-driven gene expression may at least in part be attributed to inhibition of the Tat function. The fluoroquinolone K-12 [**16.59**] acts synergistically with RT and PIs.

FURTHER READING

Advances in Antiviral Drug Design, Vol. 1, edited by E. De Clercq, pp. 1–329. London, England: JAI Press, Inc. 1993; Vol. 2, (pp. 1–233), 1996; Vol. 3, (pp. 1–237), 1999.

Rotbart, H. (2000) Antiretroviral therapy for enteroviruses and rhinoviruses. *Antiviral Chem. and Chemother.*, **11**, 261–271.

Gubareva, L., Kaiser, L. and Hayden, F.G. (2000) Influenza virus neuraminidase inhibitors. *The Lancet*, **355**, 827–835.

Chapter 17

Anticancer agents

Ingrid Kjøller Larsen and Jette Sandholm Kastrup

17.1 DNA AS TARGET FOR ANTICANCER DRUGS

The DNA molecule is essential for the growth of all living cells and so far it has been the main target for anticancer drug action. Some of these drugs act directly on the DNA molecule, either by drug-induced DNA damage or by some kind of alteration of DNA (Section 17.1.1), whereas other drugs prevent nucleic acid synthesis by inhibiting one or more of the enzymes involved in the DNA synthesis, or by disturbing the DNA function by incorporation of 'wrong pieces' into the DNA molecule (Section 17.1.2).

The DNA interacting drugs prevent cell growth, but not only cancer cell growth. Unfortunately, the growth of normal cells is also blocked. The cytotoxic effect is most serious on rapidly dividing cells, i.e. in addition to tumor cells also the cells of normal bone marrow, gut, skin epithelium, and mucosa of the mouth.

The lack of selectivity of cancer drugs is one of the main problems in cancer chemotherapy. All the known abnormal biological phenomena of cancer cells (e.g. excessive cell proliferation, loss of tissue-specific characteristics, invasiveness, and metastasis) seem to be based on normal biological functions of the cells, e.g. by use of normal enzyme systems. The abnormality of malignant tumor growth is connected to the regulation of cell growth and caused by mutations in control genes, which are converted to oncogenes. The introduction of gene therapy might be a very important step forward in the treatment of cancer in the future. In most gene therapy approaches, full, healthy genes are introduced as substitutes for wrong versions ('mutation compensation'). Inhibition of expression of unwanted genes by using DNA or RNA binding agents might also be possible (cf. Section 17.1.1.5).

It should be noticed that most anticancer drugs interfering with DNA or DNA synthesis also exhibit a variety of actions on other targets in the cells. The classification of anticancer drugs in this chapter is based on the mode of action of the specified anticancer agents, which is generally believed to be responsible for the cytotoxic activity.

All drugs with action directly on the DNA molecule affect all fast-growing cells without preference for a special phase of the cell cycle (phase non-specific agents). They are, however, usually more effective against proliferating cells than against resting cells, where no DNA replication may occur for long periods of time. Drugs interfering with one or more of the enzymes involved in DNA synthesis are most effective in one phase of the cell cycle, i.e. the S phase of the cell cycle, which is the period of DNA synthesis (S phase specific agents).

One of the very serious problems in cancer chemotherapy is the development of drug resistance. Most drugs are initially very effective, but subsequent therapy may fail because the tumor cells have become non-sensitive to the drug. In many cases, the mechanisms of resistance to antitumor drugs are known and are mentioned later in this chapter under the individual classes of drugs.

In recent years, the existence of multidrug resistance (MDR) has been recognized. The MDR is characterized by cross-resistance to a group of structurally and mechanistically distinct antitumor agents including the anthracyclines (daunomycin and adriamycin), the vinca alkaloids (vincristine and vinblastine), colchicine and podophyllotoxins, and actinomycin D. However, this resistance does not extend to all anticancer agents, for example antimetabolites (e.g. methotrexate, cytarabine, and thioguanine) and alkylating agents (e.g. carmustine and cyclophosphamide) are not affected.

There are probably several different mechanisms by which cells can be cross-resistant to multiple drugs. However, MDR is commonly associated with high levels of a membrane-associated phosphoglucoprotein (Pgp), which is a transport protein with pertinent homology to bacterial transport proteins. The Pgp functions as an energy (ATP) dependent drug efflux pump. It has been shown that the drug efflux from cells, in which the gene for Pgp is expressed, increases with resistance. The detailed mechanism by which Pgp pumps drugs out of cells is not fully understood.

17.1.1 Drugs interacting directly with DNA

The functions of the DNA molecule can be influenced by drugs in different ways. Damage to DNA, where covalent bond formation is involved, is performed by the category of compounds usually called alkylating agents, including some anticancer antibiotics (Section 17.1.1.1). *cis*-Platinum co-ordination complexes modify the DNA structure by binding of the metal ions directly to DNA (Section 17.1.1.2). Breakdown of the DNA molecule (DNA strand scission) is caused by other antibiotic agents (Section 17.1.1.3). The intercalating agents (Section 17.1.1.4) disturb DNA function by intercalating between the base pairs, but normally without bond breakage or formation. Antisense anticancer agents (Section 17.1.1.5) are designed to perform their action on nucleic acids (blocking of specified base sequences) by a combination of intercalating and alkylating abilities, in addition to hydrogen bonding and hydrophobic interactions.

17.1.1.1 Alkylating agents

At least six major classes of alkylating agents are employed in cancer chemotherapy (cf. Scheme 17.1, where representative structures are given). All these compounds undergo a reaction in which an alkyl group becomes covalently linked to some cellular constituent, preferably the DNA molecule.

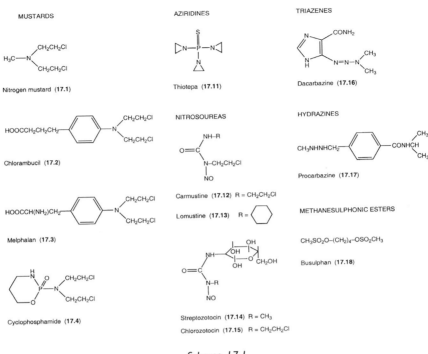

Scheme 17.1

17.1.1.1.1   Nitrogen mustards

Nitrogen mustard (**17.1**), mustine, mechlorethamine, di(2-chloroethyl)-methylamine is a volatile liquid, but it is administered clinically as the chloride. The salt is crystalline, but hygroscopic, and has to be dissolved in water immediately before use (intravenous saline infusion), because it is unstable in aqueous solution. The compound is very irritating (vesicant) to skin and mucous membranes, thus the acute side effects are severe and painful. The most serious delayed side effect is bone marrow depression, as also for all other alkylating agents. Nitrogen mustard has a very rapid alkylating effect and is therefore valuable in life-threatening situations.

Nitrogen mustard was the first drug used in cancer chemotherapy. It was discovered during the second world war that the war gas *sulphur mustard* [S(CH$_2$-CH$_2$-Cl)$_2$] and the isosterically related compound nitrogen mustard have anti-tumor activity. The sulphur mustard is too reactive and toxic for clinical use. Nitrogen mustard is also a very reactive drug with a number of toxic side effects, but it has proved to be a very useful drug and it is still in clinical use, often in combination with other drugs.

The proposed mechanism of action of nitrogen mustard is shown in Scheme 17.2. The molecule forms a reactive cyclic intermediate, an aziridinium ion, by release of a chloride ion. This aziridinium ion is an electrophile, which attacks

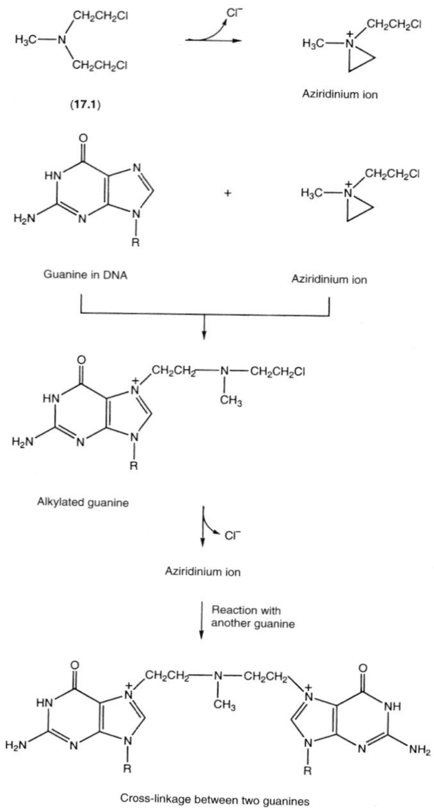

Scheme 17.2

electron-rich centers (nucleophiles) in biological macromolecules. The reaction is an S_N2 process, as the bimolecular reaction with the nucleophile is the rate controlling step, which obeys second-order kinetics. The formation of the aziridinium ion is a very fast unimolecular reaction, when CH_3 (or another alkyl group) is connected to the N-atom of the nitrogen mustard.

The nucleophilic groups, which can be attacked by the electrophile formed from nitrogen mustard, may be amino, hydroxyl, sulphhydryl or imidazole moieties in proteins and nucleic acids. The reaction of major importance in the cytotoxic effect of nitrogen mustards is the formation of a covalent bond with the N-7 atom of a guanine base of DNA. N-7 is thought to be the preferred position for purin alkylation, because it is easier accessible than N-3, and N-1 is involved in hydrogen bonding in a Watson–Crick base pair.

The other chloroethyl side chain of nitrogen mustard can undergo a similar cyclization and react with another nucleophilic group. If this second reaction involves an N-7 of a guanine base from an opposite strand of the double helix, the result is cross-linking between the DNA strands. Intra-strand cross-links can also be formed, and, in addition, reactions between monoalkylated DNA and another nucleic acid or a protein are possible. There is a good correlation between DNA cross-linking and inhibition of cell growth, and DNA cross-links are generally believed to be responsible for the antitumor activity of bifunctional alkylating agents, e.g. nitrogen mustards. However, as many cellular constituents, including membrane proteins, can be alkylated, it might be assumed that the cytotoxicity is a result of many diverse effects.

Nitrogen mustard is easily hydrolyzed. This happens when the initially formed aziridinium ion reacts with a water molecule instead of a nucleophilic group of a biomacromolecule. In this case, an inactive hydroxy form of the compound [$CH_3N(CH_2CH_2OH)_2$] is formed. A considerable amount of the injected drug is actually inactivated before reaching the biological targets.

Evidence for the formation of cross-links between two different DNA strands of the double helix has been obtained from different experiments. Alkylation of DNA bases, and especially intra- and interstrand cross-linking, disturbs the functions of the DNA molecule in different ways. The cross linkages prevent separation of the individual strands, thereby mainly inhibiting DNA replication, but DNA transcription will also be influenced. In addition, it is now accepted that alkylating agents kill tumor cells by inducing apoptosis (programmed cell death).

All living cells are able to repair DNA damage, whether accidentally arisen or due to alkylating agents, by the DNA repair system, involving several enzymes (e.g. endonucleases, repair polymerase and ligase). Drug resistance of cells treated with nitrogen mustards (or other cross-linking agents) is due to an increased ability of the resistant cells to excise the cross-linked residues in DNA and repair the defect.

Chlorambucil (**17.2**), 4-[*bis*(2-chloroethyl)amino)benzenebutanoic acid], is a synthetically prepared, crystalline compound. This aromatic nitrogen mustard was introduced at an early stage of cancer therapy. It has a milder effect than nitrogen mustard, no serious acute side effects, and it can be given orally. The long-term toxicity is bone marrow depression.

Melphalan(**17.3**), 4-[*bis*(2-chloroethyl)amino)-L-phenylalanine], is another crystalline nitrogen mustard with an aryl group attached to the N-atom. This drug was also developed as a drug with less reactivity (see below) than nitrogen mustard. In addition, it was originally synthesized in support of the idea that attachment of a mustard group to a naturally occurring carrier (in this case phenylalanine) might increase the effectiveness, because of increased affinity for certain biological sites. Since phenylalanine is a precursor for melanin, it was hoped that melphalan would preferentially accumulate in melanomas and thereby produce a selective effect. This early attempt on site-directed mustard effect was not successful, but still melphalan is a widely used drug, because of its pharmacological properties.

The mechanism of action of chlorambucil and melphalan is similar to that of nitrogen mustard (Scheme 17.2). One of the advantages of nitrogen mustards, as compared to sulphur mustard, is that the third substituent (CH_3 in nitrogen mustard) can be varied in order to introduce some variation of the reactivity of the drug. Attachment of an aromatic ring to the nitrogen atom, as in chlorambucil and melphalan, decreases the rate of alkylation. The electron withdrawing effect of the ring, and/or delocalization of the lone pair electrons, makes the nitrogen atom less nucleophilic and the rate of cyclization much slower than for alkyl nitrogen mustards. This step (formation of aziridinium ion by first order cyclization) is probably the rate limiting step in the case of aryl nitrogen mustards, and the reaction is believed to be an S_N1 type process.

The decreased reactivity of aromatic nitrogen mustards can be advantageous for several reasons. The drug can be given orally, whereas nitrogen mustard has to be be given intravenously. The higher stability allows time for absorption and wide distribution before degradation (hydrolysis) and before extensive alkylation. Finally, the acute side effects are much less severe. The biological effects are the same.

Cyclophosphamide (**17.4**), 1-*bis*(2-chloroethyl)amino-1-oxo-2-aza-5-oxaphosphoridine, is a nitrogen mustard with an oxazaphosphorine ring attached to the N-atom. It was synthesized originally as a transport form (prodrug) for nornitrogen mustard [normustine, $HN(CH_2CH_2Cl)_2$], which is also an active alkylating agent, but too toxic and with a low therapeutic index. The biochemical rationale behind this early approach to the development of a target-directed prodrug was that the compound should be enzymatically converted into the active compound *in vivo* by phosphoramidase enzymes, which were thought to be more abundant in tumors compared with normal tissue. Later it was demonstrated, however, that simple enzymatic cleavage is not the reason for the bioactivation of cyclophosphamide.

Cyclophosphamide (CPA) is one of the most effective alkylating agents with a wide application in cancer chemotherapy against many different neoplastic diseases. It can be given either orally or intravenously and its side effects are less severe and easier to control than those of nitrogen mustard (**17.1**). Immunosuppression is a side effect, which has led to its use to prevent transplant rejection. In addition, CPA has a number of undesirable side effects, some of which are probably caused by one or more of the metabolites.

Cyclophosphamide has to be metabolically activated in the body before it can alkylate cellular constituents. The CPA by itself is not cytotoxic to cells in culture (*in vitro*), but cells are killed, when incubated with both the drug and a liver homogenate, which can convert it into the active form. The mechanism of the metabolic activation of CPA has been extensively studied. The metabolic degradation pathway is considered to be as shown in Scheme 17.3. The oxidation product 4-hydroxy-CPA (**17.5a**) either undergoes further oxidation (detoxification) into 4-keto-CPA (**17.6**) or tautomerizes into the open-chain aldehyde aldophosphamide (**17.5b**). Aldophosphamide may be oxidized into carboxy-CPA (**17.7**), a detoxification reaction, or the enol form of **17.5b** may undergo a spontaneous β-elimination (reverse Michael addition) to give acrolein (**17.8**) and phosphoramide mustard (**17.9**). In addition, nornitrogen mustard (**17.10**) is formed as a decomposition product (hydrolysis, non-enzymatic) of several of the above mentioned compounds.

Phosphoramide mustard (**17.9**) is generally believed to be the final cytotoxic agent. Due to its polar nature, phosphoramide mustard is not capable of penetrating cell membranes and therefore has to be formed intracellularly. Neither of the two major urinary metabolites (**17.6**) and (**17.7**) is significantly cytotoxic and represents inactivated excretion products. Acrolein (**17.8**) and phosphoramide

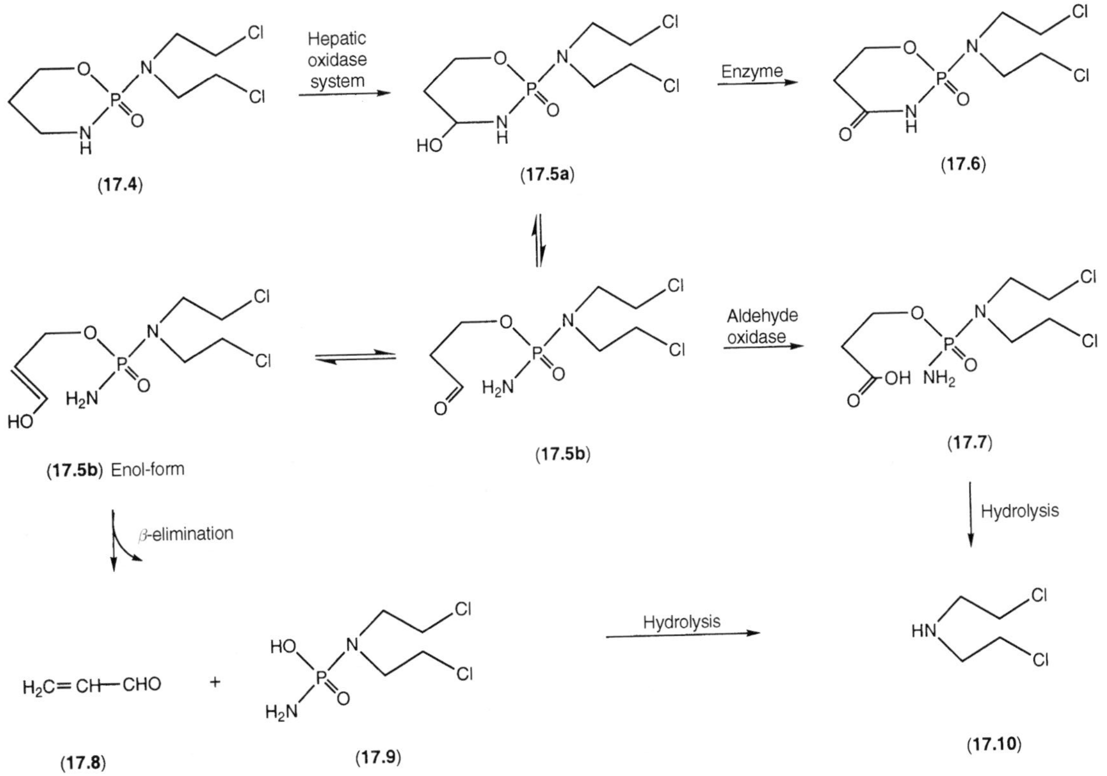

Scheme 17.3

mustard are produced in equimolar amounts during the metabolism of CPA. Because of the known toxicities of acrolein one might expect it to contribute to the final cytotoxicity of CPA. This is unlikely, however, as phosphoramide mustard is cytotoxic at levels considerably below the level of acrolein required for cytotoxicity. Some role for acrolein in the pharmacology of CPA cannot be excluded, however. Thus, the bladder toxicity observed in patients treated with CPA is caused by acrolein and can be diminished by co-administration of the drug with an alkyl sulphide (e.g. MESNA, sodium 2-mercaptoethanesulphonate), which reacts with acrolein by a Michael's reaction. The reaction product is then excreted.

Phosphoramide mustard, as well as nornitrogen mustard, are powerful cytostatic agents, also *in vitro*, and high levels of both compounds can be detected in plasma 1–10 h after CPA infusion. Phosphoramide mustard is considered to be the ultimate alkylating agent for several reasons, e.g. because it is a more powerful alkylating agent than nornitrogen mustard. In addition, nornitrogen mustard is a secondary amine and may, after formation of an aziridinium ion, deliver H^+ to solvent, thereby forming the uncharged chloroethylaziridine, which is relatively resistant to nucleophilic attack.

Phosphoramide mustard (**17.9**) is an alkylating agent because of its ability to form an aziridinium ion in contrast to CPA (**17.4**), where the withdrawing electronegative effect of the ring, and delocalization of the lone pair electrons, makes the N-atom less nucleophilic and the rate of initial cyclization very slow. In phosphoramide mustard, which is deprotonated at physiological pH (pKa of the OH group is 4.75), the nucleophilic effect of the N-atom is not decreased because of strong contributions of the resonance forms with the negative charge on the two oxygen atoms of the phosphoramide group and therefore negligible delocalization of the lone pair on the N-atom with the chloroethyl substituents.

The main biological effect of CPA is the same as that of nitrogen mustard, i.e. formation of DNA cross links by alkylation of guanine N-7. The initial phosphoramide-DNA adduct is unstable and converted to the corresponding nornitrogen mustard adduct G-nor-G. Monoalkylation also occurs. Other oxazaphosphorines used therapeutically are *ifosfamide* with one of the chloroethyl substituents positioned at the N-atom of the oxazaphosphorine ring, and *trofosfamide*, which has this substituent as a third chloroethyl group.

17.1.1.1.2   Aziridines

Thiotepa (**17.11**), triethylenethiophosphoramide, *tris*(1-aziridinyl)phosphine sulphide, is a hexasubstituted triamide of thiophosphoric acid. Thiotepa is unstable in acid and is poorly absorbed from the gastrointestinal tract. It is therefore given intravenously or used topically, e.g. to treat papillary carcinoma of the bladder. The major side effect is bone marrow depression.

Thiotepa is a trifunctional alkylating agent containing aziridine rings. It has been developed as an analog of the reactive aziridinium ion formed from nitrogen mustard, in order to obtain a deactivated alkylating agent. The aziridine ring is less attractive to nucleophiles because of the lack of a positive charge. However, if the third substituent on the N-atom of the aziridine ring is an electron-withdrawing group, some positive charge (electron deficiency) arises on the C-atoms of the aziridine ring, due to polarization of the bonds.

17.1.1.1.3   Nitrosoureas

Carmustine (**17.12**), BCNU, *N,N'-bis*(2-chloroethyl)-*N*-nitrosourea, and the structural analog *lomustine* (**17.13**), CCNU, *N*-(2-chloroethyl)-*N'*-cyclohexyl-*N*-nitrosourea, are developed as a result of the observation of promising antileukemic properties of *N*-methyl-*N*-nitrosourea in routine screening of this compound. The compounds are rather unstable in acidic and alkaline aqueous solutions. The BCNU has to be given intravenously, whereas CCNU can be administered orally.

The nitrosoureas are unionized at physiological pH and consequently they have much higher lipid solubility than the nitrogen mustards and other alkylating agents. Their ability to pass the blood–brain barrier renders them especially useful in the treatment of CNS neoplasm (e.g. brain tumors and metastases). The BCNU and CCNU both produce nausea and vomiting, and the delayed side effects are bone marrow depression, leukopenia, and thrombocytopenia. The BCNU is more toxic of the two compounds.

A number of theories on the mechanism of action of the nitrosoureas has been proposed. It is evident that these drugs are alkylating as well as carbamoylating agents and that cross-linking of DNA is a consequence of alkylation. The proposed mechanisms for the alkylation and carbamoylation outlined in Scheme 17.4 are based on the mechanism of decomposition of nitrosoureas in aqueous solution at pH 7.4. Base abstraction of the amide hydrogen atom produces an unstable intermediate, which rapidly decomposes to yield the corresponding alkylisocyanate and 2-chloroethanediazohydroxide. The isocyanate formed is capable of carbamoylating proteins, e.g. lysine and cysteine residues. By spontaneous decomposition of the diazohydroxide and reaction with a nucleophilic center, e.g. of base X, the DNA is monoalkylated. Preferably O-6 but also N-7 of guanine may be alkylated (β-chloroethylated). In a second step, an ethylene bridge is formed by reaction with the cytosine (base Y) on the complementary strand and elimination of a chloride ion. The DNA-protein cross links as well as monoalkylated nucleic acids and proteins can also occur as the result of alkylation with nitrosoureas. Resistance to nitrosoureas is caused by enzymatical removal of chloroethyl groups, thereby preventing formation of DNA interstrand cross links.

Streptozotocin (**17.14**), an anticancer antibiotic isolated from *Streptomyces achromogenes*, is a nitrosourea derivative with a glucose moiety at one N-atom and a methyl group at the other. By substitution of this methyl group with a chloroethyl group *chlorozotocin* (**17.15**) was obtained, which shows lower toxicity (myelosuppression) than streptozotocin. The drugs are retained in the β-cells of the islets of Langerhans and can be used experimentally to induce diabetes in laboratory animals. Insulin chock is a dangerous acute toxicity. Because of the β-cell effect the drugs can be used against metastatic islet cell carcinoma. The compounds probably act by alkylation of nucleophilic sites, but the precise mechanism has not been well worked out. The glucose moiety of the drugs may be of importance for the lower myelosuppression.

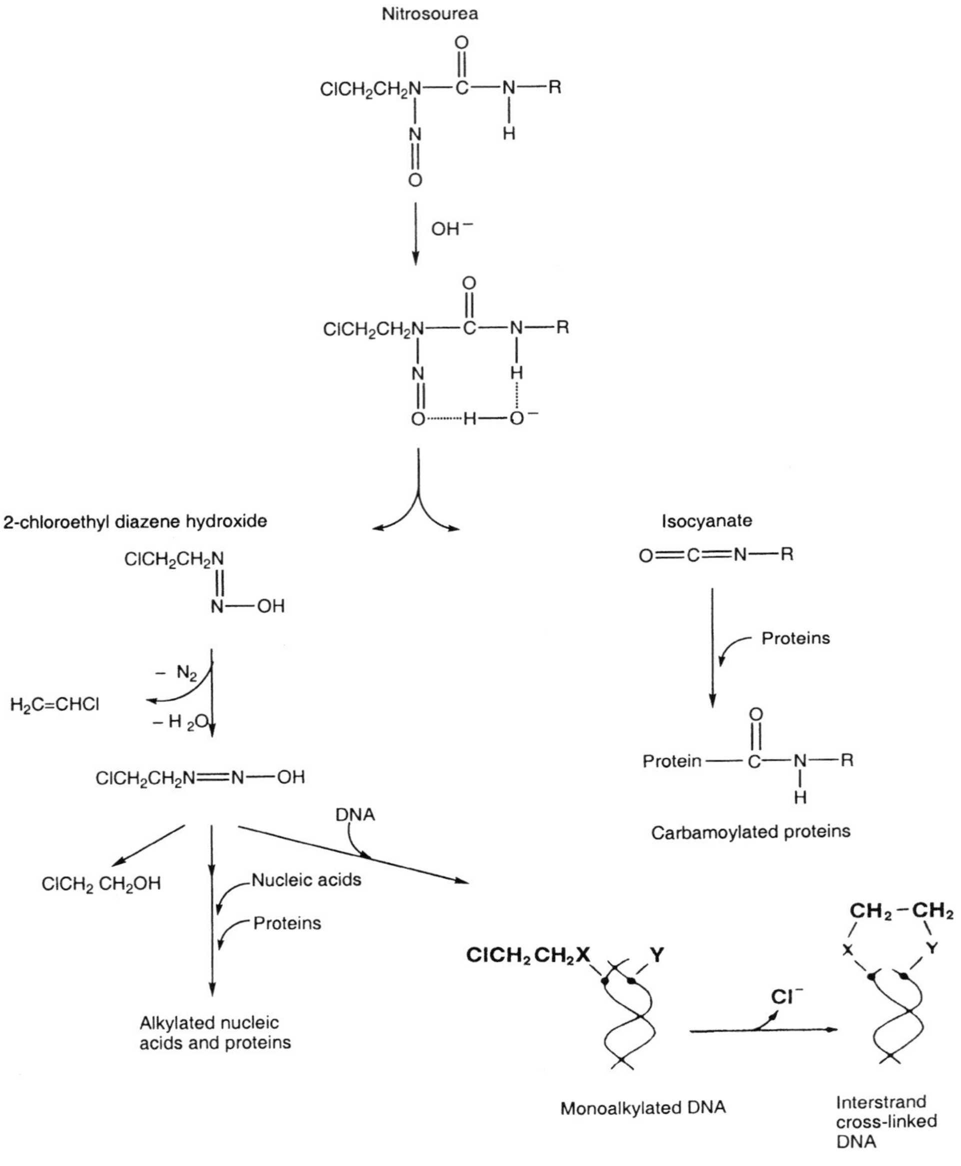

Nitrosourea

$$CICH_2CH_2N-C-N-R$$

Scheme 17.4

17.1.1.1.4   Triazenes

Dacarbazine (**17.16**), DTIC, 5-(3,3-dimethyl-1-triazenyl)-1-*H*-imidazole-4-carbox-amide, is a compound, which is stable in solution, but has to be protected against light. The drug is given intravenously and produces severe nausea and vomiting and sometimes a flu-like syndrome of fever. Dacarbazine has appeared to be particularly suitable for the treatment of malignant melanoma.

Dacarbazine was originally developed as a structural analog of 5-aminoimidazole-4-carboxamide, an intermediate in purine biosynthesis. It is, however, now known that the cytotoxicity of the drug is due to its alkylating (methylating) action, rather than to inhibition of purine biosynthesis. The generally accepted mechanism (metabolism and subsequent chemical decomposition) is shown in Scheme 17.5.

The monomethyl derivative produced via the corresponding hydroxymethyl derivative by enzymatic oxidation decomposes spontaneously (non-enzymatically) to form 5-aminoimidazole-4-carboxamide (the major metabolite excreted in the urine) and the methylating agent, which is methane diazohydroxide $CH_3-N=N-OH$. This methylating agent attacks nucleophilic groups in DNA and other cellular constituents. An important site of *in vivo* alkylation is the N-7 position of guanine, and the 7-methylguanine product has been identified in the urine of patients given ^{14}C-methyl-dacarbazine.

Many triazenes have been investigated in which the imidazole ring has been replaced by other heterocyclic systems or phenyl derivatives in a search for second-generation antitumor triazenes with enhanced selectivity and activity. The studies have shown that the nature of the aromatic moiety does not affect the activity markedly. Substitution of one of the methyl groups of the triazene moiety has no effect on antitumor activity, provided that the replacement alkyl group can undergo oxidative dealkylation (depends e.g. on chain length and bulkyness of the alkyl group). If both methyl groups of the triazene N-atom are substituted by other

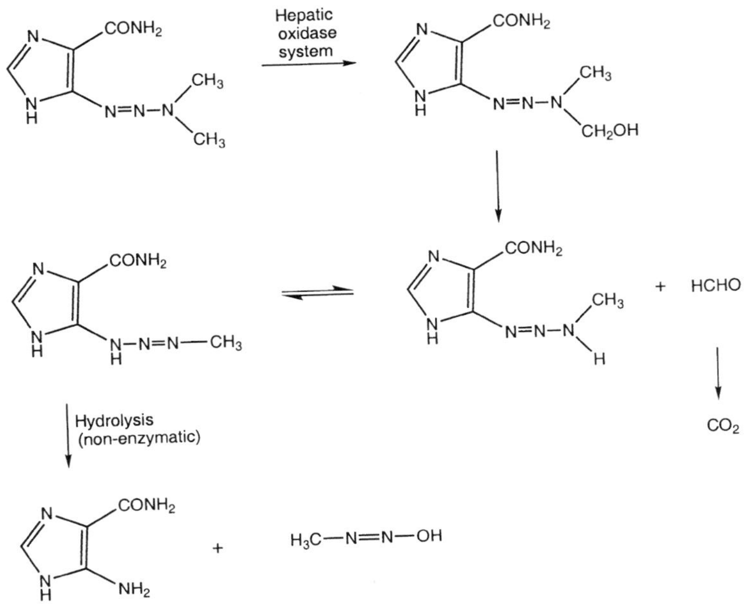

Scheme 17.5

alkyl groups, total loss of activity is observed. It is not yet fully understood why methyl substituents predispose so decisively towards the activity of the triazenes.

17.1.1.1.5 Hydrazines

Procarbazine (**17.17**), *N*-(1-methylethyl)-4-[(2-methylhydrazino)methyl]-benzamide, is used as the chloride of the hydrazine. This compound was synthesized as a potential monoamine oxidase (MAO) inhibitor, but it was later shown to have antitumor effect. It is clinically used both in combination drug therapy and in various drug protocols to treat e.g. melanoma and Hodgkin's disease. Procarbazine can penetrate into the cerebrospinal fluid and has been used to treat malignant brain tumors. Its side effects are similar to those of typical alkylating agents, but it also causes psychopharmacological effects consistent with its ability to inhibit MAO.

Procarbazine is inactive *in vitro* and requires enzymatic activation before it shows antitumor activity. *In vivo* it is rapidly converted to azo-procarbazine, $CH_3-N=N-CH_2-C_6H_4-CONHCH(CH_3)_2$, probably by hepatic microsomal enzymes. Several pathways have been proposed for the conversion of this intermediate to the major urinary metabolite *N*-isopropylterephthalamic acid, $HOOC-C_6H_4-CONHCH(CH_3)_2$. Methane is observed as a minor metabolite, and it has been suggested that methyl radicals or methyl carbocations are the biologically active methylating agent.

17.1.1.1.6 Methanesulphonate esters

Busulphan (**17.18**), myleran, 1,4-*bis*(methanesulphonyloxy)butane is unstable in aqueous solution, but can still be given orally and is well absorbed from the gastrointestinal tract. It is excreted in the urine as methanesulphonic acid and several metabolites, which are derived from the alkylating butylene moiety. It is a very mild alkylating agent with no acute side effects and it is useful mainly in the treatment of patients with chronic granulocytic leukemia. A number of long-term side effects are observed, among those bone marrow depression.

Busulphan is a bifunctional alkylating agent, which has a reactivity considerably lower than that of nitrogen mustard. The mechanism of the alkylation is believed to be similar to that of nitrogen mustards. The alkyl–oxygen bond splits with the methanesulphonate moiety as the leaving group when reacting with nucleophilic centers of the cell constituents, including N-7 of guanine bases, but also with sulphhydryl groups of cysteines in proteins. Diguanyl derivatives can be formed as a reaction product between busulfan and nucleotides, and cross-linking of DNA is believed to be the main reason for the cytotoxic activity of busulphan.

17.1.1.2 Metal complex binding to DNA

Platinum co-ordination complexes with the formula *cis*-PtA$_2$X$_2$, where X is a uninegative, readily exchangeable group, and A is ammonia or an amine, have been known for many years to exhibit antitumor properties. The initial trials were very promising, but the toxic side effects, e.g. renal toxicity, appeared to be a serious limitation of the use of the Pt-complexes as anticancer agents. Improved administration procedures have now resulted in large-scale clinical application of *cis*-Pt-complexes, especially in combination with many other anticancer drugs. It is generally believed that the antitumor properties of *cis*-Pt-complexes are mainly based on interactions of these compounds with DNA. Introduction of Pt-complexes is regarded as one of the most important acquisitions in cancer chemotherapy of the last two decades.

Cisplatin (**17.19**), *cis*-diamminedichloroplatinum(II), possesses a very broad spectrum of activity and is one of the most widely used anticancer drugs. It is routinely administered by intravenous infusion, and supplied as a lyophylized powder, because of the low solubility in water. Cisplatin is particularly used in combination therapy, e.g. with paclitaxel (taxol **17.39**), cyclophosphamide and bleomycin, in the treatment of testicular cancer, but good response in the treatment of several other cancer forms has been observed. In particular, promising results have been obtained with cisplatin in combination with paclitaxel in treatment of ovarian cancer, and there is a broad consensus that this combination represents a significant advance in the treatment of advanced ovarian cancer.

Several methods have been used in order to elucidate the mechanism of action of cisplatin and other Pt-complexes. It is known that cisplatin interacts with DNA by specific binding to the guanine N-7 sites. Binding to cytosine N-3, adenine N-1, and adenine N-7 is also possible, but is less common. A second binding interaction readily takes place on the same strand of DNA, most frequently at another guanine base being a next-neighbor. Interstrand cross-linking is also possible.

Detailed information on the nature of the binding of cisplatin to DNA has been obtained from studies of the model complexes consisting of cisplatin bound to short DNA fragments. The accurate structure in solution of the adduct *cis*-Pt(NH$_3$)$_2$-[d(GpG)] has been studied using high-resolution NMR techniques, and the solid-state structure of the very similar adduct *cis*-Pt(NH$_3$)$_2$-[d(pGpG)] was solved using X-ray diffraction (Figure 17.1). The geometry of the two adducts (in solution and in the solid-state) was shown to be substantially the same. Pt binds to the two guanine bases of the dinucleotide by co-ordination through N-7, and the conformational changes of the overall structure of the nucleotide are limited to small changes in the position of the sugar ring at the 5′ side of d(GpG) and of the dihedral angle between the guanine bases. The distortion of the DNA structure, after chelation of cisplatin to a GpG sequence, should therefore be rather small.

Molecular modeling studies suggested a helix distortion, which can best be described as a kink or a bend in the helical axis of about 40°. This has now been confirmed by the X-ray structure determination of a double-stranded DNA dodecamer containing cisplatin (Figure 17.2). The biological consequences of the

Cisplatin (**17.19**) Carboplatin (**17.20**)   Oxaliplatin (**17.21**)

A = NH$_3$ X = Cl

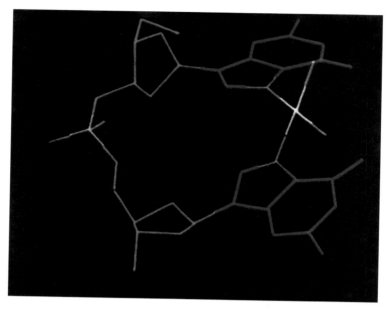

Figure 17.1 Structural model of the Pt(NH₃)₂ [d(GpG)] adduct, determined from analysis of the NMR spectra. From Reedijk, J. in *NMR Spectroscopy in Drug Research*, eds. J.W. Jaroszewski, K. Schaumburg and H. Kofod. Munksgaard, Copenhagen 1988, with permission by Munksgaard.

DNA distortion (bending and unwinding) are not quite clear, but high-mobility-group (HMG)-domain proteins seem to be involved. The ultimate result is that cell replication is hampered. The cytotoxic effects of cisplatin might, however, be considered to be due to the combined effects of various lesions.

It has been known for sometime that also *trans*-PtA₂X₂, e.g. *trans*-diamminedichloroplatinum(II), binds to DNA, but these complexes have much lower cytotoxic effect and no anticancer activity. As the binding affinities to the nucleobases are quite comparable with those of the *cis* complexes, the different activity must originate from differences related to the bifunctional binding. The NMR studies have shown that *trans*-Pt compounds can chelate to GNG sequences (N = A, T or C) through the guanine N-7 atoms, but the distortion of DNA after such *trans* binding is larger. This has prompted the hypothesis that repair enzymes recognize and remove the *trans* compound easier than the *cis* compound. It may also be possible that the distortion of DNA is of a nature that do not cause erroneous binding of HMG-domain proteins.

Several thousands of analogs of cisplatin has been synthesized and tested in order to enhance the therapeutic index and or reduce the resistance development. So far, most analogs are found to be so-called 'me too' versions of cisplatin. One of the few, which has provided definite advantage over cisplatin is *carboplatin* (**17.20**), *cis*-diammine-1,1-cyclobutanedicarboxylatoplatinum(II). Carboplatin has, however, afforded benefit in reducing some of the toxic side effects, and has now replaced cisplatin in many clinical situations. It has the same spectrum of

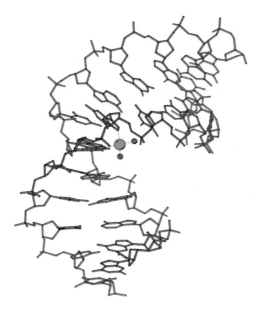

Figure 17.2 The X-ray structure of a double-stranded DNA dodecamer (shown in red) containing cisplatin (Pt ion shown in green and amine ligands in blue). The DNA structure has been modified by binding of cisplatin to two neighbouring intrastrand guanine bases. The structure is generated using the program Molscript with co-ordinates from Protein Data Bank.

anticancer activity and is not active in cisplatin-resistant cancers. Another analog of cisplatin, *oxaliplatin* (**17.21**), appears to have a somewhat different spectrum of antitumor activity. Introduction of this drug, in monotherapy as well as in combination with fluorouracil (**17.30**), represents a significant advance in the treatment of advanced colorectal cancer and is registered for this use in several European countries.

SAR studies have been performed on *cis*-platinum compounds with the following conclusions:

1 The nature of the leaving group X in PtA_2X_2 determines the rate of the substitution reactions. Strongly bound groups, such as thiocyanate, lead to inactivity in biological systems. On the other hand, very labile groups, such as H_2O or NO_3^-, give rise to very toxic compounds with little or no antitumor activity. It should be mentioned in this context that both chloride ions of e.g. cisplatin are replaced by water molecules before the binding to DNA occurs inside the cells. This does not happen outside the cells, as the concentration of chloride ions in the extracellular fluid is very high.

2 The nature of the amine group A co-ordinated to platinum also influences anticancer activity. Active compounds have at least one hydrogen atom at the N-atom of the amine ligand, which should not be too large.

3   The net-charge of the complexes has to be zero. Presumably, charged complexes are unable to cross the cell membranes.

17.1.1.3 Degradation of DNA

Anticancer agents of a wide range of structural types have been observed to produce strand breaks in DNA *in vivo* and *in vitro*. These include some of the earlier mentioned categories of compounds, e.g. nitrosoureas, but this is not the primary cytotoxic action of these compounds, as it appears to be in the case of *bleomycin*. This drug binds to DNA and causes strand scissions by an oxidative attack involving chelated iron and free radical species.

Bleomycin (**17.22**): Bleomycins are a group of related glucopeptide antibiotics iso-lated from *Streptomyces verticillus*. Bleomycin A$_2$ (Scheme 17.6) is the major compo-nent of the bleomycin employed clinically (as the sulphate). The various bleomycins differ only in their terminal amine moieties. In bleomycinic acid, which is inactive, the terminal amine moiety is replaced by a hydroxyl group.

Bleomycin (BLM) can be given by a number of parenteral routes, but it is most commonly injected intravenously. The drug is widely distributed in the tissues, except in brain tissue. Apparently BLM cannot enter the cerebrospinal fluid in any significant concentration. The highest concentrations of active drug are found in skin and lung. This is important because these two sites are very susceptible to BLM toxicity. The most common acute side effects involve the skin and mucous membranes, and the most severe, dose-limiting BLM toxicity is the pulmonary toxicity. The BLM is unique among the available antitumor antibiotics by produ-cing very little bone marrow depression. For this reason, it is particularly useful in combination therapy with nearly all major anticancer drugs.

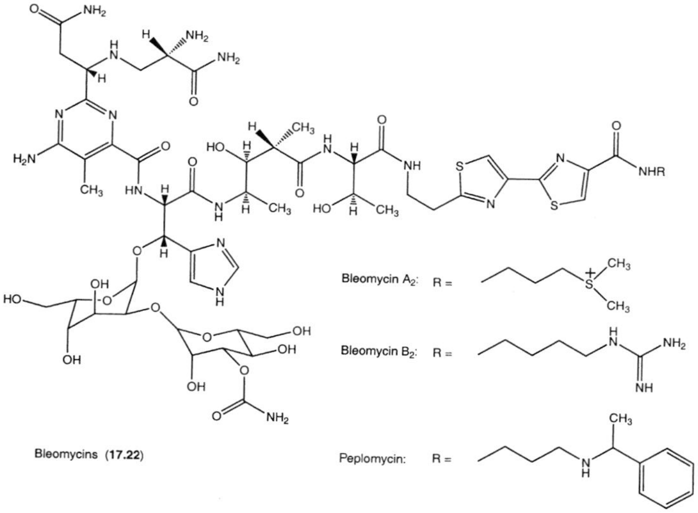

Scheme 17.6

The chemistry and biological effects and mechanism of action of BLM have been extensively studied. The glycopeptide contains several unusual amino acids and sugars, a pyrimidine ring, an imidazole ring, and a bithiazole ring system. X-ray structure determination of BLM has not been reported, and the structure shown in Scheme 17.6 is based on conventional methods and confirmed by high-resolution, 2D NMR spectroscopy.

The BLM molecule contains at least four functional domains. The left part of the molecule is the metal chelating domain, where the oxidative reaction with DNA is initiated. The bithiazole and C-terminal substituent are known to be involved in DNA binding, and the linker region (the pentapeptide) has been shown to be of importance to the efficiency of DNA cleavage by BLM. The function of the fourth domain, the carbohydrate moiety, is not well understood, but may be important for metal ion co-ordination.

The BLM binds in the minor grove of DNA with specific DNA sequences (5′GC3′ and 5′GT3′ sites) leading to sequence selectivity in DNA cleavage. Computer analysis and modeling of a DNA–BLM complex has been performed, but the structure of the complex has not yet been confirmed by X-ray analysis. The reaction by which DNA strand scission is effected by BLM has been found to require Fe(II) and O_2 as cofactors. The ultimate agent of DNA damage is an active BLM dioxygen species.

Bleomycin forms one-to-one complexes with several metals, e.g. copper, zinc, iron, and cobalt. The BLM–Cu(II) complex is the most stable complex and also the natural form produced by fermentation. It is inactive and resistant to BLM hydrolase, a BLM inactivating enzyme. The BLM hydrolase is present in cells and hydrolyses metal-free BLM, resulting in inactivation of BLM.

After injection of BLM (metal-free) it binds to Cu(II) ions in blood to form the stable BLM–Cu(II) complex. Inside the cells, the copper of the complex is removed reductively and trapped by other proteins, leaving BLM free to form the active iron complex (or to enzymatical inactivation). Thus, the Cu(II) complex of BLM protects against inactivation and provides transport and distribution of BLM in the body in an inactive form.

The structure of the Fe(II) complex of BLM is shown in Scheme 17.7. The structure of the iron complex is based on the X-ray structure of a model compound, i.e. a copper complex of a smaller part of the BLM molecule, lacking the sugar and bithiazole moieties. In the oxygenated iron complex there is strong evidence suggesting that dioxygen is the sixth ligand.

In the cells the oxygenated complex, BLM-Fe(II)-O_2, is further converted into a transient ferric species called 'activated BLM', which produces the oxidative species that initiate DNA degradation by abstraction of a H-atom at C-4′ of a backbone sugar ring. The degradation of DNA by BLM has been studied by identification of the products (DNA fragments) formed, and, while degrading the deoxyribose, BLM releases the bases undamaged. This is compatible with a site-specific generation of an oxygen radical species close to a susceptible site on the deoxyribose moiety and remote from the bases.

One of the disadvantages of BLM treatment is the development of pulmonary fibrosis. A lot of semi-synthetic BLM analogs have been prepared in order to find an active drug with lower pulmonary toxicity, e.g. *peplomycin*, a BLM with a

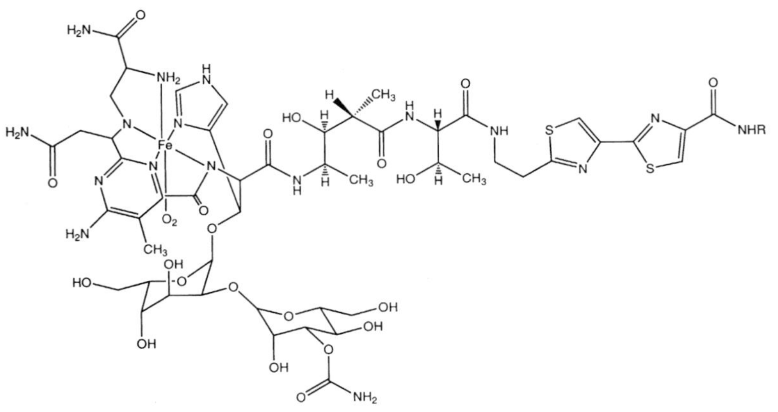

Scheme 17.7

synthetic terminal amine (Scheme 17.6). Semi-synthetic BLM analogs can be prepared by reaction of the Cu(II) complex of BLM acid with the amine in the presence of a coupling reagent for peptide synthesis. The BLM acid is prepared enzymatically from native BLM in order to avoid cleavage also of other peptide bonds in the molecule. The Cu(II) co-ordination protects the primary amino group in the α-position of the terminal β-aminoalanine moiety and prevents inter- and intramolecular coupling.

17.1.1.4 Intercalating agents

Several compounds bind reversibly to double-stranded DNA by intercalation, i.e. by squeezing in between adjacent base pairs of DNA. Such compounds have to be rather planar and are most often aromatic ring systems, which are held between the flat purine and pyrimidine rings by van der Waals' forces and charge-transfer complex formation. Some of the compounds also bind covalently, in some cases after metabolic transformation, e.g. *benzopyrene*, which is a carcinogen. Intercalating drugs can be primarily antibacterial (e.g. *aminoacridines*), antimalarial (e.g. *mepacrine*), or carcinostatic agents (e.g. *actinomycin D, daunorubicin* and *doxorubicin*). In this chapter, only the anticancer agents will be considered.

Several techniques have been used to characterize the interactions of intercalating agents with DNA. Evidence for binding to DNA can be obtained by determination of the association constant and number of binding sites. Intercalating agents give rise to increase in the length of DNA, as shown diagrammatically in Figure 17.3. This unwinding property of intercalators can be used in several ways to demonstrate that drugs bind to DNA by intercalation. One method is to investigate the effect of the drugs on the supercoiling of closed circular duplex DNA, by monitoring the rate of sedimentation, which decreases by unwinding. The anticancer antibiotic *mithramycin* is an example of a drug, which binds to DNA in a different way, as it does not change DNA supercoiling. Detailed information on the nature of the binding of intercalating agents to DNA can be obtained by studying

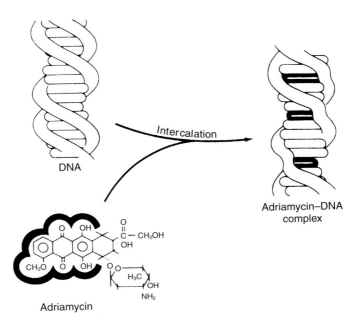

Figure 17.3 Diagrammatic model of intercalation of the flat part of the adriamycin molecule (in black) into DNA, showing local unwinding of the helical structure. From Lerman, L.S. *J. Cell. Comp. Physiol.*, **64**, Suppl. 1:1 (1964) with permission by LISS (Alan R. Liss, Inc.). New York.

model drug–DNA complexes by NMR methods or – when crystalline complexes are available – by X-ray structure determinations. In addition, molecular modeling methods have become increasingly significant in recent years.

The DNA intercalation has various biological consequences, e.g. inhibition of DNA replication and transcription, probably due to prevention of DNA/RNA polymerase activity. The cytotoxicity of intercalating agents is believed to be primarily a consequence of the DNA interaction, but DNA breakage (strand scissions), generated by some of the drugs in a reaction involving the nuclear enzyme topoisomerase II, contributes to the cytotoxicity and may play an important role in their mutagenic and carcinogenic activity.

Actinomycin D (**17.23**), d-actinomycin, AMD, is an anticancer antibiotic isolated from *Streptomyces* species. It is given by rapid flowing infusion, because injection is accompanied by severe local reaction. Additional serious side effects, both acute and delayed, have limited the clinical application, but the drug is still in use, e.g. in combined chemoradiotherapy.

The AMD molecule consists of an aminophenoxazone ring system, to which two identical cyclic pentapeptides are attached. The first and the last amino acids are linked by the formation of a lactone ring. Information on the binding of AMD to DNA was originally obtained from the X-ray structure determination of a drug–nucleoside model complex (Figure 17.4).

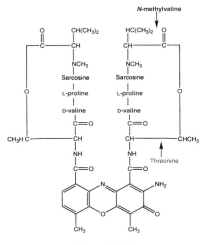

Actinomycin D **(17.23)**

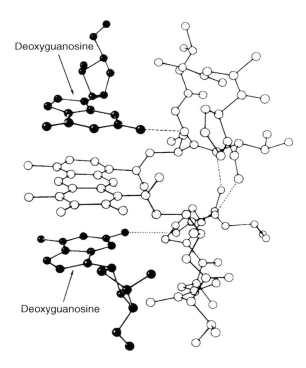

Figure 17.4 The X-ray structure of the actinomycin–deoxyguanosine complex. The two deoxy-guanosine molecules stack on alternate sides of the phenoxazone ring. Hydrogen bonds are indicated by dashed lines. (Redrawn from Sobell, H.M. *et al.* (1971), *Nature New Biol.*, **231**, 200 with permission by Macmillan Journals Ltd.).

The study showed that the planar phenoxazone ring of AMD in the model complex is squeezed in between the planar guanine bases of two deoxyguanosine molecules. Strong hydrogen bonds connect the 2-amino groups of guanine and the carbonyl oxygen of threonine residues in the cyclic peptides and contribute to the strong binding of AMD to DNA. Based on model building, the cyclic peptides were suggested to lie in the minor grove of DNA. This was confirmed by structure determination of a model complex consisting of AMD and the self-complementary double helix DNA octamer d(GAAGCTTC), Figure 17.5. The numerous van der Waals interactions between the peptide side chains and DNA contribute considerably to the tight binding of AMD.

Daunorubicin (**17.24**), daunomycin, and *doxorubicin* (**17.25**), adriamycin, are both anthracycline antibiotics isolated from various *Streptomyces* species. The compounds are unstable in alkaline and acidic aqueous solution and cannot be given orally. Although daunorubicin and doxorubicin have very similar chemical structures, doxorubicin is more cytotoxic and has a wider spectrum of antitumor activity. The reasons for these differences in activity are not quite clear. Both drugs bind tightly to DNA with comparable association constants (ca. $10^5 M^{-1}$). The differences in potency and clinical use may be due to differences in cellular pharmacokinetics, uptake, transport and distribution of the drugs.

Doxorubicin has the broadest range of clinical usefulness of the anticancer drugs in routine clinical use and has established activity against several solid tumors, which earlier were relatively unresponsive to chemotherapy. Daunorubicin is primarily used to treat acute leukemia. The side effects of the two anthracycline drugs are similar, e.g. nausea and vomiting, alopecia, myelosuppression and cardiotoxicity (cardiomyopathy). The cardiotoxicity, which is the most serious side effect limiting the doses and the duration of the treatment, is connected to the quinone moiety of the aromatic ring system, which, after reduction to a semi-quinone radical species, induces lipid peroxidation by a free radical mechanism. The involvment of iron has been suggested, and iron-chelators are considered for use as cardioprotective agents against doxorubicin-mediated cardiotoxicity. In addition, thousands of analogs have been synthesized and tested in order to find effective drugs without – or with lower – cardiotoxicity.

The anthracyclines daunorubicin and doxorubicin have a characteristic four-ring structure (rings A–D), the aglycon chromophore, which is linked, via a glycoside bond, to an amino sugar, daunosamine. The rings B–D constitute the anthracycline

Daunomycin (**17.24**) R = H
Adriamycin (**17.25**) R = OH

Mitoxanthrone (**17.26**)

$R_1 = R_2 = NHCH_2CH_2NHCH_2CH_2OH$

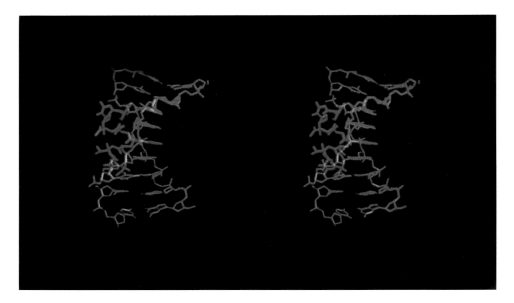

Figure 17.5 Stereoview of the AMD-d(GAAGCTTC) complex. The AMD molecule is shown in magenta, the DNA octamer in green. This side view of the complex shows the intercalation of the chromofore in the G5C5 site and the cyclic peptides of AMD in the minor groove. The structure was generated using the program SYBYL with co-ordinates from Protein Data Bank.

nucleus. The only difference between the structures of the two drugs is in the C-9 side chain of ring A, doxorubicin being the C-14 hydroxy derivative of daunorubicin.

The interaction of anthracycline drugs with DNA by intercalation has been demonstrated by several methods. Detailed information on the daunorubicin-DNA interactions has been obtained from X-ray structure determinations of several model complexes, e.g. of daunorubicin co-crystallized with the self-complementary DNA hexamer d(CGTACG). The six-base pair fragment of the double helix of DNA binds two molecules of daunorubicin (plus several water molecules and two sodium ions). The structure of part of this model compound is shown in Figure 17.6, which focuses on four base pairs of the hexamer with daunorubicin intercalated.

In the model complex, the planar anthracycline part of the daunorubicin molecule is squeezed in between the layers of C–G base pairs of the right-handed DNA double helix (B-DNA), at the CpG sites of both ends of the hexamer duplex (cf. the structure of the doxorubicin–DNA hexamer complex shown in Figure 17.7). The long axis of the anthracycline aglycon is almost perpendicular to the direction of the base pair hydrogen bonds. This is in contrast to model complexes of other drugs, e.g. *proflavine* in complex with the dinucleotide d(CpG), where the long axis is parallel to the base pairs (parallel overlap). As a result of the non-parallel intercalation of the daunorubicin aglycon, the amino sugar ring is placed in the

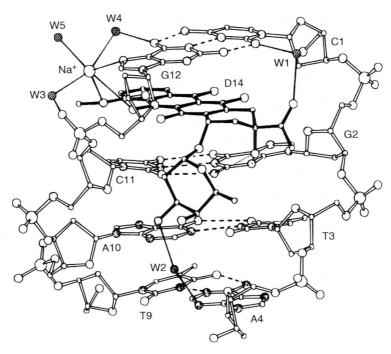

Figure 17.6 Diagram of daunomycin (D14) intercalated into the DNA hexamer. Four base pairs are shown (G12:C1, C11:G2, A10:T3, and T9:A4). Hydrogen bonds in base pairs are represented by dashed lines, other hydrogen bonds by dotted lines (those involving O-9) or thin lines (those involving bridging water molecules, W1 and W2). From Wang, H.-J. *et al.* (1987) *Biochemistry*, **26**, 1152 , with permission by The American Chemical Society.

minor groove of DNA, while the ring D of the anthracycline moiety protrudes on the major groove side. The distance between the base pairs of the intercalation site is increased from the normal 3.4 to 6.8 Å, and this can be achieved by adjusting the torsion angles of the phosphate ester backbones, resulting in a slightly distorted DNA fragment (unwinding of the DNA double helix).

The model complex shows that the cyclohexene ring A of the daunorubicin aglycon is almost planar, with the exception of C-9, which is displaced in the same direction as the amino sugar relative to the plane of the aglycon. This arrangement, in combination with the axially placed hydroxyl group at C-9, gives rise to several specific hydrogen bonding interactions, which stabilize the binding of daunorubicin. The hydroxyl oxygen atom O-9 is involved in two hydrogen bonds, both to nitrogen atoms of the guanine base G2 below the intercalator. Another hydrogen bonding system is seen on the other side of the aglycon ring system involving the C-13 oxygen atom O-13. This carbonyl oxygen is hydrogen bonded via a water molecule (W1) to a carbonyl oxygen atom of the cytosine ring C1 in the base pair above the intercalator. In this way, the OH group and the side chain at C-9 of ring A together serves as an anchor for the daunorubicin molecule and

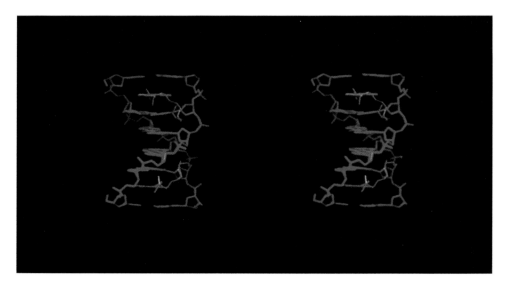

Figure 17.7 A stereoview of the adriamycin-d(CGATCG) complex. The two antibiotic molecules are shown in green, the DNA hexamer in red. The structure was generated using the program SYBYL with co-ordinates from Protein Data Bank.

contributes considerably to the stability of the binding complex, in addition to the 'stacking forces' at the intercalation site.

The amino sugar portion of daunorubicin is held in a proper orientation by the hydrogen bonding system of the C-9 substituents. It fits snugly into the minor groove, but this position excludes any interaction between the positively charged amino group of the sugar ring and the negatively charged phosphate oxygen atoms of the backbone. The X-ray results show that the sugar ring is very mobile, probably due to the lack of strong specific hydrogen bonding as well as ionic interactions. It is believed that the amino sugar is the recognition site for the enzyme topoisomerase II during the process leading to the formation of a ternay DNA–drug–enzyme complex and ultimately to enzyme-mediated DNA cleavage.

Several X-ray structures of the model complexes have now been determined. The model complexes consisting of the DNA hexamer d(CGATCG) and dauno-rubicin and doxorubicin, respectively, are almost isostructural. In both structures, the anthracycline antibiotic intercalate with d(CpG) as the intercalation site, indi-cating some sequence specificity of the drugs. Theoretical as well as experimental studies indicate that the third base pair is also of importance and should preferably be an A–T base pair (triplet recognition). In the doxorubicin complex, the O-14 hydroxyl group is hydrogen bonded to a nearby phosphate group via a water molecule.

Structure–activity studies, involving numerous synthetic, semisynthetic as well as natural anthracycline analogs, have been performed with the aim of finding structural analogs with reduced toxicity and/or a wider spectrum of activity. The testing for anticancer activity of compounds with modifications in the amino sugar moiety showed relatively low limitations for structural variations in this part of the drug molecule. The chirality of the 4′-position can be changed, *epirubicin* (4′-epidoxorubicin) has antitumor activity comparable to doxorubicin and is in clinical use. The compound has reduced cardiotoxicity when compared to doxorubicin, probably due to a more extensive metabolism (conversion to the 4′-O-beta-D-glucuronide). *Idarubicin* (4-demethoxydaunorubicin) is a highly potent antileukemic drug. A notable property of this analog is represented by its rate of cell uptake, which is distinctly higher when compared with that of the parent 4-methoxylated compound daunorubicin.

The presence of a cationic charge on the sugar ring connected to the aglycon seems to be of importance. Acylation of the amino group leads to markedly lower potency as is the case when the amino group is replaced by a hydroxy group. In all anthracycline aminoglycosides reported earlier, the amino sugar was invariably directly attached to the aglycone. However, recently a 'third generation' doxorubicin analog (MEN 10755) was reported with a disaccharide attached to the aglycone, in which the dounosamine is the second sugar ring. This compound has shown very promising antiproliferative activity when tested in a spectrum of human tumors and is undergoing clinical trials. The design of disaccharide compounds was based on the consideration that extension of the sugar moiety might increase the capacity of the topoisomerase enzyme to recognize the DNA–drug complex, and actually increased enzyme-mediated DNA cleavage was observed using MEN 10755 and enzyme preparations *in vitro*.

The anticancer agent, *mitoxanthrone* (**17.26**), is an aminoalkyl-substituted anthraquinone, i.e. a derivative in which the amino sugar, as well as ring A, are replaced by side chains with several possibilities for hydrogen bonding and protonation (hydroxy and amino functions). X-ray structure determination of a mitoxantrone–nucleotide model complex has not been published, but computer modeling and energy calculations have shown that this compound, as well as several analogs, can also bind intercalatively with DNA, and that the aminoalkyl substituents are used to anchor the molecules. Mitoxanthrone is an example of a drug designed on the basis of knowledge on drug–DNA interactions obtained from model complexes.

The methoxy group on C-4 of ring D of the anthracyclines is not required for anticancer activity, idarubicin is, as mentioned, a highly active compound. This is in accordance with the model, which shows that ring D protrudes out into the major groove without direct interaction with the DNA helix. *Carminomycin*, in which the methoxy group is replaced with an OH group, also has antitumor activity. The hydroquinone system is more sensitive to structural changes. The overlap of the rings B and C with base pairs is relatively small, but the oxygen atoms on each side of the rings may play a stabilizing role by being stacked with the bases. Methylation of the hydroxy groups results in loss of potency and lower affinity to DNA.

The geometry and substitutions of ring A are most important for the activity of anthracycline antibiotics. This is in full agreement with the model, which shows that this part anchors the molecules by hydrogen bonding to the bases on either side of the intercalator. The chirality at C-9 and C-7 cannot be changed without loss of activity. Substitution of the C-9 hydroxy group with a methyl group also leads to inactive compounds, and when the hydroxy group is removed, compounds with reduced affinity to DNA and lowered anticancer efficacy are obtained. Ring A cannot be 9,10-dehydrogenated without loss of activity, probably because the proper 'sofa'-conformation of this ring is thereby hindered. The C-9 side chain has to be of small size and with one or two oxygen atoms, which can provide for the hydrogen bonding to the base pair above the intercalator molecule.

Several drug design studies are aimed at developing sequence-specific DNA intercalators, e.g. *bis*-intercalators in which two intercalating ligands are bridged by a central linking chain, in order to obtain specific effects and stronger binding to DNA. Such compounds might become of interest in gene therapy.

17.1.1.5 Antisense agents

Nucleic acids are the targets for the so-called antisense agents, which are under design and development for e.g. anticancer and antivirus chemotherapy. The antisense gene-targeted therapeutic approach is a new and emerging technique, for selective manipulation of gene activity. In this technique an 'antisense' sequence (inverted piece of the gene code) complementary to the coding strand is used to specifically lock unto potentially dangerous genetic messengers, canceling their ability to do harm. The bad gene could be a cancer-causing oncogene, and this is one of the potential roles of antisense agents in cancer therapy.

Antisense agents normally target the gene's messenger RNA (mRNA), as they are designed to bind with and block the specific piece corresponding to the bad gene on DNA (Figure 17.8). Translation of the genetic information is thereby blocked, and the ribosomal production of the corresponding protein is prevented (the antisense strategy). Alternatively, it is possible to use the double-stranded DNA as target. In this case, the compounds (oligonucleotides, 'oligos') are called anti-gene agents, as they block the gene by binding directly to DNA, forming a local triple helix (the antigene approach).

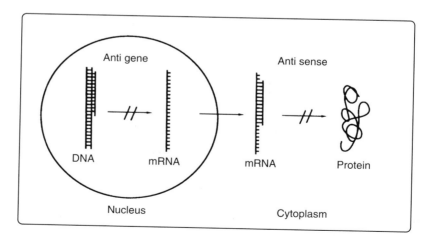

Figure 17.8 Schematic illustration of the antisense/antigene DNA principle. (The drawing was kindly provided by Professor Peter E. Nielsen, Research Center for Medical Bio-technology, University of Copenhagen, Denmark).

The major technical problems in using antisense/antigene agents as drugs are to figure out (1) how to penetrate into the cells; (2) how to prevent degradation of the oligos by nucleases; and (3) how to obtain effective binding to the target. Improvement of stability and cellular uptake of oligos have been obtained by chemical changes in the phosphodiester group. In addition, it appears that oligos with 10–15 bases are able to effectively block a gene.

Peptide nucleic acids (PNAs) are nucleic acid mimics showing a promising potential as gene-specific drugs. The PNAs are oligonucleotides in which the backbone is replaced by a peptide-like backbone of N-(2-aminoethyl)glycine units that bind with high affinity to complementary sequences of DNA and RNA. The PNAs are easy to prepare, water soluble and stable at biological conditions. The main problem is that PNAs does not readily enter the cells. The cellular uptake of PNA might be facilitated by conjugation to carrier molecules or incorporation into liposomes, and then the basis for the development of gene-specific drugs of decisive value in gene chemotherapy seems to be very good. Oligonucleotides with other modifications of the nucleotide backbone are currently being developed, e.g. phosphorothioates with a sulphur atom substituting one of the non-bridging oxygen atoms, and locked nucleic acids (LNAs) consisting of 2'-O, 4'-C methylene bicyclonucleotides, i.e. with a 'locked' normal backbone.

The new approach in anticancer, antibacterial and antivirus research, based on mRNA (or duplex DNA) as the primary drug target, is very promising and might lead to the desired goal in chemotherapy: selective cell death.

17.1.2   Drugs interfering with DNA synthesis

A number of different enzymes are involved in the synthesis of DNA and these are potential targets for anticancer (as well as antibacterial and antiviral) drug action. Inhibitors of these enzymes, which also often are called antimetabolites, block more or less crucial steps in DNA synthesis. Most of the drugs so far used in cancer chemotherapy were found by routine screening of the compounds and their mechanism of action was established later. Now, several of the structures of the enzymes involved in DNA synthesis are known from X-ray structure determinations, and new drugs are being designed and developed using this knowledge (structure-based drug design). Anticancer agents with effect as inhibitors of enzymes involved in DNA synthesis are specific for the S-phase of the cell cycle.

17.1.2.1   Inhibition of tetrahydrofolate synthesis

Folic acid analogs have for many years been used in the chemotherapy of infectious and neoplastic diseases. These drugs act by inhibiting the enzyme dihydrofolate reductase (DHFR). This enzyme, which is widely distributed in nature (from bacteria, protozoa and plants to man), converts dihydrofolic acid to tetrahydrofolic acid in the presence of NADPH as a cofactor (Scheme 17.8).

The DHFR is one of the enzymes that has been most thoroughly studied, and the 3D-structure of the protein is known from X-ray structure determinations of DHFR from many different origins (e.g. *E. coli*, *L. casei*, chicken and man). Some of the structures are known both without and with inhibitor and/or cofactor

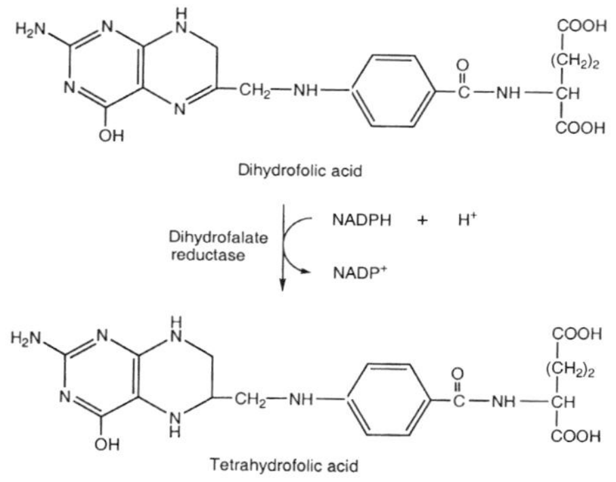

Dihydrofolic acid

Dihydrofalate reductase

NADPH + H⁺

NADP⁺

Tetrahydrofolic acid

Scheme 17.8

(NADPH) bound to the enzyme in a binary or ternary complex, showing the interactions between the drug and its 'receptor' (the biomacromolecule). Some of the inhibitors of DHFR have become useful in the treatment of cancer, e.g. *methotrexate*, others as antibacterial drugs, e.g. *trimethoprim*, while *pyrimethamine* is used as an antimalarial drug. Only the anticancer drug methotrexate is discussed in more detail. The other drugs will be mentioned for comparison in an attempt to understand the differential use of the drugs.

Methotrexate (**17.27**), MTX, is closely related to folic acid (Scheme 17.9), and the compound can be prepared synthetically. The MTX has a low aqueous solubility, and the risk of nephrotoxicity can be minimized in patients on high dose therapy by alkalinizing the urine. The MTX is widely used in cancer chemotherapy, most often in combination with other drugs. It has serious side effects, both acute effects,

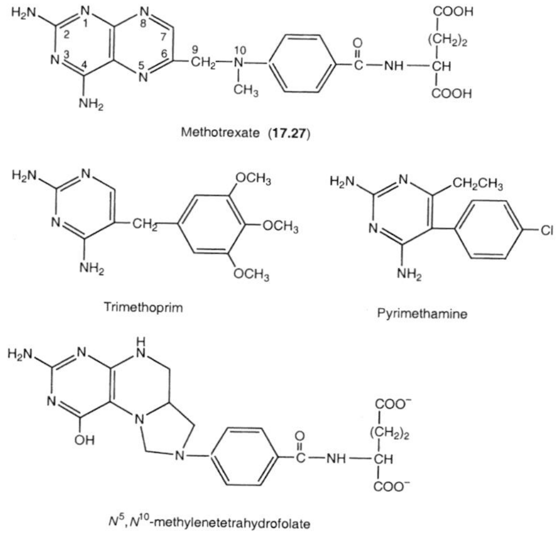

Methotrexate (**17.27**)

Trimethoprim

Pyrimethamine

N^5, N^{10}-methylenetetrahydrofolate

Scheme 17.9

e.g. ulceration, and delayed toxicities as bone marrow depression and – particularly with high doses – hepatic toxicity.

The MTX and other folic acid analogs are potent competitive inhibitors of DHFR ($K_i < 10^{-9}$ M). There are several consequences of inhibiting the synthesis of tetrahydrofolate, since this compound is further converted *in vivo* to N^5, N^{10}-methylenetetrahydrofolate (methylene-THF, Scheme 17.9), which functions as a cofactor for various enzymes involved in one-carbon transfer reactions, e.g. for the enzyme thymidylate synthase (cf. Figure 17.12). The most critical effect leading to cell death after exposure to MTX is probably the indirect inhibition of the action of thymidylate synthase and thereby blocking of the production of deoxythymidylate, which is required for the synthesis of DNA. The MTX·is actively transported into the cells, and the ability of various tumor cells to transport MTX seems to be related to their ability to respond to the drug. Increased cellular content of DHFR due to increased rate of enzyme synthesis is probably the main reason for resistance to MTX.

The amino acid sequences for a number of DHFRs (i.e. enzymes from several different sources) have been determined, and, as expected, they have common features. The sequence identity between enzymes from different vertebrates is in the region of 75–90%, between the vertebrate enzymes and the bacterial enzymes, on the other hand, only about 20–30%. Nevertheless, X-ray crystallographic studies of the DHFRs have shown that there is a high degree of resemblance in the folding of the main chains of these enzymes. As an example of this, the tertiary structures of DHFR from chicken liver and from *E. coli* are shown in Figure 17.9.

Common to these, and other known DHFR structures, is a central 8-stranded β-sheet area with the strands denoted βA–H. In addition, the molecules contain four helical regions, αB, αC, αE and αF. The molecules have a bi-lobed appearance, as the active site forms a 15 Å deep cleft in the central part of the molecule between the B and C helices. The width of this cleft has been observed to be 1.5–2.0 Å greater in the vertebrate enzymes than that in the bacterial enzymes. In addition to that, the foldings mostly differ in the loop areas at the surface of the enzyme. Nevertheless, it seems evident that the structural differences between enzymes are responsible for the highly selective inhibition of *E. coli* DHFR exhibited by trimethoprim and the particular selectivity of pyrimethamine for DHFR of the malarial protozoan *Plasmodium berghei*. Recently, the structure of the fungal pathogen *Pneumocystis carnii* DHFR has been determined, and structure-based drug design is in progress. Development of selective drugs is important, because this infective agent is critical to AIDS patients, causing the severe pneumonia that is a major cause of death.

X-ray crystallographic studies of the enzyme–inhibitor complex of e.g. DHFR from *E. coli* and MTX show the binding interactions between drug and protein (Figure 17.10A). As it appears from the figure, there are good contacts to side chains of amino acids at the active site of the protein. The pteridine ring interacts with Asp-27 through the electrostatic interactions at N-1 and the 2-amino group (salt bridges or 'charge-assisted' hydrogen bonds). The pKa value for N-1 of MTX has been shown to be much higher in the complex than in free MTX (10 and 5.7, respectively), which implies that in the complex, the pteridine ring is protonated at physiological pH. In addition to inhibitor binding, Asp-27 appears to play an

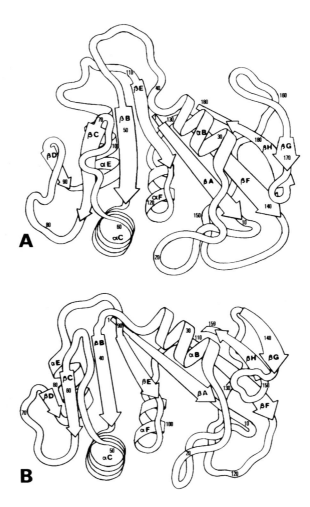

Figure 17.9 Schematic illustration of the folding of the main chain, A of chicken liver, and B of *E. coli* DHFR (From Beddell, C.R. in *X-Ray Crystallography and Drug Action*, eds. A.S. Horn and C.J. De Ranter, Oxford University Press, Oxford 1984 with permission by Oxford University Press).

important functional role in the reduction of the enzyme substrate. The 4-amino group of the pteridine ring is hydrogen bonded to backbone carbonyl groups behind the drug (not shown). The α-carboxylic group of the glutamate moiety of MTX is involved in strong hydrogen bonding (charge-assisted) with the guanidinium group of Arg-57, whereas the γ-carboxylic group is not directly bonded to the protein. The benzene moiety of MTX is sandwiched between Ile-50 and Leu-28 forming hydrophobic (or van der Waals) contacts to these residues.

In Figure 17.10B, the X-ray structure of the trimethoprim (TMP) complex with *E. coli* DHFR is illustrated. As it can be seen, there are qualitative similarities between the binding of the two drugs, MTX and TMP. The 2,4-diamino-

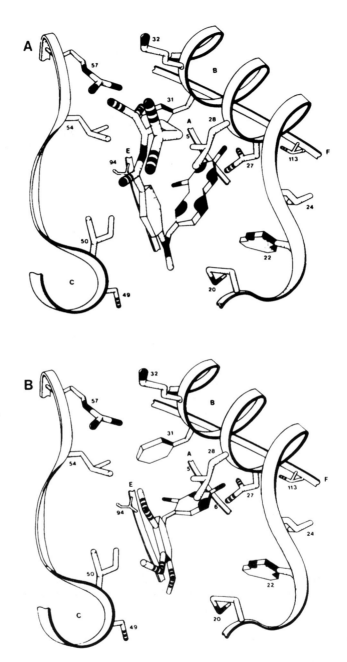

Figure 17.10 Schematic illustration of the active site of *E. coli* DHFR; A with bound methotrexate, and B with bound trimethoprim. Selected atoms of drugs and protein side chains are highlighted: oxygen by stripes, nitrogen in black, and sulphur by hatching. (From Beddell, C.R. – see legend to Figure 17.9).

pyrimidine rings bind in the same manner, the benzene rings are involved in hydrophobic interactions, and charged-assisted hydrogen bonds are formed to Asp-27 in both cases. However, TMP does not have a carboxylic group and cannot interact electrostatically with Arg-57. On the other hand, the trimethoxyphenyl ring fits very favorably into the more narrow active site cleft of *E. coli* DHFR. The relatively subtle structural differences are apparently largely responsible for the 3000-fold difference in affinity of TMP for *E. coli* DHFR compared to the chicken liver enzyme.

The structure of the *E. coli* DHFR-TMP complex has been used for modeling studies with the aim of designing analogs of TMP with higher affinities for the enzyme. This study is a very early example of structure-based drug design. The TMP analogs in which one *meta*-methoxy group was replaced by carbalkoxy substituents of varying lengths were designed (Scheme 17.10). Modeling experiments using computer graphics indicated that the compound with five methylene groups in the chain was able to interact particularly well with Arg-57 in the same way as methotrexate.

The compounds were synthesized and tested for enzyme affinity, and the compound with five methylene groups was found to be most active. X-ray structure determination of *E. coli* DHFR complexed with this carbalkoxy analog was performed in order to determine the actual position of the analog in the active site. The study shows that the compound actually is binding as modeled (Figure 17.11). Because of unfavorable biopharmaceutical properties this analog did not become a new antibacterial drug, but similar analogs are being developed.

Other methods, e.g. classical QSAR, have been used for rational design and analysis of inhibitors of DHFR. However, the most obvious approach to the design of novel inhibitors is the utilization of the 3D-structures of the enzyme. With detailed knowledge of the structure of the enzymes of different origin (vertebrate, bacterial, fungal etc.), the opportunities for rational design of selective inhibitors are optimal.

17.1.2.2 Inhibition of purine and pyrimidine synthesis

Analogs of purine and pyrimidine block one or more steps in the purine/ pyrimidine synthesis. Both categories of compounds have to be converted in the cells into the corresponding nucleotides before they become active. Several analogs of purine and pyrimidine nucleotides are important as antiviral agents and are discussed in Chapter 16.

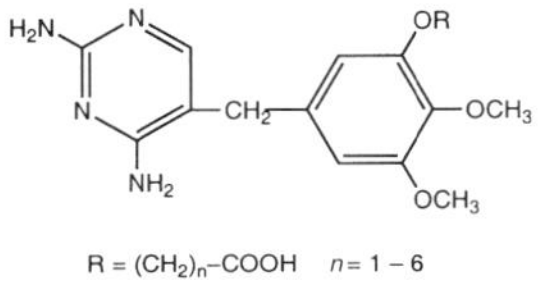

$R = (CH_2)_n-COOH$ $n = 1 - 6$

Scheme 17.10

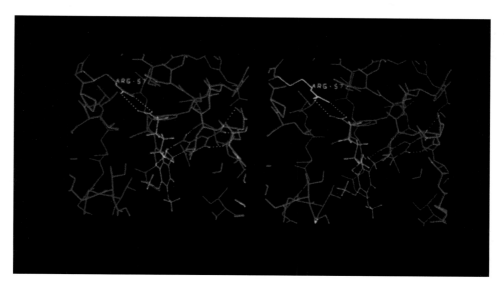

Figure 17.11 The active site of *E. coli* DHFR with an carbalkoxy analog of trimethoprim bound (C, green; H, white; N, blue; O, red). (From Hitchings, G.H. *et al.* in *Design of Enzyme Inhibitors as Drugs*, eds. M. Sandler and H.J. Smith. Oxford University Press, Oxford 1989, with permission by Oxford University Press.

6-mercaptopurine (17.28)   6-thioguanine (17.29)   5-fluorouracil (17.30)

6-Mercaptopurine (**17.28**), 6-MP, and *6-thioguanine* (**17.29**), 6-TG, are purine analogs, which can be given orally, and are used in the treatment of leukemias. Bone marrow depression is the principal toxic effect of both drugs. Allopurinol can be given to inhibit xanthine oxidase degradation of 6-MP into thiouric acid, thereby preventing renal damage.

The 6-MP acts as a normal substrate for the enzyme hypoxanthine–guanine phosphoribosyl transferase and is thus converted into the nucleotide 6-mercaptopurine ribose phosphate (6-MPRP). This nucleotide interferes with an early step in the purine biosynthesis by inhibiting the enzyme phosphoribosylpyrophosphate (PRPP) amidotransferase. In addition, several other enzymatic pathways are inhibited, and cell death may be the result of a combination of different events. The 6-TG is also converted *in vivo* to the nucleotide (6-TGRP), but it has a much weaker inhibitory effect on the enzymes involved in purine synthesis, e.g. the amidotransferase. The cytotoxic action of 6-TG seems to be primarily due to incorporation into DNA of the nucleotide 6-TGRP after further phosphorylation into the triphosphate.

Fluorouracil (**17.30**), 5-FU, is a synthetically prepared pyrimidine analog with a close structural relationship to the natural base uracil. The drug can be given orally, e.g. as the orally formulated drug tegafur/uracil (UFT), which is a combination of uracil and tegafur (5-FU linked to a dehydroxylated ribose sugar ring, that is hydroxylated *in vivo* by hepatic enzymes leading to a slow but sustained level of 5-FU in the cells). The 5-FU is effective against several types of solid tumors. In combination with oxaliplatin (**17.21**), 5-FU is now successfully used in the treatment of colorectal cancer. The 5-FU has severe side effects, both acute and delayed.

Like the thiopurines, 5-FU has to be converted *in vivo* into a nucleotide, 5-fluoro-2′-deoxyuridine-5′-monophosphate (FdUMP), before it becomes active as a cytotoxic drug. This conversion can be accomplished via different pathways involving various enzymes, and resistance to 5-FU might be due to decreased activity of some of these enzymes.

The FdUMP blocks DNA synthesis by inhibition of the enzyme thymidylate synthase (TS). This enzyme catalyzes the conversion of dUMP into dTMP, which subsequently is incorporated into DNA (Figure 17.12). The FdUMP inhibits the enzyme irreversibly after acting as a normal substrate through part of the catalytic cycle. First, a sulphhydryl group of the enzyme (cysteine-SH) reacts with C-6 of FdUMP (Scheme 17.11). The cofactor methylene-THF then adds to C-5, and, in the case of the substrate dUMP, a proton is removed from C-5 of the bound nucleotide. However, the C–F bond of the bound inhibitor FdUMP cannot be broken, and the catalysis is blocked at the stage where a ternary covalent complex is formed, consisting of enzyme, FdUMP and cofactor.

This mechanism has been confirmed by the X-ray structure determinations of TS from several sources, e.g. *E. coli*, *L. casei*, and human TS, both with and without

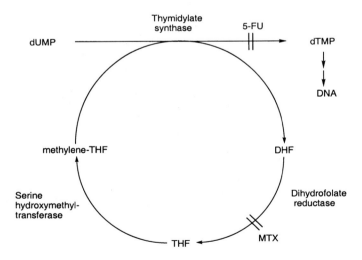

Figure 17.12 Schematic representation of the conversion of dUMP (deoxyuridine monophosphate) into dTMP (deoxythymidine monophosphate). DHF = dihydrofolate, THF = tetrahydrofolate, and methylene-THF = N^5N^{10}-methylenetetrahydrofolate. Fluorouracil (5-FU) inhibits the methylation of dUMP, and MTX blocks the regeneration of THF from DHF.

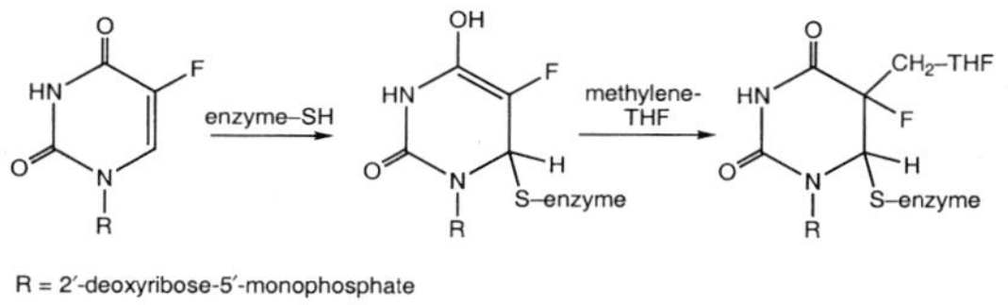

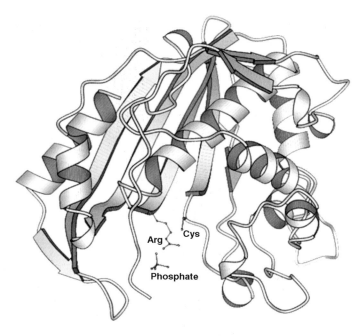

R = 2'-deoxyribose-5'-monophosphate

Scheme 17.11

inhibitor and/or cofactor or cofactor analog. In the native enzyme, the cysteine residue that reacts with C-6 of FdUMP is situated in the active site cleft with hydrogen bonding to an arginine residue (Figure 17.13) and is thereby activated (more nucleophilic). In complexes with inhibitor (or substrate) and cofactor (or cofactor analog), covalent bonds connect the inhibitor with enzyme and cofactor (short distances are observed, Figures 17.14 and 17.15).

The 5-FU has been used in cancer treatment for more than 40 years. However, TS is still an attractive target for anticancer drugs because of its central position in the pathway of DNA synthesis. Co-administration of leucovorin (5-formyl-THF) is now frequently used. Leucovorin is rapidly converted *in vivo* to 5-methyl-THF and further to methylene-THF. Excess of this cofactor ensures the tight binding of FdUMP to the enzyme, the result being optimal inhibition of TS and increased cytotoxic effect of 5-FU.

Figure 17.13 Ribbon representation of the folding of the main chain of TS. Two important residues and a bound phosphate ion in the active site cleft are shown. The figure is generated using the program Molscript with co-ordinates from Protein Data Bank.

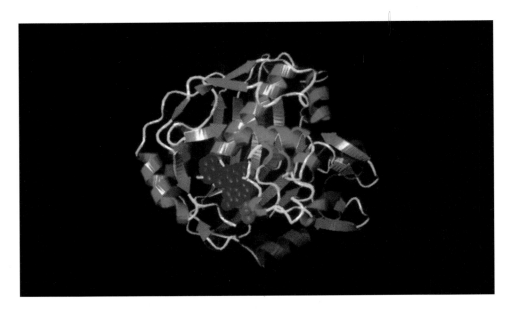

Figure 17.14 The structure of TS of *E. coli* with substrate (in magenta) and co-factor analog (in blue) bound in active site. The structure was generated using the program 'O' with co-ordinates from Protein Data Bank.

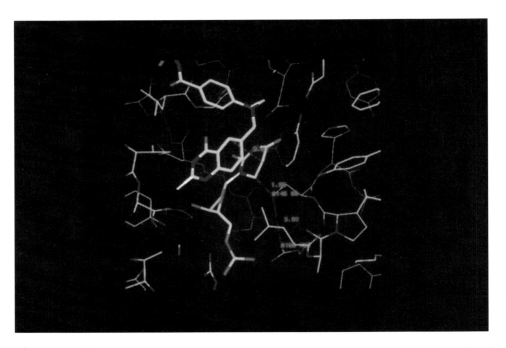

Figure 17.15 The active site of TS with substrate and co-factor analog bound (N, blue; O, red). Dashed lines indicate short distances. The structure was generated using the program 'O' with co-ordinates from Protein Data Bank.

Thymidylate synthase is extensively used for structure-based drug design. Several new cofactor analogs are being developed, some of them very promising and in clinical testing. Also other advanced computer methods are being used, e.g. screening of all compounds of a data base of commercial available compounds for molecules that fits to the active site of *L. casei* TS, using a molecular docking program (DOCK). In addition to retrieving the substrate and several known inhibitors, some previously unknown putative inhibitors were proposed, e.g. phenolphthalein analogs. These compounds, which were found to inhibit TS in the micromolar range, do not resemble the substrate dUMP. X-ray structure determinations of the TS-drug complexes showed that the compounds bind in the active site cleft at another binding region 6–9 Å displaced compared to the substrate. The phenolphthalein analogs are a novel family of tight-binding specific TS inhibitors, found by the use of the known target protein structure, which might lead to the development of new drugs in chemotherapy.

17.1.2.3 Inhibition of DNA/RNA polymerases

The DNA polymerases catalyze the step-by-step addition of deoxynucleotide units to the new DNA strand during DNA replication and are potential targets for anticancer and antiviral drug action. Very few inhibitors of DNA polymerases are in clinical use in cancer therapy, whereas several inhibitors (substrate analogs) have become useful in curing virus infections (see Chapter 16). The compounds are purine or pyrimidine analogs, and some of them are also incorporated into DNA.

Cytarabine (**17.31**), cytosine arabinoside, Ara-C, is a pyrimidine nucleoside analog with a structural change in the ribose ring. The drug is poorly absorbed orally, and it is routinely given intravenously or by continuous infusion methods because of rapid hepatic deamination by cytosine deaminase into inactive ara-U (uracil arabinoside). It is used primarily in the treatment of acute leukemias. The principal toxicities are nausea, vomiting, and bone marrow depression. Ara-C is converted *in vivo* into the active nucleotide triphosphate Ara-CTP by enzymes that treat Ara-C as a normal substrate. Ara-CTP is an analog of the deoxycytidine triphosphate substrate of DNA polymerase and inhibits this enzyme competitively. As a consequence, DNA synthesis and cell growth is inhibited. Resistance to Ara-C is probably associated with high levels of deaminase activity.

Cytarabine (**17.31**)   Vidarabine (**17.32**)

Vidarabine (**17.32**), adenine arabinoside, Ara-A, is a purine nucleoside analog with a similar mechanism of action as Ara-C, but this drug is primarily used as an antiviral agent. Structural modifications of Ara-A and Ara-C, as well as co-administration of a deaminase inhibitor, have been used in order to avoid inactivation of the drugs.

17.1.2.4 *Inhibition of ribonucleotide reductase*

The enzyme *ribonucleotide reductase* (RNR) is an essential component of all living cells. The function of the enzyme is to participate in the synthesis of DNA by catalyzing the conversion of all of the four ribonucleotides into the corresponding deoxyribonucleotides, see Scheme 17.12. This is the only pathway for the formation of deoxyribonucleotides, and the reaction is believed to be a rate limiting step in DNA synthesis. Consequently, RNR is an obvious target for anticancer as well as antibacterial and antiviral drug action. The only RNR inhibitor in clinical use is *hydroxyurea*, but other compounds are in clinical trial. Design and development of selective antiviral agents will also be possible, as some viruses (e.g. herpes simplex virus, HSV) code for their own enzyme system. Structural differences between host and virus enzymes exist and are being utilized in drug design.

Hydroxyurea (**17.33**), *N*-hydroxyurea, hydrea, is a crystalline compound, which is routinely given orally, as it is water soluble and well absorbed from the gastro-intestinal tract. It is excreted very rapidly and has to be given in very high and

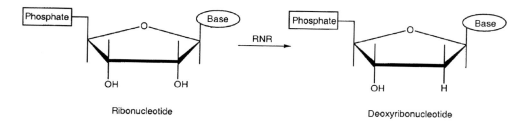

Ribonucleotide   Deoxyribonucleotide

Scheme 17.12

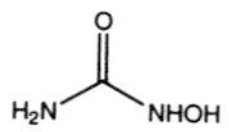

Hydroxyurea (**17.33**)

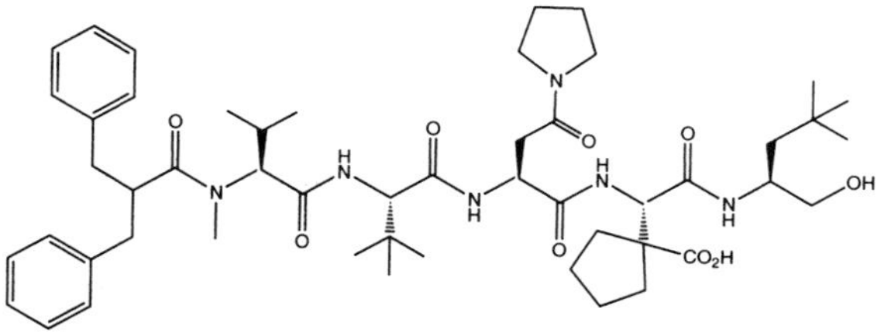

BILD 1263 (**17.34**)

frequent doses. Hydroxyurea is primarily used to treat chronic myelogenous leukemia, but has also demonstrated activity in malignant melanoma and other solid tumors. The acute side effects are mild and bone-marrow depression is the dose-limiting toxicity. Recently, hydroxyurea has been introduced in the treatment of HIV-1 infection because of its inhibitory action in viral replication and to its potentialization of the activitiy of the nucleosides, e.g. AZT (cf. Chapter 16).

Hydroxyurea inhibits RNR by interfering with the smaller of the two proteins, of which the enzyme consists (protein R2, Figure 17.16). R2 is unusual in containing a free radical group (a tyrosyl radical), which is essential for catalysis. This radical is destroyed (reduced to a normal tyrosine residue) by hydroxyurea, and the enzyme function is thereby prevented. Hydroxyurea is an iron chelator, but the iron centers of protein R2 are not affected by the drug. The function of the iron is to generate and stabilize the free radical group.

Studies on analogs of hydroxyurea have indicated that inhibitors of this type (radical scavengers) have to be rather small molecules. X-ray structure determination of protein R2 of the *E. coli* and mammalian enzymes has shown that the tyrosyl radical (and iron center) is buried in a hydrophobic pocket in R2 of *E. coli*, whereas it is more accessible in R2 of the mammalian RNR. The structure of the

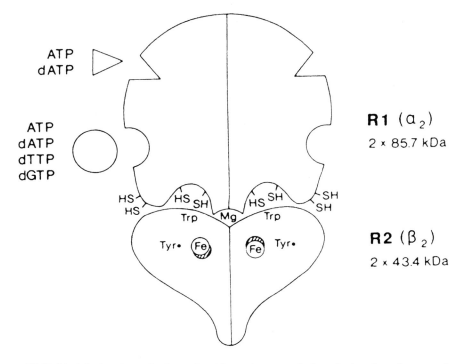

Figure 17.16 Model drawing of ribonucleotide reductase of *E. coli* showing the two homodimeric proteins, R1 and R2, the effector sites and the redox-active sulphhydryl groups on R1, and the iron centers and tyrosyl radicals on R2. (The drawing was kindly provided by Professor Britt-Marie Sjöberg, Department of Molecular Biology, University of Stockholm, Sweden).

R1 subunit of *E. coli* RNR has also been determined, and the R1R2 holoenzyme complex has been modeled on the basis of the two separate protein structures (Figure 17.17).

The carboxy terminal of R2 is known to be involved in the R1R2 association. Consequently, peptidomimetics, i.e. analogs of oligopeptides with amino acid sequences corresponding to the carboxy terminal of the R2 subunit of RNR of HSV, have been developed as selective antivirus agents. These compounds inhibit the enzyme by interfering with the interphase between the subunits, thereby preventing association of the subunits. BILD 1263 (**17.34**) was the first HSV R1R2 subunit association inhibitor published with antiviral activity *in vivo*. Other peptidomimetics are being developed, including cyclic peptide inhibitors, with effect on the mammalian RNR where the R2 carboxy terminal is different. Disruption of protein–protein interactions is a relatively new strategy of inhibitor design for the development of chemotherapeutic agents.

17.2 MITOTIC APPARATUS AS TARGET FOR DRUGS

The mitotic inhibitors act by interfering with the mitosis of cells and thereby inducing mitotic arrest. Mitosis takes place during the M phase of the cell cycle, and drugs that prevent cell division by interfering with mitosis are M phase specific. Mitotic arrest is induced because of damage to the spindle apparatus. Consequently, the chromatides, which are separated in the metaphase, are prevented from being pulled toward opposite poles in the following anaphase.

The separate threads of the spindle apparatus are built as a microtubule system. Microtubules are hollow, cylindrical structures built up of the protein tubulin, which consists of two subunits, α- and β-tubulin, with very similar amino acid sequences. The cylinder consists of 13 rows of tubulin heterodimers, the protofilaments. The microtubule cylinder can also be regarded as consisting of a helical array of alternating α- and β-tubulin subunits (Figure 17.18). Most of the mitotic inhibitors disrupt microtubule assembly by binding with high affinity to tubulin. Some of the drugs have a common binding site (the *vinca alkaloids*) and others a different, but probably common, binding site (*podophyllotoxin* and *colchicine*). *Taxanes*, on the other hand, promote the assembly of tubulin to microtubules and prevent depolymerization by binding to tubulin at a separate site.

Microtubules are found as a ubiquitous substituent in cells and have several other functions than being elements in mitosis. Microtubules are part of the cytoskeleton, and take part in intracellular transport and communication. Some of the toxic side effects of the mitotic inhibitors may be due to disturbance of these phenomena.

17.2.1 Drugs interfering with the Vinca alkaloid binding site of tubulin

Vinblastine (**17.35**) and *vincristine* (**17.36**) are constituents of the Madagascar periwinkle *Vinca rosea* Linn. Vinblastine (VBL) is found in much larger quantity than

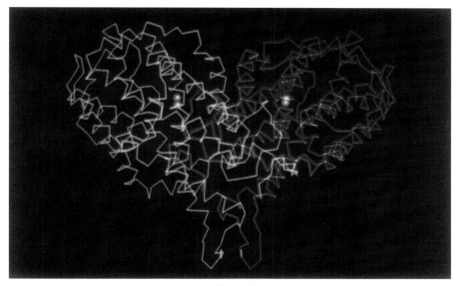

Plate (A)

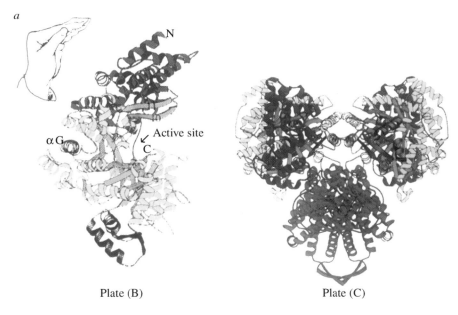

Plate (B)   Plate (C)

Figure 17.17 The structures of (A) protein R2 of *E. coli* RNR as the dimer (in green and magenta) with the iron atoms in red; (B) protein R1 of *E. coli* RNR as the monomer. The colors illustrate different domains of the protein; and (C) the R1R2 holoenzyme modeled on the basis of the separate X-ray structures of R1 and R2. The R2 dimer is colored in red. The figures were kindly provided by Professor Hans Eklund, Department of Molecular Biology, Biomedical Center, Uppsala, Sweden.

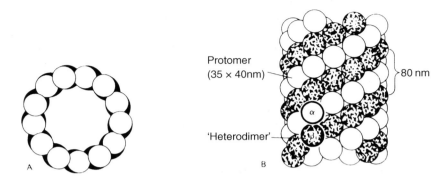

Figure 17.18 Schematic model of a microtubule, showing the pattern of tubulin subunits. A is a cross-sectional view showing the arrangement of the 13 protofilaments. B is a longitudinal view showing the surface lattice of α and β subunits. (From Bryan, J. (1974) *Fed. Proc.*, **33**, 152 with permission by the Federation of American Societies for Experimental Biology).

vincristine (VCR), but it is easily converted synthetically into the clinically more useful drug VCR (conversion of a methyl group into a formyl group). The VBL and VCR are used as the sulphates and are given intravenously because of bad and unpredictable absorption from the gastrointestinal tract. The compounds are highly irritating to tissue and great care has to be taken to avoid extravasation and contact with eyes. The dose-limiting toxicity of VBL is bone marrow depression, whereas VCR is considered to be bone marrow sparing compared to most anticancer drugs. Neurotoxicity is dose-limiting for VCR, on the other hand, while this is a less frequent and serious problem with VBL. The reasons for these differences in toxicity of the structurally very similar compounds are not fully understood.

The clinical use of the drugs is also different. The VCR is given in combination therapy to induce remission in acute lymphocytic leukemia of childhood, and it has actually revolutioned the therapy of this disease, as 90–100% of the patients are achieving complete remission. Very high percentages of remission are also achieved in the treatment of Hodgkin's disease with combinations of drugs including VCR or VBL. Both drugs are used in the treatment of several other cancer diseases.

Vinblastine (**17.35**) R = CH₃

Vincristine (**17.36**) R = CHO

The vinca alkaloids are known to bind to tubulin at a common binding site. As a result of this binding, the tubulin units cannot polymerize to form microtubules, a reversible reaction, which occurs in the presence of Mg^{2+} and GTP in addition to the microtubules-associated proteins (MAPs). Only when GTP is bound to tubulin the filament can grow, and only from one end (the plus end). Thus, the microtubules are in dynamic equilibrium with tubulin in cytosolic solution. When VBL (or VCR) is bound to tubulin, new GTP-tubulin units cannot be added to the filaments, and the growth is thereby prevented. Dissociation of tubulin units from the minus end can still occur, and the result is rapid disappearance of the spindle apparatus.

The binding site of the vinca alkaloids is located to the β-subunit of tubulin, but very little is known on the nature of the binding. In addition to the vinca alkaloids, compounds of other natural sources, and with quite different structures, share binding site with the vinca alkaloids. Some of these, e.g. the *dolastatin* peptides derived from a marine origin, are in clinical trials.

17.2.2 Drugs interfering with the colchicine binding site of tubulin

The two drugs mentioned below are not commonly used in cancer therapy, but are considered for comparison with the vinca alkaloids and the taxanes.

Podophyllotoxin (**17.37**) can be isolated from extracts of the roots of *Podophyllum peltatum* L. (American mandrake), and is primarily used in the treatment of condyloma. *Colchicine* (**17.38**) is the major alkaloid of the meadow saffron *Colchicum autumnale* L. It is an active antimitotic drug, but the toxicity of the compound has limited its use to the treatment of gout and related inflammatory disease states. However, analogs with lower toxicity are still being developed.

Like the vinca alkaloids, podophyllotoxin (PODO) and colchicine (COL) both inhibit mitosis by binding to tubulin and thereby preventing microtubule assembly. The two drugs share a common binding site, which is distinct from the VBL binding site. It has been proposed that, while VBL/VCR prevent longitudinal interactions between tubulin subunits, COL and PODO seem to prevent microtubule assembly by inhibiting lateral interactions between subunits in adjacent protofilaments. The binding of both COL and PODO to tubulin is tight, but, although practically irreversible, probably non-covalent in nature. Details on the nature of the bindings are not yet known.

Podophyllotoxin (**17.37**)   Colchicine (**17.38**)

17.2.3   Drugs stabilizing the assembly of tubulin into microtubules

Paclitaxel (**17.39**), taxol, is a plant product isolated from the cortex of the western yew *Taxus brevifolia*. The compound has a very low solubility in water, and this has caused serious problems related to its formulation. It is most often used as an emulsion with Cremophor EL (a polyethoxylated castor oil) as the surfactant, and taxol is now the trade-marked name of this formulation. However, the formulation is far from ideal and others are under investigation. The allergic reactions observed in some patients are probably caused by the solvent, but improved administration procedures, including premedication with glucocorticoides and antihistamines, have reduced this problem.

Another problem is the very low yield of paclitaxel from the cortex of *T. brevifolia*. However, the compound can be produced semisynthetically from a precursor that is obtained in higher yield. Paclitaxel is now in Phase III trials and in clinical use against ovarian cancer and breast cancer, but has also effect against a variety of other cancer diseases. The major side effect of paclitaxel, in addition to hyper-sensitivity, is neurotoxicity.

Paclitaxel is a taxane diterpenoid characterized by its ester side chain at C-13 (the *N*-benzoyl-*β*-phenylisoserine ester of the compound *baccatin III*) and by its oxetane ring D. The X-ray structure of paclitaxel has been determined, as well as of *docetaxel* (earlier taxotere that now is the trade-marked name for a formulation using Tween 80 as solvent). Docetaxel is a C-10 deacylated analog of paclitaxel with the *N*-benzoyl group replaced by a *tert*-butoxycarbonyl group. The structures clearly show a cup-like shape of the taxane skeleton (Figure 17.19). Docetaxel is also a promising anticancer drug and is progressing through clinical trials. Though very similar structures, there are significant differences in the pharmacology of the two agents.

Unlike other plant-derived antimitotic agents (colchicine, podophyllotoxin and the vinca alkaloids), which inhibit microtubule assembly, the taxanes actually promote the assembly of tubulin and stabilize the microtubules formed against depolymerization. The cytotoxicity is related to the microtubule-mediated inter-ruption of mitosis, resulting from distortion of the mitotic spindle.

The drugs bind to the *β*-subunit of tubulin, and an understanding of the binding of taxanes to microtubules has recently been obtained by the structure determin-ation of a tubulin-drug complex at low resolution (3.7 Å). Two-dimensional zinc-induced crystalline sheets of tubulin, stabilized by docetaxel, were obtained and studied by electron crystallography (Figure 17.20). The structure shows that the drug binds to *β*-tubulin in a pocket near to the lateral interaction between the

Taxol (**17.39**)

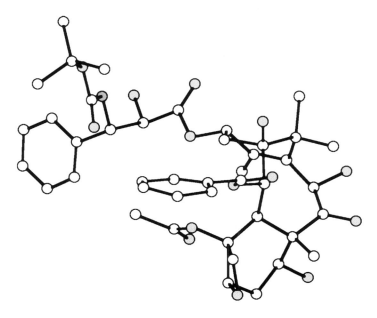

Figure 17.19 The X-ray structure of docetaxel (taxotere), generated using the program MacMimic with co-ordinates from Cambridge Structural Data Base. Oxygen atoms are light gray and nitrogen dark gray.

β-subunits. In this way, a strengthening of the lateral contacts and thereby stabilization of the protofilament adhesion may be obtained. In the α-subunit, the corresponding binding pocket is occupied by a loop, which is not present in β-tubulin. More detailed structures are still needed for the design of improved anticancer drugs.

However, some information on taxanes has been obtained indirectly by SAR studies. Beccatin III, without the ester side chain at C-13, is significantly less active than paclitaxel, indicating the importance of this side chain for the activity. An *N*-acyl group is required in the side chain (benzoyl in paclitaxel, and *tert*-butoxycarbonyl in docetaxel). Various paclitaxel analogs that lack the 3'-phenyl group of the side chain are significantly less active than paclitaxel. A free 2'-hydroxy group (or a hydrolysable ester) is required, and a change of the chirality at 2' and 3' leads to less active compounds.

Structural variations along the upper part (C-6–C-12) of the taxol molecule (e.g. acylation or removal of an OH group) do not greatly affect the bioactivity, suggesting that this region is not intimately involved in binding to tubulin. The lower part, on the other hand, including C-14, C-1–C-5 and the unusual oxetane ring at C-4–C-5, appears to be a region, which is crucial to the activity of taxol, as structural changes has major effects on activity. Opening of the oxetane ring with electrophilic reagents yields products, which are less active than paclitaxel, and also the benzoyloxy group at C-2 is required. The oxetane ring is relatively inert chemically, and it has been suggested that its role simply may be to act as a lock to maintain the

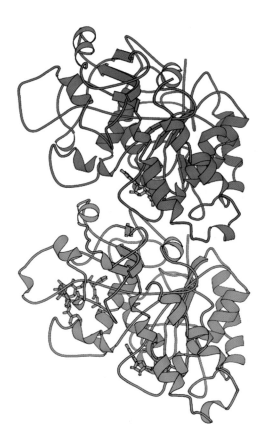

Figure 17.20 Ribbon drawing of the tubulin dimer showing the α subunit (in purple) with bound GTP (in gray) and the β subunit (in green) containing GDP (in gray) and taxotere (in red). The structure was obtained by electron crystallography and determined to 3.7 Å resolution. The figure is generated using the program Molscript with co-ordinates from Protein Data Bank.

conformation of the diterpenoid ring system of paclitaxel. The cup-like shape of the ring system is conserved in the known X-ray structures of taxanes.

FURTHER READING

Arcamone, F. (1984) Structure–activity relationships in antitumour anthracyclines. In *X-Ray Crystallography and Drug Action*, edited by A.S. Horn and C.J. De Ranter, pp. 367–388. Oxford: Clarendon Press.

Arcamone, F., Animati, F., Capranico, G., Lombardi, P., Pratesi, G., Manzini, S., Supino, R. and Zunino, F. (1997) New developments in antitumor anthracyclines. *Pharmacol. Ther.*, **76**, 117–124.

Boddy, A.V. and Yule, S.M. (2000) Metabolism and pharmacokinetics of oxazaphosphorines. *Clin. Pharmacokinet.*, **38**, 291–304.

Champness, J.N., Kuyper, L.F. and Beddell, C.R. (1986) Interaction between dihydrofolate reductase and certain inhibitors. In *Topics in Molecular Pharmacology*, Vol. 3, edited by A.S.V. Burgen, G.C.K. Roberts and M.S. Tute. Amsterdam: Elsevier.

Cody, V., Galitsky, N., Luft, J.R., Pangborn, W., Gangjee, A., Devraj, R., Queener, S.F. and Blakeley, R.L. (1997) Comparison of ternary complexes of pneumosystis carnii and wild-type human dihydrofolate reductase with coenzyme NADPH and a novel classical antitumor furo[2,3-d]pyrimidine antifolate. *Acta Cryst.*, D**53**, 638–649.

Cohen, J. (ed.) (1989) *Oligodeoxynucleotides Antisense Inhibitors of Gene Expressions*. London: The Macmillan Press.

Danenberg, P.V., Malli, H. and Swenson, S. (1999) Thymidylate synthase inhibitors. *Semin. Oncol.*, **26**, 621–631.

Dedon, P.C. and Goldberg, I.H. (1992) Free-radical mechanisms involved in the formation of sequence-dependent bistranded DNA lesions by the antitumor antibiotics bleomycin, neocarzinostatin, and calicheamicin. *Chem. Res. Toxicol.*, **5**, 311–332.

Friedman, O.M., Myles, A. and Colvin, M. (1979) Cyclophosphamide and related phosphoramide mustards. Current status and future prospects. In *Advances in Cancer Chemotherapy*, Vol. 4, edited by A. Rosowsky, pp. 143–204. New York: Marcel Dekker.

Hardy, L.W., Finer-Moore, J.S., Montfort, W.R., Jones, M.O., Santi, D.V. and Stroud, R.M. (1987) Atomic structure of thymidylate synthase. Target for rational drug design. *Science*, **235**, 448–455.

Hecht, S.M. (2000) Bleomycin: new perspectives on the mechanism of action. *J. Nat. Prod.*, **63**, 158–168.

Iwasaki, S. (1993) Antimitotic agents: chemistry and recognition of tubulin molecule. *Med. Res. Rev.*, **13**, 183–198.

Joshua-Tor, L. and Sussman, J.L. (1993) The coming age of DNA crystallography. *Curr. Opin. Struct. Biol.* **3**, 323–335.

Judson, I. and Kelland, L.R. (2000) New developments and approaches in the platinum arena. *Drugs*, **59** (Suppl. 4), 29–36.

Kingston, D.G.I. (1994) Taxol: the chemistry and structure–activity relationships of a novel anticancer agent. *TIBTECH*, **12**, 222–227.

Kingston, D.G.I. (2000) Recent advances in the chemistry of taxol. *J. Nat. Prod.* **63**, 726–734.

Knudsen, H. and Nielsen, P.E. (1997) Application of peptide nucleic acid in cancer therapy. *Anti-Cancer Drugs*, **8**, 113–118.

Kuyper, L.F. (1989) Inhibitors of dihydrofolate reductase. In *Computer-Aided Drug Design. Methods and Applications*, edited by T.J. Perun and C.L. Propst, pp. 327–364. New York: Marcel Dekker.

Larsen, I.K. (1990) Inhibition of the enzyme ribonucleotide reductase. In *Frontiers in Drug Research. Crystallographic and Computational Methods*, edited by B. Jensen, F.S. Jørgensen and H. Kofod, pp. 47–57. Copenhagen: Munksgaard.

Liehr, S., Barbosa, J., Smith, A.B. and Cooperman, B.S. (1999) Synthesis and biological activity of cyclic peptide inhibitors of ribonucleotide reductase. *Org. Lett.*, **I**, 1201–1204.

Liuzzi, M., Déziel, R., Moss, N., Beaulleu, P., Bonneau, A.-M., Bousquet, C., Chafouleas, J.G., Garneau, M., Jarmillo, J., Krogsrud, R.L., Lagacé, L., McCollum, R.S., Nawooy, S. and Guindon, Y. (1994) A potent peptidomimetic inhibitor of HSV ribonucleotide reductase with antiviral activity *in vivo*. *Nature*, **372**, 695–698.

Lown, J.W. (1983) The chemistry of DNA damage by antitumour drugs. In *Molecular Aspects of Anti-Cancer Drug Action*, edited by S. Neidle and M.J. Waring, pp. 283–314. London: The Macmillan Press.

McCormick, J.E. and McElhinney, R.S. (1990) Nitrosoureas from chemist to physician: classification and recent approaches to drug design. *Eur. J. Cancer*, **26**, 207–221.

Mirkes, P.E., Brown, N.A., Kajbaf, M., Lamb, J.H., Farmer, P.B. and Naylor, S. (1992) Identification of cyclophosphamide-DNA adducts in rat embryos exposed *in vitro* to 4-hydroperoxocyclophosphamide. *Chem. Res. Toxicol.*, **5**, 382–385.

Nielsen, P.E., Egholm, M. and Buchardt, O. (1994) A DNA mimic with a peptide backbone. *Bioconjugate Chemistry*, **5**, 3–7.

Nogales, E., Whittaker, M. Wolf, S.G. and Downing, K.H. (1998) Structure of the $\alpha\beta$-tubulin dimer by electron crystallography. *Nature*, **391**, 199–203.

Nordlund, P. and Eklund, H. (1993) Structure and function of *Escherichia coli* ribonucleotide reductase protein R2. *J. Mol. Biol.*, **232**, 123–164.

Pratt, W.B. and Ruddon, R.W. (eds.) (1979) *The Anticancer Drugs*. Oxford: Oxford University Press.

Reedijk, J. (1988) Structure determination of platinum antitumour compounds and their adducts with DNA. In *NMR Spectroscopy in Drug Research*, edited by J.W. Jaroszewski, K. Schaumburg and H. Kofod, pp. 341–357. Copenhagen: Munksgaard.

Shoichet, B.K., Stroud, R.M., Santi, D.V., Kuntz, I.D. and Perry, K.M. (1993) Structure-based discovery of inhibitors of thymidylate synthase. *Science*, **259**, 1445–1450.

Sugiura, Y., Takita, T. and Umezawa, H. (1985) Bleomycin antibiotics: metal complexes and their biological action. In *Metal Ions in Biological Systems*, Vol. 19, edited by H. Sigel, pp. 81–108, New York: Marcel Dekker.

Takahara, P.M., Rosenzweig, A.C., Frederick, C.A. and Lippard, S.J. (1995) Crystal structure of double-stranded DNA containing the major adduct of the anticancer drug cisplatin. *Nature*, **377**, 649–652.

Wang, A.H.-J. (1992) Intercalative drug binding to DNA. *Curr. Opin. Struct. Biol.*, **2**, 361–368.

Weiss, R.B. and Christian, M.C. (1993) New cisplatin analogues in development. *A review. Drugs*, **46**, 360–377.

Wilman, D.E.V. and Connors, T.A. (1983) Molecular structure and antitumour activity of alkylating agents. In *Molecular Aspects of Anti-Cancer Drug Action*, edited by S. Neidle and M.J. Waring, pp. 233–282. London: The Macmillan Press.

Index